Mechanisms of Microbial Disease

Mechanisms of Microbial Disease

Edited by

Moselio Schaechter, Ph.D.

Distinguished Professor and Chairman
Department of Molecular Biology and Microbiology
Tufts University School of Medicine
Boston, Massachusetts

Gerald Medoff, M.D.

Professor
Departments of Medicine and Microbiology and Immunology
Director, Infectious Diseases Division
Washington University School of Medicine
St. Louis, Missouri

David Schlessinger, Ph.D.

Professor
Department of Microbiology and Immunology
Washington University School of Medicine
St. Louis, Missouri

Illustrated by

Christo M. Popoff, LL.D.

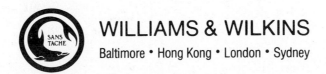

WILLIAMS & WILKINS
Baltimore • Hong Kong • London • Sydney

Editor: John N. Gardner
Associate Editor: Linda Napora
Copy Editor: Elia A. Flanegin
Design: Dan Pfisterer
Illustration Planning: Wayne Hubbel
Production: Theda Harris

Copyright © 1989
Williams & Wilkins
428 East Preston Street
Baltimore, MD 21202, U.S.A.

Accurate indications, adverse reactions, and dosage schedules for drugs are provided in this book, but it is possible that they may change. The reader is urged to review the package information data of the manufacturers of the medications mentioned.

Printed in the United States of America

Library of Congress Cataloging in Publication Data

Mechanisms of microbial disease/edited by Moselio Schaechter, Gerald Medoff, David Schlessinger.
    p. cm.
    Includes index.
    ISBN 0-683-07607-8
       1. Bacterial diseases—Pathogenesis.   2. Communicable diseases—Pathogenesis.
I. Schaechter, Moselio. II. Medoff, Gerald, 1936-   III. Schlessinger, David.
    [DNLM: 1. Bacteria—pathogenicity. 2. Communicable diseases—microbiology.
3. Communicable diseases—physiopathology. 4. Fungi—pathogenicity.
5. Viruses—pathogenicity. QW 700 M4856]
QR201.B34M43 1989
616.9—dc 19
DNLM/DLC
for Library of Congress   88-17430
                                             CIP

89 90 91 92 93   10 9 8 7 6 5 4 3 2 1

*To Judith, Alice,
and the memory of Barbara*

PREFACE

Medical sciences, with one major exception, deal with a single species, *Homo sapiens*. The exception is the science of infectious diseases, which involves hundreds of bacteria, viruses, fungi, and protozoa. This poses a special problem to students and teachers of this subject alike.

Obviously, the impact of microbial disease cannot be overstated. We live with the constant menace of these diseases, most mild or treatable, but invariably made more threatening when our defense mechanisms are weakened. We must cope with organisms that have developed resistance to antimicrobial drugs. In addition, we become aware of new or newly recognized diseases: AIDS, Legionnaires' disease, Lyme disease, and others. Many diseases are on the wane—some, such as smallpox, because of human intervention, others, for unknown reasons. Altogether, there is a staggering number of facts about microbial agents and the diseases they cause. What are we, beginners or veteran students, to do?

Traditionally, the teaching of this subject has been based too much on the memorization of facts (the "bug parade"), frequently with little distinction of what is important. We propose that there is a better approach, based on the use of two principles:

• Material about microbial agents and how the host responds to them is presented solely for the purpose of understanding the mechanism of infectious diseases. Aspects of microorganisms that are not important in the causation of disease are left for other books.

• Focusing on the common features of all host-parasite relationships facilitates learning and recall. Necessary facts can then be organized on a predictable conceptual framework.

We believe that our presentation should derive directly from relevant biological and medical phenomena. For this reason, we have made extensive use of clinical case presentations. This helps introduce both biological and clinical realism and, more important, suggests what questions need to be discussed. The cases presented, for the most part, have a favorable clinical outcome; this is generally realistic and makes them more suitable for discussion.

This textbook is intended to be used in courses on medical microbiology and infectious diseases for medical students and other health professionals, graduate students, and advanced undergraduates. In medical schools the topic is often divided between two courses: one on microbiology and another on infectious diseases (frequently embedded within a pathophysiology course). Our intent is to bridge the contents of these two courses by discussing first the major infectious agents as biological models (sections I and II), then presenting ways in which the major systems of the body are affected by infectious diseases (section III). Since the purpose of this book is to develop a conceptual framework, it highlights certain infectious agents and diseases and does not attempt to present the material in exhaustive fashion. It is not intended as a reference manual; the depth of coverage is left purposefully uneven.

Students using this book should be generally familiar with basic aspects of molecular and cellular biology, but we have tried to minimize medical and technical jargon.

Moselio Schaechter
Gerald Medoff
David Schlessinger

ACKNOWLEDGMENTS

This book arose from our dissatisfaction and that of many of our colleagues and students with the ad hoc syllabi produced in many medical school microbiology departments in lieu of a textbook that adequately combines medical microbiology and infectious diseases. We were encouraged by the logic and charm of Mims' monograph, "The Pathogenesis of Infectious Disease" (Academic Press, New York, 3rd ed.) and Taussig's book, *Processes in Pathology and Microbiology* (Blackwell Scientific Publications, Oxford, 2nd ed.), which helped us in formulating our approach.

We are pleased to thank the contributors to this book, who were willing to accept the additional responsibility connected with a novel approach. We are also indebted to many of our medical students, graduate students, and colleagues who patiently and creatively read portions of the manuscript and who contributed useful comments and suggestions. Reviewers included Elliot Androphy, Irwin Arias, Peter Brodeur, Arthur Brody, John Coffin, David Faling, David Feingold, Bernard Fields, Eugene Foster, Jeffrey Gelfand, Michael Gill, William Goldman, Sherwood Gorbach, David Hecht, Takashi Ikejima, Ralph Isberg, Mark Klempner, Carol Kumamoto, Sol Langemann, Sidney Leskowitz, Douglas Lowy, Michael Malamy, Zell McGee, Cody Meissner, Robert Mitchell, Claire Moore, Patrick Murray, Cynthia Needham, Thomas North, Miercio Pereira, Andre Plaut, Naomi Rosenberg, Debra Rowse, Thomas Russo, Abraham Sonenshein, Stephen Straus, Emanuel Suter, Andrew Wright, and Susan Ziegler. The original and thoughtful help of Eric Rubin and Douglas Braaten deserves special thanks. We thank Gretchen Hester for her help with word processing. We accept the responsibility for errors that remain and will be grateful to readers who may wish to point them out.

We also thank our publisher, Williams & Wilkins; the president of its book division, Sara Finnegan, for the trust placed in us and our untried notions; and our editors, John Gardner and Linda Napora, whose patience and understanding helped bring this effort to fruition.

CONTRIBUTORS

Michael Barza, M.D.
Professor
Department of Medicine
Division of Geographic Medicine and Infectious Diseases
Tufts University School of Medicine and New England Medical Center
Boston, Massachusetts

John M. Coffin, Ph.D.
Professor
Department of Molecular Biology and Microbiology
Tufts University School of Medicine
Boston, Massachusetts

David T. Durack, M.B., D.Phil.
Professor
Departments of Medicine, Microbiology, and Immunology
Division of Infectious Diseases
Duke University Medical Center
Durham, North Carolina

Gerald Keusch, M.D.
Professor
Department of Medicine
Division of Geographic Medicine and Infectious Diseases
Tufts University School of Medicine and New England Medical Center
Boston, Massachusetts

George S. Kobayashi, Ph.D.
Professor
Department of Microbiology and Immunology and Department of Internal
    Medicine
Washington University School of Medicine
St. Louis, Missouri

Donald J. Krogstad, M.D.
Associate Professor
Departments of Pathology and Medicine
Washington University School of Medicine
St. Louis, Missouri

Zell A. McGee, M.D.
Professor
Center for Infectious Diseases, Diagnostic Microbiology, and Immunology
University of Utah School of Medicine
Salt Lake City, Utah

Gerald Medoff, M.D.
Professor
Departments of Medicine and Microbiology and Immunology
Director, Infectious Diseases Division
Washington University School of Medicine
St. Louis, Missouri

Cody Meissner, M.D.
Associate Professor
Department of Pediatrics
Tufts University School of Medicine and New England Medical Center
Boston, Massachusetts

Andrew Plaut, M.D.
Professor
Department of Medicine
Tufts University School of Medicine and New England Medical Center
Boston, Massachusetts

William Powderly, M.D.
Assistant Professor
Department of Medicine
Infectious Diseases Division
Washington University School of Medicine
St. Louis, Missouri

Edward N. Robinson, Jr., M.D.
Assistant Professor
Department of Medicine
Division of Infectious Diseases
University of Louisville School of Medicine
Louisville, Kentucky

Eric Rubin
Department of Molecular Biology and Microbiology
Tufts University School of Medicine
Boston, Massachusetts

Moselio Schaechter, Ph.D.
Distinguished Professor and Chairman
Department of Molecular Biology and Microbiology
Tufts University School of Medicine
Boston, Massachusetts

David Schlessinger, Ph.D.
Professor
Department of Microbiology and Immunology
Washington University School of Medicine
St. Louis, Missouri

Arnold L. Smith, M.D.
Professor
Department of Pediatrics
Division of Infectious Diseases
University of Washington School of Medicine and Children's Medical Center
Seattle, Washington

David R. Snydman, M.D.
Associate Professor
Departments of Medicine and Pathology
Tufts University School of Medicine and New England Medical Center
Boston, Massachusetts

John K. Spitznagel, M.D.
Professor and Chairman
Department of Microbiology and Immunology
Emory University School of Medicine
Atlanta, Georgia

Gregory A. Storch, M.D.
Assistant Professor
Departments of Pediatrics and Medicine
Washington University School of Medicine
St. Louis, Missouri

Stephen E. Straus, M.D.
Medical Virology Section
Laboratory of Clinical Investigation
National Institute of Allergy and Infectious Diseases
National Institutes of Health
Bethesda, Maryland

Francis P. Tally, M.D.
Lederle Laboratories
Pearl River, New York

Donald M. Thea, M.D.
Department of Medicine
Division of Geographic Medicine and Infectious Diseases
Tufts University School of Medicine and New England Medical Center
Boston, Massachusetts

Victor L. Yu, M.D.
Professor
Department of Medicine
University of Pittsburgh
Infectious Disease Section
Veterans Administration Medical Center
Pittsburgh, Pennsylvania

H. Kirk Ziegler, Ph.D.
Associate Professor
Department of Microbiology and Immunology
Emory University School of Medicine
Atlanta, Georgia

CONTENTS

II. THE INFECTIOUS AGENTS 185

Bacteria

Viruses

Fungi

Animal Parasites

SECTION

Principles

I

CHAPTERS:

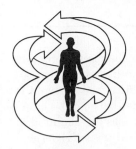

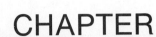

The Establishment of Infectious Diseases

1

M. Schaechter

As a student and as a physician you are going to face a large number of facts about infectious agents and the diseases they cause. How can you learn this much material? Given the magnitude of the task, trying to deal with all the pieces of information singly and in isolation would be difficult and unproductive. Fortunately, there are features that characterize all forms of parasitism, making it possible to develop a conceptual framework on which to hang the multitude of facts. These common features of all infections fall into two generalizations:

1. The following events take place in all infectious diseases:
   Encounter: The agent meets the host.
   Entry: The agent enters the host.
   Spread: The agent spreads from the site of entry.
   Multiplication: The agent multiplies in the host.
   Damage: The agent, the host response, or both cause tissue damage.
   Outcome: The agent or the host wins out, or they learn to coexist.

2. All these steps require the breaching of host defenses. What distinguishes one parasite from another is the manner in which each elicits and combats these host defenses.

ENCOUNTER

Most of us first encounter microorganisms at birth. Microbiologically speaking, we lead a sterile existence while in our mother's womb. This is true for two reasons: First, the unborn is well shielded from the microorganisms of the exterior environment by the fetal membranes. Second, there is little chance that the unborn will acquire foreign organisms from the mother. The mother's blood carries infectious agents only sporadically and in small numbers. Also, the placenta is a formidable obstacle to the passage of any microorganisms that may be circulating in the mother. Still, passage is possible and some diseases are acquired in just this way. Examples of these so-called congenital infections are rubella (German measles), syphilis, or toxoplasmosis.

First Encounters

The first encounter with environmental microorganisms usually takes place at the moment of birth. During parturition the newborn comes in contact with microorganisms present in the mother's vaginal canal and on her skin. Thus, the newborn faces from the very beginning the challenge of living in the intimate company of a bewildering number of microorganisms. However, the mother does not send the newborn into the world totally unprotected. Through her circulation she endows the fetus with a vast repertoire of specific antibodies. Some of this immunological inheritance is further provided by the mother's milk, which also contains maternal antibodies. Sooner or later, however, these acquired defenses wane and the child must learn to cope on its own. The microbial challenge is renewed time and again as all of us come in contact with new organisms for the rest of our lives. Most of these organisms rapidly disappear from the body, whereas others are adroit colonizers and will become part of the normal flora for extended times. A few will cause disease.

Endogenous vs. Exogenous Encounters

Microbial diseases may be contracted in two general ways, exogenously and endogenously: (*a*) Exogenously acquired diseases refer to those that result from the encounter with agents in the environment. Thus we "catch" a cold from others, or we get sick with typhoid fever from eating or drinking contaminated food or water. Disease-causing agents can be acquired from outside in various ways: food, water, air, objects, insect bites, or other humans or animals with whom we share our environment. Many agents are readily transmitted among human beings through the exchange of bodily fluids, for instance by sneezing, touching, or sexual intercourse. The way we encounter the disease agent often suggests a mode of prevention (Table 1.1). Note also that prevention has been successful for many of the serious epidemics, at least in the developed countries of the world. With the exception of vaccination, most preventive measures involve better sanitation and raising the standard of living, rather than employing medical procedures. (*b*) Endogenously acquired diseases refer to those that result from encounters with agents in or on the body. Members of the microbial flora that are normally present on our skin or mucous membranes may cause disease, usually when they penetrate into deeper tissues. A cut may lead to pus caused by the staphylococci that inhabit the healthy skin. Here the encounter with the agent took place long before the disease, namely at the time of colonization of the skin by the staphylococci. A distinction must be made at the onset between *colonization* and *infectious disease*. Colonization denotes the presence of microorganisms at a site of the body, and does not necessarily imply that this leads to tissue damage and to signs and symptoms of disease. It does suggest, however, that the microorganisms have invaded that site of the body and can multiply there.

Table 1.1
Examples of encounters and prevention

Type of Contact	Example	Type of Agent	Source	Strategy for Prevention
Inhalation	Common cold	Virus	Aerosol from infected persons	None
	Coccidioido-mycosis	Fungus	Soil	None
Ingestion	Typhoid fever	Bacterium	Water, food	Sanitation
	Salmonella food poisoning	Bacterium	Food	Sanitation
Sexual contact	Gonorrhea	Bacterium	Person	Social behavior
Wound	Surgical infections	Bacteria	Normal flora, surroundings	Aseptic techniques
Insect bite	Malaria	Protozoan	Mosquito	Insect control

The difference between endogenous and exogenous infections is sometimes quite sharp, as shown by the preceding examples. However, in many other instances the demarcation becomes less clear because it may be difficult to define precisely what constitutes the "normal flora" (see Chapter 9). For example, some people harbor certain strains of virulent streptococci in their throats for a considerable time but only rarely come down with strep throat. Now, before any symptoms arise, we may ask, "Was the streptococcus a member of the normal flora?" The answer is yes if by "normal flora" we mean organisms in or on our body that are not in the process of causing disease. The answer is no if we consider that this kind of streptococcus is not found in the throats of about 95% of all healthy people and that when it is present it frequently causes disease. There is no easy way out of this ambiguity, and the terms must be defined operationally. Obviously, if we cannot define precisely what the normal flora is, we cannot always distinguish between endogenous and exogenous infections.

Another reason why the distinction is so vague is that exposure to highly virulent agents does not always lead to disease. For example, even at the height of the deadly black plague and typhus epidemics, only about half of the population became sick, although most people were likely to have encountered the disease agent.

Thus, the encounter of humans and microbe is quite varied. Each bacterium, virus, fungus, or animal parasite has its quirks. For that matter, each human being displays an idiosyncratic pattern of responses. Even within one individual the pattern usually changes with age, nutritional state, and many other factors.

ENTRY

Much of what is commonly considered to be the inside of the body is topologically connected with the outside (Fig. 1.1). For instance, the surfaces of the lumen of the intestine, the alveoli of the lung, the bile canaliculi, and the tubules of the kidney are in direct connection with the exterior. In fact, almost all the organs contained within the thorax and the abdomen have this topological characteristic. In principle, a crawling insect could go from the mouth to the anus without

Figure 1.1 The regions of the body in direct contact with the exterior. Note that they include the outer aspect of the digestive, respiratory, and urogenital systems. These systems account for most of the organs of the thorax and abdomen. The main systems that do not have such direct connections are the musculoskeletal, nervous, circulatory, and endocrine. Not included in the drawing is the biliary tree and, in women, the peritoneal cavity, which is connected to the outside via the fallopian tubes.

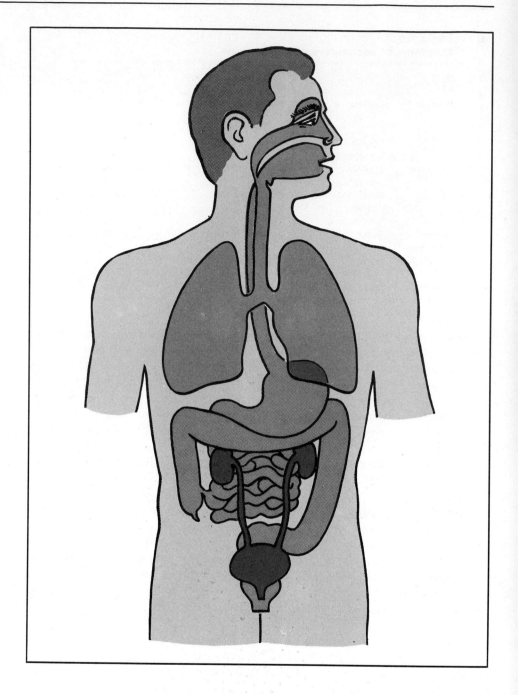

penetrating any mucous membrane, although it would have to go through several sphincters and valves. In reality, these "external" sites of the body have powerful mechanisms that keep out invading microorganisms. With the exception of much of the digestive tract and the lower reaches of the genitourinary system, these sites are normally sterile. Yet, for our purposes, an organism that resides on the lumen side of the intestine or the lung alveoli cannot be said to have *penetrated* the body.

Entry, then, means either the *ingress* of microorganisms into body cavities that are contiguous with the outside, or the *penetration* into deeper tissue after crossing an epithelial barrier. We will discuss both aspects of entry in some detail.

Ingress: Entry Without Crossing Epithelial Barriers

Obviously microorganisms get into the intestine by being eaten and into the lung, by being inhaled. There is not a comparable term for the process that allows ingress into the urinary tract or the genital system, which can also become populated by external microorganisms. It must also be kept in mind that microorganisms can cause serious diseases without getting deep into the tissue. Examples of serious infectious diseases that take place without bacterial penetration through epithelial surfaces are cholera, whooping cough, and infections of the urinary bladder.

Inhalation

To enter the respiratory system, microorganisms face a series of aerodynamic and hydrodynamic obstacles. Microorganisms are inhaled in the aerosol droplets or the dust particles contained in the air we breathe. The air column is not uniform but is buffeted by complex anatomic structures (nasal turbinates, oropharynx, larynx). Accordingly, the surgical removal of the larynx (with its nooks and crannies) predisposes to diseases of the lower respiratory tract. Those microorganisms that arrive in the lower reaches of the respiratory tree face the powerful upward sweeping action of the ciliary epithelium. As expected, persons in whom this is impaired (e.g., heavy smokers) are more likely to get sick with pneumonia. The colonization of these sites by microorganisms requires that they be able to stick to the epithelial surface. Once again, such organisms may cause disease without penetrating the epithelial barrier.

Ingestion

When contaminated food or water is ingested, microorganisms face a powerful host defense, the acid in the stomach. The stomach is a chemical disinfection chamber where many microorganisms are destroyed. Its effectiveness in microbial killing is not always the same since it is determined by the length of time microorganisms spend in the stomach, which depends on the nature and amount of the food eaten. Even under conditions of greatest destruction, some bacteria and yeasts escape alive, although their original number may have been reduced one million-fold or more. This may seem like a lot of bacterial killing, but be aware that some diseases, such as bacillary dysentery, can be acquired from just a few hundred organisms.

Bacteria, fungi, parasites, and viruses that escape this barrier enter the duodenum. Here they meet the enzymes of the pancreatic juice, the bile salts, and the strong sweeping force of peristalsis. Not unexpectedly, very few get a foothold at this site or anywhere else in the upper reaches of the small intestine. Toward the ileum, the situation is more favorable to bacterial life, but even here, the few organisms that gain a foothold must avoid being washed away. Indeed, bacteria found in this region have special mechanisms that allow them to adhere to the epithelial cells of the intestinal mucosa. As will be discussed in Chapter 2, several surface components of these bacteria serve as "adhesins." The main ones are the hair-like pili and the surface polysaccharides. As mentioned already, bacteria at this site may cause disease without penetrating through the mucosal epithelium. Cholera, and its milder relative, "travelers' diarrhea," are the manifestations of the local production of powerful toxins in the intestine that affect the epithelial cells. The bacteria that produce these toxins need not enter the host cells at all.

Penetration: Entry into Tissues After Crossing Epithelial Barriers

Penetration into tissues takes many forms. Some microorganisms can pass directly through epithelia, especially mucous membranes that consist of a single cell layer. To penetrate the skin, which is tough and multilayered, most infecting agents must be carried across by insect bites or await breaks in the surface. On the other hand, certain worms can burrow unaided through the skin and invade the host. Hookworms, for example, are parasites that may be acquired by walking barefoot on contaminated soil.

To penetrate through mucosal epithelia, many microorganisms first interact with specific receptors on the surface of the host cell. This phenomenon has been studied intensively with viruses, some of which have a complex mechanism for attachment and internalization. For instance, influenza viruses have surface components that bind to receptors on the surface of sensitive host cells. Binding is soon followed by the uptake of the virus particles by the cells. In the case of bacteria these two functions, attachment and internalization, are also being studied. In fact, recently it has been possible to clone a bacterial gene that confers the ability to enter cells into strains of *Escherichia coli* that are normally noninvasive.

Microorganisms may also be actively carried into tissue by white cells (macrophages) that lie topographically outside of the body. There are, for instance, macrophages that reside in the alveoli of the lungs and are known as "dust cells," which can pick up infectious agents by phagocytosis. Most of the time they carry them upward on the ciliary epithelium, but occasionally these macrophages can reenter the body and carry their load of microorganisms into deeper locations. Such a mechanism of cell-mediated entry may function at other mucous membranes as well. It is thought, for example, that acquired immunodeficiency syndrome (AIDS) may be sexually transmitted by the penetration of virus-laden macrophages from semen.

Insect Bites

Insect bites may lead to the penetration of viruses (viral encephalitis or yellow fever), bacteria (plague, typhus), protozoa (malaria, sleeping sickness), or worms (river blindness, elephantiasis). In the case of protozoa and higher animal parasites, residence in the insect is part of complex life cycles. The life stage of the parasite in the insect is often quite different from that found in the person. Insects also spread diseases by carrying microorganisms on their surfaces and contaminating foodstuff or the skin. A particularly unsavory example is that of the so-called reduviid bug, which defecates at the same time it bites. Parasites contained in the insect's feces are then introduced by scratching the bite area. A very serious protozoal infection, Chagas' disease, is transmitted in this manner.

Cuts and Wounds

Penetration from cuts and wounds is a common occurrence that is usually unnoticed because it does not usually lead to symptoms of disease. For example, brushing one's teeth or vigorously defecating causes minute abrasions of bacteria-laden epithelial membranes. Bacteria can then be found in small numbers in the blood, but they are rapidly removed by the filtering mechanisms of the reticuloendothelial system. However, if internal tissues are damaged, the defense mechanisms are partially disrupted and circulating bacteria may gain a foothold and cause serious diseases. An example is subacute bacterial endocarditis, a disease that was devastating before the availability of antibiotics. This infection was usually caused by oral streptococci that became implanted on heart valves damaged by a previous disease, usually rheumatic fever.

Organ Transplants and Blood Transfusion

There is yet another way for organisms to penetrate into deeper tissue, namely, as the unfortunate consequence of organ transplants or blood transfusions. For instance, transplants of corneas have been known to result in the infection of recipients with a virus that causes a slow degenerative disease of the central nervous system (Jakob-Creutzfeldt disease). Kidney transplants sometimes result in infections by an agent called cytomegalovirus, possibly because the virus resided in the transplanted kidney. A transplanted organ is not necessarily the source of infection since the immune response of transplant recipients must be suppressed in order to avoid graft rejection. In such a patient an endogenous virus may now be able to multiply.

Of the infectious agents that may be acquired via blood transfusions, none causes greater concern than the virus of AIDS. However, many others, such as hepatitis B virus, can also be transmitted in this manner. Screening of blood in blood banks has become an imperative.

Inoculum Size

The likelihood that organisms from the flora of the skin or mucous membranes might cause disease depends on many factors. Among them is the size of the inoculum, meaning that a few organisms are unlikely to result in an infection; it usually takes many infecting agents to overcome the local defenses. An example is what happens when people take baths in contaminated hot tubs. At times the water can become a veritable culture broth with as many as 100 million bacteria per milliliter. Bacteria that are normally harmless can now overcome the normal defenses of the skin and cause boils all over the body. Clearly, what a surgeon tries to achieve in "prepping" an area before making an incision is to reduce the number of bacteria that may invade a surgical wound. Infections are almost inevitable if large numbers of microorganisms are deposited in deeper tissues, either from dirty skin or from contamination by soil or other microbial-rich material. This requires a great deal of attention in the treatment of patients with open wounds, even in the modern era of powerful antimicrobial drugs.

SPREAD

The term "spread" also has two shades of meaning. It suggests direct, lateral propagation of organisms from the original site of entry to contiguous tissues, but it can also refer to dissemination to distant sites. Either way, microorganisms spread and multiply only if they overcome host defenses. It should be kept in mind that spread sometimes precedes and sometimes follows microbial multiplication in the body. For instance, the parasite that causes malaria enters the body through a mosquito bite and is distributed throughout the bloodstream before it has a chance to increase in numbers. On the other hand, staphylococci that infect a cut must multiply locally before spreading to distant sites.

Understanding the role of host defenses in impeding the spread of microorganisms requires a fair knowledge of the immune response and of the innate defense mechanisms. They are presented in detail in Chapters 4 and 5 and are a central theme of this book. For now, it is important to keep in mind the dynamic nature of host-parasite interactions: For every defense mechanism in existence, microbes develop strategies to try to overcome it; the host, in turn, adapts to such new challenges, which elicits yet different responses from the agents. This intricate counterpoint is played out, sometimes over extended periods of time, until one of three things happens: (a) The host wins out, (b) the parasite overcomes the host, or (c) they learn to live with one another in an uneasy truce.

Anatomical Factors

The pattern of spread of microorganisms from a given site is often dictated by anatomical considerations, so that a knowledge of human anatomy often helps understand infectious diseases. Consider a localized infection, a bacterial abscess of the lung, as an example. The abscess may burst open and allow the organisms to escape into the bronchial tree or, if pointed outwards, to the pleural cavity. Spread in one or the other direction will have different consequences: In the first case it may lead to a more generalized involvement of the lung; in the second, to pleurisy. Another example is the infection of the middle ear, a condition common in children but rare in adults. This age difference is explained in part by developmental changes that take place in the eustachian tubes with growth. These conduits are nearly horizontal in children and become more steeply inclined with age. For this and other reasons, the eustachian tubes of children do not drain as well as those of adults. Note how knowledge of human anatomy helps us to understand a disease process.

Spread of microorganisms is greatly influenced by fluid dynamics. Thus, infected fluids in the interior of the body tend to flow along fascial planes. For example, infection of one site of the meninges will usually result in generalized meningitis, since there are no barriers to impede the spread of the infected cerebrospinal fluid. The same is true for the pleura, the pericardium, and the synovial cavities. Of course, the most extensive liquid system of the body, the blood, is replete with defense mechanisms. All the liquids of the body (blood, lymph, cerebrospinal fluid, synovial fluid, urine, tears, etc.) contain different antimicrobial defense factors that, if overcome, result in disease.

Active Participation by Microorganisms

Infectious agents are not always silent partners in the process of spreading. Some contribute to it by actively moving. Worms wiggle, amoebas crawl, many bacteria swim. Some of these movements seem random; other movements are probably in response to chemotactic signals, a point that has not been extensively investigated. Spreading can also be facilitated by chemical rather than mechanical action. For instance, streptococci manufacture a variety of extracellular hydrolases that let them break out of the walling-in force of the inflammatory response. They make a protease that breaks up fibrin, a hyaluronidase that hydrolyzes hyaluronic acid of connective tissue, and a deoxyribonuclease that reduces the viscosity of pus caused by the release of DNA from lysed white cells. Other bacteria make elastases, collagenases, or other powerful proteases. Such organisms can break through some of the natural surface barriers or can penetrate through thick viscous pus that would otherwise impede their spread. On a more superficial level, fungi that cause athlete's foot make keratin-hydrolyzing enzymes that help them spread through the horny layers of the skin. These factors confer clear selective advantagees on the microorganisms that produce them.

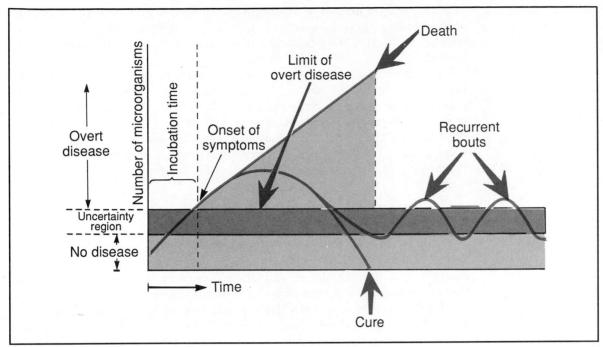

Figure 1.2 Microbial multiplication and clinical manifestations of disease. The number of microorganisms present in a patient must exceed a given threshold to cause disease. If the number is below this threshold, no signs and symptoms of disease will be apparent. In some cases, the numbers will oscillate above and below the threshold, resulting in recurrent bouts of disease. Note that this is an idealized schematic drawing. In reality, the threshold of overt disease is not fixed but varies with the physiological state of the host.

MULTIPLICATION

Rarely do infectious agents cause disease without first multiplying within the body. The number of microorganisms we inhale or ingest (the size of the inoculum) is usually too small to produce symptoms directly. Infectious agents must grow before their presence is felt. (Fig. 1.2) Of course the ingestion of bacterial toxins such as those of botulism or staphylococcal food poisoning leads to disease directly, but these conditions are intoxications, not infections.

In most cases, symptoms are manifested a period of time after the organisms enter the body. This *incubation period* reflects the time needed for the infectious agents to overcome early defenses and to grow to a certain population size. The subject of the host defenses against microbial multiplication is a lengthy and varied one. Later in this chapter we will bring up some of their less obvious manifestations: Not infrequently, defense mechanisms go overboard and contribute to tissue damage in infections.

Microbial Nutrition

As microbial nutrition goes, the body would seem to be a rich medium. Body fluids such as plasma contain sugars, vitamins, minerals and other substances that can be used for growth by bacteria, fungi, and animal parasites. Still, if plasma were inoculated with a culture of bacteria, their growth would be sparse. The major reason is the inhibitory effect of antimicrobial substances such as lysozyme and constituents of the complement system.

Plasma and many other body fluids contain very little free iron since this metal is combined with extremely avid iron-binding proteins. This point, which has been studied in detail, appears to be significant in limiting the growth of bacteria in the body. Bacteria need iron for the synthesis of their cytochromes and other enzymes. In fact, the body sequesters iron to defend itself against bacteria.

When a sufficient number of organisms enters the body it causes the outpouring of iron-binding proteins into plasma and tissue fluids. In other words, the body tries to limit further the availability of free iron by sequestering an ever greater amount of it.

The spectrum of nutritional requirements of microorganisms associated with the body reflects their ecological habits. For instance, many of the bacteria that grow on the human body but not in many other places, such as the staphylococci or certain streptococci, require several amino acids and vitamins. Organisms that are found both within the body but also in soil or water are usually much less picky and can fulfill their organic requirements with simple carbon compounds. Examples are *E. coli* or many *Pseudomonas* that can grow in laboratory "minimal media."

Physical Factors

The physical environment of the body selects for microorganisms that grow within certain ranges of temperature, osmotic pressure, and pH. For example, most of the pathogenic bacteria and viruses have a temperature optimum around that of the body of their host. Some have strict requirements. For instance, poliovirus will not grow just a few degrees over normal human body temperature. Fever, then, may be a defense mechanism that may serve to limit the disease. (Do you want to think again before prescribing two aspirins and asking the patient to call you in the morning?) Fungi that cause athlete's foot do not grow well above around 30°C and are found only on the cooler body surfaces. It follows that in most circumstances they cannot cause internal diseases. As with nutritional requirements, the breadth of the temperature range for growth is often dictated by the organism's habits. Organisms that are almost always found in association with their host tend to have a narrow temperature optimum. Organisms that are also found in the environment, such as *Pseudomonas*, also grow well at lower temperatures.

DAMAGE

There are nearly as many kinds of damage as there are infectious diseases. The type and intensity of the damage depend on the tissues and organs affected, which makes it difficult to make generalizations. Damage in infectious processes may be loosely categorized as due to (*a*) mechanical causes, (*b*) cell death, (*c*) pharmacological alterations of metabolism, and (*d*) vehement host responses. These manifestations are interrelated, and several are usually seen at one time.

Mechanical Causes

If infectious agents are large enough and present in sufficient numbers, they may obstruct vital passages. Such a mechanical obstruction happens, although rarely, in children with an overload of worms in the intestine. A heavy infestation with the large roundworm *Ascaris* (15–35 cm long and about 0.5 cm thick) may result in the occlusion of the intestinal lumen. A single worm may also migrate into the common bile duct and obstruct the passage of bile.

More often, mechanical obstruction results not from the infectious agents alone but from the inflammatory response of the host elicited by their presence. An example is the disease elephantiasis, an enormous swelling of limbs or the scrotum caused by small worms, the filariae, becoming lodged in lymphatics. Their presence sets off a tissue reaction that occludes the vessels, causing swelling and hypertrophy.

Almost any duct or tube-like organ, thick or thin, may be obstructed by infections, sometimes with life-threatening consequences. Some examples are the inflammation of the epiglottis, which may impede the passage of air; the spread of inflammation from the middle ear, which can result in hydrocephalus, a dilatation of the cerebral ventricles due to obstruction of the flow of cerebrospinal fluid; infection of the prostate, which may obstruct the flow of urine from the bladder; and an inflammatory reaction to the eggs of a liver fluke, which may result in severe disturbances of local circulation.

Cell Death

The effect of cell death depends on (a) which cells are involved, (b) how many are infected, and (c) how fast the infection proceeds. If the cells belong to an essential organ, such as the heart or the brain, the outcome is likely to be serious and may even be fatal. Myocarditis, for example, the infection of the heart muscle, is sometimes a fulminating disease when it is caused by an agent called coxsackievirus. On the other hand, myocarditis is usually a chronic condition when the infecting organism is a less virulent parasite, as with the trypanosome of Chagas' disease. Coxsackievirus is thought to kill the insulin-producing cells of the islets of the pancreas and appears to be one of the causes of infantile diabetes.

Sometimes the effects of cell death are easily seen. For instance, in patients with gas gangrene, lysis of red blood cells and the outpouring of hemoglobin may result in a reddish or burgundy appearance of serum and urine. Rocky Mountain spotted fever derives its name from the skin rash produced by blood spilled when endothelial cells of small vessels are killed by infecting rickettsiae. In both examples the cells break open and liberate the infectious agents into the bloodstream.

Some bacteria kill cells by poisoning them with toxins. Sometimes toxins function in the immediate surroundings of the bacteria that produce them. For example, the bacteria that cause dysentery kill nearby epithelial cells of the intestinal mucosa. Other bacteria produce toxins that act at great distances. An example is diphtheria, where bacteria in the throat produce a toxin that affects the heart and the nervous system. Toxins produced by bacteria are among the most powerful cell poisons known and work at extraordinarily low concentrations. It has been estimated that a single molecule of diphtheria toxin is sufficient to kill a sensitive cell. Considerable knowledge has been gathered about how these toxins work and will be presented in the chapters on individual organisms and in Chapter 7.

Pharmacological Alterations of Metabolism

Certain infectious diseases do not involve the direct killing of cells at all. Among these are some of the most severe ones, such as tetanus, botulism, or cholera. They are caused by bacterial toxins that alter important aspects of metabolism in ways that resemble the action of hormones or other pharmacological effectors. Tetanus toxin works on motor cells, leading to a spastic paralysis. Botulism toxin interferes with the release of acetylcholine at cholinergic synapses and neuromuscular junctions, resulting in a flaccid paralysis. Cholera toxin increases the level of cyclic AMP in intestinal cells, which leads to a massive diarrhea because of loss of water and electrolytes. In all these cases, the affected cells remain intact.

Damage Due to Host Responses

Almost invariably the symptoms of infectious diseases are not produced by the microorganisms alone but also by the response of the host to their presence. In almost no case is the host response so finely tuned that it does just what is desired of it. Its overemphatic expression may well help the host survive in the long run, but it contributes greatly to the immediate signs and symptoms. There are two manifestations of this, damage due to inflammation and damage from the immune response.

Inflammation

The most familiar example of inflammation is pus, which consists of a mixture of dead and live white blood cells, bacteria, and exudate. Pus results from the rapid migration of neutrophils to a site where bacteria are present. Neutrophils are called up by chemotactic substances, some produced by the bacteria themselves, and some by tissue and serum components. When neutrophils die they release powerful hydrolases from their lysosomal granules. These enzymes damage surrounding tissues, extending the lesion to adjacent areas.

When pus is walled off, the lesion is called an *abscess*. An example is a boil, the familiar furuncle that most people have experienced on their skin. It is caused by the stoppage of a sebaceous gland, which gives staphylococci normally present on the skin an initial opportunity for sheltered growth. Organisms do, however, advertise their presence, and neutrophils arrive at the scene to join battle. Pus may be damaging locally, but note that this is a small price to pay for containing the infection. Patients with genetic defects in neutrophil function pay a very heavy price, in the form of severe recurrent infections. Despite antibiotic treatment, many such patients do not survive into adolescence. It should be noted that the anatomic location of this battlefield is all-important. An abscess in the skin may be painful, but one in the brain could be fatal.

As mentioned before, the presence of bacteria in tissues also elicits a generalized reaction known as the *acute phase response*. Bacteria set off the outpouring of a powerful protein called *interleukin 1*, which acts on the fever centers to raise body temperature. Interleukin 1 stimulates the synthesis of substances called prostaglandins, which work on the thermoregulatory center of the brain. Prostaglandins are also responsible for the feeling of malaise, that ill-defined but well-known sensation of "feeling sick" that besets us when we have the common cold. Aspirin and acetaminophen interfere with the production of prostaglandins, thereby reducing fever and malaise.

With many common bacteria, the so-called Gram negatives, the acute phase response is elicited by a major component of their surface, a lipopolysaccharide known as *endotoxin*. In small amounts endotoxin elicits fever and mobilizes certain defense mechanisms. In large amounts, it results in shock and intravascular coagulation. Thus, the body response to the presence of these bacteria depends entirely on the amount of endotoxin present.

The Immune Response

The immune response is complex and has multiple manifestations. There are many ways in which it may go awry and cause damage. Immune responses are usually classified as "humoral," related to circulating antibodies, and "cellular," elicited by special cells of the immune system. Both may cause damage.

Humoral Immunity

Infecting agents elicit the formation of specific antibodies. In the circulation and in tissues, antibodies combine with the infecting agents or with some of their soluble products. These antigen-antibody complexes elicit an inflammatory response. How do they do this? The answer requires knowledge of a complex set of serum proteins, the *complement system*. In the presence of antigen-antibody complexes these proteins become activated by a series of proteolytic reactions, the so-called *classical pathway* of activation. Complement can also be activated by the presence of microorganisms alone, resulting in the *alternative pathway*. The products of these proteolytic cleavages are pharmacologically active. Some work on platelets and white cells to produce substances that increase vascular permeability and vasodilation. The result is edema, the outpouring of fluids into tissues. Other complement factors act on white blood cells, some as chemotaxins, others to make bacteria more easily phagocytized. The result of these activities is, on the one hand, the mobilization of powerful defenses against invading microorganisms, and, on the other hand, inflammation.

Antigen-antibody complexes sometimes are deposited on the membrane of the glomeruli of the kidneys, resulting in impairment of kidney function, a condition called glomerulonephritis. This condition is seen as the aftermath of certain streptococcal and viral infections. Similar effects also take place in blood vessels, leading to visible skin rashes.

Cellular Immunity

A different type of response is expressed via special cells of the immune system and is called *cell-mediated immunity* (CMI). This complex phenomenon leads to the activation and mobilization of macrophages, the powerful phagocytic cells that participate in the later stages of inflammation to clean up debris and remaining microorganisms.

CMI is associated with chronic inflammation, the histological changes that limit the spread of infections but also cause lesions in tissues. These damaging activities are characteristic of chronic infections, often caused by intracellular microorganisms and viruses. An example is chronic tuberculosis, where the main damage to tissue is due to CMI. It is elicited by the tubercle bacilli, which have the ability to persist in cells for a long time. As the result, pathological changes associated with CMI lead to the production of *tubercles* or *granulomas*, and eventually to destruction of tissue cells.

It is worth repeating that although the immune responses may cause tissue damage, the price is well worth it. The point is illustrated in people who have genetic or acquired defects in their immune system. Unfortunately, such people are no longer a medical rarity. The advent and spread of AIDS has placed hundreds of thousands of persons in this category. The result is that these patients are ravaged and even killed by microorganisms that cause little or no disease in healthy persons. In the immunocompetent person, for example, active tuberculosis causes much damage and may even kill the patient, but usually only after many years. In the immunocompromised patient the disease can become rampant in a much shorter period.

CONCLUSION

There is nothing simple about infectious diseases, be they mild or life threatening. A large number of properties of the invading agent and the host lead to an intricate and ever changing interplay. It is not always possible to figure out the relative role of the known properties, leave aside those that still await discovery. To complicate matters, humans are beset by a huge number of possible invaders. New ones emerge apparently under our very eyes, to be added to the long list.

The student of medical microbiology therefore faces a demanding challenge. The fascination of each topic may not suffice to overcome the problems in studying so much detail. We suggest that a student is helped by resorting to a conceptual framework such as the one used in this chapter, based on the fact that all host-parasite interactions have steps in common. As we indicate at the beginning of this chapter, parasites and host must encounter, the parasite must enter the host, spread and multiply, and eventually cause damage. All these steps require the breaching of host defenses. If these facts are kept in mind the myriads of facts will fall into place logically. May you thereby be able to enjoy one of the liveliest and important subjects in all of biology and medicine!

SUGGESTED READINGS

McNeill WH: *Plagues and Peoples.* Garden City, NY, Anchor Books, 1976.
Mims CA: *The Pathogenesis of Infectious Diseases,* ed 3. New York, Academic Press, 1987.
Taussig MJ: *Processes in Pathology and Microbiology,* ed 2. Boston, Blackwell Science Publications 1984.

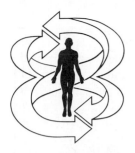

CHAPTER

Biology of Infectious Agents

2

D. Schlessinger
M. Schaechter

WHAT DO WE WANT TO KNOW ABOUT MICROORGANISMS?

Mainly, we want to know how pathogenic microorganisms harm the host and what we can do about it. This requires understanding more than just how they cause lesions in specific diseases. For example, features of bacterial anatomy and metabolism have suggested targets for the successful development of powerful antibiotics. Similarly, unraveling details of viral structures and metabolism has led to the development of protective vaccines and to the beginnings of antiviral therapy.

An analysis of microbial life must also extend beyond the disease state, since many microorganisms appear to be harmless passengers on the body or are found in habitats very different from human tissues. Not infrequently, these organisms reveal their opportunistic capacity and cause disease, especially in debilitated persons. From the point of view of students of infectious diseases, the life cycle of microorganisms may be critical to understand their capacity to cause disease. For example, figuring out the etiology of Legionnaires' disease required an analysis of bacterial survival in the cooling water towers of large hotels. Analogously, control of malaria is based on knowing that a critical density of both the mosquito vector and infected people is required for the spread of the parasite.

PROCARYOTIC AND EUCARYOTIC PATHOGENS

The world of pathogenic microbiology spans the largest cleft in the living world, that between the procaryotes and the eucaryotes. Bacteria belong to the

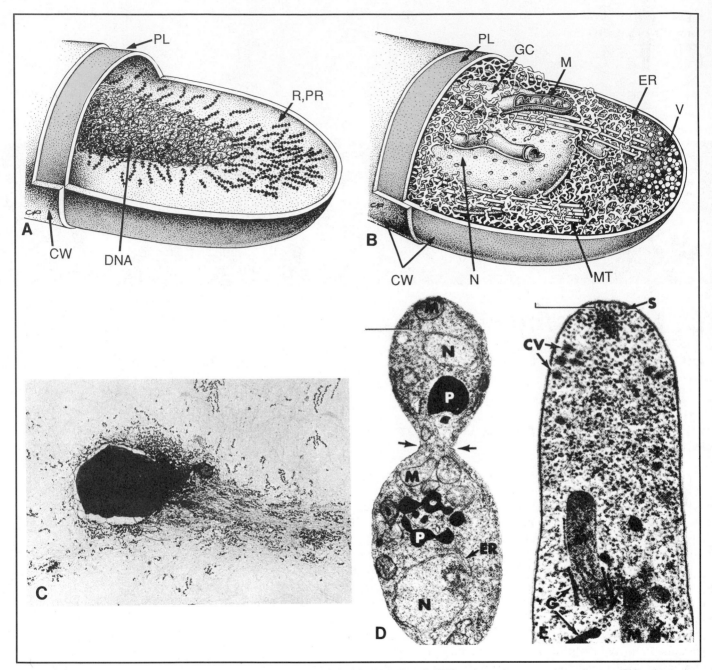

Figure 2.1. Ultrastructure of typical bacterial and fungal cells. *A*, Inside the cell wall (CW) and membrane or plasmalemma (PL), a bacterium is filled with ribosomes (R), polyribosomes (PR), and proteins. DNA fibrils cluster near the center of the cell in a coiled mass. *B*, The cell wall (CW) and plasmalemma (PL), of a hyphal tip surround the Golgi complex (GC), mitochondria (M), vacuoles (V), endoplasmic reticulum (ER), and nucleus (N) characteristic of the eucaryotic cell. The DNA in the nucleus and the ribosomes and proteins of the cytoplasm are not indicated, for clarity. *C*, Contents of an *E. coli* cell released by osmotic shock of a ''spheroplast''. Note polyribosomes attached to DNA via ''nascent'' mRNA molecules. *D*, Electron microscopy of a yeast cell with a uninucleate bud (''P'' is a granule of polyphosphate) and the tip of a mycelium G, the Golgi equivalent; S, an accumulation of vesicles at the growing point). The fungal sections are of *Histoplasma capsulatum*. (*C*, Courtesy of O.L. Miller Jr. and B. Hamkalo, *D*, from Kobayashi GS et al. In Szaniszlo PJ (ed): *Fungal Di-morphism*. New York, Plenum.)

Table 2.1
Composition of a typical procaryote and eucaryote.

	% Dry Weight		No. Molecule/Cell		Molecular Weight	
	E. coli	Yeast	E. coli	Yeast	E. coli	Yeast
Wall	10	40				
Membrane	10	7				
Mitochondria		0.2		1–50		
DNA	2	0.16	1	17–18	2×10^9	10^{10} total
RNA		(8)				
mRNA	2	0.4	6,500	36,000	4×10^5	7×10^5
tRNA	3	1.2	160,000	3.2×10^6	2.5×10^4	2.5×10^4
rRNA (ribosome)	30	6.4	20,000	105,000	2×10^6	3.9×10^6
Soluble protein	42	40	10^6	4.4×10^7	5×10^4	5.5×10^4
Small metabolites		5	6.5×10^6	1.5×10^9	200	200

procaryotes, whereas fungi, protozoa, and worms are eucaryotes. Procaryotes lack nuclei and other internal membrane-bound organelles. They do not carry out endocytosis and are incapable of ingesting particles or liquid droplets. Procaryotes differ from eucaryotes in important biochemical details, such as the composition of their ribosomes and lipids (Fig. 2.1). Procaryotes are usually haploid, with a single chromosome and extrachromosomal plasmids; eucaryotes have a diploid phase and many chromosomes.

Differences in organization between procaryotes and eucaryotes have important consequences for the way they synthesize certain macromolecules. For instance,

Table 2.2
Transcription/processing of mRNA.

	Procaryotes	Eucaryotes
Transcription		
Gene regulation developmental	Operon-polycistronic mRNA	Single genes; block of genes
Copies of genes	Single-gene copy	Single-gene copy plus repetitive DNA
Chromosomes	One	Many
Ploidy	Haploid	Haploid/diploid cycle
"Cytoplasmic"DNA coding	Plasmids	Mitochondria kinetoplasts
Colinearity of gene/mRNA differences	Precise; one form of each protein	Introns within gene sequence; organ
Locus of regulation	Mostly transcriptional	Often posttranscriptional Regulation by protein turnover, etc.
Relation of transcription and translation	Coupled	Uncoupled
Processing of mRNA at double-stranded sites in mRNA	Rare; some cleavages	Poly(A) at 3'-end Cap 5'-end. Splicing, functional domains
Stability of mRNA	Unstable	Range of stability; some very stable mRNA
Translation		
First amino acid	Formylated methionine	Methionine
Signal for start	Ribosome binding site preceding AUG	Binding to 5'-end, use of first AUG along mRNA
Initiation factors	Three	>6
Ribosomes	30S + 50S = 70S	40S + 60S = 80S
	Characteristic inhibitors	Characteristic inhibitors

not having a nuclear membrane allows procaryotes to carry out protein synthesis using chains of messenger RNA that are themselves being synthesized. In other words, translation can be coupled to transcription and begin rapidly on new mRNA chains. In eucaryotes the two processes cannot be directly linked. Transcripts of heterogeneous nuclear RNA must first be processed in the nucleus before they are transported across the nuclear membrane to the ribosomes in the cytoplasm. Only then can eucaryotic protein synthesis take place.

Table 2.1 shows differences in composition between *Escherichia coli*, the paradigm of a bacterium, and the best known of the lower eucaryotes, a yeast. A comparison of the regulation of expression of their genes is presented in Table 2.2. A review of basic biochemistry and molecular biology may be appropriate to understand this material.

PROBLEMS OF UNICELLULARITY

Free living organisms face constant challenges in their environment. The demands made on microorganisms fall into three general categories: nutrition, related to the intermittent availability of food; occupancy, related to the need to remain in a certain habitat; and resistance to damaging agents.

A Life of Feast or Famine

Frequently in their existence, microorganisms run out of food. Consider a bacterium such as *E. coli* that lives in the large intestine of human beings. Every so often, some 20 times a day on average, the ileocecal valve opens and nutrient-rich contents squirt from the small intestine into the cecum. Here a large bacterial flora rapidly uses the nutrients, soon making the environment fallow. Clearly, the different kinds of bacteria normally present at this site have adapted to a life of feast and famine. On the one hand they are able to utilize rapidly nutritional substrates when they become available, and to compete efficiently with their microbial neighbors. On the other hand they must be able to adapt to the lack of nutrients during periods of starvation, and also be poised for action whenever food again becomes plentiful. Two themes emerge in the evolution of such cells: *efficiency* and *adaptability*. We will see how these two properties are manifested in bacteria.

Colonization and Occupancy

Not all problems in the microbial world are nutritional. In certain environments, survival depends on being able to remain in a given place and avoid being swept away by liquid currents. Many species of bacteria ensure their occupancy by developing devices for sticking to surfaces. For instance, bacteria attach to the surface of our teeth by elaborating gooey polysaccharides. When built up sufficiently, they form dental plaque. Likewise, in our intestine there is an abundant microbial flora that adheres to the epithelial wall and that is different from the one that is living free in the lumen. Note that the "wall" flora faces different nutritional problems from the "lumen" flora. The selective pressure on these two populations is very different.

Coping with Damaging Agents

Microorganisms often encounter chemical or physical agents that threaten their existence. Not unexpectedly, they have evolved mechanisms that allow them to cope with these life-threatening challenges. Among the better studied are structural devices and physiological responses that protect them (up to a point) from such environmental insults as membrane-damaging chemicals, heat, or DNA-damaging radiation. Microorganisms also use genetic strategies to withstand antibiotics and can develop resistance to these substances in a number of ways. Attempts by the physician to rid tissues of pathogenic organisms are counteracted by the mechanisms developed by the organisms to thwart these efforts.

SMALL SIZE PROMOTES METABOLIC EFFICIENCY

The microbial world is composed of small entities, generally below the range of what the unaided human eye can see. Consequently, large numbers can be packed in small volumes. Typical bacteria are of the order of 1 μm in diameter and, if they were stacked neatly as tiny blocks, 10^{12} would occupy 1 cm^3 and weigh about 1 g. In suspension the turbidity contributed by such small particles is so minuscule that a clear fluid such as urine only becomes visibly cloudy when the bacteria present exceed about 1 to 10 million per ml. It will not surprise you that each of us is currently carrying a load of some 10 to 100 trillion bacteria in our large intestine, greatly surpassing the number of our own eucaryotic cells.

Being small allows high metabolic rates because the surface-to-volume ratio increases as the size of cells decreases. Ultimately, biochemical reactions are limited by diffusion, and the smaller the cells, the less limiting it is. Consequently, bacteria are in intimate contact with external nutrients and are capable of metabolic rates in orders of magnitude higher than those of eucaryotic cells. They can grow extremely fast and many double as often as once every 15 minutes under optimal conditions. One measure of the rapidity of their metabolic flux is that small metabolites (amino acids, sugars and nucleotides—the building blocks of macromolecules) constitute about 1% of their total dry weight. Some microbial eucaryotes, such as yeasts and other fungi, have comparable efficiency.

The amazing speed with which these small cells convert food into energy and biosynthetic building blocks requires the coordination of metabolic activities. This subject is reviewed below, first for bacteria, then for yeast cells. Features of cell structure and macromolecular synthesis help us to understand how individual species of bacteria maximize their chance for survival and suggest how we may intervene therapeutically against pathogenic organisms and anticipate their defenses.

BACTERIA HAVE COMPLEX ENVELOPES AND APPENDAGES

Bacteria are surrounded by a complex set of envelopes and appendages, different in individual species. Some of these structures are useful in certain environments only and are dispensable under laboratory conditions. These components often determine whether an organism can survive in a particular environment and cause disease.

Like all cells, bacteria have an indispensable structure, the cytoplasmic membrane. Most bacteria also form elaborate structures outside the membrane, namely a cell wall and some, an "outer membrane", flagella, pili, and a capsule. These structures can amount to 10% to 20% of the dry weight of the cell (as in other organisms, the "wet weight" is about two-thirds water). The reason for the extra layers outside the cell membrane becomes clear if one considers the stresses that

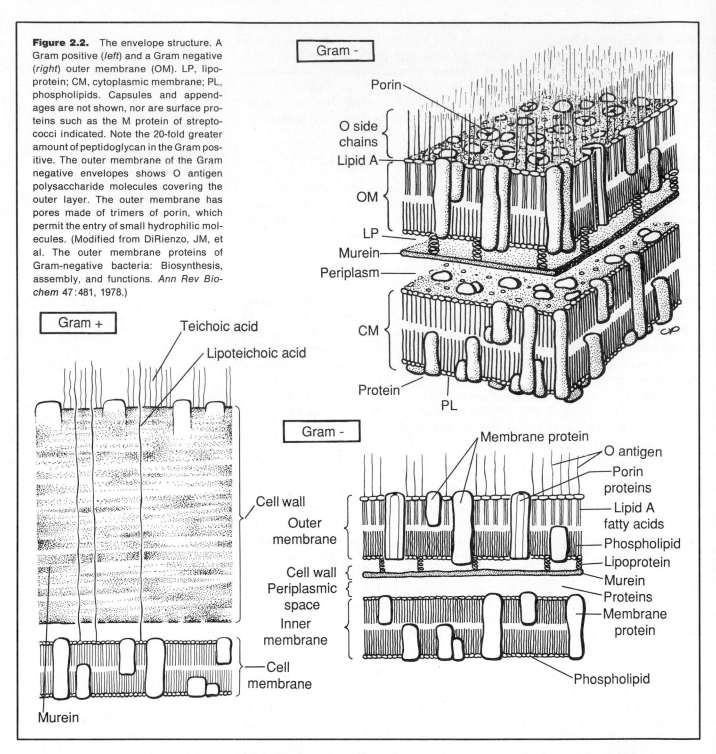

Figure 2.2. The envelope structure. A Gram positive (*left*) and a Gram negative (*right*) outer membrane (OM). LP, lipoprotein; CM, cytoplasmic membrane; PL, phospholipids. Capsules and appendages are not shown, nor are surface proteins such as the M protein of streptococci indicated. Note the 20-fold greater amount of peptidoglycan in the Gram positive. The outer membrane of the Gram negative envelopes shows O antigen polysaccharide molecules covering the outer layer. The outer membrane has pores made of trimers of porin, which permit the entry of small hydrophilic molecules. (Modified from DiRienzo, JM, et al. The outer membrane proteins of Gram-negative bacteria: Biosynthesis, assembly, and functions. *Ann Rev Biochem* 47:481, 1978.)

bacteria must face in natural surroundings. For example, intestinal bacteria such as *E. coli* are exposed to bile salts that would dissolve an unprotected cell membrane. Envelope layers and appendages are used by bacteria to stick to surfaces and for protection from phagocytes and other defense mechanisms. Virulence is often determined by the presence or absence of these cell-bound constituents.

The surface components of bacteria are what the host senses first during infection. Consequently, many of the properties of the surface components are relevant both to the establishment of infection and to the response of the host to the organisms. The strongest antibody response to bacterial antigens is usually directed to surface components.

PROTECTION OF THE CYTOPLASMIC MEMBRANE

Bacteria have three principal ways to protect their cytoplasmic membrane from environmental stresses, such as low osmotic pressure or the presence of detergents. These solutions are represented by the Gram positive, Gram negative, and acid-fast bacteria. Figure 2.2 illustrates the first two.

The Gram stain (named after an early Danish microbiologist) divides most bacteria into two groups, nearly equal in number and importance. This staining procedure is central in microbiology and must be learned by every medical student in due course. In brief, it depends on the ability of certain bacteria (the Gram positives) to retain a complex of a purple dye and iodine when challenged with a brief alcohol wash (Table 2.3). Gram negatives do not retain the dye and can later be counterstained with a dye of a different color, usually red. This distinction turns out to be correlated with fundamental differences in the cell envelope of these two classes of bacteria.

Table 2.3
Gram stain procedure.

Gram Stain	Acid-Fast Stain
1. Stain with crystal violet (purple).	1. Stain with hot carbol-fuchsin (red).
2. Modify with potassium iodide.	2. Decolorize with acid: alcohol; only acid-fast remain red.
3. Decolorize with alcohol; only Gram positives remain purple.	3. Counterstain with methylene blue: Acid-fast remain red; others become blue.
4. Counterstain with safranin: Gram negatives become pink; Gram positives remain purple.	

The Gram Positive Solution

Gram positive bacteria protect their membrane with a thick cell wall. The major constituent of the wall is a complex polymer of sugars and amino acids called *murein* or *peptidoglycan* (Fig. 2.3). Murein is the critical component in maintaining the shape and rigidity of both Gram positives and Gram negatives, but plays a bigger role in protecting the cell membrane of Gram positives. It is a polymer unique to bacteria. How does it contribute to the defense of cell integrity? Murein is composed of glycan (sugar) chains that are cross-linked to one another via peptides. The overall structure is similar in all cases, but differs somewhat in chemical details (see for example Figure 2.4). This polymeric fabric consists of many layers wrapped around the length and width of the bacteria, to form a sac the size and shape of the organisms. Depending on the shape of the murein sac, bacteria may have the appearance of *bacilli* (rods), *cocci* (spheres), or *spirilla* (helices). The rigid murein corset allows bacteria to survive in media of lesser osmotic pressure than that of their cytoplasm. In the absence of a rigid corset-like structure to push against, the membrane bursts and the cells lyse. This can be demonstrated experimentally by removing the murein with a hydrolytic enzyme present in many

Figure 2.3. Structure of murein. The basic repeating unit of alternating N-acetylglucosamine (GlcNAc) and substituted muramic acid (N-acetyl glucosamine connected to an O-lactyl ether and the pentapeptide).

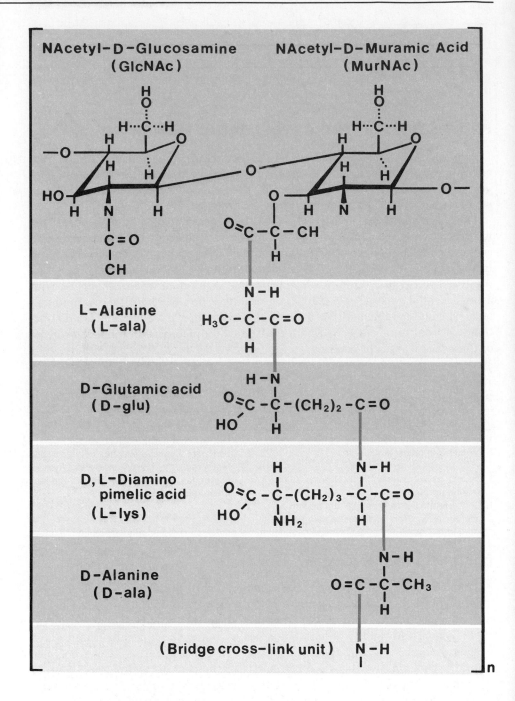

human and animal tissue fluids, *lysozyme*. Treatment with lysozyme causes bacteria to lyse in a low osmotic pressure environment. If lysozyme treated bacteria are kept in an isoosmotic medium, they do not lyse but become spherical. Such structures are called *spheroplasts*.

The cell wall of Gram positives is made up of many layers of the sac-like murein, so thick that it impedes the passage of hydrophobic compounds. This is because the sugars and charged amino acids make murein highly polar and surround the cells with a dense hydrophilic layer. Thus, many Gram positives can withstand

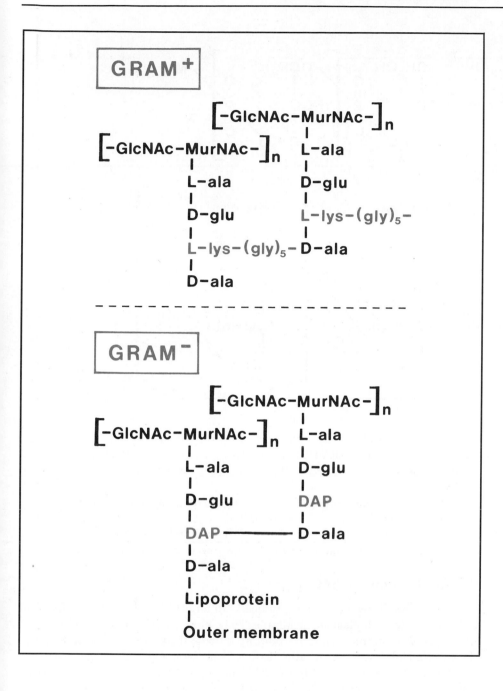

Figure 2.4. Typical structure of murein in Gram positive and Gram negative bacteria. In the Gram positives, peptide chains are cross-linked through a peptide bond between the free amino group of lysine and the terminal carboxyl group of a D-ala residue. In the Gram negatives, the cross-link is between diaminopimelic acid and D-ala. Other D-ala residues are linked to a lipoprotein that is attached to the outer membrane.

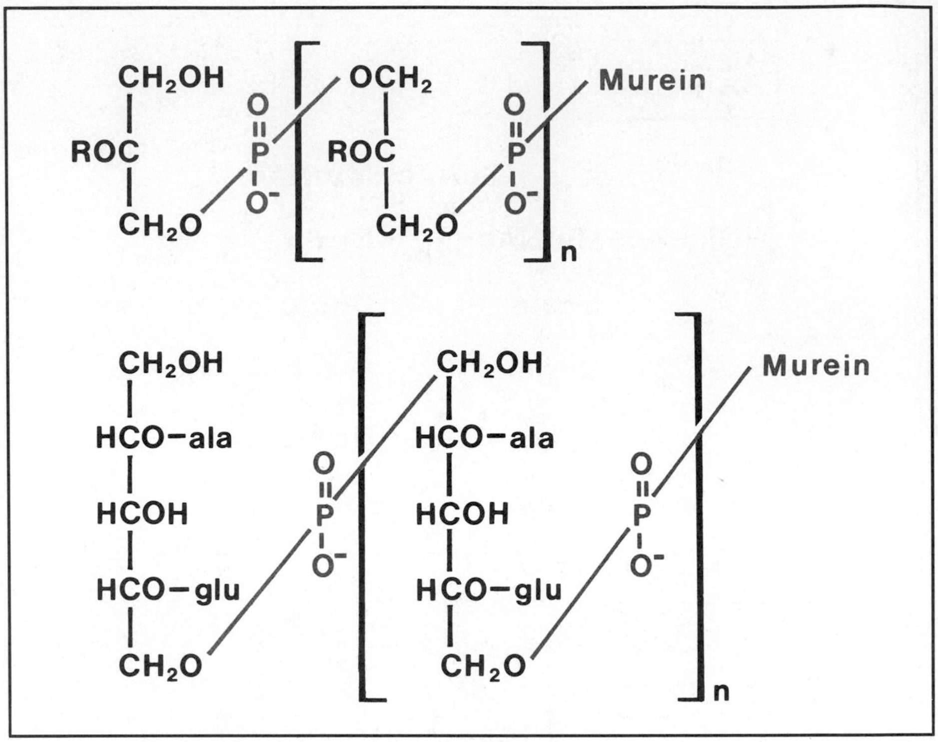

Figure 2.5. Teichoic acid structure. The repeating unit of ribitol and glycerol teichoic acids are shown. The chains in Gram positive organisms vary in length and amounts.

certain noxious hydrophobic compounds, including the bile salts in the intestine. The feature that makes bacteria Gram positive, the ability to retain the dye-iodine complex, also seems to depend on the characteristic murein structure of the Gram positive wall.

Gram positive walls contain other unique polymers, for example, *teichoic acids*, which are chains of ribitol or glycerol linked by phosphodiester bonds (Fig. 2.5). Teichoic acids will be discussed in connection with individual groups of bacteria, since at least some of them appear to play a role in pathogenesis.

The Gram Negative Solution

Gram negatives have adopted a radically different solution to the problem of protection of the cytoplasmic membrane. They make a completely different structure, an *outer membrane*, which is built up outside the murein cell wall (Fig. 2.2). The outer membrane is chemically distinct from the usual biological membranes and has built into it the ability to resist damaging chemicals. It is a bilayered structure, but its outer leaflet contains a unique component in addition to phospholipids. This is a *bacterial lipopolysaccharide* (LPS), a complex molecule not found elsewhere in nature.

Bacterial Lipopolysaccharide

LPS consists of three portions (Fig. 2.6):

• The first component is a lipid called *lipid A*, and anchors LPS in the outer leaflet of the membrane. Lipid A is an unusual glycolipid composed of disaccharides to which are attached short-chain fatty acids and phosphate groups.

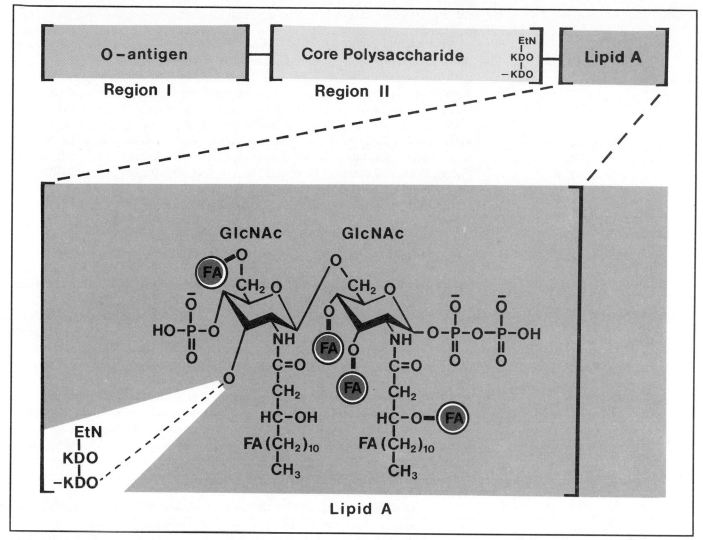

Lipid A

Figure 2.6. The structure of lipopolysaccharide. In a typical *Salmonella*, region I consists of a characteristic series of sugars in the polysaccharide. The sugars vary between organisms. Region II also shows some variation, but always ends with ketodeoxyoctanoate (KDO). The molecules of fatty acid (FA) attached to the sugars vary with the organisms, but are always a major source of the hydrophobicity of the molecule. The circles indicate O-linked fatty acids.

- The second component is a short series of sugars, the *core*, whose structure is relatively constant among Gram negative bacteria and includes two characteristic sugars, *ketodeoxyoctanoic acid* (KDO in Fig. 2.6) and a heptose.

- The third component is a long carbohydrate chain, up to 40 sugars in length, the *O antigen* (Fig. 2.6). The hydrophilic carbohydrate chains of the O antigen cover the bacterial surface and exclude hydrophobic compounds. The importance of the O antigen chains is shown with mutants deficient in their biosynthesis. Mutants that make either no O antigen or merely shortened chains become sensitive to compounds such as bile salts and antibiotics to which the wild type is resistant.

Thus, exclusion of hydrophobic compounds in Gram negative bacteria, as in Gram positive bacteria, relies on surrounding the cells with hydrophilic polysaccharides, different in structure and organization in the two groups. Because of its lipid nature, the outer membrane could be expected to exclude hydrophilic compounds as well. Seemingly nothing could then cross the outer membrane. By solving the problem of protection of the cytoplasmic membrane the Gram negative bacteria appear to have created a new one. How do they transport their nutrients? Are the active transport devices of the cytoplasmic membrane copied in the outer membrane? This would not only be wasteful but probably incompatible with the protective role assigned to the outer membrane. Once again, bacteria have found an interesting solution: The outer membrane has special channels that permit the passive diffusion of hydrophilic compounds such as sugars, amino acids, and certain ions. These channels consist of protein molecules with holes, aptly called *porins*. Porin channels are narrow, just right to permit the entry of compounds up to 600 to 700 daltons (Fig. 2.2). The channels are small enough that hydrophobic compounds would come in contact with the polar "wall" of the channel and thereby be excluded.

Certain hydrophilic compounds that are sometimes necessary for survival are larger than the exclusion limit of porins. These larger molecules include vitamin B_{12}, sugars bigger than trisaccharides, and iron in the form of chelates. Such compounds cross the outer membrane by separate, specific permeation mechanisms that utilize proteins especially designed to translocate each of these compounds. Thus the outer membrane allows the passage of small hydrophilic compounds; excludes hydrophobic compounds, large or small; and allows the entry of some larger hydrophilic molecules by especially dedicated mechanisms.

The dual membrane system of Gram negative bacteria creates a compartment called the *periplasmic space*, or *periplasm*, on the outside of the cytoplasmic or inner membrane. This compartment contains the murein layer and a gel-like solution of components that facilitates nutrition. These include degradative enzymes (phosphatases, nucleases, proteases, etc.) that break down large and impermeable molecules to "digestible" size. In addition, the periplasm contains so-called binding proteins that help soak up sugars and amino acids from the medium. It also contains enzymes that inactivate certain antibiotics, like those that work against penicillins and cephalosporins, the β-lactamases. The Gram positive bacteria do not have a defined periplasmic compartment and secrete analogous enzymes into the medium.

The outer membrane barrier constitutes both an advantage and a disadvantage to Gram negative bacteria. For example, some bacteriophages use proteins in the outer membrane as attachment sites for infecting their host bacteria. On the other hand, the outer membrane confers considerable resistance to many antibiotics. Broadly speaking, Gram negative bacteria are more resistant to some of the antibiotics, especially penicillin.

The Gram negatives' peculiar solution to the problems of protecting the cytoplasmic membrane has unexpected biological consequences. The lipopolysaccharide of the outer membrane is highly reactive in the host. The lipid A component has a large number of biological activities. It elicits fever and activates a series of immunological and biochemical events that lead to the mobilization of host defense mechanisms. In large doses, this compound, also known as *endotoxin*, can cause shock and even death (see Chapter 7 for details). The O antigen portion, as the name denotes, is highly antigenic. O antigens come in many varieties, each defining a species or a subspecies of Gram negative bacteria.

The Acid-Fast Solution

A few bacterial types, notably the tubercle bacillus, have developed yet another solution to the problems of environmental challenge to the cytoplasmic membrane. Their cell walls contain large amounts of *waxes*, which are complex long-chain hydrocarbons with sugars and other modifying groups. With such a protective cover, these organisms are impervious to many harsh chemicals, including acids. If a dye is introduced into these cells, for instance, by brief heating, it cannot be removed by dilute hydrochloric acid, as would be the case in all other bacteria. These organisms are therefore called *acid fast*, or acid resistant (Table 2.3).

The waxy coat is interlarded with murein, polysaccharides, and lipids. It enables the organisms to resist the action of many noxious chemicals as well as killing by white blood cells. All this is at a cost; these organisms grow very slowly, possibly because the rate of uptake of nutrients is limited by their waxy covering. Some, such as the human tubercle bacillus, divide once every 24 hours.

MUREIN AND ANTIBIOTICS THAT INHIBIT ITS SYNTHESIS

The uniqueness of bacterial murein makes it a natural target for antibiotics. Drugs that block its formation lead to lysis and death of susceptible bacteria. It is not surprising, therefore, that some of the clinically most effective antibiotics, the penicillins and the cephalosporins, act by inhibiting murein synthesis. They are among the most unequivocally bactericidal antibiotics and among those least toxic to humans. The critical steps in their mode of action are presented in Figures 2.7 and 2.8.

Murein, like many other polysaccharides, is synthesized from nucleotide-bound building blocks. These monomeric units are composed of uridine diphosphate plus either N-acetylglucosamine (GlcNAc) or N-acetyl muramic acid (an unusual sugar, the 3-O-D lactic acid derivative of GlcNAc). The latter has a peptide chain attached to it (Fig. 2.3). The monomeric units are made in the cytoplasm and transferred from uridine-diphosphate to a *lipid carrier* in the membrane (Fig. 2.7). Disaccharides are then linked to a growing chain of murein. This step is inhibited by the antibiotic vancomycin. Regeneration of the lipid carrier is inhibited by another antibiotic, bacitracin.

The final reaction in murein synthesis is transpeptidation. The long chains of disaccharides are cross-linked to make a two-dimensional network (Fig. 2.8). The cross-linking reaction consists of forming a peptide bond between D-alanine on one chain and the free N-end of a lysine or a diaminopimelic acid on the other chain. The linkage is formed with the *subterminal* D-alanine, and the *terminal* D-alanine is cleaved away in the process. Thus, the reaction is the exchange of one peptide bond (that between the two D-alanines) with another—a true transpeptidation. Cycloserine is an antibiotic that inhibits the ligation of the two D-ala residues and also inhibits the racemase that forms D-ala from L-ala, the common constituent of proteins. The amino acids that make up the peptides vary in different organisms, but the D-alanine cross-bridge to either lysine or diaminopimelic acid is universal. This reaction is inhibited by most penicillins and cephalosporins.

The reason why penicillin inhibits transpeptidation may lie in its stereochemical similarity with the D-alanine-D-alanine dimer (Figs. 2.8 and 2.9). In the presence of the drug, the transpeptidase becomes confused: Instead of synthesizing an intermediate D-alanine-enzyme complex, it makes a lethal penicilloyl-enzyme complex.

Antibiotics that inhibit murein synthesis almost invariably kill bacteria by lysing them. In contrast with lysozyme, these drugs do not affect murein itself, only its synthesis. How then do they cause lysis? Cells treated with these drugs continue to synthesize their cytoplasmic components and increase in mass. The enlarged cytoplasm is not restrained by a properly cross-linked murein sac, with

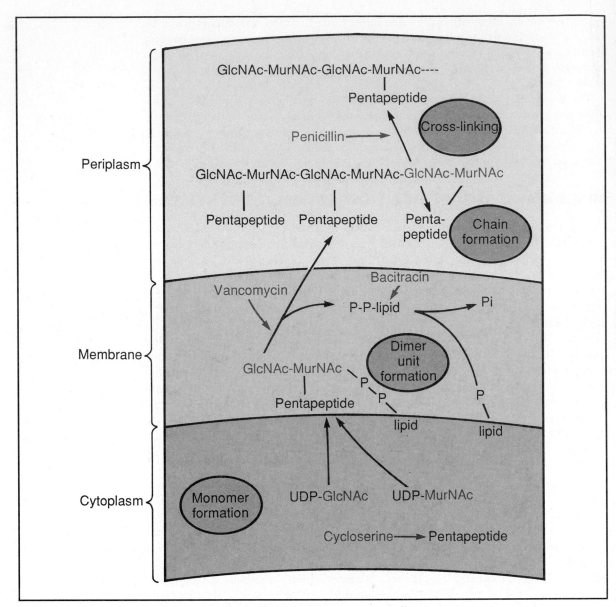

Figure 2.7. Biosynthesis of murein, indicating the site of action of a number of antibiotics. The successive steps occurring in the cytoplasm, at the cytoplasmic membrane, and outside the membrane (in the periplasm of Gram negatives; in the murein layer of Gram positives) are indicated, along with the points of attack of cycloserine, bacitracin, vancomycin, and penicillin.

the result that the cell contents extrude and the cells lyse. Cells that are not growing are not lysed by penicillin—they are not increasing in mass. Consider: Would it be advisable to administer an antibiotic that inhibits cell growth at the same time that the patient is receiving penicillin?

Penicillins and cephalosporins have an unusual property; they bind covalently to certain proteins of the cytoplasmic membrane, the so-called *penicillin binding proteins* (PBPs). These drugs are especially reactive because they have a highly strained β-lactam ring that can be readily hydrolyzed. Individual species of bacteria have a characteristic set of PBPs, each with a different affinity for a given penicillin. These proteins are thought to be involved in the cross-linking of murein. At least three types of PBPs have been distinguished: One seems to be especially involved in the generalized cross-linking that occurs at many points in the periphery of the cell. Another may participate in the special cross-linking at the junc-

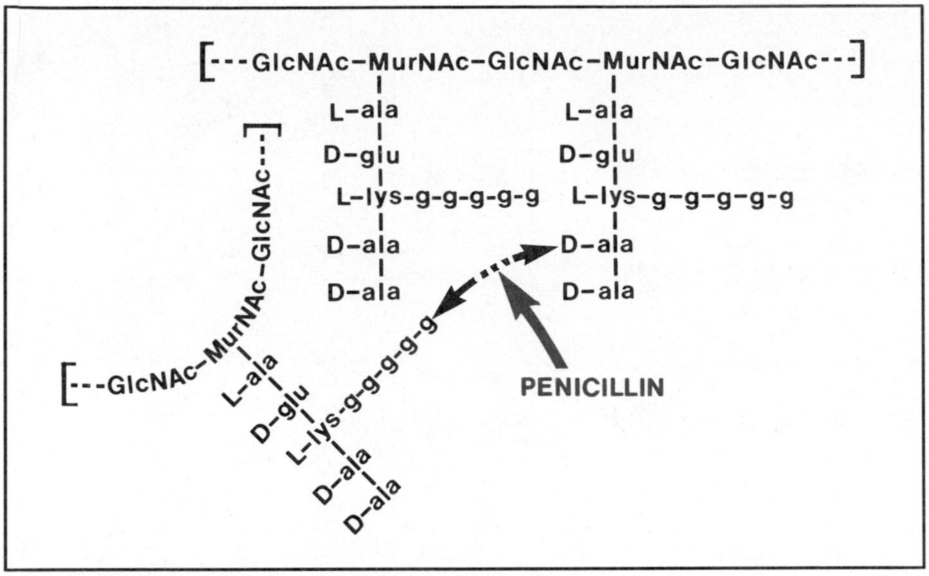

Figure 2.8. Formation of cross-links in murein, and the point of penicillin action in detail. In this case of a typical Gram positive murein structure, a cross-link forms between the last glycine residue (g) in one chain and the penultimate D-alanine in another chain, as indicated by the *double-headed arrow.* At that point, penicillin intervenes.

tion (septum) between separating daughter cells. The third appears to function at points where the nascent murein "turns corners" to determine cell shape. The functional distinction between PBPs has been facilitated by a penicillin called *mecillinam*, which binds to only one of these proteins (Fig. 2.10). Mecillinam blocks only parts of murein cross-linking, and leads to the release of constraints on the cell shape of *E. coli*. This results in the formation of large, unstable spherical cells that slowly lyse. In mutants resistant to mecillinam this particular PBP is modified and no longer binds β-lactam antibiotics. The mutants remain suscepti-ble to other penicillins which bind to other PBPs.

This simple view, that cells lyse by outgrowing their coats, runs into some difficulties. First, in cultures treated with penicillin there is usually a small num-ber of "persisters", bacteria that stop growing but do not lyse. Second, for some

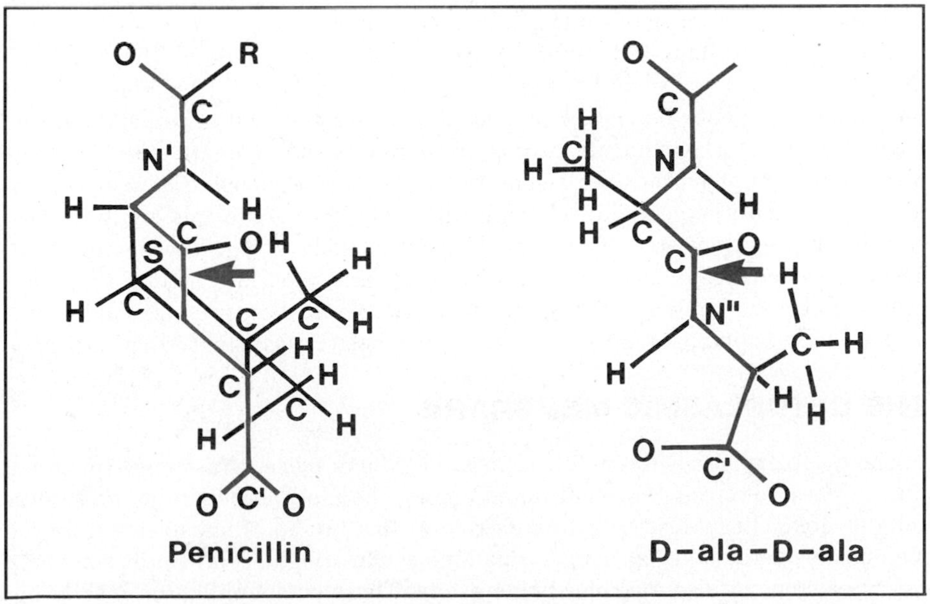

Figure 2.9. The resemblance of part of the penicillin structure to the backbone of D-ala-D-ala is indicated, with the *ar-rows* at the bonds broken during cova-lent attachment to the enzyme involved. (From Blumberg P, Strominger JL. Inter-action of penicillin with the bacterial cell wall: Penicillin-binding proteins and penicillin-sensitive enzymes. *Bacterial Rev* 38: 291–335, 1974)

Figure 2.10. Binding of penicillin to membrane proteins (PBPs) of wild-type and mecillinam-resistant *E. coli*. Radioactive penicillin binds to a number of proteins. In the resistant mutant, the only protein to which mecillinam binds is missing. ^{14}C labeled benzylpenicillin (A–D) or mecillinam (E–H) were bound to cell envelopes from a wild-type strain and one resistant to mecillinam. The inner membranes were solubilized in detergent and the radioactive proteins separated by gel electrophoresis and detected by autoradiography. Benzylpenicillin binds to six PBPs in wild-type cells (A–B) and five in the mutant (C, D); mecillinam binds only to one protein in the wild type (E, F) and not at all in the mutant (G, H). (From Spratt B: Distinct penicillin binding proteins involved in the division, elongation and shape of *Escherichia coli* K12. *Proc Natl Acad Sci USA* 72: 2999, 1975.)

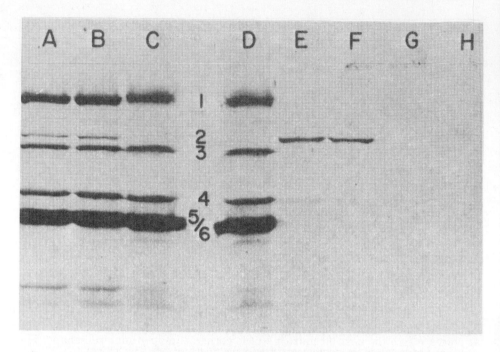

types of bacteria, penicillin is bacteriostatic, not bactericidal. These bacteria are called "tolerant". How do we explain "persisters" or "tolerant" bacteria? It appears that tolerant organisms are deficient in an *autolysin*, a bacterial enzyme that cleaves murein. Bacteria use such an enzyme to break open some bonds of murein at the septum, which permits the separation of daughter cells during cell division. Normally the activity of autolysin is tightly controlled. Treatment with penicillin may arouse it to more unrestrained action. The role of autolysin in penicillin-induced lysis is well illustrated with pneumococci, which are extraordinarily easy to lyse by many means. Autolysin-defective mutants are found among penicillin-resistant derivatives; these mutants are not lysed even by strong detergents. Thus, bacteria do not burst easily. Rather than a spontaneous explosion, lysis involves active steps of self-destruction.

There are exceptions to the universal use of murein to maintain bacterial cell integrity. The *mycoplasmas* have no murein and consequently are not rigid and have almost no defined shape. As expected, they are resistant to penicillin. Some, such as an agent of pneumonia, *Mycoplasma pneumoniae*, contain sterols in their membrane, an unusual feature among procaryotes. It is puzzling how mycoplasmas cope well without a rigid cell wall. Although these organisms are quite delicate in culture, they are common in the human body and in the environment. There are other exceptions to the ubiquity of mureins, especially among a separate group of bacteria known as the Archaeobacteria. Thus, there are unorthodox and as yet poorly understood means by which some bacteria safeguard their integrity.

THE CYTOPLASMIC MEMBRANE

The cytoplasmic membrane of bacteria is a busy place. It assumes functions that in eucaryotic cells are distributed among the plasma membrane and intracellular organelles. Most critical is its role in the uptake of substrates from the medium. Bacteria take up mainly small-molecular-weight compounds and only rarely macromolecules and phosphate esters. These compounds are usually hydrolyzed by enzymes in the periplasm or the surrounding medium, and the result-

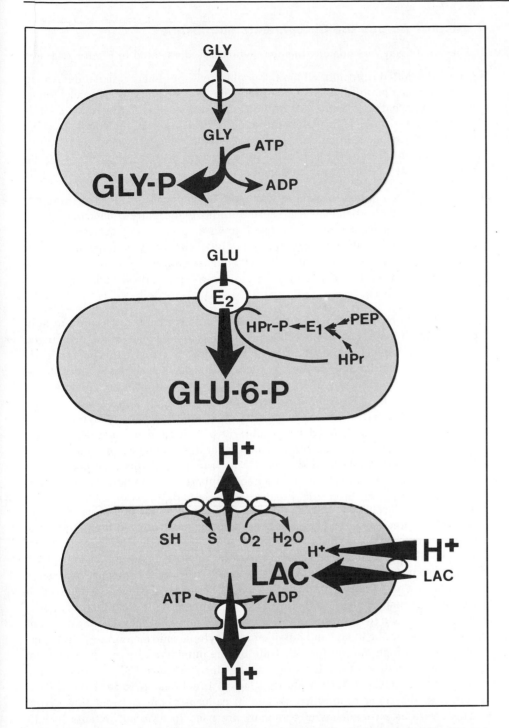

Figure 2.11. Mechanics of transport. Three types of transport in *E. coli* are shown. Facilitated diffusion; group translocation; active transport with the lactose permease. (From Kaback HR: Ion gradient coupled transport. From Andreoli TE, Hoffman JS, Sanastil DD, *et al*: *Physiology of Membrane Disorders*. New York: Plenum Pub. 1986, pp. 387–407.)

ing breakdown products (peptides, oligosaccharides, nucleosides, phosphate, etc.) can then be transported across the cytoplasmic membrane.

The cytoplasmic membrane contains specific carrier proteins called permeases that facilitate the entry of most metabolites. In some cases the carrier facilitates the equilibration of a compound inside and outside the cell (Fig. 2.11). However, in most cases carrier-mediated transport requires the expenditure of energy. This permits the internal concentration of certain substances to be as much as 10^5 higher than that in the medium surrounding the cell.

Transport Across the Cytoplasmic Membrane

The three main versions of transport, which are illustrated in Figure 2.11, are:

- *Carrier-mediated diffusion*, which takes place without energy demands. An example of a compound that is transported this way is glycerol. This mechanism does not concentrate compounds in the inside of the cells relative to the outside environment. Uptake is driven by intracellular utilization of the compound. For instance, the concentration of free glycerol inside cells is lowered by its phosphorylation to glycerol-3-phosphate. More glycerol is then taken up to equilibrate with the outside concentration.

- *Phosphorylation-linked transport*, which is a mechanism used for the transport of certain sugars. Substances transported in this manner are chemically altered in the process, which is why it is also known as *group translocation*. The example of glucose is shown in Figure 2.11. The sugar binds to a specific carrier in the membrane (e.g., "enzyme 2"). The glucose-enzyme 2 complex interacts with an enzyme called HPr-P, to yield glucose-6-phosphate, which can then be further metabolized.

- *Active transport*, in which energy is utilized to drive the accumulation of substrate. A substrate, for instance the sugar lactose, is concentrated unchanged inside the cell, which makes the transport of additional molecules energetically unfavorable. In order to drive the transport of lactose, the cells use energy stored in an electrochemical gradient of protons, the *proton motive force*. This gradient is generated by the extrusion of protons from the cell (Fig. 2.11), resulting from the oxidation of metabolic intermediates such as NADH or by hydrolysis of ATP. Lactose is accumulated intracellularly by coupling its energetically unfavorable transport with the energetically favorable reentry of protons into the relatively acidic cytoplasm of the cell. Thus, transport of this type takes place via a *synport*, which allows the simultaneous uptake of molecules, H^+ and sugar.

Each type of transport system involves specific protein molecules. Some of these aid the process by modifying or concentrating substrates in the periplasmic space of Gram negatives. These *binding proteins* are specific for sugars, nucleotides, etc. The periplasmic space also contains nucleosidases, nucleases, peptidases, proteases and other hydrolytic enzymes. The actual transport process is carried out by membrane-bound carriers called *permeases*, which are involved in the types of transport mentioned above. We do not have a physical picture of how permeases respond to the proton gradient, but we know that they assume different configurations on the inside and outside of the cytoplasmic membrane. Thus, permeases have a high affinity for substrate on the outside and low affinity on the inside. However they work, they are essential for transport. For example, in the much studied lactose system, cells that lack a functional permease remain impervious to the sugar even when soaked in concentrations approaching syrup!

These various mechanisms of transport are used to different extents by different bacteria. In general, few substrates equilibrate across membranes without the expenditure of energy. Among the energy-requiring mechanisms, "group translocations" are used to a different extent: *E. coli*, for instance, transports a wide variety of sugars in this way, whereas strictly aerobic bacteria use it little. All in all, active transport dominates the repertoire of transport mechanisms in bacteria, especially when nutrients must be concentrated from the medium in order to support cell growth.

Uptake of Iron

The uptake of iron deserves special mention. Iron is not available in free form in the blood and many tissues because it is bound by proteins such as transferrin or ceruloplasmin, yet is essential for the growth of bacteria. Many bacteria that inhabit the human body have developed ingenious mechanisms to obtain the amounts of this element they need for growth. They excrete chelating compounds known as *siderophores* that bind iron with great avidity. Each organism can take up its own particular form of complexed iron; individual complexes are .unique enough to be less digestible for other organisms. However, in response to the competition for iron, many bacteria have multiple siderophores and uptake systems, thus trying to gain an edge on the other organisms in the same environment; some can efficiently extract iron from transferrin, an advantage at our own expense.

Other Functions of the Bacterial Membrane

The cytoplasmic membrane of bacteria is also the site where cytochromes are located and where oxidative metabolism is carried out. It thus performs the role of the mitochondria of eucaryotic cells. Another function of the bacterial membrane is to act like a primitive mitotic apparatus. It is thought that bacterial DNA is attached to the cell membrane, with each newly replicated molecule sticking to one side of the septum made during cell division. When the bacterium divides, each half receives one of the daughter chromosomes.

The membrane is also the location of nascent proteins destined either for secretion or for incorporation in the membrane itself. Some bacteria secrete as much as 10% of all the proteins they make. The nascent peptide chains, containing the hydrophobic "signal sequences" at the N-termini, are translocated from ribosomes across the cytoplasmic membrane by an energy-requiring mechanism. Proteins that are to be secreted are released into the environment while those that become part of the membrane structure are retained within it. Note that in the Gram negative bacteria there is an added problem, that of transporting proteins to the outer membrane. It is not known how this takes place.

Bacteria have also the exceptional ability to take up huge DNA molecules. Although uptake of very large molecules is usually regarded as a property of eucaryotic cells only, at least for the case of DNA uptake, the phenomenon was first demonstrated by genetic transformation of pneumococci and occurs among other bacterial species. Some, such as *E. coli*, must be coaxed to take up DNA by the addition of calcium ions. Very little is known about the mechanism of uptake of DNA by bacteria but it appears that, like active transport, it depends on the proton motive force.

In spite of its versatility and range of activities, the cytoplasmic membrane of bacteria is rarely the site of action of useful antibiotics (see Chapter 3). May this be due to its overall similarity in structure to the membranes of eucaryotic cells?

DNA AND CHROMOSOME MECHANICS

The genome of bacteria consists of a single circular chromosome of double-stranded DNA. For all its importance, it accounts for only some 2% of the cellular dry weight. The chromosome of *E. coli* has a molecular weight of about 3×10^9, or about five million base pairs. This codes for about 2000 to 3000 genes, about half of which have been identified. The total description of the *E. coli* genome seems only a few years away, making this the genetically best known of all living organisms.

Bacteria must solve a demanding topological problem in organizing their DNA, since it is long and thin. If stretched out it would be about 1000 times the length of the cell. If a bacterium were to be magnified to the size of a human being, its DNA would be about a mile long. The DNA is coiled in a central irregular structure called the *nucleoid*. Its physical state is unknown and somewhat mysterious because in the test tube a solution 100 times more dilute is a gel! About all that is known about the physical state of the DNA is that it is twisted into supercoils and that this condition is indispensable for its organization, its replication, and the transcription of a number of genes. Supercoiling is thought to be achieved by the balance of the action of two topoisomerases. One of these, *DNA gyrase,*

Figure 2.12. Replication of DNA in slow and fast-growing *E. coli*. Replication begins at a specific site, the origin, and proceeds in both directions towards a terminus. The process takes about 40 minutes at 37°C. In a culture doubling every 20 minutes, this requires that the process initiate every 20 minutes, that is, before the previous round of replication has terminated. In such cultures the DNA is undergoing multifork replication.

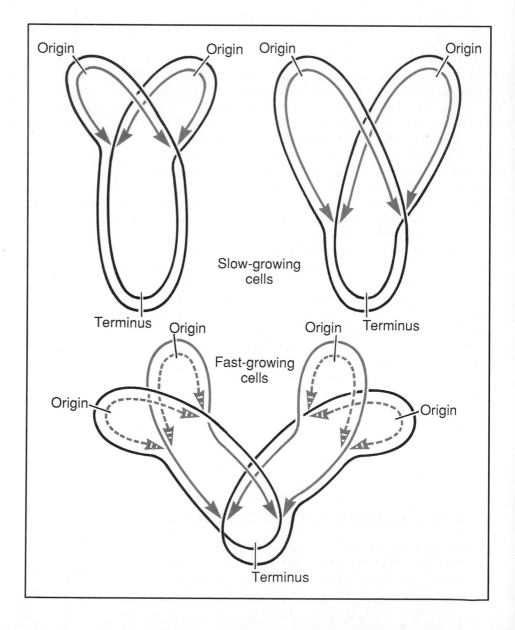

introduces supercoils into circular DNA, an action counteracted by a second enzyme, *topoisomerase I*, which relaxes the supercoils by making single-strand nicks.

Like all macromolecular synthesis, DNA replication has three phases: initiation, elongation, and termination. Replication takes place bidirectionally; that is, DNA synthesis starts at a precise place on the chromosome, the replicative origin, and proceeds away from it in both directions. The two moving polymerase complexes meet halfway around the chromosome. In order to replicate, the DNA helix in *E. coli* must unwind and rotate at some 6000 rpm. One wonders how this can take place without entanglement of the tightly coiled nucleoid.

The timing of chromosome replication is a highly regulated process and is coupled to growth and cell division. At a given temperature the rate of DNA polymerase movement is independent of the growth rate of the cells. In *E. coli*, DNA replication takes 40 minutes, whether the cells are growing slowly or fast. In slowly growing cells, e.g., those dividing once every 100 minutes, one round of synthesis occurs in each division cycle, and no DNA is synthesized during the remaining 60 minutes. In very fast growing cells (dividing, for example, every 20 minutes), initiation of rounds of replication is adapted to produce new chromosomes as often as the cell divides (Fig. 2.12). Since each chromosome requires 40 minutes to be synthesized, replication will initiate again on a strand, long before its own replication has completed. Thus chromosome replication in bacteria is regulated by how often the process gets started, i.e., by the frequency of initiation of DNA synthesis.

How Do Antibiotics Inhibit DNA Metabolism?

Most inhibitors of DNA replication bind to DNA and are too toxic for clinical use. An interesting exception is *metronidazole*, a drug that is itself inert but that can be selectively modified to an active form by some bacteria. This compound contains a nitro group that must be partially reduced to render the molecule active. Full reduction to the amino state makes the molecule inactive again. Partial reduction is achieved by anaerobic bacteria but only rarely by the cells of the human body or by aerobic bacteria.

Partially reduced metronidazole is incorporated into the DNA of the bacteria. This is an example of lethal synthesis since the metronidazole-containing DNA molecules are unstable. It follows that metronidazole and related drugs are particularly useful against anaerobic bacteria and against amoebas, which also grow anaerobically. These drugs, however, are not ideal. To a small extent, the partial reduction to active agents occurs in normal tissue, leading to possible mutagenesis and perhaps carcinogenesis as well.

Other DNA inhibitors act selectively by binding to specific enzymes. *Nalidixic acid*, for example, inhibits DNA gyrase and is bactericidal. Whether it binds to the counterpart human enzyme in vivo is not known, but it is relatively nontoxic.

GENE EXPRESSION: THE UNIQUENESS OF PROCARYOTIC RNA POLYMERASE AND RIBOSOMES

The bacterial cytoplasm is composed largely of proteins (about 40% of the dry weight, with about one million molecules per cell) and RNA (up to 35% of the dry weight in rapidly growing cells). Bacterial ribosomes have smaller subunits (30S and 50S vs. 40S and 60S) and smaller RNA molecules than do their eucaryotic counterparts. Bacterial ribosomal RNAs have sedimentation values of 16S and 23S, which, combined with 21 and 35 different proteins respectively, make up the ribosomal subunits. These join together in the 70S ribosomes, which move along messenger RNA molecules to synthesize proteins.

The large requirement for proteins makes their synthesis the principal biosynthetic activity of rapidly growing bacteria. A large proportion of a bacterium's energy and metabolic building blocks is devoted to the assembly of the protein-synthesizing machinery, including ribosomes and RNA polymerase. Over a considerable range of growth rates, the production rate of RNA is proportional to the number of RNA polymerase molecules engaged in the process of transcription. Likewise, the rate of protein synthesis is proportional to the cellular concentration of ribosomes. This suggests that the rate of polymerization of single chains of RNA or protein is the same in cells growing either rapidly or slowly, and cannot be increased. Remember that this is also true for DNA replication (see "DNA and Chromosome Mechanics"). Thus, the synthesis of the principal macromolecules of bacteria is *regulated by the frequency with which each chain is initiated* and not by altering their rate of manufacture of each molecule (the speed of chain elongation).

Cells growing rapidly increase the frequency of initiation of RNA or protein synthesis by an analogous mechanism to that used to generate chromosomes more often than once every 40 minutes. As one RNA polymerase molecule moves away from the start site on the DNA, another can become engaged, so that a single gene can be transcribed concurrently into many RNA molecules. Likewise, a single mRNA can be translated by many ribosomes simultaneously, creating a structure called a polyribosome or polysome.

Antibiotics That Inhibit Transcription and Translation

Antibiotics may act selectively at initiation or elongation of macromolecular synthesis. For example, *rifampin*, a powerful inhibitor of bacterial transcription, acts at the initiation step. How does it recognize this step? This drug binds strongly to molecules of RNA polymerase that are floating freely in the cytoplasm, but much less well to polymerase molecules that are bound to DNA. As a result, a polymerase that is bound to DNA and has initiated RNA synthesis will not be inactivated by rifampin until it completes its round of RNA synthesis and is released from the DNA. Rifampin is clinically useful, particularly in case of tuberculosis and leprosy, in part because it is relatively nontoxic. The reason is that mammalian RNA polymerases do not bind rifampin.

The largest class of clinically useful antibiotics, apart from the β-lactams, consists of those that inhibit protein synthesis. Some of them work by binding to ribosomes, either to the large or the small subunit (Table 2.4). Among them are *chloramphenicol*, *lincomycin* and *erythromycin*, which block the formation of peptide bonds by binding at or near the aminoacyl tRNA binding site on the large ribosomal subunit. After some time, the previously synthesized peptidyl tRNA is released and hydrolyzed. The ribosomal subunits are then released from the mRNA and are free to rejoin other mRNA molecules to start another abortive cycle. This leads to a truncated version of the ribosome cycle (Fig. 2.13). As a result, when these antibiotics are withdrawn, many free ribosomes are present and ready to resume normal protein synthesis. This explains why the action of these drugs is reversible and why these antibiotics are bacteriostatic and not bactericidal. It should be pointed out that this does not necessarily diminish their usefulness. When bacteria are kept in check by bacteriostatic drugs, they are usually cleared from tissues by the body defense mechanisms.

Table 2.4
Mechanisms of action of commonly used antimicrobial agents

β-lactams: Murein synthesis inhibitors Penicillins & cephalosporins	Interfere with cell wall biosynthesis through interaction with penicillin-binding proteins; autolysis.
Polyenes: Inhibitors of membrane function (Amphotericin B)	Bind to sterols in eucaryotic cell membranes, leading to membrane leakiness and, at high levels, lysis.
Sulfonamides: Folate antagonists Sulfanilamide	Competitive inhibitor of dehydropteroate synthesis. Blocks synthesis of tetrahydrofolate, and cell-linked metabolic pathways.

Aminoglycosides: Protein-synthesis inhibitors
  Streptomycin
  Kanamycin
  Neomycin
  Gentamicin
  Amikacin
  Tobramycin
	Bind to 30S subunit of bacterial ribosome. Cause translational misreading and inhibit elongation of protein chain. Kill by blocking initiation of protein synthesis.

Other protein-synthesis inhibitors
  Chloramphenicol
  Erythromycin
  Lincomycin
	Bind to ribosome 50S subunit. Inhibit protein synthesis at chain elongation step.

Fusidic acid	Blocks protein synthesis by interaction with soluble elongation factor G (the translocation factor).
RNA synthesis inhibitors Rifampin	Binds to bacterial RNA polymerase and blocks transcription (synthesis of RNA) at initiation step.

DNA synthesis inhibitors
  Nitrofurans
  Metronidazole
	Partially reduced nitro groups give addition products on DNA that lead to cidal strand breakage.

Nalidixic acid
  Novobiocin
  Ciprofloxacin
	Interfere with DNA replication by inhibiting the action of DNA gyrase.

Mercury salts, organomercurials	Inhibit protein function by interaction with sulfhydryl groups.

One important group of protein synthesis inhibitors, the *aminoglycosides*, is bactericidal. How they kill bacteria has not yet been satisfactorily explained, but we have some hints. Aminoglycosides, such as streptomycin, kanamycin and neomycin, are taken up by bacteria and bind to the smaller 30S ribosomal subunit. This is their critical site of action, as demonstrated by the finding that a single amino acid change in a mutated 30S ribosomal protein leads to resistance to these drugs. Binding of aminoglycosides has many effects on ribosome function; for instance, the interaction of the 30S and 50S subunits becomes tighter, and the elongation of peptide chains is inhibited. Typical of the action of this group of antibiotics is the accumulation of free ribosomes as aberrant 70S particles and

Figure 2.13. Antibiotic blockage of the ribosome cycle. The normal cycle of 30S and 50S subunits in and out of polysomes is recalled, with the assembly of a 70S initiation complex, elongation of the polypeptide chain as the ribosome moves across the mRNA, and release of all components on completion of the polypeptide. Points of blockage by antibiotics are shown. Tetracycline inhibits aminoacyl tRNA binding; cidal aminoglycosides provoke formation of "dead" aberrant initiation complexes; fucidin blocks translocation by elongation factor G; and others block elongation, leading to premature dissociation of the active complex.

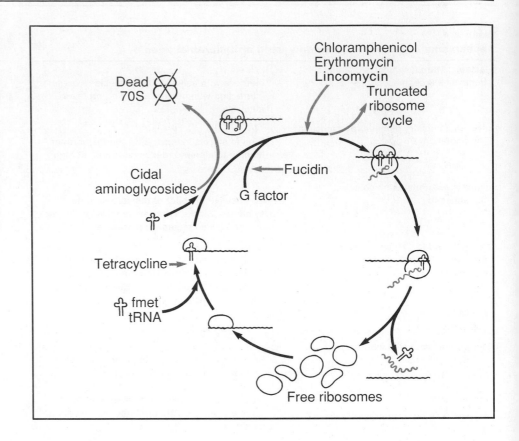

not as subunits. This coincides with cell death. These accumulating 70S ribosomes result from abortive attempts to initiate protein synthesis and do not function appreciably in protein synthesis. However, they bind to mRNA and thus block the function of ribosomes that are still unaffected by the drug. The inhibition of protein synthesis by aminoglycosides is apparently irreversible because once the drug is taken up it cannot be removed. Thus, cells treated with these drugs cannot recover, which is one possible way to explain why the aminoglycosides are bactericidal; but the reason for the extraordinary irreversibility of uptake remains imperfectly understood.

CAPSULES, FLAGELLA, AND PILI: HOW BACTERIA COPE IN CERTAIN ENVIRONMENTS

The morphological variety of bacteria is not limited to walls and membranes. Some bacteria, but by no means all, have other exterior structures such as capsules, flagella, and pili. These components are dispensable, that is, they are important for survival under certain circumstances but not others. The capsule is a slimy outer coating found in some bacteria. Under laboratory conditions the capsule is not needed and bacteria may grow well without it. Capsules usually consist of high-molecular-weight polysaccharides that make the bacteria very slippery and difficult for white blood cells to phagocytize. As you will see, pneumococci, meningococci and other bacteria that are likely to encounter phagocytes during their infective cycle are indeed encapsulated. In the laboratory, colonies of encapsulated bacteria on agar plates are viscous and shiny. Colonies of nonencapsulated organisms appear dull.

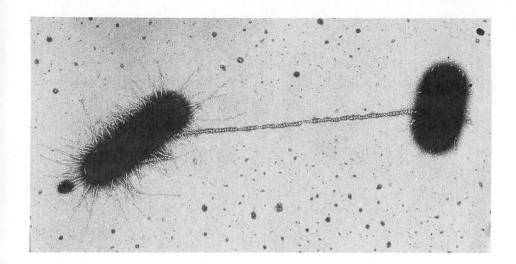

Figure 2.14. *Escherichia coli* mating. The cell covered with numerous append-ages (pili) is a genetic donor connected to a recipient cell (without appendages) by the so-called F pilus. The F pilus is a specialized structure (sex pilus) itself controlled by genes on the fertility, or F plasmid. The F pilus has been labeled by special virus particles that infect do-nor cells via the F pilus. The other pili surrounding the cell have no role in con-jugation but are required by *E. coli* for colonization and pathogenicity in the in-testinal and urinary tracts of humans and animals. (Electron micrograph courtesy of Drs. C. C. Brinton and J. Carnham.)

Protruding through the surface layers of many bacteria are two kinds of fila-ments, flagella and pili (also called fimbriae) (Fig. 2.14). Flagella are long, helical filaments that endow bacteria with motility. Many successful pathogens are motile, which probably aids their spread in the environment and possibly in the body of the host. Depending on the species, a single bacterial cell may have one flagellum or many flagella (Fig. 2.15). In some, the flagella are located at the ends of the cells (polar) and in others at random points around the periphery (peritrichous, or "hairy all over"). This distinction is useful in taxonomy and in diagnostic micro-biology. Pili are involved in the attachment of bacteria to cells and other surfaces (see "Bacterial Adhesion and the Pili").

Figure 2.15. Arrangement of flagella in some types of bacteria.

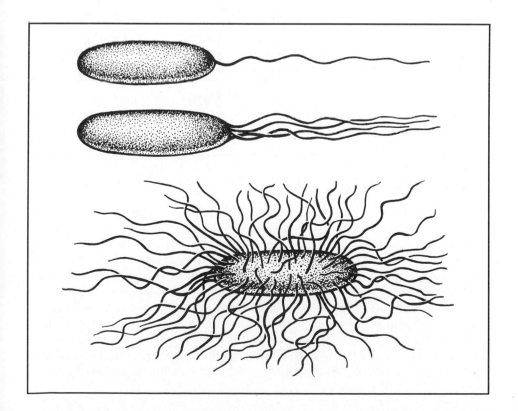

Figure 2.16. Flagellar arrangement and motility. *A*, A bacterium moving smoothly right to left when its single polar flagellum rotates counterclockwise; this is the same direction as the thread of the helix formed by the flagellin molecules in the flagellum. *B*, The same bacterium tumbles generally left to right when the flagellum rotates clockwise. *C* and *D*, With a peritrichous bacterium, counterclockwise rotation (*C*) produces a coherent bundle of flagella and smooth movement; the tumbling produced by clockwise rotation is extreme (*D*). (Adapted from Boyd RF, Hoerl BG: *Basic Medical Microbiology*. Boston, Little Brown & Co., 1986.)

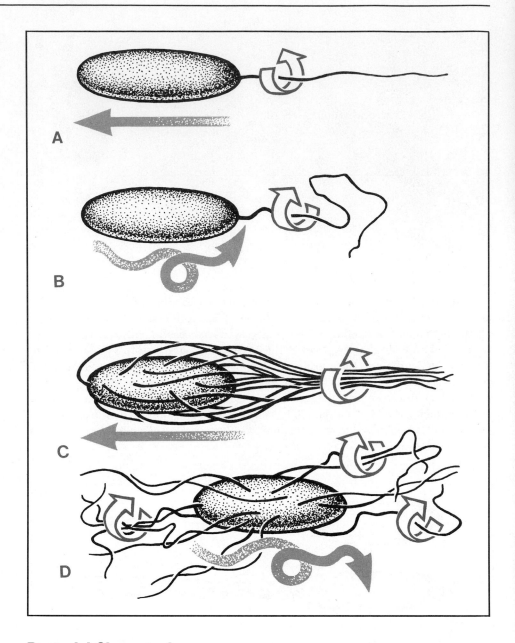

Bacterial Chemotaxis

The movement caused by flagella is used by bacteria for chemotaxis, i.e., movement toward substances that attract and away from those that repel. Considerable research has shown that bacterial chemotaxis is based on the following sophisticated mechanism: Flagella spin around from their point of attachment at the cell surface. Each flagellum has a counterclockwise helical pitch and when there are several on a bacterium, they array themselves in coherent bundles as long as they all rotate counterclockwise. When the flagella are arranged in these bundles, they beat in the same sense and the bacteria swim in a straight line (Fig. 2.16). However, when flagella rotate clockwise they get in each other's way and cannot form bundles. As a result, the bacteria tumble in random fashion. The two types of motion, swimming and tumbling, account for bacterial chemotaxis. In the absence of attractants or repellants, bacteria alternate indifferently between swimming and tumbling. When an attractant is sensed, swimming lasts longer than tumbling, whereas swimming stops more quickly when a repellant is present. The net result is movement toward attractants and away from repellants. Little is known about the role of chemotaxis in pathogenesis, but it would be surprising if it were not important in some instances in guiding bacteria toward cellular targets or possibly away from white blood cells.

Bacterial Adhesion and the Pili

Whether by active chemotaxis or more passive mechanisms, microorganisms home in on specific tissues. Sometimes this *tissue tropism* results from the selective survival of the organism in a particular environment; for example, the fungi that cause athlete's foot cannot grow at 37°C, which explains why they are found only on the skin and not in the interior of the body. In other cases, tropism involves attachment of surface components of the organisms to specific receptors present on the cells of certain tissues. The bacterial structures most often involved in attachment are the pili. These are filaments shorter than flagella and distributed, often in large numbers, over the surface of some bacteria. Bacteria that can conjugate have, in addition, specialized *sex pili*. These are rather different structures from the "common pili". They are much longer and link the donor (male) and recipient (female) cells during transfer of DNA by conjugation.

Pili allow bacteria to adhere to the surface of host cells, or, in the case of sex pili, to other bacteria. The *E. coli* strains that cause traveler's diarrhea adhere through pili to cells of the small intestine where they secrete a toxin that causes the symptoms of the disease. Likewise, pili are essential for gonococci to infect the epithelial cells of the genitourinary tract.

Pili have other roles in disease. Like capsules, they can be antiphagocytic. They are also highly changeable and permit some organisms to put on a succession of disguises that enable them to outflank the immune system. This has been studied in detail in the gonococcus. Gonococci have a large number of genes that code for variants of the protein, *pilin*, that polymerizes to form pili. Each version of pilin is antigenically distinct and elicits the formation of different antibodies. In the presence of antibodies to one type of pilin, there is rapid selection for variants of gonococci that have switched to the synthesis of another antigenic type of pilin. Thus they keep one step ahead in this quick-change scenario. Only one (or a few) of the large repertoire of pilin genes is active at any time. The molecular basis for the shift from one pilin to another is that pilin genes contain two types of sequences: One codes for a constant portion of the pilin protein that is not very antigenic, the second codes for a variable region that is highly antigenic. At intervals, a constant region will recombine with a variable region to form a gene that codes for a complete pilin protein. The result is that many varieties of pilin genes can arise and be expressed, allowing the organisms to survive for long times in the face of the host immune response. It is easy to see why attempts to immunize against gonococci using a particular pilin vaccine have failed so far.

Such specific rearrangements of portions of genes are not unique. A comparable shuffling of constant and variable portions of genes gives rise to the magnificent variety of antibodies made by the body. In microorganisms, analogous mechanisms have been found in yeast, in the bacteria that cause relapsing fever (*Borrelia*) and in the protozoa that cause sleeping sickness (trypanosomes). By a related mechanism organisms that cause food poisoning and other illnesses, the

Salmonella, undergo rapid changes between expression and nonexpression of genes that code for the protein of flagella. This change in flagellar synthesis is called *phase variation* and is based on the control of a gene for flagellar protein. The gene can be inverted on the chromosome and can only be read in one of the two orientations.

NUTRITION AND ENERGY METABOLISM

Bacteria survive and grow in a large variety of ecological niches. Whatever their habitat, they must synthesize cellular constituents in a coordinated manner in order to grow. The required building blocks must either be provided at suitable levels in the medium or be synthesized in proper amounts by the organisms themselves. With regard to their nutritional requirements, bacteria can be divided into two large groups: In one are the photosynthetic or chemosynthetic bacteria that subsist on CO_2 and minerals, using either light or chemical energy. The other includes all the organisms that need preformed organic components. All pathogenic microorganisms fall in the second group, but within it they have many gradations of nutritional needs. Some, like *E. coli*, are satisfied with glucose and some inorganic material (Table 2.5). Other pathogenic bacteria, like their human host, are unable to make one or more essential metabolites—vitamins, amino acids, purines, pyrimidines, etc., which must be supplied as growth factors.

Bacteria also have a wide range of responses to oxygen. At the extremes are the *strict aerobes*, which must have oxygen to grow. An example is the tubercle bacillus, which thrives in the portions of the body that are better oxygenated, such as the lungs. At the other extreme are the *strict*, or *obligate*, *anaerobes*, bacteria that cannot grow in the presence of oxygen, such as the organisms that cause botulism and tetanus. The largest number of bacteria that are medically important can grow whether or not oxygen is present. They are called *facultative anaerobes*, and include *E. coli* and other intestinal bacteria.

These differences in the response to oxygen mirror the way bacteria oxidize substrates to obtain energy. Strict aerobes carry out *respiration* only, the process in which the final electron acceptor in a series of coupled oxidation-reductions is molecular oxygen. Strict anaerobes carry out *fermentation*, where the final hydrogen acceptor is an organic molecule. Examples of organic electron acceptors are pyruvate, which is reduced to lactate in the lactic acid fermentation, or acetyl-CoA, which is reduced to alcohol in ethanol fermentation. Facultative anaerobes are capable of either form of metabolism, depending on whether oxygen is present or absent. Thus, they will respire in its presence and ferment in its absence.

Respiration yields more energy per molecule of substrate oxidized. Therefore, fermentative organisms must turn over more substrate to obtain the same amount

Table 2.5
Glucose minimal medium

Per liter:	g	Main Source of
Na_2HPO_4	6	P, buffering power, osmotic strength
KH_2PO_4	3	P, buffering power, osmotic strength
NH_4Cl	1	N
$MgSO_4$	0.012	Mg, S
$CaCl_2$	0011	Ca
Glucose	2	Energy, carbon-building blocks

of energy. The industrial microbiologist takes advantage of this for the purpose of maximizing either the yield of cell mass or the amount of metabolic products formed. Under what conditions of oxygenation would you grow yeast in a fermentation tank if the intended product were (a) yeast cake, or (b) alcohol?

We have mentioned that *E. coli* can use glucose as its sole organic source. It can also utilize other compounds, such as lactose, fructose, or one of several amino acids. The list includes some 30 known substances, but this is not particularly impressive compared with species of *Pseudomonas*, which can grow on any of several hundred organic compounds. No wonder these nearly omnivorous organisms have been used by genetic engineers to construct strains for use in the degradation of environmental pollutants. No wonder *Pseudomonas* species are omnipresent in the water supply and the soil, and often infect wounds and burns.

Although these bacteria can manage on meager solutions of glucose and a few salts, they do not disdain richer fare. When *E. coli* is given a mixture of amino acids, sugars, vitamins, etc., it will use the compounds provided rather than making them endogenously. The result is sparing of energy and biosynthetic potential, and faster growth. In the laboratory it is possible to culture bacteria in media that are truly spartan, the so-called *minimal media*, which are water solutions of glucose, ammonia, phosphate, sulfate, and other minerals (Table 2.5). Conversely, they can be grown in a rich medium, a *nutrient broth* that contains meat extract and soluble partial hydrolysates of complex proteins. Add agar to these solutions and you have the corresponding solid media.

Some bacteria can grow only in complex media and have nutritional requirements that rival or exceed those of humans. The organisms are said to be *nutritionally fastidious*. This is characteristic of highly parasitic species that are found in close association with the rich environment of the human body. Examples of these organisms are the staphylococci or the streptococci which can grow only if provided with a long list of compounds. As expected, bacteria that can get by with only a few nutrients, *E. coli* or *Pseudomonas*, are found also in less enriched habitats, like bodies of water. The ecology of an organism usually gives good hints of its nutritional requirements.

GROWING AND RESTING STATES

When bacteria find themselves in a suitable environment they grow and eventually divide. The time it takes for a bacterium to become two is called the *generation time*, or doubling time. For example, *E. coli* requires about 20 minutes to double in rich nutrient broth and 1 to 2 hours in minimal medium at 37°C. Growth will go on until the population reaches a certain density when the nutrients in the environment become exhausted or toxic metabolites accumulate. Until this occurs, the bacteria grow in an unhindered manner and are physiologically all alike. This condition is called *balanced growth*, since all cell constituents will increase proportionally over the same period of time. Such a steady state does not exist for long in nature since the environment usually undergoes rapid changes.

The Measurement of Bacterial Growth and a Few Definitions

How is bacterial growth measured? The most direct way is to take samples at different times and count the number of bacteria under a microscope using a hemocytometer chamber. This tedious procedure has been superseded by electronic particle analyzers that detect bacteria as little semiconductors in an electric field. Either of these procedures measures the number of bacteria as physical particles. In other words, they give the body count, with no discrimination between living and dead bacteria. This is known as the *total count*. The total count can also be conveniently estimated by measuring a property proportional to the number of bacteria present, for instance, the turbidity of a liquid culture.

Often it is important to determine the number of living, or viable, bacteria. This number is determined by a *colony count*, which is carried out by placing an appropriate dilution on solid growth medium. Since colonies arise from living bacteria, the number of colonies multiplied by the dilution factor is the number of *colony forming units* (cfu's) originally present. Note that if bacteria grow in clumps, like staphylococci, or chains, like streptococci, the number of cfu's is an underestimate of the total number of living bacteria present.

The Law of Growth

Balanced growth can be described mathematically as follows. Let N be the number of bacteria and t the time, then

$$dN/dt = Nk$$

where k is the *growth rate constant*. By integration we obtain the growth law:

$$N_t = N_0 e^{kt}$$

where N_t is the number of bacteria at time t and N_0 is the initial number of bacteria at time $= 0$. This describes a geometric progression, which holds for many natural phenomena. In situations that lead to cell death (for instance, sterilizing heat or antiseptic chemicals) the decrease in viable bacteria is described by the same equation, but with a negative constant. The same equation also describes the decay with time of a radioactive isotope or the kinetics of degradation of unstable messenger RNA molecules in cells.

Growth in the Real World

If balanced growth went unchecked, a single bacterium dividing twice an hour would produce a mass as large as that of the earth in just 2 days. Instead, when bacteria grow to a certain density, they either exhaust required nutrients or they accumulate toxic levels of metabolites (Fig. 2.17). They may run out of the carbon source, a required inorganic compound, or essential amino acids or vitamins. For aerobic bacteria, crowding leads to the exhaustion of oxygen since it is poorly soluble in water. Toxic metabolites may be hydrogen peroxide for some anaerobes that lack catalase, or acids formed by fermentation, which results in a pH too low to be compatible with growth. Which of these factors actually slows down growth first depends on the strain of bacteria and on the composition of the culture medium. For example, in a well-buffered medium *E. coli* may exhaust nutrients before the pH drops, while the converse may be true in poorly buffered media. The stage of the culture where growth stops is known as the *stationary phase*.

The explosiveness of exponential growth means that even a small number of bacteria may initiate an infection. An example of unhampered growth that leads to dangerous illness is acute bacterial meningitis in a child. Bacteria that cause this disease, like the meningococcus, grow so rapidly in the patient that the physician may have to intervene immediately to avoid a fatal outcome. On the other

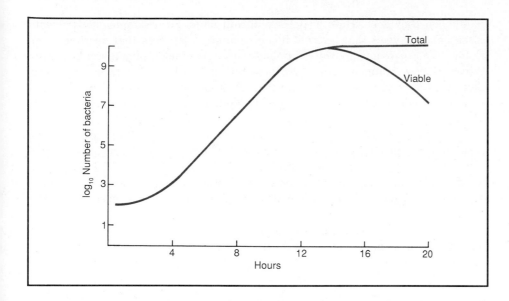

Figure 2.17. The growth of a bacterial culture. Bacteria in the inoculum sometimes resume growth slowly (lag phase, hours 0–5). They then enter the *exponential phase* of growth (hours 5–10). When foodstuff is exhausted or toxic material accumulates, they enter the *stationary phase* (hours 10 onwards). During the stationary phase bacterial cultures sometimes lose their viability, as reflected in the *viable count*, often without losing cell integrity (maintaining a constant *total count*).

hand, not all pathogens grow fast. For example, tubercle bacilli divide every 24 hours or so even under optimal conditions. The disease they cause is chronic and takes considerable time to be manifested.

In the tissues of the body, bacteria are often stressed by nutritional limitations or by the damaging action of the defense mechanisms. Consequently, bacterial populations in the body are rarely fully viable. To permit them to adapt to such conditions, bacteria do not cease all metabolic activities when they stop growing. Instead, they may cease net growth but continue some synthetic activities that permit them to make specific constituents needed for adaptation. To use a laboratory example, when *E. coli* cultures exhaust glucose they continue to carry out a low level of protein synthesis, sufficient to adapt to the utilization of other nutrients, such as other sugars, that may be present. Energy and building blocks are supplied by turnover of cell material that is not needed in the stationary phase. A major source of amino acids are ribosomes and preexisting proteins that are present in excess under these conditions. Their breakdown products can also be oxidized to supply energy. This process of feeding on itself allows adaptability and postpones death, which might otherwise occur by random degradative events in the absence of synthetic activities.

Bacteria are exposed to countless kinds of injury and have developed special adaptive mechanisms to cope with many of them. For example, damage to the DNA of *E. coli* by ultraviolet light activates a set of genes that code for proteins capable of repairing this damage. This is known as the *SOS response*. Other protective responses are turned on when bacteria are starved for the source of carbon, nitrogen, or phosphorus; when the temperature is raised abruptly; or when anaerobic cultures are suddenly exposed to oxygen. In each case, the rapidity of adaptation is a tribute to the powers of bacterial adaptation.

Even when they are not growing, bacteria can still cause damage to their host. In the first place, nongrowing bacteria are still immunogenic and can elicit immune responses with both beneficial and detrimental results. In the second place, production of toxins often starts or accelerates when bacteria enter the stationary phase. In some cases, we can fathom the reason for this timing because toxin production provides certain bacteria with nutrients. For example, some streptococci make enzymes that lyse red blood cells and proteases that degrade hemoglobin. The organisms are thus supplied with amino acids plus a source of iron. Why do these organisms make their hemolysins mainly in the stationary phase? Clearly, as long as they are growing they must already be supplied with enough iron and needed amino acids. Why should they then expend energy to make hemolysins?

Cessation of growth of some bacteria initiates *sporulation*. This results in the production of metabolically inert spores that are extraordinarily resistant to chemical and physical insults. During sporulation the "mother cell" is eventually lysed. The cytoplasmic contents that are released sometimes contain large amounts of toxins. This happens in tetanus, gas gangrene, and other diseases caused by sporulating bacteria.

The relationship between microbial growth and pathogenesis is far from simple but should be kept in mind when attempting to understand the etiology and course of infections.

PLASMIDS: A POWERFUL MECHANISM OF ADAPTATION OF PATHOGENS

Plasmids are among the most powerful elements of bacterial adaptation to environmental changes. They are small, autonomously replicating double-stranded DNA circular molecules. They are a dispensable addition to the genome of most bacteria but encode properties that make a lot of difference for survival in certain environments. They differ in size, but most are large enough to encode between 5 and 400 proteins. Some have the capacity to mediate DNA transfer between conjugating bacteria.

Plasmids are of great importance in medicine for two reasons:

• They are frequently responsible for antibiotic resistance. Indeed, most drug-resistant bacteria isolated in hospitals carry plasmids with resistance genes (see Chapter 3 for details).

• They frequently encode traits that contribute to bacterial pathogenicity.

"Virulence plasmids" involved in human disease were first discovered in *E. coli* strains that colonize the surface of the small intestine, where they provoke massive diarrhea. These strains contain plasmids with genes for adhesion to the intestinal wall and for the production of a powerful enterotoxin. Many other types of virulence plasmids are known. For example, in other *E. coli* strains plasmids code for factors that make them resistant to the bactericidal activity of serum or that facilitate uptake of iron. In other organisms as well, the genes for toxins and other virulence factors are plasmid borne.

The power of plasmids does not lie only in coding for virulence factors or antibiotic resistance. Many of them, but not all, have another important property: They may acquire genes from the chromosome of bacteria and then transfer these genes from cell to cell. Plasmids often contain *insertion sequences*, stretches of DNA that are homologous to sequences found at a number of points on the bacterial chromosomes. As a result, they may integrate into the chromosome by undergoing *homologous recombination* (also known as "crossing over"). In a reverse process, the plasmid DNA may loop out, become excised and again form a plasmid. In the process it may pick up chromosomal genes, which it can now transfer to other cells.

Plasmids have a second way of picking up genes from the chromosome or from other plasmids. They can move in and out of the chromosome or other plasmids through the action of *transposons*, or *jumping genes*. These elements permit plasmids to enter the chromosome at almost any point, often even without sequence homology. Again, in the process of becoming excised, plasmids may pick up chromosomal genes.

Plasmids are also involved in the phenomenon of *conjugation* between bacterial cells. In *E. coli* a plasmid called *F factor* codes not only for the genes needed for its own replication but also for the *sex pilus*, the structure that enables direct cell contact between mating cells. In this fashion, F factor and other plasmids may spread rapidly in a bacterial population, transferring genes from cell to cell. Note that plasmids may also be transferred by *transduction*, being carried in a bacteriophage, or directly by DNA *transformation*. The mobility of plasmids contributes to the genetic diversity of bacteria. The rate at which they pick up genes is not particularly high, about that of spontaneous mutations. However, it is easy to see that when bacteria are under intense selective antibiotic pressure, genes that confer resistance to the drug may rapidly spread through the population.

HOW DO YEASTS DIFFER FROM BACTERIA?

Many of the general properties critical for the growth and pathogenesis of bacteria apply to eucaryotic pathogens as well. We will consider fungi as examples and pick yeasts as typical representatives. There are two reasons for doing this. In the first place, some of the principal fungal infections are caused by species of yeasts or yeast-like fungi. In the second place, brewer's and baker's yeast, *Saccharomyces cerevisiae* is rapidly becoming one of the best studied of all eucaryotic cells.

Like the pathogenic bacteria, yeasts live on complex nutrients and do not carry out photosynthesis. Yeasts and other fungi also have a rigid cell wall that encloses the cytoplasmic membrane. Here too, the wall is made of polysaccharide polymers, usually *cellulose* and *chitin*. The cell wall comprises as much as 40% of the dry weight of the cells and is composed more as a series of overlapping, noncovalently attached belts that girdle the cell than a rigid sac-like structure. There are no inhibitors of cell wall synthesis in fungi as powerful as penicillin. The role of surface components in pathogenesis is also less well understood in the fungi than in bacteria. This is a promising subject for study; it may explain why some fungi have a definite tissue tropism or can grow in macrophages.

Concerning most of their properties the yeasts are typical eucaryotic cells. With regard to size, they are about 10 times smaller in volume than typical human cells and 10 to 100 times more bulky than most bacteria. Their cell structure is typically eucaryotic and they possess organelles bound by separate membrane systems (nucleus, mitochondria, Golgi apparatus, endoplasmic reticulum.) Their permeases are less specific than those of bacteria.

Fungal cells differ from both bacteria and animal cells in one important respect. Their membrane contains a sterol, *ergosterol*, which is unlike that of the cell membrane of higher eucaryotes, cholesterol. With the exception of the mycoplasma, bacteria have no sterols in their membranes. This difference makes ergosterol the target of antibiotic action. Certain antibiotics, notably one called *amphotericin B*, bind specifically to sterols. At low concentrations, this drug reversibly permeabilizes fungal membranes, and at a higher level it induces lysis. Another class of antifungal agents also affects membrane function. An example is *ketoconazole*, and a prevailing theory is that its target is also ergosterol, affecting its synthesis rather than its function. According to this view, the precursor of ergosterol, lanosterol, accumulates in the membrane but is less effective in maintaining its integrity.

Yeasts contain only a few mitochondria, two to five per cell, but these suffice for their oxidative metabolism. Yeast mitochondria contain a small amount of circular DNA, about 1300 base pairs long. The yeast nucleus has about 10,000 times more DNA, divided into nearly 20 chromosomes. Mitochondrial DNA replication can be selectively inhibited by the drug ethidium bromide. This "curing" results in cells defective in mitochondria that can only obtain their energy by fermentation. The genome of mitochondria encodes for part of the cytochrome complement of the oxidative chain. It also encodes mitochondrial ribosomal RNA and transfer RNA, and at least one ribosomal protein. The ribosomes of mitochondria have many of the characteristic features of those of bacteria. Thus, they are susceptible to streptomycin and chloramphenicol, typical bacterial protein synthesis inhibitors. These attributes suggest that mitochondria represent the evolutionary vestige of a bacterial endosymbiont of an earlier eucaryotic cell.

The cytoplasmic ribosomes of yeast cells are of the larger, eucaryotic variety, with correspondingly larger RNA chains. No clinically useful antibiotics act on yeast cytoplasmic ribosomes, probably because they would also inhibit human ribosomes. As in bacteria, soluble proteins make up a large amount of the yeast cytoplasm, about 35% of the dry weight. Small metabolites make up somewhat larger pools than those of bacteria (about 5% of the dry weight), consistent with the lower rate of flow of building blocks into macromolecules.

In general, the features that most distinguish yeasts from bacteria are their intracellular membrane systems (Fig. 2.1). In addition to mitochondrial membranes, these include the endoplasmic reticulum and the Golgi apparatus on which secretory proteins are synthesized and modified, the nucleus and a prominent vacuole. The compartmentalization results in profound differences in cell physiology. For example, RNA formation and processing are essentially complete before a chain of mRNA arrives in the cytoplasm to direct protein synthesis (Table 2.2). The same features that distinguish fungi from procaryotes also hold for protozoa and multicellular parasites as well.

SELF-ASSESSMENT QUESTIONS

1. What distinguishes procaryotes from eucaryotes? Compare a typical bacterium and a typical fungal cell.

2. Discuss the physiological and structural consequences of bacteria being small.

3. What are the structural features of a "typical" bacterium? What distinguishes Gram positives from Gram negatives?

4. Describe the outer membrane of Gram negatives and discuss its role in bacterial ecology and virulence.

5. How does penicillin work?

6. What are the principal mechanisms used by bacteria to take up substrates?

7. Discuss DNA replication in *Escherichia coli*.

8. Is it clear to you why some protein-synthesis inhibiting antibiotics are bacteriostatic? Discuss why some others are bactericidal.

9. Discuss the role of bacterial flagella and pili in growth and pathogenesis.

10. What are the main ways in which bacteria derive their energy? What is the relation between this and how they cope with oxygen?

11. Discuss the law of bacterial growth and some of its consequences in the real world.

12. What makes plasmids so powerful in bacterial pathogenesis?

SUGGESTED READINGS

Ingraham JL, Maaloe O, Niedhardt FC: *Growth of the Bacterial Cell.* Sunderland, MA, Sinauer Assoc., 1983.

Neidhardt FC *et al*: *Escherichia coli and Salmonella typhimurium.* Washington, DC, American Society of Microbiology, 1987, vols 1 and 2. (This is an encyclopedic treatise on the structure, function and heredity of these organisms.)

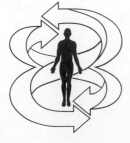

Biological Basis for Antimicrobial Action

3

D. Schlessinger

Killing microorganisms is relatively simple as long as it does not have to be done selectively. They can be killed by heat, radiation, strong acids, etc. To target them specifically, without damaging host cells and tissues, is much more difficult. According to the formulation originally made by Paul Ehrlich in 1906, what we want is a "specific chemotherapy."

We are indebted to the microorganisms themselves for many such chemotherapeutic agents, the antibiotics. We discussed how antibiotics act in Chapter 2; the principles of their clinical use are presented in Chapters 28, 37, and 38. Here we will discuss the biological basis for the usefulness of these drugs, including how microorganisms defend themselves against them.

WHERE DID ANTIBIOTICS COME FROM AND WHEN?

Organisms in the environment—soil, water, or areas of the human body—attempt to get an edge on others by secreting specific chemicals. Some do it directly by excreting antibiotics. Others carry this out in more subtle ways. In Chapter 2 we mentioned that microorganisms secrete iron-chelating compounds and are capable of reabsorbing their own iron-bearing product. In this manner, the iron concentration is reduced to a level that is incompatible with the growth of other organisms. Thus, in complex environments, competition for nutrients combines with the action of antibiotic substances to produce a balanced microbial ecology.

In the last 30 years, we have taken advantage of this natural warfare for our own purposes. We borrow antibiotics from one organism to combat others. This has resulted in a medical revolution of immense proportions. Figure 3.1 shows the

52

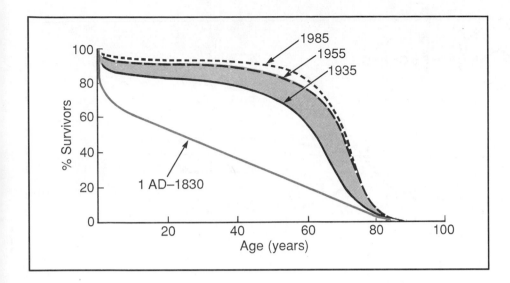

Figure 3.1. Survival of human populations as a function of age. Average life expectancy (50% level) remained at 25 until 1830. Between then and 1935, the impact of sanitation, public health, and immunization extended the life expectancy. Antibiotics (along with nutrition and health education) added an average of another 8 years. Note that the more recent medical breakthroughs have not extended average life expectancy very much. (Adapted from Strehler BL: Implications of aging research for society. *Federation Proc* 34:6, 1975.)

increase in human longevity since the introduction of antibiotic therapy. Since we all take for granted the use of antibiotics, it is hard to recapture the early impact of modern chemotherapy. You might ask older family members how they feared the loss of a loved one from pneumonia or postoperative infections; or talk to older physicians about how powerless they were when treating children with meningococcal meningitis or subacute bacterial endocarditis. There is a price to pay for our therapeutic progress. The selective pressure exerted by antibiotics on bacteria is so great that within one human generation they have responded most vigorously by becoming resistant, often to several antibiotics.

The first important antimicrobial agents were not antibiotics but synthetically made "antimetabolites." Ehrlich's seminal work derived from his own findings that dyes used in histochemistry became bound to cell-specific receptors. "Why then," he asked, "should not such dyes be made to be toxic for specific organisms?" Ehrlich's intuition was validated by workers in the mammoth German chemical industry, who systematically synthesized thousands of compounds and tested them for biological effects. In 1934, Domagk found that one of these, Prontosil, cured a fatal streptococcal infection in mice. It was then shown that Prontosil was inactive on pure cultures of bacteria in vitro but was hydrolyzed in vivo to the active drug, *sulfanilamide*. Cures with this first of the sulfa drugs were soon reported. These findings gave impetus to the efforts to purify penicillin, a true antibiotic that had been detected as the product of a mold by Fleming in 1928. The new era had arrived; the search for new antimetabolites and antibiotics has continued uninterrupted ever since.

WHAT IS THE BASIS FOR SELECTIVE ANTIMICROBIAL ACTION?

The Example of Sulfonamides

Early on it was found that extracts from yeast contain a substance that antagonizes the action of sulfonamides. When purified, this proved to be para-aminobenzoic acid (PAB; Fig. 3.2), a component of folic acid. Sulfanilamide was therefore the first structural analogue of a natural metabolite; the first *antimetabolite*. The similarity in the structure of the two compounds is obvious in this case. Following this lead, hundreds of thousands of antimetabolites have been tested for possible

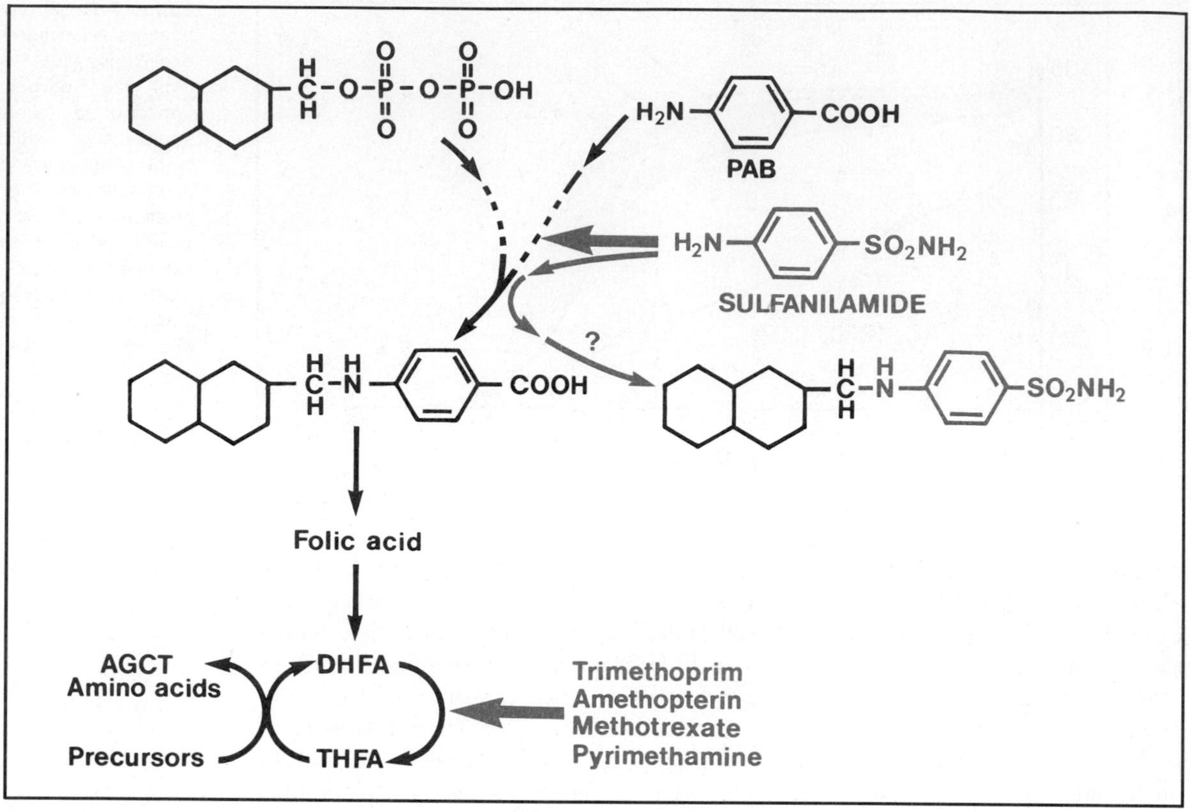

Figure 3.2. Blockage of folic acid syntheses (by sulfa) and function (by other antibiotics). The analogue of PAB may form a "lethal product," as well as inhibit folate formations. Dihydrofolate (DHFA) reductase catalyses the periodic reduction to tetrahydrofolate (THFA) after each oxidative transfer of a methyl group from 5–10 (methyl)THFA during the synthesis of nucleic acid bases and 6 amino acids. (Adapted from Gale EF et al: *The Molecular Basis of Antibiotic Action*, ed 2. New York, J. Wiley & Sons, 1981.)

therapeutic value. In the sulfa class alone, thousands of derivatives with small and large modifications have been studied; about 25 of them are still in use.

The competition between sulfonamide and PAB in their action on bacteria is illustrated in Figure 3.3; when more drug is added, proportionally more PAB is required to counteract its action. This type of antagonism is called *competitive inhibition*. The mechanism of action of sulfanilamide was clarified when the function of PAB became better known. Since PAB was found to be a constituent of folic acid (Fig. 3.2), it was inferred that sulfa drugs inhibit the synthesis of this vitamin, and thereby of the coenzymes that contain it. The main coenzyme is tetrahydroformyl folic acid, which functions in the reactions that add one carbon unit during the synthesis of nucleosides and certain amino acids (Fig. 3.2). So, it was reasoned that (*a*) folic acid should suppress the action of sulfa drugs, and that (*b*) if bacteria were given enough folic acid to satisfy their growth requirement, no amount of an inhibitor of folic acid synthesis could suppress their growth. Unlike the case of PAB, antagonism of sulfas by folic acid is *noncompetitive*. This expectation was confirmed (Fig. 3.3).

Is the competition between PAB and sulfa drugs enough to explain the efficiency of these drugs? Not quite. There is a problem with all competitive inhibitors. Even if a drug has greater affinity for a target enzyme than does the natural substrate, its inhibitory action will be reversed as the cells make more and more of the natural substrate for the enzyme. In the case of sulfa drugs, this reversal should be particularly rapid because these drugs have a *lower* affinity for the biosynthetic enzyme than PAB. Why then are sulfa drugs so effective? We still do not have an unequivocal answer to this question. There is some evidence that,

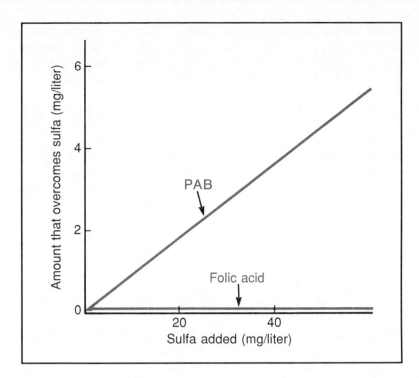

Figure 3.3. PAB overcomes sulfa addition competitively; folic acid, noncompetitively.

in addition to their competitive action, sulfas also act noncompetitively by a separate mechanism: They are slowly incorporated into an analogue of folic acid that is itself poisonous to the bacteria. The drug thus becomes a potent metabolic poison by being used for a *lethal synthesis*.

There is another reason why the effectiveness of sulfa drugs is surprising. Our cells require preformed folic acid, which explains why they are unaffected by sulfonamides, which inhibit the synthesis of this compound, not its utilization. On the other hand, the folic acid we require must be present in the circulation and in tissues. Why then can't bacteria use it, and escape sulfonamide action? The reason seems to be that many bacteria that make folic acid lack a system for the uptake of preformed folic acid and cannot benefit from its presence in the environment. Thus they must make their own folic acid, which makes them susceptible to sulfa drugs. Folic acid everywhere, and not a molecule to save them!

WHAT LIMITS THE EFFICACY OF ANTIMICROBIAL DRUGS?

The mechanism of action of a drug is only one of the properties that determines its potential usefulness. You will learn of many others, e.g., pharmacodynamics, cost, likelihood of patient compliance (see Chapter 28). Here we will consider briefly three kinds of limitations on the efficacy of antimicrobial drugs that are related directly to their mode of action: the speed with which the drugs work, the sensitivity of the microbial target, and the side effects on the host.

1. How fast drugs stop bacteria in their tracks sometimes determines their practical efficacy. The case of sulfanilamide is instructive: When the drug is given to a culture of susceptible bacteria, they keep growing for about two to four

generations of growth before they are inhibited. The reason for this delay is that each bacterium contains enough preformed folic acid to meet the demand of up to 16 daughter cells. Only after that many cells are formed does the drug become bacteriostatic. Inhibition by sulfonamides, then, is dependent on their continued presence.

Other things being equal, a *bactericidal* agent, one that kills microorganisms rapidly, is preferable to a bacteriostatic one that inhibits growth reversibly. Organisms that remain alive in the presence of a drug may still be harmful to the host, either by continuing to produce toxins or by becoming resistant to the drug and eventually resuming growth. Nevertheless, even the preference for bactericidal agents is conditional. For example, an inhibitor of protein synthesis, such as erythromycin, is bacteriostatic but stops the synthesis of protein toxins abruptly. In contrast, penicillin kills bacteria but not immediately: During the lag before the drug exerts its cidal lytic effect, the organisms continue to produce toxins. In experimental infections of mice with an agent of gas gangrene, *Clostridium perfringens*, a static drug protected the animals better than a cidal one. In practical terms, static antibiotics are also generally effective. Ultimately, inhibition of bacterial growth gives the defense mechanisms of the body the chance to get rid of the organisms.

The distinction of *static vs. cidal* should not be taken as absolute. First, the action of a drug may differ in different organisms. For example, the modified aminoglycoside spectinomycin is static for *Escherichia coli* and cidal for gonococci. Some drugs show odd kinetics of action that make them difficult to classify. For example, rifampin rapidly kills 99% of *E. coli* cells in vitro, but is static for the remaining 1%, perhaps because they are particularly resistant during a phase of their cell cycle. In other cases, a combination of two static drugs may achieve a cidal action. Despite these ambiguities, the criterion of static vs. cidal is generally useful in considering the outcome of drug therapy.

2. The efficacy of antimicrobial drugs depends on the degree of sensitivity of the intended target organisms. Every agent is effective against a defined range or *spectrum* of organisms. Broad-spectrum antibiotics, effective against a wide range of bacteria, might, a priori, be thought to be preferable to drugs with narrow spectra. Several practical considerations argue against the widespread use of broadside antibiotics (see Chapter 28). These drugs should be reserved for appropriate situations, as in cases when the etiological agent cannot be determined before therapy begins, or for immunocompromised patients who may be subject to simultaneous infection by several agents.

The spectrum of microbial susceptibility depends not only on the organisms but also on the conditions of the infection. For example, aminoglycosides are taken up poorly by all bacteria under anaerobic conditions. Thus, these drugs are ineffective against anaerobes. Also, the level of a drug achievable at the site of infection places limits on its usefulness. For example, nitrofurantoin is concentrated in the urine and is effective in many cases of urinary tract infections. On the other hand, the rapid excretion of this drug also means that it does not reach effective levels in tissues or blood.

3. A most important limitation comes from side effects on the host. In antimicrobial chemotherapy, as in daily life, there is no such thing as a free lunch. One tries to optimize the *therapeutic index*, the ratio between the effective and the toxic dose. It must be kept in mind that the degree of selectivity allowed depends on the plight of the patient. Sulfa drugs, for example, are relatively nontoxic. Other inhibitors of folic acid metabolism, such as methotrexate, are very toxic in humans but are used as anticancer agents. Sometimes there is no choice.

Infectious agents that do not penetrate into deep tissues provide special cases in therapy. Topical applications for skin infections are less likely to produce side effects. This permits extensive use of agents such as the antibacterial drug polymixin and the antifungal antibiotic nystatin, that can harm host cell membranes. This also applies to drugs against intestinal worms, which topologically are also located exterior to body tissues (Chapter 44).

Astute clinical observation sometimes can turn side effects to advantage, sometimes outside the field of antimicrobial pharmacology. Some derivatives of sulfonamides cause blood acidosis and alkaline urine, and have a diuretic effect. These effects are weak, but they led to the synthesis of an important group of modern diuretics. Similarly, some sulfa drugs produce hypoglycemia, which led to the development of new drugs for the treatment of diabetes.

THE MANY WAYS IN WHICH ANTIBIOTICS ARE SELECTIVE

In the case of sulfa drugs, selectivity is based on the fact that bacteria, but not humans, have the need to synthesize folic acid. Any step in metabolism, unique to microorganisms or not, is a potential target for antimicrobial action. All that is needed is selective toxicity. In the same pathway as that affected by sulfonamides, the drug *trimethoprim* blocks the *function* rather than the *synthesis* of folic acid (Fig. 3.2). It inhibits the enzyme dihydrofolate reductase that catalyzes the reduction of dihydrofolate to tetrahydrofolate. This enzyme is absolutely necessary for human cells as well as for bacteria, but the amount needed to cause 50% enzyme inhibition is 0.005 mM for bacteria, 0.07 mM for protozoa, and 250 mM for mammals! Thus the drug can be used against bacteria and protozoa without causing harm to humans.

This is an example of efficacy based on the relative insensitivity of the host compared with bacterial targets. In another instance, e.g., tetracycline, the target of both host cells and bacteria is sensitive, but bacteria, unlike mammalian cells, *concentrate* the antibiotic. As the result, tetracycline is effective even against intracellular organisms (e.g., chlamydiae).

The armamentarium of antimicrobials includes drugs that affect the synthesis or function of every class of microbial macromolecules. Extreme selectivity is achieved when the biochemical target is absent in the host cells. The best examples are the penicillins, which affect the biosynthesis of the murein layer of the bacterial cell wall (Chapter 2). No comparable structure exists in mammalian cells, which are totally insensitive to the action of these antibiotics. Nonetheless, even penicillins can have two undesirable side effects. Some individuals cannot take them because they have a strong allergic reaction. Also, administration of ampicillin, one of the most widely used of the penicillins, may lead to the destruction of the normal bacterial flora, particularly of the gut. This sometimes leads to colitis, overgrowth by fungi, and other complications. Thus, even a nearly perfect antibiotic comes with a price tag.

HOW DO PATHOGENS CIRCUMVENT THE ACTION OF ANTIBIOTICS?

The power of antibiotics is so pervasive that within years of their introduction resistant organisms may supplant susceptible ones. At what point in the action of antibiotics does resistance come into play? The activity of antimicrobial drugs can be broken into a sequence of three steps: First, the drugs must associate with the bacteria and penetrate their envelope. Second, they must be transported to an intracellular site of action. Third, they must bind to their specific biochemical target. Resistance to drugs may occur at each of these steps. Pathogenic microorganisms act like sophisticated biochemists and have developed a multitude of ways to do this. The clinically relevant mechanisms of resistance include

• Preventing access to the target site by inhibiting uptake or increasing excretion of the drug;

• Modifying the target site;

• Reducing the physiological importance of the target site;

• Competitively binding the drug; and

• Synthesizing an enzyme that inactivates the drug.

All these mechanisms have been recognized in clinical pathogens, but the most common is the last one. Some of the examples introduced in Chapter 2 are treated more fully below.

β-Lactams and Resistance to Them

In Chapter 2 we summarized the effects of the antibiotics penicillins and cephalosporins on cell wall formation and their consequences for bacterial survival. This is a large group of drugs, and for various reasons, their efficacy varies greatly.

In general, these antibiotics contain a β-lactam ring (Fig. 3.4). Particular side chains permit the drugs to penetrate the outer membrane of Gram negative bacteria and thus to extend the list of susceptible organisms. They become "broad spectrum antibiotics". Other substitutions make these drugs more easily absorbed or more resistant to stomach acid, thus making them effective oral chemotherapeutic agents.

An example of drug development is the transformation of cephalosporin. The original drug is more resistant to β-lactamase than penicillin but is less potent. The addition of new side chains created a so-called second generation of cephalosporins with markedly greater potency, especially against Gram negatives. A

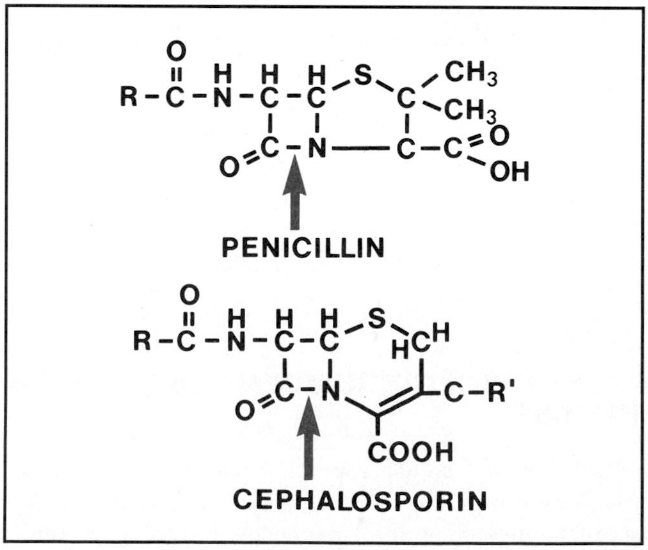

Figure 3.4. Core structure of penicillins and cephalosporins. The R groups specify the particular antibiotic; *arrow* indicates the bond broken during function and during inactivation by β-lactamases.

third generation with a somewhat different spectrum has been synthesized by replacing the sulfur in the ring nucleus with an oxygen (Fig. 3.4). Cephalosporins in this class have two important advantages. First, they extend the spectrum of activity to organisms like *Pseudomonas* and *Haemophilus influenzae* that were resistant to most of the previous ones. Second, unlike the previous cephalosporins, they penetrate well into the central nervous system. This has made them especially useful in the treatment of Gram negative meningitis.

The action of the β-lactam antibiotics requires the following steps:

1. Association with the bacteria;

2. In Gram negatives, penetration through the outer membrane and the periplasmic space;

3. Interaction with penicillin-binding proteins on the cytoplasmic membrane;

4. Activation of an autolysin that degrades the cell wall murein.

The principal mechanism of resistance to the β-lactams is the elaboration of inactivating enzymes, the *β-lactamases*. So far, more than 100 β-lactamases have been identified, a small number of which account for most of the clinically encountered resistance. They can be divided into two categories, the penicillinases and the cephalosporinases. There is a fair degree of crossing over, i.e., a cephalosporinase may also inactivate a penicillin and vice versa—but with different efficiency.

In general, Gram-positive bacteria such as the staphylococci produce extracellular β-lactamases. Being secreted into the medium, these enzymes destroy the antibiotic even before it comes in contact with the bacterial surface. Gram-positive β-lactamases are often made in large amounts after induction by the corresponding antibiotic. Adding more drug only induces the formation of greater amounts of enzyme, and as a result, resistance cannot usually be overcome even with massive doses. In the Gram negatives, β-lactamases are found in the periplasm or bound to the inner membrane. They are often constitutive; that is, they are produced at a constant rate that does not increase with the addition of the drugs. In clinical terms, this means that resistance in these organisms can sometimes be overcome with higher doses of antibiotic.

β-Lactamase–dependent resistance to penicillins and cephalosporins is widespread among pathogenic bacteria. It has become so common in staphylococci, both those acquired in hospitals and in the community, that infecting strains of these organisms must be considered penicillin resistant unless proven otherwise by antibiotic susceptibility tests.

The history of β-lactam resistance among the Gram negatives is different. With few exceptions, like the gonococcus, they are resistant to the first drug of this group, the original penicillin G. However, when challenged with the newer drugs to which they are susceptible, the Gram negatives have been more slow to develop resistance. For example, prior to 1974, *Haemophilus influenzae*, an important pathogen in meningitis and pulmonary infections, was universally susceptible to the penicillin derivative ampicillin. This antibiotic was considered the drug of choice in treatment of *H. influenzae* infections. However in 1975, it became apparent that 10–20% of the isolates of *H. influenzae* elaborate an ampicillin degrading β-lactamase. This enzyme is encoded in a highly promiscuous plasmid, which probably accounts for the rapid spread of ampicillin resistance in this organism.

A similar reversal has occurred with the gonococcus. This organism used to be universally susceptible to penicillin, although higher levels of the drug have been gradually required over the last 30 years. In 1976, highly penicillin-resistant strains were isolated in two widely separated areas of the world. The gene coding for this resistance is carried on a transposon, which is likely to hop to other strains of gonococci and to other aerobic Gram negatives. Thus, we may no longer be able to rely on penicillin as the universal agent for the treatment of gonorrhea.

These examples illustrate the role of transferable genetic elements in the spread of penicillinase resistance. Plasmids and transposons have increased in importance since the early days of the antibiotic era. The first strains that became antibiotic resistant harbored chromosomal genes and only later were they replaced by strains with plasmidborne resistance. The result is an increase in the spread of resistance to what previously were enclaves safe for antibacterial therapy. Thus, not only is there increased resistance in *H. influenzae* and gonococci, but there are scattered reports of resistance in other previously highly susceptible organisms, such as the pneumococci. If this pattern were to spread further and include other important β-lactam susceptible pathogens like the meningococci and certain streptococci, it would be a serious blow to our ability to treat some important infectious diseases.

Other mechanisms of resistance to β-lactams have been reported. In a few instances, bacterial resistance has been attributed to poor penetration of the drugs into the periplasmic space or to mutations in the penicillin binding proteins. This type of staphylococcal resistance sometimes takes on global proportions. Some strains become resistant to most of the known penicillins and cephalosporins, including a rather different one called methicillin. For this reason, these strains have the blanket designation of methicillin resistant *Staphylococcus aureus*, or MRSA. They are responsible for some of the worst outbreaks of hospital-acquired infection in recent history.

Finally, certain strains of pneumococci and staphylococci are inhibited rather than killed by certain levels of β-lactams. This results in a form of partial resistance called *tolerance*. In the case of tolerant pneumococci the drugs are bacteriostatic and not bactericidal because these strains lack high enough levels of the suicidal autolysin. Bacterial tolerance may possibly explain some of the relapses in treating staphylococcal and streptococcal infections. However, compared with drug inactivation by β-lactamases, this accounts only for a small percentage of clinically important resistance.

Antiribosomal Antibiotics: Effectiveness and Resistance

The effectiveness of the second largest class of antibacterial agents, the antiribosomal antibiotics, is based on structural differences between the ribosomes of bacteria and of eucaryotic cells. In higher cells, ribosomes have larger RNA molecules and more protein components. Typical drugs of this group, such as streptomycin or erythromycin, bind to bacterial but not to mammalian ribosomes. The difference is not always absolute and does not completely explain the selective toxicity of all the drugs. In the first place, some antibiotics like tetracycline work in vitro as well on mammalian as on bacterial ribosomes. Secondly, mammalian cells have bacteria-like ribosomes in their mitochondria, and these are sensitive to many of the drugs of this class. The reason why these drugs are not toxic is thought to be that they cannot pass through the plasma membrane. However, some patients experience damage to their bone marrow after treatment with chloramphenicol. We may speculate that this results from the selective uptake of the drug into the mitochondria of highly oxidative bone marrow stem cells.

Other toxic side effects of these antibiotics cannot be anticipated from their mechanism of action. Examples are chelation of magnesium by tetracyclines with attendant bone and tooth malformation in children, or toxicity of various aminoglycosides for the eighth cranial nerve. Another significant complication is the inhibition of the normal bacterial flora, as seen in the diarrhea that results from treatment with some of these drugs.

Tetracycline

Resistance to the antiribosomal antibiotic can take many forms because these drugs must go through many steps to reach their targets. Tetracycline, for example, must

1. Bind to the cytoplasmic membrane, which, in the case of Gram negatives, requires passage through the outer membrane and the periplasmic space.

2. Be transported across the cytoplasmic membrane by an active transport mechanism. This has been shown to have two components, an initial rapid uptake and a second phase of slower uptake.

Resistant strains do not accumulate tetracycline within the cell. The reason is not, as might be expected, failure to take up the drug. Rather, the intracellular concentration is kept low by an exit mechanism that actively excretes the drug. Tetracycline resistance has been found in almost all bacteria, including Gram positives, Gram negatives, aerobes, and anaerobes.

Chloramphenicol

Many kinds of bacteria have become resistant to chloramphenicol since its introduction. Recent examples of resistance to this drug have been in outbreaks of bacillary dysentery and typhoid that occurred in Central America and Mexico in the late 1960s and the early 1970s. Since this was considered the drug of choice for these diseases, it was widely administered. Patients did not respond to the treatment and many died.

Bacterial resistance to chloramphenicol is mediated by two mechanisms. First, a bacterial enzyme *acetylates* it to an acetyl or diacetyl ester. The acetylated derivatives are biologically inert because they cannot bind to the ribosomes. The enzyme, *acetyl transferase*, is responsible for the widespread resistance to chloramphenicol in aerobic bacteria, both Gram positives and Gram negatives. The genes coding for this enzyme are also plasmidborne. The second mechanism for chloramphenicol inactivation has been demonstrated in anaerobic bacteria, which reduce a *p*-nitro group on the molecule.

The Macrolides

The macrolide antibiotics, another important group, are represented in clinical medicine by erythromycin, lincomycin, and clindamycin. The target of these drugs can be modified in a particularly interesting way, by *methylation* of 23S ribosomal RNA of susceptible Gram-positive bacteria. This modification makes the 50S ribosomal subunits resistant to the drugs. The *methylase* involved is usually made from a plasmid gene and little is formed during normal bacterial growth. It has been suggested that the synthesis of this enzyme is regulated by an illuminating but complicated mechanism. Here we go: The mRNA for the enzyme starts with a *leader sequence* that encodes a short polypeptide. This sequence can adopt

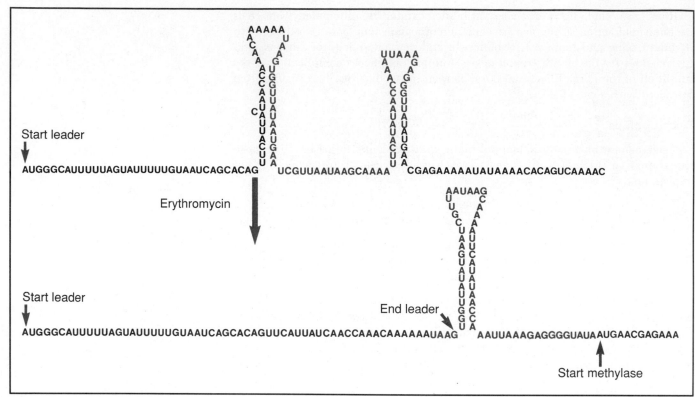

Figure 3.5. Model for the induction of plasmid-borne erythromycin resistance in *S. aureus*. The beginning of the methylase mRNA is shown. In the absence of erythromycin, ribosomes translate the leader peptides; the start of the methylase sequence is blocked in a double-stranded stem. When drug is added, ribosomes stalled in the leader sequence preempt one secondary structure and promote the alternate stem shown, with the start of the methylase gene now exposed for ribosome loading and translation. (Adapted from Mayford M, Weisblum B: Messenger RNA from *Staphylococcus aureus* that specifies macrolide-lincosamide-streptogramin resistance. *J Molec Biol* 185:772, 1985.)

alternate double-stranded conformations, exposing different start codons (Fig. 3.5). This resembles the phenomenon of *attenuation* seen in the biosynthesis of certain amino acids such as tryptophan. In the presence of erythromycin, ribosomes *stall* in this leader region. A second start codon, specific for methylase production, is thereby exposed and becomes available for interaction with ribosomes. Thus, erythromycin induces resistance to itself. Why don't other inhibitors of protein synthesis induce erythromycin methylase? A small number of methylated ribosomes are always present before the antibiotic is added. These are specifically resistant to macrolide antibiotics but not to others. Ergo, when other inhibitors are added, no further protein synthesis can take place and no methylase will be formed.

Ribosomes of lincomycin-resistant staphylococci also fail to bind the drug. Curiously, there is cross resistance between erythromycin and lincomycin, although they have different chemical structures. It appears that these drugs bind at overlapping or conformationally related sites on the ribosomes.

The Aminoglycosides

Perhaps the most complex mechanism of action of all antiribosomal antibiotics is that of the aminoglycosides. They must go through the following steps:

1. Penetration of the outer membrane of Gram negatives.

2. Association with a two-stage active transport system. This is a one way irreversible system, unlike that of tetracycline or most metabolites.

3. Binding to the 30S ribosome subunit to inhibit protein synthesis, primarily at or near the initiation step, and to increase "miscoding" by the ribosomes that still manage to function. Miscoding results in "nonsense proteins."

Two major mechanisms of resistance to aminoglycosides have been recognized in Gram negative bacteria. The first is the *inactivation of their active transport*; this is the mechanism of resistance in anaerobic bacteria. The second uses inactivating enzymes, and is the most common mechanism in clinical isolates. Twelve distinct enzymes that inactivate these drugs have been identified in coliforms, pseudomonads, and staphylococci. Each one can inactivate more than one aminoglycoside, but usually not all of them. Thus, a given strain can become resistant to, say, streptomycin, kanamycin, and tobramycin, but remain fully susceptible to amikacin. Usually, the aminoglycoside inactivating enzymes are encoded by genes carried on plasmid or transposons, and more than one enzyme may be carried by one plasmid.

Selectivity and Limitations of Antifungal Agents

As we move up phylogenetically and consider eucaryotic pathogens, the differences between host and parasite begin to narrow. For example, most of the

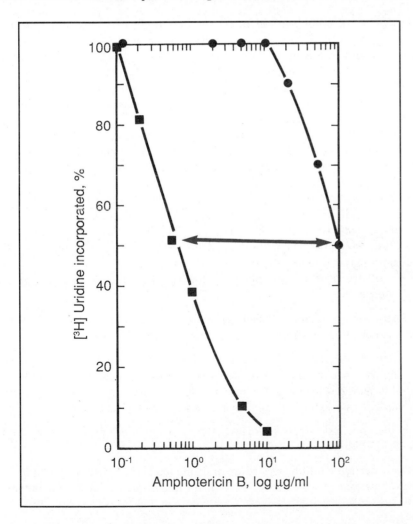

Figure 3.6. Inhibition of RNA synthesis in cultured *S. cerevisiae* (■) or human HeLa cells (●) by increasing doses of amphotericin B. RNA synthesis was measured by the incorporation of [³H] uridine into acid-insoluble RNA during a 10-minute pulse in replicate samples in the presence of the indicated amounts of antibiotic. (From Kwan CN et al: Potentiation of the antifungal effects of antibiotics by amphotericin B. *Antimicrob Agents Chemother* 2:61, 1972.)

antibiotics that inhibit fungal ribosomes are active against human ribosomes and therefore useless. Therapeutic agents against fungi, viruses and animal parasites are often quite toxic. Nervertheless, there are antifungal agents with selective toxicity.

Especially interesting examples are the polyenes (see Chapters 2 and 38), which bind more avidly to the ergosterol in the membranes of fungi than to cholesterol in the membranes of higher eucaryotes. The margin of safety is depicted in Figure 3.6, which shows that yeasts are about 200-fold more sensitive to the polyene amphotericin B than are cultured human cells. Amphotericin B is one of the few antifungal compounds that is sufficiently nontoxic to be used systematically. Yet its efficacy is limited: At the higher effective doses it also damages membranes of kidney cells.

Griseofulvin, a second potent antifungal agent (Chapters 2 and 38), binds tightly to newly formed keratin and is effective against many superficial skin and nail infections. The required levels are nontoxic enough that the drug can be ingested orally for extended periods, although at higher levels cytotoxicity and carcinogenesis have been demonstrated in animal studies.

IF ONE ANTIBIOTIC IS GOOD, ARE TWO BETTER?

A recurrent and potent argument for counteracting drug resistance in microorganisms can be made for the administration of several antibiotics at once. Mutants resistant to a drug occur with frequencies of 10^{-6} to 10^{-9} per generation. Thus, outgrowth of resistant bacteria can easily take place and be a significant risk. Let us assume that resistance to drug A has a frequency of 10^6 per generation. If drug B has a similar frequency of resistant mutants and is given simultaneously, the chance of a single bacterium becoming resistant to both antibiotics is 10^{-6} times 10^{-6}, or 10^{-12}, which is vanishingly small.

An excellent example of this concept in practice is the combined therapy with sulfamethoxazole and trimethoprim. Although both drugs act on one-carbon metabolism, their sites of action are different and resistance to one does not influence resistance to the other. Another example is antifungal therapy by the joint administration of amphotericin B and 5-fluorocytosine. The two act synergistically because 5-fluorocytosine is highly toxic in high doses, but can be used effectively at lower blood levels if the fungal membrane is selectively perturbed to become more permeable (Fig. 3.7).

The use of drugs in combination is not without problems. In fact three outcomes are possible:

1. *Synergism.* For example, when penicillin is given along with streptomycin, the penetration of streptomycin is often enhanced.

2. *Antagonism* by one of the two drugs. Thus, when chloramphenicol is given along with penicillin, it blocks protein synthesis, preventing the cell growth that is required for penicillin to cause lysis. The result is dominance by the weaker, bacteriostatic drug in some cases.

3. *Indifference.* Each drug works no better and no worse alone or in combination with the other.

There are further cautions regarding multiple drug administration. Thus, drugs may show *synergism in toxicity*, as well as in antimicrobial action (an exam-

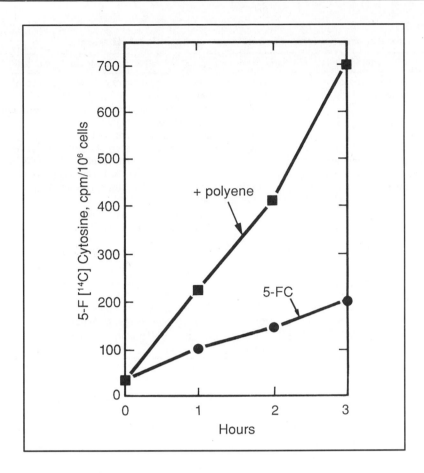

Figure 3.7. Uptake of labeled 5-fluorocytosine into growing *C. albicans* in presence (■) or in the absence (●) of 0.2 μg/ml amphotericin B. The uptake into cells was measured as acid-insoluble [^{14}C]5-F-cytosine. (From Medoff G et al: Potentiation of rifampicin and 5-fluorocytosine as antifungal antibiotics by amphotericin B. *Proc. Natl Acad Sci USA* 69:196, 1972.)

ple is the heightened damage to the kidney by the joint administration of vancomycin and an aminoglycoside). Finally, in a hospital setting, the main sources of drug resistance are the members of the resident bacterial flora. Therefore, the choice of whether to administer multiple drugs and which ones to pick should be governed by the spectrum of multiple drug resistance of the dominant organisms in that hospital.

ARE SUPERGERMS A THREAT?

Many of the genes that lead to antibiotic resistance are chromosomal and part of the patrimony of the bacterial species. Others are plasmidborne and acquired from other bacteria. Many important examples of antibiotic resistance are listed in Table 3.1.

Resistance genes, both chromosomal and on plasmids, predate the use of antibiotics. They have been found in strains frozen away before the introduction of the drugs or in isolates from areas where antibiotics have never been knowingly introduced. The selective pressure of the widespread use of antibiotics has resulted in an increasing frequency of resistant bacteria. In broad terms, the spread of resistance genes increases with the usage of drugs in a particular geographic area or medical center. Both rapid spread and the accumulation of

Table 3.1
Most common mechanisms of resistance to antimicrobial agents

Agent	Plasmidborne	Resistance Mechanism
Penicillins and cephalosporins	Yes	Hydrolysis of β-lactam ring by β-lactamase
Chloramphenicol	Yes	Acetylation of hydroxyl groups of chloramphenicol transacetylase; interference with transport into cell
Tetracyclines	Yes	Exit pump pushes drug out of cell
Aminoglycosides (streptomycin, kanamycin, gentamicin, tobramycin, etc.)	Yes	Enzymatic modification of drug by R plasmid encoded enzyme; drug has reduced affinity for ribosome, and transport into cell is reduced
Sulfanilamides	Yes	Sulfanilamide-resistant dihydropteroate synthase
Trimethoprim	Yes	Trimethoprim-resistant dihydrofolate reductase
Erythromycin	Yes	Enzymatic modification (methylation of 23S ribosomal RNA)
Lincomycin	Yes	RNA of susceptible cells converts ribosome to drug resistance (unable to bind inhibitor)
Mercury (merthiolate)	Yes	Enzymatic reduction of mercury salts to metallic state and vaporization
Nalidixic acid, rifampin, nitrofurans, etc.	Not known	Resistance arises by spontaneous mutation of gyrase, other target enzymes
Methicillin	Not known	Change in PBP (not in β-lactamase)

multiple resistance genes in a single strain come about effectively by gene transposition. This process could lead to the emergence of "supergerms", microorganisms resistant to a large number of antimicrobial agents. Near supergerm status has been achieved by occasional isolates that are resistant to 15 or more antibiotics!

Not all species have the potential to become supergerms. Some species have probably not developed an effective system of DNA transfer. Others have a transfer system that is limited in its capacity to spread multiple drug resistance. For example, staphylococcal plasmids usually do not bear multiple drug resistance genes. They are usually transferred by phage transduction; this mode of transmission may restrict the size of the DNA that can be transferred. In any case, meningococci, group A streptococci, and the spirochete of syphilis by and large remain as susceptible to penicillin today as they were when the drug was first used.

The threat of accumulating resistance factors is nevertheless quite real. During the 6 years that followed the introduction of penicillin, resistant hospital isolates of *Staphylococcus aureus* climbed from a very low level to more than 80% of the total. As mentioned above, drug resistant strains of gonococci, *H. influenzae*, and penumococci have been found recently. With the successive accumulation of resistance to many penicillinase-resistant penicillins, other agents of greater toxicity, such as vancomycin, have been reluctantly restored to clinical use.

The countermeasures taken against resistant organisms include the continued development of more effective antibiotics (see the example of cephalosporins). In addition, some ways in which antibiotic effectiveness can be preserved are discussed in Chapter 28. Certainly the war between therapy and resistance mechanisms is unlikely to abate, but the battles must continue to be won. The alternative would be to give up what many physicians and historians of science regard as the difference between modern medicine and the Dark Ages.

SELF-ASSESSMENT QUESTIONS

1. Prepare yourself to give a short talk to laymen about the history and importance of antibiotics in medicine.

2. Discuss the mode of action of sulfonamides. What is meant by competitive and noncompetitive inhibition? What is the basis of their selective toxicity?

3. Distinguish between bactericidal and bacteriostatic drugs. Under what conditions is one type preferable to the other?

4. What are the general mechanisms for bacterial resistance to antibiotics? Give examples of each class.

5. Discuss the steps required for β-lactam antibiotic activity. Which steps are commonly modified in resistant mutants?

6. Describe the mode of action of the following protein-synthesis-inhibiting antibiotics: tetracycline, chloramphenicol, macrolides, and aminoglycosides. What steps become modified in resistant mutants?

7. Discuss the basis for the selective toxicity of some commonly used antifungal agents.

8. Discuss two reasons for the use of multiple antibiotics to treat a patient. Why is it sometimes undesirable?

SUGGESTED READING

Gale EF, et al: *The Molecular Basis of Antibiotic Action.* New York, John Wiley & Sons, 1981.

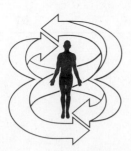

CHAPTER 4

Constitutive Defenses of the Body

J. K. Spitznagel

DEFENSES AGAINST THE ENCOUNTER WITH THE PARASITE

We humans have a unique ability to shape our environment. In good part, our sanitary lifestyle determines the extent of encounter with exogeneous microorganisms, including potential pathogens. Our degree of health is influenced by our material wealth and how it determines cleanliness and nutrition. Thus, defenses against infectious diseases begin with the way we affect our environment and one another. The children of the very poor, living in crowded, inadequately ventilated housing and eating a diet lacking in proteins are much more likely to contract infectious diseases such as, for example, tuberculosis. The reason is twofold: poor nutrition diminishes the effectiveness of body defenses, and crowding makes the encounter with tubercle bacilli more frequent. The adults in such families may already have tuberculosis and, in close quarters, become a ready source of contagion. This chain of circumstances, poor nutrition and greater exposure, makes it likely that the child will be infected, contract the disease, and, in time, become a source of further infection. Defenses against these events are clear; they include good nutrition, adequate housing, and treatment of the ill. While these favorable conditions occur readily in an affluent society, they have to be fostered with care and sacrifice in developing countries.

Our environmental defenses against infectious diseases are only partly medical. Good food in sufficient quantity, uncontaminated water, freedom from insects and rodents—all these are primary concerns of the sanitary engineer and the social scientist. Some activities, on the other hand, are directly related to medicine, such as immunization, or treatment of human carriers or patients likely to contribute to the spread of disease.

We will leave this subject to the chapter on epidemiology (Chapter 60). For now we will continue with the body's own defense mechanisms.

THE BARRIERS TO ENTRY

Defenses intensify as microorganisms encounter the skin and the mucous membranes. Throughout life the body surfaces tolerate a rich and complex flora that is usually harmless but capable of causing opportunistic infections. In contrast, domains of the body just a few micrometers beneath the epidermis or the mucous membranes are usually sterile. In this and the next chapter we will ask how the body maintains this microbial gradient, from bacteria-associated surfaces to aseptic intercellular and intracellular tissue domains. The question is important because a breakdown of this gradient is usually what infection is about.

Before microorganisms can enter the normally aseptic regions of the body they must pass through the barriers of the skin, the conjunctivae of the eye, or the mucous membranes of the respiratory, alimentary, or urogenital tracts.

Each surface has its own protective mechanisms (Table 4.1). The skin is bathed with oils and moisture from the sebaceous and sweat glands. These secretions contain fatty acids that are inhibitory to bacterial growth. The skin further cleans itself of adherent microorganisms by desquamation, as the keratinized squamous cells are steadily sloughed off and replaced with new layers. This formidable barrier is seldom breached except by injuries such as burns, cuts, or wounds.

Table 4.1
Constitutive defenses: Barriers to infection

System or Organ	Physical Cell Type	Clearing Mechanism
Skin	Squamous epithelium	Desquamation
Mucous membranes	Columnar nonciliated (e.g., gastrointestinal tract)	Peristalsis
	Columnar ciliated (e.g., trachea)	Mucociliary movement
	Cuboidal ciliated (e.g., nasopharynx)	Tears, saliva, mucus, sweat
	Secretory (various)	Antimicrobial compounds

System or Organ	Chemical Source	Substances
Skin	Sweat, sebaceous glands	Organic acids
Mucous membranes	Parietal cells of stomach	Hydrochloric acid, low pH
	Secretions	Antimicrobial compounds
	Neutrophils	Lysozyme, peroxidase, lactoferrin
Lung	A cells	Pulmonary surfactant
Upper alimentary	Salivary glands	Thiocyanate
	Neutrophils	Myeloperoxidase
		Cationic proteins
		Lactoferrin
		Lysozyme
Small bowel and below	Liver via biliary tree	Bile acids
	Gut flora	Low-molecular-weight fatty acids

Once across the skin, microorganisms encounter powerful defenses in the underlying soft tissues. However, these do not work at full capacity under all conditions. For instance, abrasions or lacerations impair the local vascular and lymphatic circulation and interfere with soluble and cellular defense mechanisms to render the underlying connective tissue vulnerable. When this occurs, substantially fewer microorganisms are required to cause infection. This effect is seen in chronically debilitated patients who suffer from decubitus ulcers (bed sores), which become contaminated and are constantly infected with normally harmless organisms on the skin. When an injury introduces foreign bodies, such as splinters or particles of soil, the impairment of the defensive mechanisms is even more profound.

Mucous Membranes

The mucous membranes of the mouth, pharynx, esophagus, and lower urinary tract comprise several layers of epithelial cells, whereas those of the lower respiratory, gastrointestinal, and upper urinary tracts are delicate single layers of epithelial cells, often endowed with specialized functions. Membranes of the alveoli and the intestine are very thin since they serve as exchangers of gases, fluids, and solutes. They are easily traumatized, especially when subjected to high pressures or abrasions. In fact, this happens daily in the colon during defecation and in the mouth during vigorous toothbrushing.

Many mucous membranes are covered by a protective layer of mucus, that provides a mechanical and chemical barrier, yet permits proper function. Mucus is a giant, cross-linked gel-like structure made up of glycoprotein subunits, each with a molecular weight of 530,000. It entraps particles and prevents them from reaching the mucous membrane. Mucus is hydrophilic and allows passage of many substances produced by the body, including antimicrobial enzymes such as lysozyme and peroxidase. Its rheological properties enable it to bear substantial weight and yet be readily moved by the motion of the cilia of the underlying cells.

Thus, each region of the body surface is endowed with physical and chemical barriers to microbes that otherwise may do harm in deep tissues. These special barriers will be dealt with in more detail in the chapters on infections of the systems and regions of the body (Chapters 45–52).

Asepsis of deep tissues depends heavily on complex antimicrobial mechanisms, some of which are constitutive, and others, inducible. The constitutive systems are known collectively as the *inflammatory response* and the inducible systems as the *immune response*.

CONSTITUTIVE DEFENSES IN DEEP TISSUES: AN INTRODUCTION

When a microorganism crosses the protective epidermis of the skin or the epithelia of mucous membranes it encounters defense mechanisms that are *constitutive* in the sense that they do not require previous contact with the invading microorganisms (Table 4.2). The most powerful of these defenses is not manifested in all tissues at all times but must be called up. It is *inflammation*, or the *inflammatory response*. It is elicited by a complex set of alert signals and pharmacological mediators, many of which are part of an intricate collection of interacting serum proteins called the *complement system*. This system, never completely inactive, is normally in an idling state. Its activity is greatly increased, usually

Table 4.2
Constitutive defenses: Humoral mediators

Ions and Small Molecules	Source	Function
Reduced oxygen species, OH·, H_2O_2 O_2^-, OH·H_2O_2	Phagocytes, occasionally bacteria	O_2 tension in tissues influences microbial growth. Reduced oxygen molecules are antimicrobial
Chloride ion	Body fluids	Cl^- combines with myeloperoxidase and H_2O_2 to form a potent antimicrobial system
Hydrogen ion	Phagocytes (and other cells)	Antimicrobial in high concentrations
Fatty acids	Metabolites (of phagocytes and other cells)	Most antibacterial at low pH

Single Protein Systems	Source	Function
Lactoferrin	Neutrophil granulocytes	Binds iron
Transferrin	Liver	Binds iron
Interferons	Virus-infected cells of many types	Limit virus multiplication
Interleukin-1	Macrophages	Induces fever and acute phase proteins some of which are antimicrobial. Makes vascular endothelium sticky
Lysozyme	Neutrophils, macrophages, tears saliva, urine	Antimicrobial for many bacteria (degrades murein)
Fibronectin	Macrophages, fibroblasts	Opsonin for staphylococci

Complex Protein Systems	Source	Function
Complement cascade	Macrophages, hepatic parenchymal cells	Products increase vascular permeability, cause smooth muscle contractions. Chemotaxis Opsonization of bacteria Bactericidal action
Coagulation system		
Kinins	Proteolytic enzymes	Increase vascular permeability, vasodilatation, pain
Fibrinopeptides	Fibrinogen	Chemotaxis
Hageman factor	Clotting cascade	Triggers several inflammatory events in the coagulation system
Platelet-activating factor	Inflammatory	Induce secretion of platelets and neutrophils. Induce aggregation of both platelet and neutrophils. Affects smooth muscle and permeability

locally, by the presence of microorganisms in tissues. The most important consequence of these activities is the recruitment of *phagocytes*, which are white blood cells that are able to ingest and often kill invading bacteria and other microorganisms.

Early investigators believed that constitutive mechanisms lack the potency of the inducible immune response. It was gradually learned that the two responses are interrelated: The inducible response cannot be expressed in the absence of constitutive mediators. It is now clear that these mediators sound the alarm for the inducible response and in the meanwhile they hold the invading microorganisms at bay. The two systems act synergistically to provide a magnificently enhanced defense system. The body then becomes: "*A Fortress built by Nature for herself against Infection . . .*", to appropriate what Shakespeare said (in a distinctly different context).

INFLAMMATION

Inflammation is the sum of the changes that occur in tissue as the reaction to injury. At first it is a purely local happening, manifested by pain, swelling, or both, and a sense of heat and throbbing of the injured part. The inflamed site appears red and shiny, hot and painful to the touch as the result of alterations in local blood vessels and lymphatics. These changes are dynamic and undergo predictable and continued evolution. The tissues may return to normal or they may become scarred. The outcome depends on the extent of damage done by trauma, by the infecting microorganisms, or by the inflammatory response itself. These rapid changes characterize *acute inflammation*. If acute inflammation does not cure the problem, it may change character and become a *chronic inflammation*. Both processes are essential for defense and both can damage the structure and function of tissues. A more detailed description can be found in pathology textbooks.

What are the underlying changes in acute inflammation? Briefly, the *blood supply to the affected part increases due to vasodilatation and capillaries become more permeable*, allowing fluid and large molecules to cross the endothelium. This is important because antibodies and complement components normally tend to remain within the vasculature. Inflammation allows them to enter the tissues. White blood cells, especially neutrophils, and monocytes accumulate on the increasingly sticky endothelium of inflamed capillaries. In greater and greater numbers white blood cells cross the capillary endothelia by *diapedesis*, migrate into surrounding tissue, and move by chemotaxis toward the injured site. Thus, redness and increased heat are due to greatly increased blood flow in the area. Swelling is caused by the outpouring of fluid and white blood cells. In mild inflammation the fluid has a low protein content, as in the contents of a blister; this is known as the *serous exudate*. In severe inflammation, the fluid is known as *fibrinous exudate*, is rich in fibrinogen and other proteins, and eventually clots because of fibrin formation. Pain is caused by the release of chemical mediators and by the mechanical compression of nerves.

An important consequence of inflammation is that the pH of inflamed tissues is lowered. This is due to the production of lactic acid by the inflammatory cells that enter the area. Low pH itself is antimicrobial and results in the killing, for instance, of *Escherichia coli*. Moreover, the antimicrobial action of small-molecular-weight organic acids such as acetic and lactic acids is enhanced at low pH. Low pH may alter microbial sensitivity to antibiotics and antimicrobial tissue peptides, making them either more resistant or more sensitive. The oxygen tension in inflamed tissue also changes, first increasing when circulation is increased by vasodilation, then decreasing when circulation is impaired by edema, necrosis, or vascular spasm.

The Molecular Basis of the Inflammatory Response and the Acute Phase Response

Inflammation due to microorganisms often starts with the activation of complement or of the blood clotting cascade. This sets off the production and release of a number of the *chemical mediators of inflammation* that are responsible for vascular permeability, vasodilation, and pain. The complement and the clotting systems are interactive, since either one can set off the other. In general, however, clotting is seen when the acute inflammatory response is severe.

Among the best known chemical mediators is *histamine*, which dilates the blood vessels and increases their permeability. It has many other activities which are described in textbooks of pharmacology. Three small peptides called *anaphylatoxins C3a, C4a,* and *C5a,* produced by activation of the complement system, stimulate the release of histamine from mast cells (Table 4.3).

Other inflammatory mediators include the so-called *kinins,* small basic peptides that alter vascular tone, increase permeability, and initiate or potentiate the release of other mediators from leukocytes. The best known one is *bradykinin,* whose potency in increasing vascular permeability rivals that of histamine. Kinins are produced by cleavage of larger proteins, the *kininogens,* by activation of enzymes produced during the clotting cascade or released from granulocytes. These enzymes are known as *kallikreins.* A key compound in these complex interactions is the *Hageman factor,* which induces the production of the mediators mentioned above after becoming activated during inflammation. One of the compounds that elicits the activation of Hageman factor is the endotoxin (lipopolysaccharide) of Gram negative bacteria (see Chapter 7 for details). Hageman factor also plays an important role in blood coagulation, an important aspect of the tissue changes observed during inflammation.

Another class of mediators, the leukotrienes and the prostaglandins, acts on the motility and metabolism of white blood cells. Leukotrienes, prostaglandins, and certain phospholipids also cause the aggregation of blood platelets, an important step in arresting bleeding. Prostaglandins formed in the hypothalamus also act on the thermoregulatory centers of the brain and cause fever. Aspirin and indomethacin prevent the synthesis and the effects of these substances by inhibiting the cyclooxygenase pathway by which they are synthesized. Note that in preventing the synthesis of these compounds, these drugs remove not only an important warning sign that infection may be present but also interfere with an antimicrobial mechanism.

During inflammation, certain proteins are released, chiefly from the liver, and their concentration increases in serum. Collectively, their rise is known as the *acute phase response.* Some of these proteins, for example, the so-called *C reactive protein* and *serum amyloid A protein,* increase 1000-fold or more in concentration. Others, such as α_1-*antitrypsin* and *complement factor B,* increase by two- or three-fold. These proteins appear to play different roles in the inflammatory response. For instance, C reactive protein (so called because it reacts with the C polysaccharide of pneumococci and with antigens of other bacteria, see Chapter 13) may enhance the inflammatory response by activating complement. 1-antitrypsin inhibits proteases that function in inflammation. Another important class of proteins mobilized during the acute phase response are those that avidly bind iron and other metals. This reduces the availability of required ions for invading microorganisms and helps inhibit their growth.

Evidence suggests that the acute phase response is generated primarily by proteins formed by "activated monocytes". Two proteins have been implicated in eliciting this response, *interleukin-1* (IL-1) and *tumor necrosis factor* (TNF), which are also called **cytokines**. IL-1 and TNF are distinct proteins but appear to have some functions in common. IL-1 is also known as *endogenous pyrogen* because it causes fever by stimulating the production of prostaglandins. IL-1 is also involved in stimulating the proliferation of cells involved in the immune response. One of its more important activities is to enhance the stickiness of the inside surface of vascular endothelia to neutrophils, thus facilitating their recruitment to a particular area.

Tumor necrosis factor was given that name because it has antitumor activity in some experimental situations. It is also called *cachectin* because it causes weight loss (cachexia in its extreme form), which is a severe problem in certain chronic infections, such as tuberculosis, as well as in some cancers. Both of these

Table 4.3
Components of the complement system

Alternative Pathway	Molecular Weight	Serum Concentration, μg/ml	Biological Role
C3b (from C3)	185,000	Trace	Component from C3 convertase cleavage of C3 in an autocatalytic system
Factor B	95,000	225	Cleaved to Bb (component of C3 convertase)
Factor D	25,000	1	Serum activator of C3
Properdin	190,000	25	Stabilizer for the $\overline{\text{C3bBb}}$ C3 convertase.

Classical Pathway	Molecular Weight	Serum Concentration, μg/ml	Biological Role
C1q	410,000	70	Fixed to Fc of IgM, IgG, and to various bacterial glycolipids, polysaccharides
C1r	190,000	34	Binds to C1q to form protease, splitting C1s
C1s	85,000	31	Activated by C1r to enzyme, activating C4
C4	117,000	25	Activated by C1s to C4b, which binds to cells and activates C2 to C2a and to C4a with anaphylatoxic action
C2	206,000	600	Activated C2a is part of $\overline{\text{C4b2a}}$, the classical C3 convertase
C3	195,000	1,200	Pivotal protein cleaved by C3 convertases to C3b and C3a in an autocatalytic system. C3b is involved in all central complement conversions and in opsonization. C3a is anaphylatoxic.

Proteins of the Membrane Attack Complex (MAC)	Molecular Weight	Serum Concentration, μg/ml	Biological Role
C5	180,000	85	Split to C5b and C5a by C5 convertases. C5b initiates membrane attack complex. C5a is chemotactic and anaphylatoxic.
C6	128,000	0.60	Bound into complex with C5b, C7, C8, and C9
C7	120,000	55	See C6
C8	150,000	55	See C6
C9	79,000	60	See C6. Note that multiple C9 molecules assemble to form pore in membrane

Control Proteins	Molecular Weight	Serum Concentration, μg/ml	Biological Role
C1E1	105,000	180	Inhibits C1 esterase (C1q1r1s complex)
C4bp	560,000		Binds C4b in fluid phase permitting cleaving by Factor I
Factor H	150,000	500	Dissociates C3b and Bb, thus down-regulates C3 cleavage. Co-factor in inactivating C3b by factor I
Factor I	90,000	34	C3b/C4b inhibitor cleaves fluid phase C4b bound to C4bp, downregulating C4b

proteins play a major role in the shock that is elicited during some bacterial infections (see also Chapter 7). Both are made in response to the presence of microorganisms.

The list of cytokines is rapidly becoming longer (see Table 5.3 for details). Interleukin-2 is also involved in the proliferation of immunologically important cells and has been used therapeutically to treat certain tumors. Skipping a few numbers, interleukin-6, or hepatocyte stimulating factor, is apparently involved in the synthesis of acute phase response proteins by the liver.

COMPLEMENT

A visit to the complement system must include the somber warning that this is a complex subject (Table 4.3). It has many components that are known by unfamiliar names, it mediates a large number of biological effects, and it interacts with other complex systems, such as blood clotting and specific immune responses. Yet, the complement system plays an essential role in health and disease, thus some familiarity with it is needed. It will be presented here in abbreviated form. For greater detail, consult an immunology textbook.

The system derives its name from the original belief that it complements, or completes, the immune response. Only later was it realized that it plays a crucial role even in the absence of specific antibodies. The complement system is constitutive and, in the immunological sense, nonspecific. Normally, the complement system "ticks over" slowly. It must be *activated* in order to become a significant part of the defense mechanisms (Fig. 4.1). Once activated, it enhances the antimicrobial defenses in several ways:

• By making invading bacteria susceptible to phagocytosis;

• By lysing some of them directly;

• By producing substances that are chemotactic for white blood cells;

• And, as we have already seen, by *promoting the inflammatory response.*

The complement system can be activated in one of two ways, which start out separately but eventually converge to make the same end products. In either case, activation results from proteolytic cleavage of inert larger proteins. Some important steps depend on the function of complexes made by binding together several of the cleaved fragments. The two activation pathways are known as classical and alternative. (Fig. 4.1) The classical pathway is usually set in motion by the presence of antigen-antibody complexes (Fig. 4.2). It is the most noticeable of the two and was described first, hence its name. The alternative pathway is elicited independently of antibodies (Fig. 4.3), often by bacterial surface components, such as lipopolysaccharides.

Nomenclature

The complement system comprises as many as 26 proteins, most of them in serum and a few that are part of cell membranes. The nomenclature of complement components is complicated by their sheer numbers and by the chronology of their discovery. The major components of the classical pathway are designated by the letter C followed by a number, for example, C3. When the component is

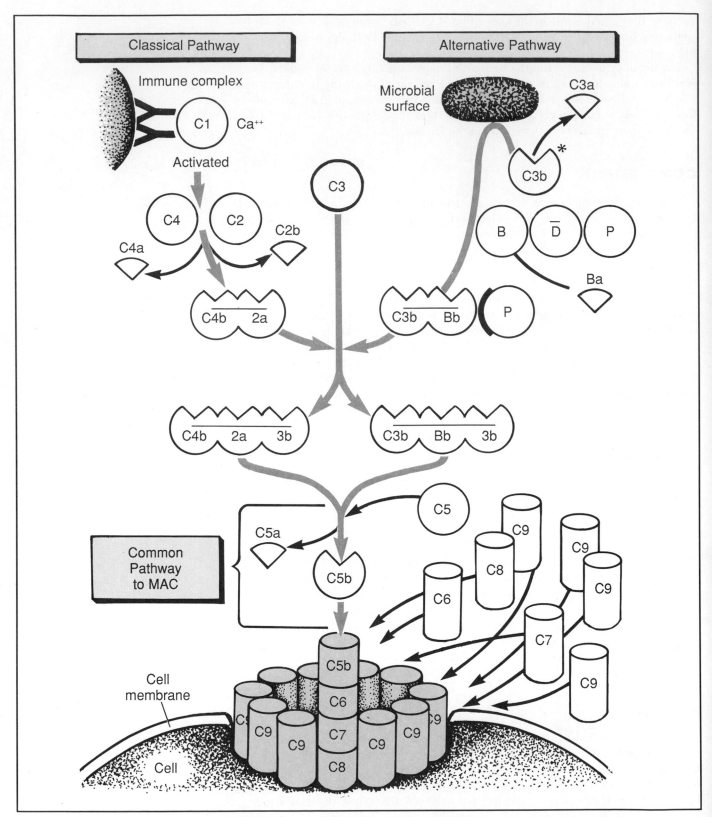

Figure 4.1. Activation of complement through the classical and alternative pathways. See text for more details.

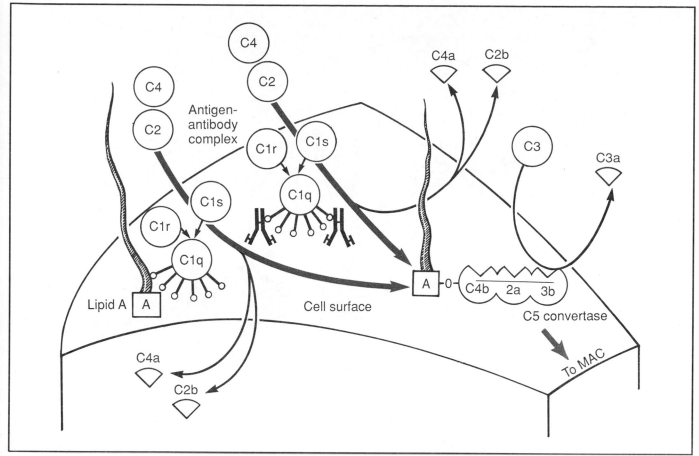

Figure 4.2.   The classical pathway (early steps). (Here we show a Gram-negative bacillus defective in the synthesis of the O antigen of the lipopolysaccharide. It was chosen to demonstrate the point that the classical pathway of complement may be activated in the absence of antibodies by lipid A molecules exposed on the surface of these mutants.) First, the C1 component of fluid phase complement is bound via C1q to the bacterium. C1r is bound and activated by C1q. C1r in turn binds and activates C1s. C1 binds and activates C4, splitting it into a small peptide, C4a, that can act as an anaphylatoxin. The other fragment, C4b, covalently binds to the bacterial surface, binds and activates C2, producing C$\overline{4b2a}$. C$\overline{4b2a}$ is then able to convert C3 to C3b and C3a. C3a is also an anaphylatoxin. Multiple C3s are cleaved. Thus, both the classical and alternative pathway C3 convertases are formed. In addition, C3b bound to the microbe acts as opsonin and C4a and C3a that diffuse away in the fluid phase modulate vascular and cellular inflammatory actions. Finally, some of the C3bs complex with C4b2a on the cell surface to form C$\overline{4b2a3b}$, the C5 convertase. The C5 convertase initiates the formation of the membrane attack complex (MAC).

cleaved in the process of activation, its pieces receive an additional letter, a or b. Thus, C3a and C3b are the products of proteolytic cleavage of C3. The "a" usually designates a small soluble peptide, whereas "b" denotes a larger peptide that may bind to cell surfaces. When cleavage products form an active enzyme, this is indicated by a superscript bar, for example C$\overline{4b2a}$. Components of the alternative pathway are designated by letters, such as B, D, P, except for C3b, which is formed by either pathway. Control proteins for the classical pathway are known by a combination of letters and numbers, while those for the alternative pathway are called H and I (Tables 4.3 and 4.4). What an alphabet soup this is!

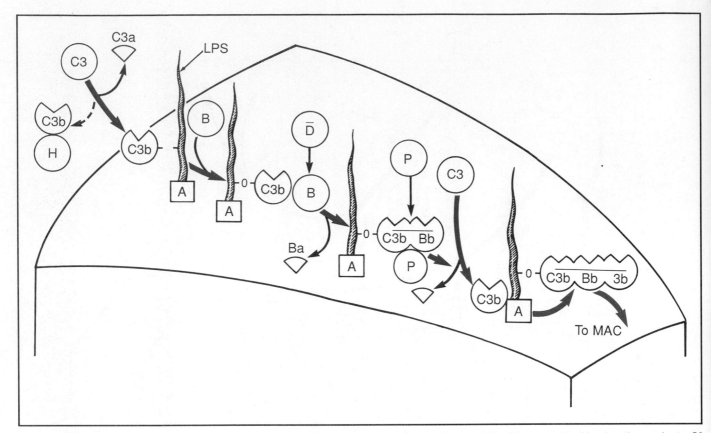

Figure 4.3. The alternative pathway (early steps). Proteinases in the blood or tissue cleave C3 to C3b and C3a randomly. C3b covalently binds to various kinds of microbial polysaccharides. Failing such binding, "fluid phase" C3b binds H, an inhibitor protein, and becomes inactive. Surface-bound C3b binds B, which is cleaved to Bb by D̄, a protease specific for C3Bb. This forms C3̄bB̄b (the C3 convertase). The pivotal event, covalent binding of C3b to a solid phase with a suitable surface, occurs when the formation of C3b takes place very close to strands of microbial polysaccharides or glycolipids. This permits stabilization of C3̄bB̄b by properdin, P. The functional alternative pathway C3 convertase is now a part of the bacterial surface. It cleaves many C3 to C3b in close proximity to the microbial surface where they also bind. There they can bind more B molecules, leading to proliferation of C3̄bB̄b sites or functioning alone as opsonins. C3a anaphylatoxic molecules diffuse away in sufficient numbers to have a significant effect on surrounding smooth muscle fibers and on the permeability of blood vessels. It is important to note the requirement that C3b form in close range of microbial surfaces to which it can bind. Then the convertase can be formed and stabilized by properdin. The formation of C3̄bB̄b is autocatalytic and amplifying. These events can be triggered by binding of C3b to IgA molecules, but the usual binding sites are glycosyl groups of microbial surface polysaccharides.

Role of Complement in Host Defenses: An Overview

Activation of the complement system is involved in several important aspects of host defenses. Patients genetically unable to manufacture some of the crucial complement components are particularly susceptible to bacterial infections. In some cases, this results in life-threatening conditions. These patients are also subject to unusual noninfectious disease (Table 4.5). Genetic defects in some of the components of the alternative pathway are not known to occur, suggesting that they may be indispensable for survival.

Two activities of complement are specifically directed toward enhancing phagocytosis, which is probably the most effective of the constitutive defenses against

Table 4.4
Receivers for complement-derived ligands[a]

Component	Molecular Weight	Cell Types
C1q		Neutrophil, monocyte, null cells, stimulates oxidative metabolism cytotoxicity, in neutrophils
CR1	250,000	Erythrocyte: C3b receptor, immune adherence, immune complex clearance
		Neutrophil: Enhanced phagocytosis
		Monocyte macrophage: Enhanced phagocytosis, absorptive endocytosis
		Eosinophil: Enhanced phagocytosis
		B lymphocyte
		T lymphocyte
		Glomerular podocyte
CR2	72,000	B lymphocyte
		Null cells: Enhanced ADCC?
CR3	?	Same as Cl
Factor H	?	Peripheral blood, B lymphocyte
C3a and C4a		Mast cells, tissue T cells
		Secretion of leukotrienes with concomitant release of leukotriene causing smooth muscle contraction secretion, leukotriene synthesis
C5a		Neutrophil: Chemotaxis, secretion, increased stickiness, increased C3b receptor expression.
		Monocyte: Chemotaxis, secretion, spreading leukotriene synthesis.

[a] Adapted from Paul: *Fundamental Immunology*. New York, Raven Press, 1984.

Table 4.5
Inherited deficiencies in complement-related protein[a]

Deficient Protein	Observed Pattern of Inheritance at Clinical Level	Reported Major Clinical Correlates[b]
C1q	Autosomal recessive	Glomerulonephritis, systemic lupus erythematosus
C1r or C4	Probably autosomal recessive	Syndrome resembling systemic lupus erythematosus
C1s	Found in combination with Clr deficiency	Systemic lupus erythematosus
C2	Autosomal recessive, HLA-linked	Systemic lupus erythematosus, juvenile rheumatoid arthritis, glomerulonephritis
C3	Autosomal recessive	Recurrent pyogenic infections, glomerulonephritis
C5, C6, C7, or C8	Autosomal recessive	Recurrent disseminated neisserial infections, systemic lupus erythematosus
C9	Autosomal recessive	None identified
Properdin	X-linked recessive	Recurrent pyogenic infections, fulminant meningococcemia
Factor D	?	Recurrent pyogenic infections
C1 inhibitor	Autosomal dominant	Hereditary angioedema, increased incidence of several autoimmune diseases
Factor H	Autosomal recessive	Glomerulonephritis
Factor I	Autosomal recessive	Recurrent pyogenic infections
CR1	Autosomal recessive[b]	Association between low numbers of erythrocyte CR1 and systemic lupus erythematosus
CR3	Autosomal recessive[c]	Leukocytosis, recurrent pyogenic infections, delayed umbilical cord separation

[a] From Frank MM: Complement in the pathophysiology of human disease. *N Engl J* Med 316:1525–1530, 1987.
[b] Note that many people with complement deficiencies, especially of C2 and the terminal components, are clinically well. A substantial number of patients with defects in C5 through C9 have had autoimmune disease.
[c] Low but not absent levels of leukocyte CR3 are detectable in both parents of most CR3-deficient children.

Figure 4.4. Chemotactic action of C5a diffusing from bacteria toward a postcapillary venule. See text for details.

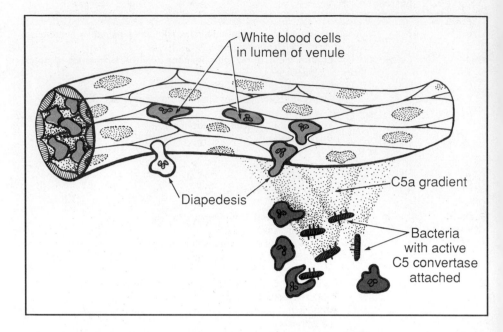

microorganisms. They are the recruitment of white cells by chemotactic proteins or *chemotaxins* (Fig. 4.4), and the facilitation of phagocytosis by proteins called *opsonins* (Fig. 4.5).

Other components of complement are responsible for the lysis of bacteria, some viruses, and foreign cells. They may even lyse infected tissue cells that appear alien because they contain viral or other foreign proteins in their cell membrane.

Figure 4.5. Opsonization enhances phagocytosis. This is a schematic representation of *Escherichia coli* opsonized with immunoglobulin (IgG) and complement component C3b. The Fc and C3b ligands on the bacteria attach to the phagocyte through specific receptors. The mechanism of this interaction probably resembles that of a zipper or of Velcro. Thus, sequential binding leads to the ingestion of the bacteria by the phagocytic membrane, until the vesicle formed is pinched off as a new organelle inside the phagocyte. Meanwhile, degranulation, the fusion of granules with the phagocytic vesicle, forms a destructive chamber for the bacteria. The secondary granules (SG) and the azurophil granules (AG), also known as primary granules, fuse their membranes with that of the nascent phagosome, thus making a phagolysosome. Phagocytes tend to be sloppy eaters, so there is some "drooling" and the enzymes and surfactant proteins enter the surrounding fluid, contributing to the tissue changes of inflammation.

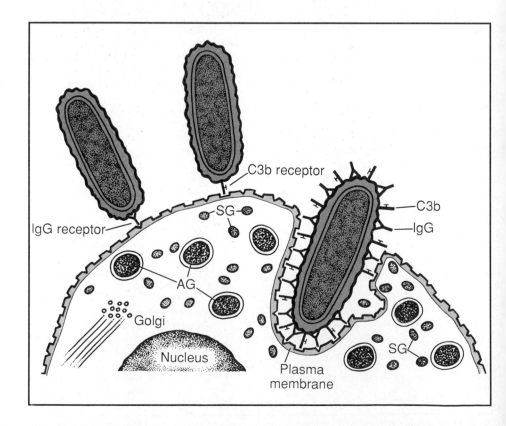

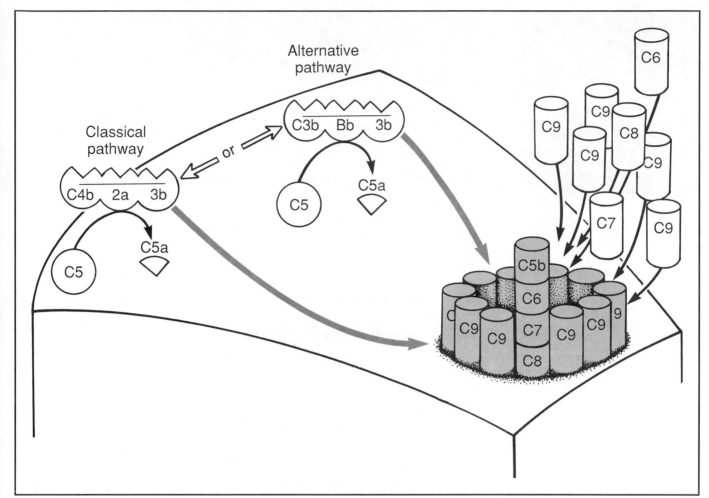

Lysis is carried out by a so-called *membrane attack complex*, which has the ability to insert itself into membranes and to alter their permeability (Figs. 4.6 and 4.7). This activity is particularly important with bacteria that resist phagocytosis, such as meningococci and gonococci. Indeed, genetic deficiencies of the proteins involved in the formation of the membrane attack complex make individuals prone to infections by these particular organisms (Table 4.5).

Lastly, complement activation induces the inflammatory response via the formation of interleukin-1, TNF, and anaphylatoxins (Figs. 4.2 and 4.3). These activities can be considered beneficial, insofar as the inflammatory response helps fight invading microorganisms. However, they also have negative manifestations that at times are quite severe. In persons with hypersensitivity disorders the inflammatory response damages sensitive tissues, especially by causing leukocytes to secrete their lysosomal enzymes. These diseases include rheumatoid arthritis, serum sickness, and infective endocarditis.

Figure 4.6. Formation of the membrane attack complex. Both the alternative and the classical pathway C3 convertases on the bacterial surface split C5 molecules to C5b and C5a. C5b molecules fix to the bacterial surface and form aggregates with C6, C7, and C8. This aggregate in turn assembles multiple C9 molecules, enabling them to insert into the outer membrane of the bacterial cell, forming 140-angstrom holes. This destroys the microbial permeability barrier and the bacteria are killed. C5a peptides are potent chemotaxins and anaphylatoxins and contribute to the inflammatory response.

The Crucial Step in Complement Activation: Cleavage of C3

The two pathways of complement activation converge at a biochemical step, the *cleavage of component C3* (Figure 4.1); thereafter, the remaining steps are the same. The enzymes responsible for this activity, C3 convertases, yield fragments

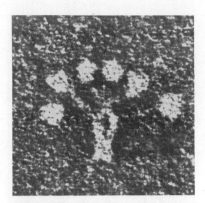

Figure 4.7. Electron micrograph of complement component C1q (× 500,000). In this lateral view, six terminal subunits are connected to a central subunit by fibrillar strands. (From Knobel HR, Villinger W, Isliker H: Chemical analysis and electron microscopy studies of human C1q prepared by different methods. *Euro J Immunol* 5:78–82, 1975.)

C3a and C3b. Both of these two components are pharmacologically active. C3a is an anaphylatoxin. C3b has several functions: It is an opsonin, and it binds to platelets to make them release mediators of inflammation. C3b also becomes part of the C3 convertase of the alternative pathway to make more of itself and participates in the further steps of complement activation.

The action of either C3 convertase is potentially dangerous, since it produces mediators of inflammation. It is not surprising, therefore, that the body contains powerful inhibitors of the convertases (discussed under "Regulation of Complement").

C3 Convertase of the Alternative Pathway

How is the alternative pathway activated? C3 is constantly cleaved by proteolytic enzymes throughout the body, but most of the C3b fragments formed are inactivated by specific inhibitors. Some C3b fragments survive by binding covalently to sugars on the surface of bacteria. This surface-bound C3b is protected from inactivation and can participate in subsequent complement reactions. Thus, the alternative pathway is elicited by the stabilization of C3b, which may be caused by the presence of bacteria.

C3 Convertase of the Classical Pathway

Activation of complement by the classical pathway usually occurs in the presence of antigen-antibody complexes and thus is set off as the result of an induced immunological response. It may, however, be elicited in the absence of antibodies. The classical pathway involves a protein complex called C1 and two proteins, C2 and C4. C1 is unusual in structure and function: It is composed of three proteins, C1q, C1r, and C1s. C1q is made up of six subunits, each shaped like a tulip (Fig. 4.7).

Complement activation by this pathway proceeds as follows: The globular "head" of C1q binds to the Fc portion of antibodies in antigen-antibody complexes. This binding takes place with immunoglobulins IgG and IgM but not with the others. Other substances may bind to C1q in the absence of antibodies, including bacterial glycolipids and polysaccharides and urate crystals. Binding of C1q to antigen-antibody complexes, or to the other substances mentioned, activates C1r to become a protease that carries out the next step in the pathway, the cleavage of C1s. The activated enzyme C1s in turn cleaves C2 and C4 and its fragments $C\overline{4b,2a}$ become the C3 convertase of the classical pathway.

The process strongly resembles the formation of the alternative pathway C3 convertase in that C4b, like C3b, binds covalently to nearby membranes. This process is also subject to positive feedback, and the production of this convertase may also be amplified as more and more C4 molecules are converted. Even further amplification takes place when this convertase cleaves C3 molecules to make C3b.

Late Steps in Complement Activation

Once C3b is formed by either pathway, further steps in complement activation can take place (Fig. 4.6). Both C3 convertases combine with C3b fragments to become C5 convertases, which cleave C5 to produce two important fragments, C5a and C5b. Like C3a, C5a is an anaphylatoxin, but has other activities as well. It is a powerful chemoattractant for phagocytes. The other fragment, C5b, is involved in making the final product of the complement cascade, the membrane attack

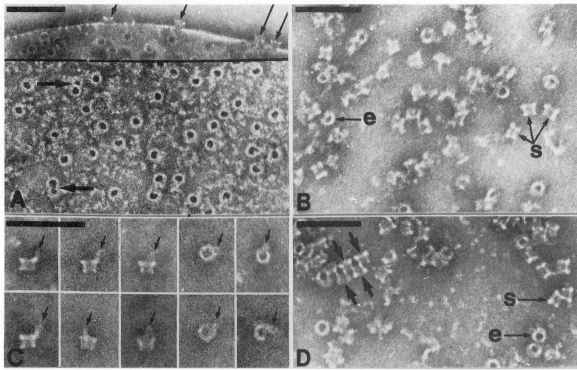

Figure 4.8. Membrane attack complex (MAC) seen directly under the electron microscope. *A,* MACs inserted into complement-lysed red blood cell membranes. MACs are shown in their lateral projections. *B,* Isolated MACs in a detergent solution. **e,** end view; **s,** side view. *C,* MACs showing a small stalk that carried the C5 and C6 determinants. *D,* Oligomers of C9 made by incubation of purified C9 component. Note their resemblance to MACs, except for the absence of the stalk. **e,** end view; **s,** side view. Scale *bars* indicate 100 μm. (From Bhakdi S, Tranum-Jensen J: Mechanism of complement cytolysis and the concept of channel-forming proteins. *Phil Trans Roy Soc London B* 306:311, 1984.)

complex, consisting of C5b, C6, C7, C8, and C9. This is an armor-piercing weapon that can punch holes in bacteria and, in some cases, in tissue cells (Fig. 4.8). Damage to cells and bacteria results from inserting in their membranes the donut-shaped molecules of C9, assembled with the help of the other components. The resulting hole makes cells permeable to ions and sugars. Water enters the cells and raises their pressure, which eventually kills them.

Regulation of Complement

The complement system is programmed to destroy. It must, therefore, be strictly regulated. Unbridled activation in body fluids is prevented by three regulatory proteins: H, C1 inhibitor, and I (Table 4.3). They prevent the formation and release of the C3 convertases, each in its own way: H prevents the binding of B to C3b, C1 inhibitor inhibits the production of C3b, and I cleaves C3b. Protein H is appropriated by some bacteria to defend themselves against opsonization. Note that if bacteria bind sufficient inhibitor protein H, the convertase will not form and the opsonin C3b will not accumulate. The action of protein I merits particular attention because it works only on cell membrane bound C3b. Since most of the bound C3b molecules are on red blood cells, protein I may serve to protect cells in the circulation from complement activation.

The importance of these inhibitory proteins is seen in persons who lack them due to genetic defects (Table 4.5). For example, C1 inhibitor deficiency is associated with a seriously debilitating disease, angioedema, which causes death by asphyxiation due to airway obstruction. H protein deficiency is associated with a form of glomerulonephritis, and lack of I protein, with recurrent pyogenic infections. These conditions arise from faulty regulation, which leads to the imbalance in the concentration of other complement components.

MICROBIAL VIEW OF COMPLEMENT AND OTHER DEFENSES IN SERUM

Serum prepared from fresh blood kills many types of bacteria and other microorganisms. This is due largely to complement and the omnipresent enzyme, lysozyme. Of the two, complement is more important because it kills a wider variety of bacterial species. It also paves the way for lysozyme to degrade many bacteria.

Complement kills bacteria by inserting the membrane attack complex. Enveloped viruses are also sensitive to the pore-forming complex. Not surprisingly, sensitive bacteria have evolved countermeasures, which are discussed in Chapter 6.

Lysozyme

This enzyme is found in most body secretions and is present in blood in large amounts (4 μg/ml). It specifically cleaves bacterial cell murein at its sugar backbone, as well as chitin of fungi (and invertebrates). Lysozyme is the only enzyme with this activity present in vertebrates. It may well represent an adaptive mechanism that keeps animals from becoming deposits of murein and chitin. This is fortunate because these two compounds activate complement and are therefore highly inflammatory.

Lysozyme acts mainly on Gram positive bacteria, although many species have evolved resistant modifications of their cell wall chemistry. Gram negative bacteria are resistant because their murein substrate is shielded by their outer membranes. Thus, lysozyme may work synergistically with complement. If the outer membrane of Gram negatives is disrupted by the membrane attack complex of complement, murein could then become available for degradation by lysozyme. Despite the impressive effects of complement and lysozyme, it should be emphasized that many bacteria are resistant to them. This does not diminish the importance of the so-called serum bactericidal activity in destroying invading bacteria. As stated already, complement-deficient patients are particularly prone to bacterial infections. Lysozyme deficiency in humans has not been described, thus it is difficult to assess the real importance of this enzyme.

LEUKOCYTE CHEMOTAXINS—SOUNDING THE ALARM

We have already seen that a product of complement activation, C5a, is an attractant for neutrophils and monocytes. It is not the only one; chemically distinct chemotaxins are also made by bacteria and by nucleated blood cells. Prominent among them are the leukotrienes, which are lipid products of cell membrane metabolism.

The chemotaxins made by bacteria have an interesting origin. You may remember that many bacterial proteins "mature" after their synthesis, when a peptide is clipped off from their N-terminus. These peptides begin with N-formylmethionine, the initiator amino acid in procaryotic protein synthesis (Table 2.2). Remarkably, these cleaved peptides are recognized by the host as strong chemoattractants for phagocytes. They differ in activity depending on their amino acid sequence, but some are remarkably potent. N-formylmethionyl-leucyl-phenylalanine, for example, is active at concentrations of 10^{-11} molar! Thus, living bacteria loudly advertise their presence when they synthesize proteins.

Chemotaxins enhance and direct the motility and, to a limited extent, the oxidative metabolism of phagocytic cells. As we will see later, this is important in the killing of bacteria. Chemotaxins diffuse away from the microorganisms that make them. This creates a concentration gradient in the surrounding tissues. If the tissues are inflamed, neutrophils are already poised for action on the vascular endothelia, which were made sticky by interleukin-1 produced by activated macrophages. When they sense the chemotaxins, the neutrophils travel along the gradient, cross the endothelial cells, and move in tissues toward the microorganisms. This chemical homing mechanism guides the neutrophils precisely and efficiently to their targets.

OPSONIZATION AND OPSONINS: THE HOST RESPONSE TO MICROBIAL COUNTERDEFENSES

Bacteria and fungi have evolved effective strategies for escaping phagocytosis (see Chapter 6). Some, for instance, build capsules around themselves that make them too slippery for the phagocytes to ingest. The body defenses, in turn, have mechanisms to cope with these obstacles. Chief among them are the opsonins, the substances that enhance the ability of phagocytes to ingest microorganisms. "Opsonin" is related to the Latin *opsonium*, "relish", an apt term for what makes bacteria more appetizing to phagocytes.

Several substances normally serve as opsonins, among them are antibodies and the C3b component of complement. C3b binds covalently to the surface of bacteria, thus providing a ligand that is recognized by receptors on neutrophils, monocytes, and macrophages. Microorganisms coated with C3b become anchored to the surface of phagocytes, which facilitates their uptake. There are at least three white blood cell receptors for C3b and its various cleavage products. These receptors are called CR1, CR2, and CR3, for "complement receptor". Children who are deficient in one of them, CR3 (the receptor for C3bi, a cleavage product of C3b), are highly vulnerable to bacterial infections (Table 4.5).

In a following section we will discuss how antibodies may also function as opsonins, and how all these substances alter the metabolism of phagocytes to make them more effective in taking up and killing microorganisms.

PHAGOCYTES: THE MAIN LINE OF CONSTITUTIVE DEFENSE

Of all the constitutive antimicrobial defenses of the body, the most potent is the cellular response. It consists of the influx of neutrophils, eosinophils, and monocytes into infected tissues. You should be versed in the properties of these cell types (Table 4.6) and may wish to review an appropriate textbook.

Neutrophils

Neutrophils are actively motile phagocytic cells produced in the bone marrow (Table 4.6). They differentiate from stem cells over a period of about 2 weeks. During this time they produce two kinds of microscopically visible granules, first

Table 4.6
Constitutive defenses of the white blood cells

Phagocyte	Source	Function
Neutrophil	Bone marrow via stem cells to peripheral blood	Adherence, chemotaxis, diapedesis Phagocytosis Degranulation Antimicrobial action, oxidative and nonoxidative
Eosinophil	Similar to neutrophil	Antiparasitic action, nonoxidative and possibly oxidative
Monocyte	Bone marrow via stem cells Promonocyte to peripheral blood	Adherence chemotaxis Diapedesis Phagocytosis Antimicrobial actions
Macrophage	Monocytes of the peripheral blood	As for monocytes. Synthesis of important molecules, including complement components lysozyme, IL-1, plasminogen activator, other proteases, undefined mediators and important cell membrane components including MHC class I and II product (see Chapter 5). Immunologic functions include, but are not limited to, antigen processing, antigen presentation, tumor necrosis factor, etc.

the azurophil, and later the specific granules (Table 4.7). When they mature—
in numbers of about 10^{10} per day—they emerge into the peripheral blood and
circulate for an average of 6.5 hours. They then disappear into the capillary bed
where they "marginate", that is, they adhere to the endothelium of blood vessels,
the stickiness caused by interleukin-1. When summoned by chemotaxins, they

Table 4.7
Substances associated with the azurophil and specific granules of neutrophils

Granule Type	Antimicrobials		Other
	O₂ independent	O₂ dependent	
Azurophil	CAP57[a] CAP37 BPI[b] Elastase Cathepsin G Defensins[c] Lysozyme	Myeloperoxidase[d]	
Specific	Lactoferrin Lysozyme	NADPH oxidase[e] cofactors	C5a receptors, bacterial chemotaxin (F-met-leu-phe) receptors, collagenase, gelatinase, vitamin B12-binding protein

[a] CAP signifies cationic antimicrobial proteins.
[b] Bacterial permeability-inducing protein.
[c] Low-molecular-weight cationic antimicrobial proteins.
[d] Myeloperoxidase together with C1 and hydrogen peroxide form a potent antimicrobial system.
[e] This enzyme complex forms with fusion of specific granule membranes with the cytoplasmic membrane. The specific granules are believed to contribute the cytochrome component of the complex and the flavoprotein, while the neutrophil cytoplasmic membrane contributes an NADPH oxidase to the complex.

become "unglued" and cross the endothelium by diapedesis through the cell junctions, traverse the basement membrane, and enter the extravascular tissue spaces (Fig. 4.4).

In a healthy person, this activity is most vigorous in the submucosa of the alimentary tract. The alimentary tract has an enormous microbial population just one cell layer away from the host's aseptic tissues. These abundant flora generate large amounts of chemotaxins, recruiting the bulk of the normally available neutrophils. Thus, the submucosa of the gut is in a constant state of inflammation, which keeps the microbial flora of the lumen in check. Failure of the bone marrow to make neutrophils due to toxic chemicals or radiation, or for any reason at all, results in infections that emanate from the gut.

Monocytes and Macrophages

Slower to arrive at the sites of microbial invasion are the monocytes. These circulating members of the mononuclear family eventually settle down in tissues and become known as the resident tissue macrophages. While monocytes and macrophages share a common progenitor with the neutrophils, their kinetics of maturation and appearance are substantially different. Unlike the neutrophils, monocytes continue essential aspects of their differentiation after they leave the bone marrow. Most important, monocytes and macrophages represent both constitutive and inducible defense mechanisms, a point that will be elaborated further (Chapter 5). Suffice it to mention that these mononuclear cells become involved in cooperative interactions with the cells of the immune system and play a crucial role in cell-mediated immunity. In general, monocytes and macrophages come into play slowly, often days after neutrophils have been active in combating invading microorganisms. This delay is seen in patients that become neutropenic as a result of chemicals or radiation. If the neutropenia develops slowly, there is time for monocytes to take the place of the disappearing neutrophils. The risk of infection is much smaller in these patients than in those with an abrupt onset of neutropenia.

It is important to realize that tissue or resident macrophages exist throughout the body. They have different names and functions, depending on the tissue. Thus, they are called Kupffer cells in the liver, alveolar macrophages in the lungs, osteoclasts in the bone, microglia in the brain, etc. They can and do phagocytize invading microorganisms. Tissue macrophages contribute greatly to the inflammatory response by releasing IL-1, which enhances sticking of neutrophils to the capillary endothelia, and TNF, which turns on newly arrived neutrophils. These tissue macrophages are replenished by the arrival and differentiation of monocytes from the bone marrow. The most active macrophages arise from monocytes delivered to sites of inflammation.

How Do Neutrophils Kill Microorganisms?

Once near their microbial target, neutrophils must do several things to carry out their antimicrobial action. They must attach and ingest the organisms, either spontaneously or with the aid of opsonins, and then kill (Figs. 4.9 and 5.5).

The granules of the neutrophils may be considered as enlarged lysosomes, packed with large amounts of powerful hydrolytic enzymes and other active substances. They are contained within unit membranes (Figs. 4.10 and 4.11). The *azurophil*, or *primary granules*, contain lysozyme, elastase, a chymotryptic-like

Figure 4.9. Phagocytosis of *Escherichia coli* by a neutrophil. Neutrophils were incubated with *E. coli*. After 60 seconds, one bacterium is partially engulfed into a phagosome and a cluster of bacteria are attached to the neutrophil surface. Scanning electron micrograph, × 19,000. (From MacRae EK, Pzyzwansky KB, Cooney MH, Spitznagel IK: Scanning electron microscopic observations of early stages of phagocytosis of *E. coli* by human neutrophils. *Cell Tissue Res* 209: 65–70, 1980.) See Fig. 26.3 for an electron micrograph of phagocytized *Legionella*.

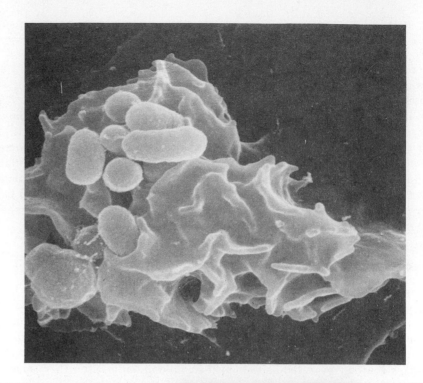

Figure 4.10. NADPH oxidase catalyzes the formation of bactericidal O_2^- and transforms it to H_2O_2. A portion of the phagolysosome showing the relationship between the enzyme (oxidase) that catalyzes oxidation of reduced pyridine nucleotides (NADPH) and reduction of O_2 to O_2^-, H_2O_2 and formation of free hydroxyl radicals that gain access to phagolysosome. The H_2O_2 reacts with myeloperoxidase and chloride ion to form hypochlorous acid. This highly cytotoxic substance is lethal for microorganisms. Curiously, the phagocytic vacuole seems to be able to contain these highly toxic reactions, protecting the phagocyte long enough to accomplish its mission.

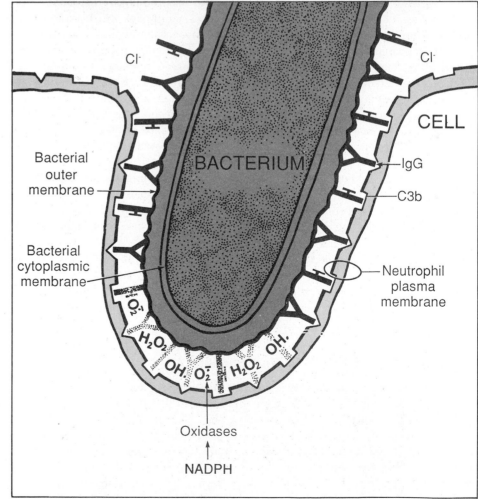

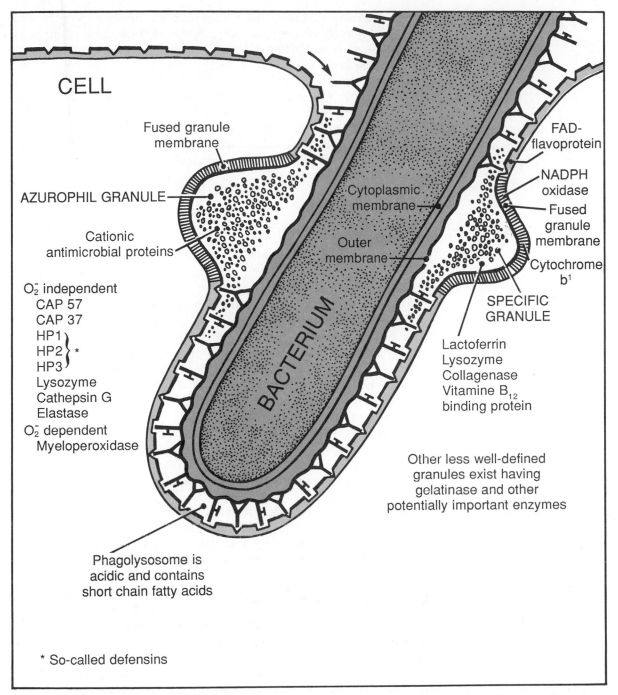

Figure 4.11. Fusion between the phagosome and the granules. As noted in Figure 4.10, fusion between the membranes of the specific granules and the cytoplasmic membrane completes the enzyme complex that generates reduced oxygen species, including the H_2O_2 that forms antimicrobial compounds, with chloride and myeloperoxidase. Fusion of the specific and azurophil granules with the phagosome activates the oxygen-independent antimicrobial mechanisms. Specific granules seem to fuse first. They deliver several proteins to the phagolysosomes; lysozyme will attack the murein of many bacteria and lactoferrin will find iron tenaciously, denying bacteria this essential metal. Lactoferrin bound to iron also has direct antimicrobial action. The azurophil granules release highly complex mixtures including cationic antimicrobial proteins CAP57, CAP37, and the defensins. Two proteolytic enzymes, cathepsin G and elastase, as well as lysozyme, are also delivered by azurophil granules. Finally, oxygen independent antimicrobial action is also mediated by hydrogen ion and short chain fatty acids produced by the glycolytic metabolism of the neutrophil.

protease, myeloperoxidase, and several cationic proteins that are also powerfully antibacterial (Table 4.7). The *specific*, or *secondary*, granules contain a cytochrome, the iron-binding protein lactoferrin, a protein that binds vitamin B_{12}, and a collagenase.

The membrane of neutrophils contains the receptors for chemotaxins and opsonins. After chemotaxins bind to them, the receptor molecules are internalized and replaced with new ones. What makes chemotaxis so effective is that neutrophils are unusually motile. They move by rearranging together their cytoplasmic microfilaments and their microtubules. Actin and myosin in microfilaments are affected by a protein, gelsolin (which invites the comparison of neutrophils with muscle cells). During chemotaxis, portions of the neutrophils that face upstream in the chemotactic gradient form a structure called a *lamellipodium*, where the cytoplasm is densely packed with microfilaments. The portions of the cell that face downstream in the gradient form a knob-like structure, the *uropod*.

Phagocytosis differs from pinocytosis, in that particles rather than just liquids are taken up. Phagocytes enfold bacteria or other particles of suitable size in a pouch-like structure, the *phagosome*, which invaginates, displacing the nucleus and the granules toward the uropod (Figs. 4.9 and 5.5). The cytoplasmic granules soon discharge their contents into the phagosome by fusion of their membranes, forming a new structure known as the *phagolysosome*. The phagolysosome quickly pinches off and becomes a separate cytoplasmic organelle. By the time the pinching off is completed, the fusion of the granules is well under way and bacteria can already be seen to be coated with antibacterial proteins. Thus, like poisonous snakes that disable their prey before swallowing it, neutrophils kill bacteria before they completely ingest them.

The bacteria become enfolded into the plasma membrane of the neutrophils by a zipper-like action, with the receptors on the phagocyte surface progressively attaching to the ligands on the bacterial surface (Figs. 4.5 and 4.9). This binding stimulates two mechanisms that lead to killing of bacteria by phagocytes: One is set in motion by a vigorous burst of oxidative metabolism that leads to the production of hydrogen peroxide and other compounds lethal to microorganisms (Fig. 4.10). This is the oxygen-dependent killing. Phagocytosis also results in the discharge of toxic compounds from the granules into the phagosome. This is known as oxygen-independent killing.

Oxygen-Dependent Killing

How does oxygen-dependent killing take place? Fusion of the specific granule membranes with the phagosome membrane (which is derived from the plasma membrane) brings together three components: NADPH oxidase of the plasma membrane (characterized as an FAD-flavoprotein cytochrome reductase) joins a unique cytochrome b in the membrane of specific granules. This complex, in the presence of a quinone, reduces oxygen (O_2) to superoxide anion, O_2^-. The superoxide ion is changed to hydrogen peroxide by the following reaction: $2\,O_2^- + H_2O \longrightarrow H_2O_2 + O_2$, in a very rapid reaction catalyzed by an enzyme called *superoxide dismutase*.

The importance of these oxidative processes in killing bacteria is illustrated in children with a congenital defect called *chronic granulomatous disease* (CGD), which results in the failure to make the superoxide anion. These children have a decreased amount of one of the essential components, the cytochrome b. Although their neutrophils can phagocytize normally, they do not efficiently oxidize NADPH and kill via the oxidative pathway. The reason this is a condition of childhood is that it results in such severe infections that patients seldom survive into adulthood, even with the use of antibiotics.

The principal form of CGD is X-linked (X-CGD) and the mutation that causes it maps to the X chromosome. Cytochrome b of normal neutrophils is composed of two subunits, a 90,000-molecular-weight glycoprotein and a 22,000-molecular-weight nonglycosylated peptide. The gene for the large subunit is missing in X-CGD patients. The absence of the gene for the larger subunit was measured by hybridization with DNA probes obtained by cloning. There are also autosomally inherited forms of the disease, some of them resulting from deficiency in the 22,000-molecular-weight protein. The availability of DNA probes may well permit the prenatal diagnosis of this disease. Cloned genes may conceivably be introduced into marrow stem cells as a therapeutic regimen.

How does the oxidative process kill microorganisms? This is a complex business, involving several different radicals and chemical species. Hydrogen peroxide plays an important role because, with the help of an enzyme called myeloperoxidase, it converts chloride ions into the highly toxic hypochlorous ions, the same chemical found in common bleach (Fig. 4.10 and Table 4.7). Myeloperoxidase is delivered to the phagolysosome by fusion of the azurophil granules. In some cases, hydrogen peroxide is produced by the bacteria themselves. For instance, pneumococci release a lot of H_2O_2 because they lack the enzyme catalase that can destroy this compound. Thus, pneumococci literally commit suicide inside the phagocytic vacuole. Accordingly, pneumococci are not particularly dangerous to patients with CGD, who do not make enough hydrogen peroxide.

Oxygen-Independent Killing

Oxygen-independent killing mechanisms are also triggered by binding opsonized bacteria to the plasma membrane of neutrophils (Fig. 4.10, Table 4.7). Specific granules seem to fuse first. They deliver several bactericidal proteins, including lysozyme and lactoferrin. The azurophil granules discharge antimicrobial cationic proteins into phagosomes. Some of these proteins are "amphipathic" (partly hydrophilic and partly hydrophobic) and resemble other cationic surface-active agents such as the antibiotic polymyxin B. Apparently they disrupt the outer membrane of Gram-negative bacteria and kill them by causing leakage of vital components. Each of these substances has a unique antimicrobial spectrum, but they tend to affect Gram negatives more than Gram positives. These proteins may account for the survival of some of the children with CGD.

The oxygen-independent mechanism also accounts for bacterial killing under the highly anaerobic conditions found in deep abscesses. Interestingly, no patient with deficiencies in cationic proteins of neutrophils has been described. Perhaps such a defect is lethal. A genetic disease known as the Chédiak-Higashi syndrome is due to the premature fusion of neutrophil granules while the cells are still in the bone marrow. Thus, when mature neutrophils of these patients phagocytize bacteria, their granules have already been spent, substantially reducing the killing power of these cells.

How do various kinds of bacteria differ in their sensitivity to the two bactericidal mechanisms of neutrophils? In general, the organisms found in the gut, such as Gram-negative rods, are readily killed by the oxygen-independent mechanism. Gram-positive bacteria of the kind found on the skin and in the upper respiratory epithelia tend to be resistant to oxygen-independent killing and are killed chiefly by the oxygen dependent pathway. Does this reflect the abundance of oxygen in the skin and its absence in the gut?

Eosinophils

The eosinophils parallel the neutrophils in lifestyle and function. However, their attention is not directed so much at bacteria as it is to animal parasites. Indeed, the increase of these cells in the circulation, *eosinophilia*, is the hallmark of parasitic diseases such as schistosomiasis or trichinosis. The reason for this specificity is not known. It has been shown that the cytoplasmic granules of the eosinophils carry large amounts of an enzyme known as eosinophil peroxidase, as well as specific cationic proteins. These compounds have the power to kill certain parasites. Thus, eosinophils have an anti-infectious armamentarium similar to that of neutrophils, but specifically targeted to certain higher parasites.

Killing by Monocytes and Macrophages

Together, monocytes and macrophages serve to mop up what is left at the scene of the battle between microorganisms and neutrophils. They phagocytize the microorganisms and the debris that is left by the neutrophils. Their mechanisms of chemotaxis, phagocytosis, and microbial killing resemble those of the neutrophils, although they have not yet been studied in the same detail. An important point is that these cells, unlike the neutrophils, continue to differentiate after they leave the bone marrow and, under proper stimulation, change into a state of activation. Activated macrophages phagocytize more vigorously, take up more oxygen, and secrete a large quantity of hydrolytic enzymes. In general, they are better prepared to kill microorganisms and, appropriately, have been called the "angry" macrophages. Macrophage activation is elicited by substances made in response to the presence of microorganisms, like complement fragment C3b or interferon. They may also become activated by a variety of other compounds, such as endotoxin of Gram negatives, or a tetrapeptide derived from immunoglobulins, known as tuftsin. Although some bacteria, fungi, and protozoa can grow within unstimulated macrophages, in general they tend to be killed when these cells become activated.

Perhaps the most important property of macrophages is their capacity to participate in the induction of specific immune responses. In this role of living garbage collectors they help rid the body not only of invading microorganisms but also of tumor and other foreign cells. They do this by stimulating the development of the lymphocytes involved in the immune response. In turn, they respond to signals from some of these lymphocytes that stimulate differentiation and activation of macrophages. In this way, macrophages and the cells of the induced immune system "talk" to each other. In fact, they carry out an animated conversation that results in a strong interaction between the constitutive and the induced systems of defense.

SUGGESTED READINGS

Dinarello CA: Interleukin-1 in the pathogenesis of the acute phase response. *N Engl J Med* 311:1413–1418, 1984.
Dinarello CA: The biology of interleukin-1 and comparison to tumor necrosis factor. *Immunol Lett* 16:227–232, 1987.

Frank MM: Complement in the pathophysiology of human disease. *N Engl J Med* 316:1525–1530, 1987.

Hugli TE, Morgan EL: Mechanisms of leukocyte regulation by complement-derived factors. Regulation of leukocyte function. *Contemp Top Immunobiol* 14:109–154, 1984.

Joiner KA, Brown EJ, Frank MM: Complement and bacteria: chemistry and biology in host defenses. *Ann Rev Immunol* 2:461–490, 1984.

Klebanoff SJ, Clark RA: *The Neutrophil: Function and Clinical Disorders*. New York, Elsevier-North Holland, 1978.

Larsen GL, Henson PM: Mediators of inflammation. *Ann Rev Immunol* 1:335–359, 1983.

Rotrosen D, Gallin JI: Disorders of phagocyte function. *Ann Rev Immunol* 5:127–150, 1987.

Silberberg A, Meyer FA: Structure and function of mucus. *Adv Exp Med Biol* 144:53–74, 1982.

Spitznagel JK: Nonoxidative antimicrobial reactions of leukocytes. *Contemp Top Immunobiol* 14:283–343, 1984.

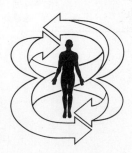

Induced Defenses of the Body

H.K. Ziegler

SELF- AND NONSELF DISCRIMINATION

Immunological defenses are based on the ability to recognize self from nonself and in that way maintain the individuality and integrity of the organism. Self may be defined as the tissues, cells, and molecules present as an integral part of the organism, encoded by the genome. Nonself is everything else. The general rule in immune defenses is that the immune system recognizes entities in the nonself world, known as antigens, and responds in a way that eliminates the antigens from the self-environment. In people, if the nonself entity is a pathogenic microorganism, the process is directed toward the successful resolution of an infection.

The maintenance of individuality or integrity of an organism is a fundamental need. This is why we are all different. Immunological defenses are normal biological phenomena common to all living organisms, including microorganisms. Bacteria use nucleases to fight invading DNA that could contaminate their genome, and elaborate toxic substances to conquer their immediate environment; the struggle among microbes is reflected in antibiotics and antibiotic resistance mechanisms. Some parasites use camouflage by coating themselves with host antigens. Even viruses ensure their survival by using such tricks as hiding in host DNA and eliciting the production of antiviral substances, such as interferon, to block infectivity of other viruses. When the survival needs and defenses of microbes conflict with ours, we have the pathology of infectious disease. Or, as Lewis Thomas said, "Disease usually results from inconclusive negotiations for symbiosis, an overstepping of the line by one side or the other, a biological misinterpretation of the boundaries." From a microbial point of view, there is little to be gained by causing disease. Pathogenicity is the side effect of the border dispute. In fact, many of the symptoms of infection are caused not by the presence of the microbe, but rather by the immune defense mechanisms invoked. Our arsenal for fighting a microbe is so powerful we are possibly in more danger from ourselves than from the microbe. We live in a war zone in the midst of exploding devices; we are mined.

What is the cost of maintaining individuality via defense reactions? Perhaps we pay the price by getting old and dying: One explanation of aging is that tissue degeneration is caused by the protracted battle of self and nonself with the resulting accumulation of damage. The immune system makes occasional mistakes in discriminating self from nonself (autoimmune reactions). Effector molecules activated during border disputes with microbes can damage host cells and tissues, and sacrificing a few cells for the good of the organism, as occurs with the "mini-amputations" that take place in the destruction of virus-infected cells, is a sound but ultimately damaging strategy.

Thus, the challenge of the immune system is to provide an efficient and powerful means for recognizing the millions of different components of the nonself-world and to respond with minimal damage to our own tissues. For this, nature has provided higher animals with highly specific immune defenses that are evoked only when needed. This is called *specific acquired immunity*.

INNATE VERSUS ACQUIRED IMMUNITY

As discussed in the previous chapter, innate immune responses are those that do not depend on prior exposure to the invading agent and, in general, do not increase after exposure to the nonself-entity. For the most part, such mechanisms are relatively nonspecific and supply the initial lines of defense against invading pathogens.

In contrast to innate immunity, specific acquired defense reactions are highly selective for the nonself-entity and are qualitatively altered by antigenic exposure. The two salient hallmarks are *specificity* and *memory*.

IMMUNITY AND MEMORY: THE CONCEPT OF IMMUNIZATION

To illustrate the concept of immunization, consider an experimental infection in mice with a microbial pathogen (Fig. 5.1). Groups of immunologically naive (normal) mice are injected with different numbers of organisms and their survival is noted after an appropriate period of time. With 10^4 bacteria, one-half of the animals die, thus defining a so-called lethal dose 50% ($LD_{50} = 10^4$). If the same experiment is performed with the animals that have recovered from the first infection (e.g., those animals receiving 10^3 organisms), immunity or resistance to the lethal effects of the infection is illustrated by the finding that it now takes 10^7 microbes to kill half the animals. Thus, these animals have acquired enhanced resistance or immunity to the pathogen by prior antigenic exposure, i.e., they remember their previous history. The specificity of this acquired immunity is illustrated by the observation that such animals are no more resistant to an antigenically unrelated pathogen than are normal controls. Thus, the immune system has remembered the specific prior insult and has successfully adapted to maintain the health of the organism. This capacity is termed *immunological memory*.

Immunity can be broadly classified as either *humoral* or *cellular*. This distinction is based on the ability to transfer resistance to normal animals or humans

Figure 5.1. Specific acquired immunity. In this experiment, groups of animals were injected as indicated with antigenically unrelated pathogenic microorganisms designated A and B. The percentage of animals killed by the infection is plotted as a function of the number of microorganisms injected into each animal. Note that animals that receive a first injection with microbe A are resistant or immune to secondary challenge with microbe A.

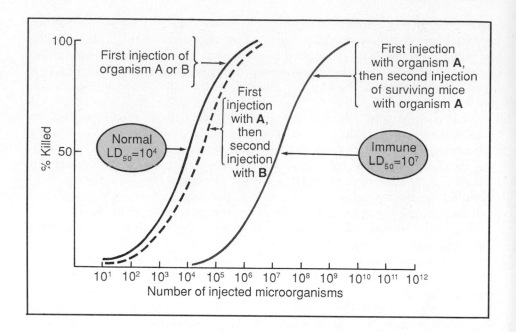

using either the serum (humors) or the cells of the immune donor. Specific humoral immunity results from the action of proteins in serum called *antibodies*, while cellular immunity is mediated by antigen-specific *T lymphocytes*. Both antibody (the product of B lymphocytes) and T lymphocytes contribute to immunity, but the relative importance of humoral and cellular immunity varies with the type of pathogen and the site of infection. For example, resistance to a toxin is usually predominantly humoral, as antibodies bind to and neutralize the injurious activity of the toxin. Also, antibody binds to antigen, which makes it easier for phagocytic cells to ingest it and to activate the complement systems (Chapter 4). In contrast, pathogens that can multiply within host cells are not accessible to antibody. Immunity to such microbes requires the cooperative efforts of T lymphocytes and macrophages. This reaction is mediated by the secretion of soluble factors called *lymphokines*, which are released by T cells. Certain lymphokines called *macrophage-activating factors* enhance the cytocidal functions of macrophages, allowing them to kill intracellular microbes. Also, cell-mediated immunity can be expressed by the direct action of a subset of T cells termed *cytotoxic T lymphocytes*. These cells recognize antigens on the surface of infected cells. For example, cytotoxic T lymphocytes can lyse virus-infected cells early in the virus-infection cycle, that is, before mass production of virus progeny occurs. Thus, specific acquired immunity is expressed either by direct cell-cell interaction or secretion of antibodies and lymphokines.

The specific memory of acquired immunity is mediated by *lymphocytes* and their receptors through a process of *clonal selection* (Fig. 5.2). There are millions of different lymphocytes, each with receptors specific for a particular antigen. These lymphocyte surface receptors consist of an *immunoglobulin* on B lymphocytes and a related protein on T lymphocytes called the *T cell receptor*. When an antigen binds to its specific receptor on a lymphocyte, that particular lymphocyte proliferates and differentiates. This results in the clonal expansion of the lymphocytes of that specificity. Thus, specific immunological memory is due to the predominance of clones of lymphocytes of a particular specificity. In the example described above (Fig. 5.1), the specifically immune mice can handle a larger num-

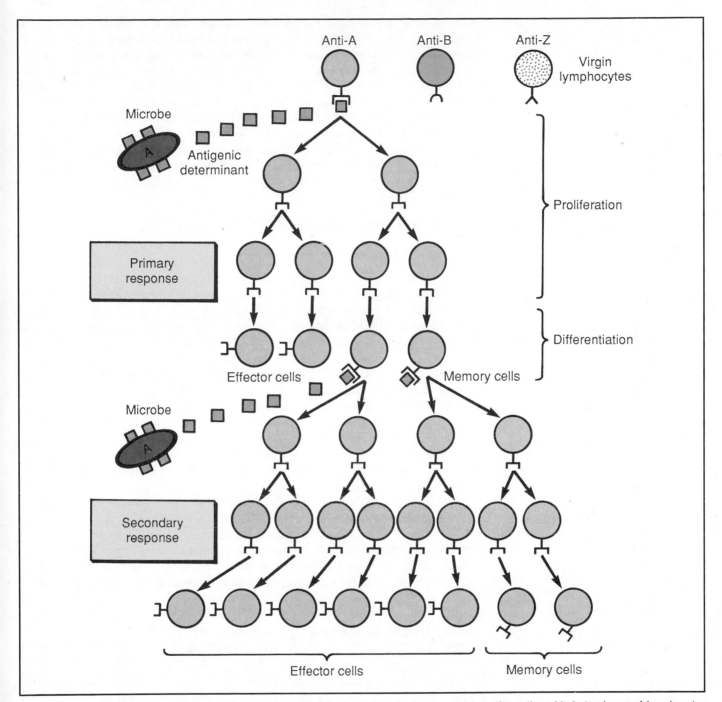

Figure 5.2. Clonal selection. When an antigen (*squares*) is introduced into the immune system, the antigen binds to clones of lymphocytes with receptors for that antigen, and this initiates the proliferation and differentiation of the lymphocytes indicated. As such, antigen is said to *select* certain clones for proliferation. Note that upon secondary contact with the same antigen, a relatively larger number of clones (memory cells) can interact with the antigen. This accounts for specific immunological memory. This process occurs with B and T lymphocytes. For simplicity, the function of antigen-presenting cells and many other cellular and molecular interactions are not shown.

ber of microbes because they now have many more lymphocytes with receptors specific for the microbial antigens.

In many ways the immune system is analogous to the nervous system. Both are complex, and both comprise very large numbers of phenotypically distinct cells. These cells interact in positive and negative ways, and this cellular network is dispersed throughout the body to patrol and guard its identity. Both systems are involved in pattern recognition. With a keen sense of touch, the immune system has the precise capacity for discrimination. It can distinguish proteins that differ in only one amino acid and can perceive differences between isomers of simple chemicals. Collectively, the cells of the immune system have intelligence and morality in telling the good (self) from the bad (nonself), with a memory that lasts a lifetime. Both systems rely on effective intracellular communication via synaptic transmission of chemical signals. However, unlike the hard wiring of the nervous system, the immune system employs transient mobile interconnections among cells with a dynamic and renewable capacity.

CELLULAR BASIS OF IMMUNE RESPONSES

Lymphocyte Function

To supply strong and appropriate immune defenses, nature has imposed a division of labor among the lymphocytes. B lymphocytes, when stimulated by antigens and the appropriate products of other lymphocytes and macrophages, proliferate and then differentiate into plasma cells whose sole purpose is to synthesize and secrete antibody molecules. Each of these antibody factories can secrete 2000 molecules per second. These terminally differentiated cells are so committed to synthesis and secretion that they are incapable of further growth and die after several days. In general, the specificity of the secreted antibody is identical to the blueprint present on their cell surfaces as the antigen receptor. Thus, B lymphocytes with a given receptor specificity expand clonally to increase their numbers, which then undergo differentiation to plasma cells. These cells are capable of secreting a large number of similar yet functionally specialized antibodies—what a well-designed system for acquiring heightened reactivity to the nonself-world!

In contrast to B cells, antigen activation of T lymphocytes does not lead to the production of secreted forms of antigen-receptor molecules. Rather, differentiated T cells express their functions through direct cell-cell interaction and via the secretion of lymphokines. There are several functionally distinct subsets of T cells. *Helper T cells* help other cells perform optimally; they help B cells make antibody, T cells become cytotoxic, and macrophages kill microbes. *Cytotoxic T*

Table 5.1
Human T lymphocyte markers[a]

Surface Marker		Cellular Distribution
T Designation[b]	Cluster Designation[b]	
T_6	CD1	Immature (Cortical) Thymus Cells
T_{11}	CD2	All T cells
T_3	CD3	Mature T cells
T_4	CD4	Helper/Inducer T cells
T_8	CD8	Cytotoxic/Suppressor cells

[a] Adapted from Shaw S: Characterization of human leukocyte differentiation antigens. *Immunol Today* 8: 1–3, 1987.
[b] This is a simplifed version of T and CD designations.

cells recognize and destroy cells infected with microbial pathogens such as viruses. *Suppressor T cells* downregulate the activity of B cells and other T cells. Thus, the functional diversity of T lymphocytes is expressed by separate subsets of cells.

Lymphocytes are all morphologically similar, but can be identified by surface markers (Table 5.1). These markers are also known as *differentiation antigens* since they appear at certain stages of lymphocyte differentiation. Human T cells express the characteristic proteins called T_1, T_{11}, and T_3. Helper T cells bear the T_4 protein. Cytotoxic T lymphocytes (CTL) and suppressor T cells express the T_8 marker. In peripheral blood, about 45% of the lymphocytes are T_4 positive and 30% are T_8 positive. (The rest are null cells [more later] and B cells.) These markers can be used for diagnostic purposes. Patients with acquired immunodeficiency syndrome (AIDS), for example, have low numbers of T_{4+} cells, which indicates an immunodeficiency.

Lymphocyte Development

Lymphocytes are found in the blood, lymphoid tissues, the lymph, and in smaller numbers in tissues throughout the body, especially at sites of inflammation. The total number of lymphocytes in humans is large (about 2×10^{12}) and the total mass of the immune system is comparable to that of the liver or the brain. Like other blood cells, lymphocytes are derived from the pluripotent hemopoietic stem cells in the fetal liver and the bone marrow of adults. Lymphocyte development occurs by two major pathways corresponding to the two major subsets, B and T lymphocytes. (Fig. 5.3).

By one pathway, the progeny of stem cells migrate from the bone marrow and enter the thymus. In this *central or primary lymphoid organ*, the development of thymus-derived (T) lymphocytes takes place. Here they "learn" to express receptors for antigens and to select appropriate specificities. This "thymic education" involves poorly understood mechanisms. Molecules produced by thymic epithelial cells and macrophages play important roles in T cell maturation. During development in the thymus, there is an ordered expression of surface markers such as T_{11}, T_6, T_4, and T_8. As T cells leave the thymus, T_6 is lost and cells express either T_4 or T_8 and then begin to express T_3. At this point these T cells are functionally mature. Upon exiting the thymus, the lymphocytes travel to the *secondary or peripheral lymphoid organs*, where responses to foreign antigen occur and mature lymphocyte function is expressed. The peripheral lymphoid organs include the spleen, lymph nodes, and gut-associated lymphoid tissue (Peyer's patches, appendix, tonsils, and adenoids).

The other major lymphocyte population, the B cells, are so named because in birds their development is dependent upon maturation in a central lymphoid organ termed the bursa (B) of Fabricius. Mammals have no bursa of Fabricius; so B cell development probably occurs in the hemopoietic tissue or in secondary lymphoid organs.

While lymphocyte development is dynamic and continues throughout the life of mammals, the importance of primary lymphoid organs is most easily demonstrable in young animals. For example, removal of the thymus at birth prevents the development of T cells and results in severely impaired immune responses in the adult. However, if the thymus is removed from adult animals, little if any deficit in immune responsiveness occurs. This is because lymphocytes are relatively long-lived and possibly because other sites of lymphocyte development take over in adults.

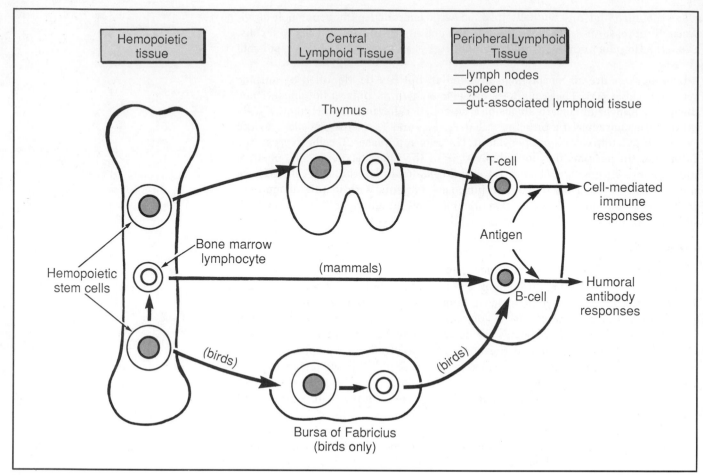

Figures 5.3. Lymphocyte development. The development of functional T
and B lymphocytes occurs in primary
lymphoid organs and the response to
antigen takes place in peripheral lymphoid tissue. B and T lymphocytes have
different pathways of development

The separate developmental pathways of B and T lymphocytes in humans were
first illustrated in naturally occurring abnormalities. Genetically caused immunodeficiencies, such as one called DiGeorge syndrome, result in a selective decrease
of T lymphocytes, while patients with X-linked agammaglobulinemia (Bruton's
disease) have normal T cell function but cannot make antibodies.

Lymphocyte Circulation

Lymphocytes patrol the body from their home bases in the lymphoid organs.
A great majority of T cells, and some B cells, continuously recirculate between
the blood and lymph. They leave the bloodstream by traversing specialized endothelial cells in venules and enter the tissues. After passing through the tissues
and cruising for intimate contact with antigens, these lymphocytes travel via the
fluid flow and accumulate in lymphatic vessels that connect to a series of downstream lymph nodes. From there they enter progressively larger lymphatic vessels
and eventually complete their round trip by passing back into the blood via the
thoracic duct. This recirculation promotes the contact of lymphocytes with antigens and ensures that information about a localized antigenic insult is dispersed
throughout the body. Thus, systemic immunity is produced.

The pattern of lymphatic circulation and structure of lymph nodes play important roles in immune responsiveness. Consider a microbe that has penetrated the defenses of the skin and is present in the extracellular fluid in the tissues. Through the inflammatory response, the microbe will be swept by the fluid flow into the blind-end afferent lymphatics present in almost all tissues (notable exceptions include the central nervous system and the placenta). The lymph is deposited into a meshwork of lymphoid cells that have the efficient ability to bind and ingest the microbe. These cells are collectively referred to as the *reticuloendothelial system* (RES), which includes macrophages and comparable cells with different names, depending on their characteristics and anatomical locations. These sticky cells are arranged in a filter-like array interspersed with lymphocytes and are the site where the antigen is trapped. The immune system has the invading microbe right where it wants it, bound by cells capable of "processing" and "presenting" the antigen and surrounded by the lymphocytes poised to engage it with specific receptors. ("Go ahead, make my day.") As a consequence of the filtering action of the lymph node, the lymph exiting the node via the efferent lymphatic vessel and ultimately emptying into the blood is microbe free, in other words sterile. The antigen trapped in the lymph node then initiates the immune response.

Figure 5.4. Cellular interactions. The processing, presentation, and recognition of antigen by lymphocytes are illustrated. Note that both macrophages and B cells express class II MHC gene products and can present antigen to helper T cells. Activated helper T cells (T_H) produce a shower of lymphokines that have powerful and diverse effects on the cells of the immune system. Following these events, intense lymphocyte proliferation and differentiation take place.

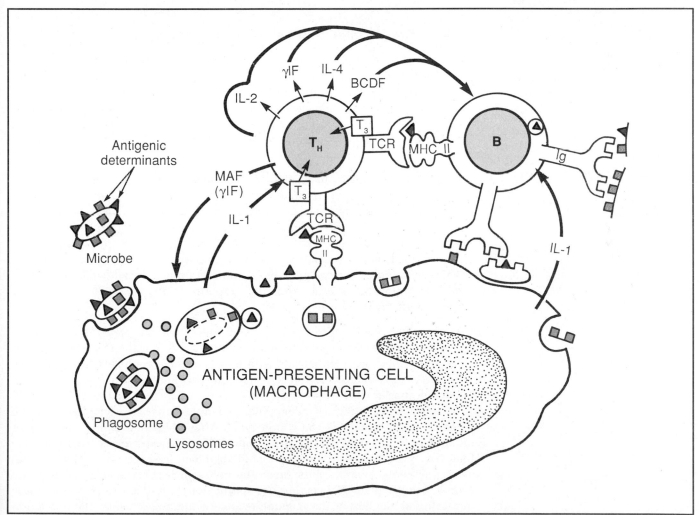

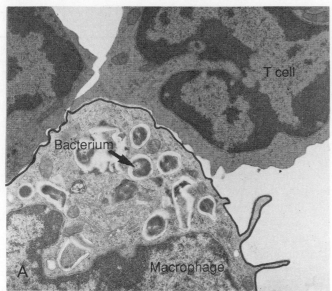

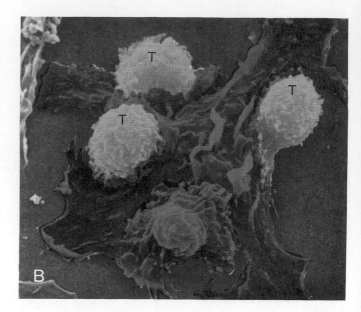

Figure 5.5. T cell–macrophage interactions. In these micrographs, T cells are recognizing bacterial antigens on the surface of macrophages. Transmission electron microscopy is used in **A** and scanning electron microscopy is used in **B**. Note the bacteria present in the phagosomes of macrophages (*A*) and the extensive membrane–membrane interaction between T cells and macrophages. This interaction is antigen specific (i.e., mediated by the T cell receptor) and requires the expression of class II MHC gene products by the macrophage. See Figure 5.4 for schematic view of molecular interactions. (Courtesy of Ziegler K, Cotran R, and Unanue E.)

Cellular Cooperation and Lymphocyte Activation

Most immune responses require intimate cellular cooperation among the lymphocytes, macrophages, and other accessory cells. These cells "talk" to each other by direct cell-cell interactions and by secreting lymphokines (Fig. 5.4). Electron micrographs of lymphocyte-macrophage interactions are shown in Figure 5.5.

To differentiate into antibody-secreting cells, B lymphocytes must interact with T lymphocytes and be stimulated by their lymphokines. The probable steps involved are

1. Binding of antigens to B cells via their immunoglobulin receptors.
2. Processing and "presentation" of the antigen to T cells. This is thought to involve the partial proteolysis of protein antigens in lysosomes or endocytic vesicles, and the transfer of resulting antigen fragments to the B cell surface, where they can be recognized by receptors on T cells (TCR in Fig. 5.4).
3. Direct delivery of T-cell derived lymphokines to B cells by cell to cell contact. This combination of signals drives the proliferation of B cells and their differentiation into plasma cells. Thus, by presenting antigens on their surface, B cells get efficient help from T cells.

Macrophages also contribute to lymphocyte activation by elaborating interleukin-1 and by processing and presenting antigens to T cells. The resulting activated T lymphocytes communicate with B cells and macrophages via the release of a variety of lymphokines. These include growth factors such as interleukin-2 (IL-2) and interleukin-4 (IL-4).

All this activity in the secondary lymphoid organs alters the lymphocyte traffic patterns and structure of the lymph node. After antigen trapping, there is an initial period (about 24 hours) of decreased flow of lymphocytes from the node followed by an increased flow. Vessels dilate, blood flow increases, and lymphocytes proliferate. These events cause the nodes to become enlarged, hence the classic "swollen glands". Lymphocytes specific for the antigen in question appear to localize at the site of the immune response, the nodes where the antigen is trapped.

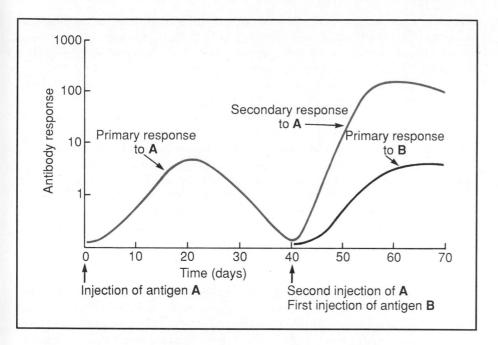

Figure 5.6. Primary and secondary immune responses. The antibody response to antigens A and B is shown as a function of time after primary and secondary stimulation with the antigens as indicated. Note the faster and stronger secondary response to antigen A.

IMMUNOLOGICAL MEMORY: PRIMARY VERSUS SECONDARY RESPONSES

When an antigen is encountered for the first time, the immune system makes a primary immune response (Fig. 5.2). The subsequent encounters are called secondary responses. If one measures the amount of antibody generated in a primary and a secondary response, marked differences are noted (Fig. 5.6). The secondary response occurs after a shorter lag period; it is of greater intensity and it has a longer duration. In addition, different kinds of immunoglobulins are produced in the secondary response.

The faster and stronger secondary response (also called the *anamnestic* or *memory response*) results from clonal selection and differentiation that occur during the initial contact with an antigen. The clonal proliferation of lymphocytes is followed by a dual pathway of differentiation of both B and T cell lineages. By yet unknown mechanisms, some of the progeny become *effector cells*—cells capable of causing an immediate effect, whereas others become *memory cells*. In general, effector cells express their function for a finite and usually short period of time. For example, plasma cells are the effector cells of the B cell lineage; cytotoxic cells are the effector cells of the CTL lineage. Immunological memory is due to the fact that the memory lymphocytes are long-lived and can persist for years. They are capable of rapid differentiation into effector cells when stimulated with antigen. For the B cell lineage, memory cells are poised to rapidly secrete large amounts of antibody when appropriately activated by secondary contact with antigen.

IMMUNOLOGICAL TOLERANCE

A major question in immunology is, How does the immune system distinguish self from nonself? There are two possibilities. One is that the genes coding for the antigen receptors specific for self-molecules are simply not present in the genome. The other (and correct one) is that the immune system is intrinsically capable of responding to both self- and nonself-entities but that mechanisms exist to prevent potentially disastrous reactions to self. The existence of *autoimmune diseases* (immune responses to self-components that result in pathology) indicates that at least some self-recognition can occur.

Several experimental observations indicate that the immune system "learns" not to respond to self-components early in development. For example, if an antigen is injected into a mouse at birth, a time when the immune system is still immature, it will not respond to that antigen as an adult. A similar phenomenon occurs in genetically different twins that have shared a common circulation before birth. They do not react to the tissue antigens of their partner. Thus, the immune system can learn to tolerate a normally foreign antigen as if it were a self-component. The state of antigen-specific immunological unresponsiveness is called *acquired immunological tolerance*. Immunological tolerance may be thought of as "negative immunological memory"; prior exposure to antigen results in a decreased response (rather than a heightened one) to the antigen. Like immunological memory, immunological tolerance is an active response that requires antigenic exposure and is mediated by lymphocytes.

Under special circumstances, and with some difficulty, immunological tolerance can be demonstrated in immunologically mature animals. Induction of tolerance is favored by intravenous injection of soluble protein antigen in either very large or in repeated small amounts. Also, the use of immunosuppressive treatments, such as X-irradiation or certain immunosuppressive drugs, can promote the induction of tolerance. Both T cells and B cells can be "tolerized" experimentally, but T cell tolerance is easier to achieve and may be more relevant to the natural tolerance to self-antigens.

Whenever tolerance to self breaks down, autoimmune disease may result. For example, in systemic lupus erythematosus (SLE), patients produce antibodies to their own nucleic acids, and in myasthenia gravis, to acetylcholine receptors. Both result in severe chronic illnesses. Multiple sclerosis, a disease characterized by chronic demyelination of the central nervous system, is thought to result from T cell reactivity to the myelin-associated self-proteins. The onset of certain autoimmune disorders is often associated with microbial infections, which allows us to speculate that microbial products may somehow alter self-components or modulate the processes that normally maintain tolerance to self-components.

The precise mechanisms of immunological tolerance are not known. There are three major possibilities for which experimental evidence exists. (*a*) Clones of lymphocytes potentially reactive to a particular antigen may be eliminated. For the T cell lineage, this *clonal abortion* is thought to occur in the thymus during T cell maturation. In fact, many newly made T cells do not leave the thymus, perhaps they represent the "forbidden" self-reactive clones. The well-established importance of thymic education in the development of the T cells receptor repertoire adds credence to this concept. (*b*) Specific clones may be present but may have received negative signals through their receptor systems and thus may be less responsive to antigen. Immature B lymphocytes behave in this manner. This has been termed *clonal anergy*. (*c*) The response of lymphocyte clones may be actively inhibited by the action of suppressor T cells. These issues are of obvious importance in organ transplantation, since the immune response represents a major barrier to graft survival. Also, intelligent intervention in the control of disease caused by too much immune reactivity (autoimmunity and hypersensitivity), or too little (immunodeficiencies and infections), will require a thorough understanding of these regulatory pathways.

ANTIGENS

Any organic macromolecule can potentially act as an antigen. In descending order of antigenicity, proteins, polysaccharides, lipids, and nucleic acids, have all been shown to be antigenic under the correct circumstances. The portions of an antigen that combine with the antigen-binding site of lymphocyte receptors are called *antigenic determinants* or *epitopes*. The size of an antigenic determinant may be 10 amino acids or five to six sugar molecules. Since most antigens are large molecules, they can have many epitopes and thus can stimulate many different lymphocyte clones. Such a response is said to be *polyclonal*. When one is dealing with the response of a single clone of cells—a situation achievable only under special circumstances—the response is called *monoclonal*.

Antigens are classified according to the relative thymus dependency of the antibody response. While all B cell responses are enhanced by the action of helper T cells, certain antigens can elicit antibody production without T cells. Such antigens, referred to as *T cell–independent antigens*, have many repeats of an epitope, and/or have the ability to cause B cells to proliferate. Many of these antigens are associated with bacterial cell envelopes; lipopolysaccharide from Gram-negative bacteria and pneumococcal capsular polysaccharide are two examples. This direct elicitation of antibody may play an important role in the rapid response to bacterial invasion.

Antigenicity or *immunogenicity* is the capacity of a molecule to elicit an immune response. This is an operational definition and depends on many factors. In general, large molecules with multiple antigenic determinants are better antigens than small-molecular-weight substances. Very small compounds, called *haptens*, can elicit an immune response but only when coupled to a larger molecule called a *carrier* Examples of haptens are simple sugars, certain drugs (e.g., penicillin) and chemical side chains such as dinitrophenyl groups, which are used experimentally. Also relevant are the dose of antigen, the route of immunization, and the presence of adjuvants, which are agents that enhance the immune response. From a microbiological view, live microorganisms are generally better antigens and make better vaccines than dead ones. Most relevant to antigenicity is the degree of difference between the antigen molecule and any analogous structure present as self. In general, the greater degree of phylogenetic difference between self and nonself, the greater the immune response.

IMMUNOGLOBULINS

Structure and Function

The term antibody is usually used for immunoglobulins that have specific antigen binding capacity. Immunoglobulins play two roles and exist in two structurally different forms: as membrane receptors on resting B lymphocytes and as major secretory products of fully differentiated plasma cells. Antibody can bind antigen and then mediate several other activities or functions in the interaction with other cells and molecules of the immune system.

Antibody molecules fall into several different yet related classes. Consider the secreted immunoglobulin of the G class (IgG) as the prototypical structure (Fig. 5.7). It is a Y-shaped protein with identical antigen-binding sites at the tip of each arm. With these two binding sites this structure is called *bivalent*. The proteolytic enzyme papain cuts antibody into functionally distinct Fc and Fab fragments. The cleaved arms of the Y represent fragments with antigen binding ability

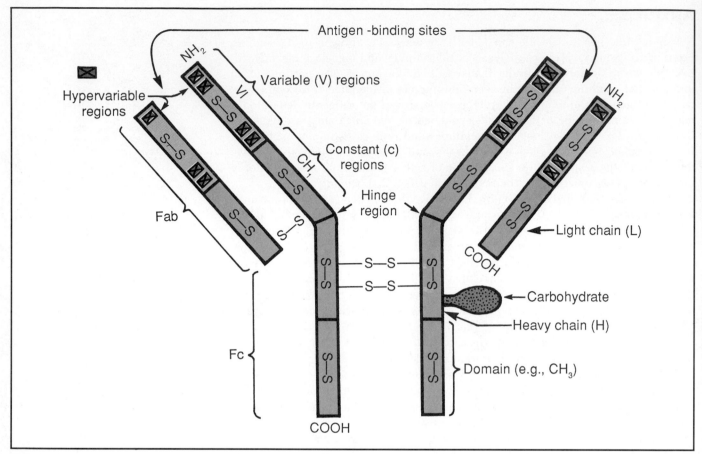

Figure 5.7. Structure of IgG. Immunoglobulin of the IgG class is composed of two heavy and two light chains. Note that portions of the amino terminal regions of both heavy and light chains form the antigen combining sites. The Fc part is formed by the heavy chains alone.

and are called Fab fragments. The tail of the Y is called the Fc because it is the fragment that is easily crystallizable. The Fc portion directs important functions of antibody other than antigen binding. These *effector* functions include complement activation and interaction with specific Fc receptors (Chapter 4). Different classes of antibody molecules may have identical antigen-binding sites but different Fc parts, therefore supplying different functions.

The multiple binding sites of an antibody molecule give it the ability to cross link soluble antigen molecules into a large lattice, provided the antigen has three or more antigenic determinants. When this complex of antigens and antibodies reaches a certain size, it comes out of solution. This is called *immunoprecipitation*. Antigen binding and cross-linking reactions are aided by the flexibility of the parts of the molecule where the arms meet the tail, the so-called *hinge region*. Within a lattice of bound antigens and antibodies, there is a multiple display of the Fc parts. They can then work cooperatively in a multivalent fashion that enhances their binding avidity to cells with Fc receptors and to the C1 component of complement.

Immunoglobulin IgG consists of four polypeptide chains, two identical light chains (each about 220 amino acids) and two identical heavy chains (each about 440 amino acids). The chains are held together both by covalent interchain disulfide bonds and noncovalent interactions. Each antigen-binding site is formed

Table 5.2
Human immunoglobulins

Isotype	Structure	Molecular Weight	Concentration in Serum, mg/ml	No. of Heavy Chain Domains	Placental Transfer	Binding to Mast Cells and Basophils	Activates Complement	Opsonin: Binds to Phagocytes	Distinguishing Features or Functions
IgM		~970,000	1.5	5	−	−	+ +	−	The first in development and response
IgD	B cell	~180,000	0.03	5	−	−	−	−	B cell receptor
IgG	B cell	~150,000	13.5	4	+	−	+(IgG4−)	+(IgG1 IgG3)	Opsonin, ADCC
IgE	Mast cell or basophil	~190,000	0.00005	5	−	+	−	±	Allergic response
IgA	SC	~390,000 ~160,000	3.5	4	−	−	±(Only alternative pathway)	−	In secretions (GALT)

by a portion of both a heavy chain and a light chain. The Fc part is composed of the carboxy-terminal halves of the two heavy chains.

Both heavy and light chains are made up of repeating segments or domains which fold independently to form compact functional units. Each domain, about 110 amino acids long, has one intrachain disulfide bond and a characteristic three dimensional structure called the immunoglobulin fold. Each domain is a sandwich of three and four antiparallel polypeptide strands in a β-sheet configuration.

In mammals, there are five major immunoglobulin classes or isotypes. The classes of antibody differ in structure and function, as summarized in Table 5.2. Classes are based on differences in the heavy chains. The isotypes are called IgM, IgD, IgG, IgE, and IgA and their respective heavy chains are designated by the Greek letters, μ δ γ ϵ α. There are two different types of light chains, λ and κ. The heavy chains determine the unique biological activity of the different isotypes. A single antibody molecule has only one type of heavy chain; it can have either two κ or two λ light chains but never one each. This ensures that both antigen-binding sites are identical.

IgG

IgG is the major class in the blood. It is produced in greater amounts in the secondary response than in the primary response. IgG can activate complement, bind to "professional" phagocytes via its Fc part, participate in antibody-dependent cell-mediated cytotoxicity (ADCC) with killer (K) cells (see "Null Cells"), and cross the placenta to supply some protection to neonates. In humans, there are four major subclasses of IgG: IgG1, IgG2, IgG3, and IgG4. These differ in their ability to activate complement (IgG4 does not), and to bind to macrophage Fc receptors (IgG1 and IgG3 do).

IgM

IgM is the major product in the primary immune response and is the predominant antibody produced in response to thymus-independent antigens. Secretory IgM consists of five copies of the basic four-chain unit (two light plus two heavy chains) and therefore has 10 antigen-binding sites. This multivalency promotes its ability to cross link, while its multiple Fc parts make it a very efficient activator of complement. IgM also contains an extra protein called J (joining) chain that aids in the polymerization process within plasma cells. The large molecular weight of IgM (about 970,000) confines it to the blood and it is not found in substantial quantities in tissues.

Membrane IgM is an important antigen receptor on B cells. It is an integral membrane protein, anchored by a hydrophobic carboxy terminus. Unlike secreted IgM, but resembling IgG, membrane IgM is a four-chain structure with two antigen-binding sites. Its heavy chain is the first to be produced during B cell development. It may be important in the receiving of "tolerogenic" signals that lead to clonal anergy and immunological tolerance. Membrane IgM may be constitutively expressed on both resting and memory B cells. Plasma cells do not express a membrane form of immunoglobulin.

IgD

IgD is another membrane immunoglobulin predominantly found on resting B cells. Human IgD is also a four-chain molecule like IgG, but with a very long hinge region. Its very low concentration in the blood may be explained by its sensitivity to proteolysis at the hinge region and the rarity of IgD-secreting plasma cells. Its only function may be as a membrane receptor for antigen. During B cell ontogeny, IgD is expressed after IgM. The appearance of IgD renders the B cell functionally mature, thus it can no longer be easily "tolerized" upon contact with antigen.

IgA

IgA is present in seromucous secretions such as milk, tears, saliva, perspiration, and secretions of the lung and gut. Small amounts are also found in the blood. In secretions, IgA molecules consist of two copies of IgG-like molecules covalently attached via disulfide bonds with an intervening J chain. They are also associated with another protein called secretory component which is synthesized by epithelial cells. The secretory component is a portion of an integral membrane protein known as the poly Ig receptor, which plays a key role in the transport of IgA across the epithelial cells into the lumen. Secretory component, which is attached to secreted IgA, also acts as a stabilizer and protector against the proteolytic activity present in secretions. IgA is synthesized at a very high rate in the lymphoid tissue of the gut, especially the Peyer's patches. The body produces amounts of IgA equal or greater to those of any other immunoglobulin class. IgA can neither activate complement nor bind well to Fc receptors, but it may play an important role in preventing the attachment and subsequent invasion of pathogenic microbes, a kind of strategic defense initiative at external surface.

IgE

IgE is the antibody class responsible for the clinical manifestations of allergies such as hay fever, asthma, and hives. Its Fc region specifically binds to very high-affinity receptors present on the surfaces of mast cells and basophils. Cell-bound IgE then serves as a receptor for antigen. The cross linking of these receptors by antigen causes the release of a variety of biologically active agents. One such agent, histamine, causes smooth muscle contraction and increases in vascular permeability. These effects may have some protective function by enhancing the influx of cells, antibodies, and complement into the site of inflammation. IgE is also important in the response to parasitic infection (principally by worms) as it is often greatly elevated in the serum of patients with these diseases. IgE participates in antibody-dependent cell mediated killing of parasites by macrophages and eosinophils, which are cells that possess low affinity Fc receptors specific for IgE. Is the price for allergy worth paying because IgE defends us against parasites?

Membrane and Secreted Immunoglobulins

With the possible exception of IgD all immunoglobulins exist in two versions: a membrane form and a secreted form. The membrane form has an extra carboxy-terminal portion on the heavy chain that anchors it to the membrane and perhaps plays a role in signal transduction. For example, memory B cells that are "ready" to secrete IgG contain a membrane form of IgG. Upon activation by antigen the switch from a membrane form to a secreted form occurs via an alteration of mRNA mediated by differential RNA processing.

Structural Basis of Antigen-Binding Specificity

Each class of antibodies includes millions of different molecules, each with unique antigen-binding specificity and amino acid sequence. No other known family of proteins has so many members. This diversity provides the variety of functions of each isotype, and the multitude of specific antigen-binding sites required for a sophisticated mobile defense system. All this presents formidable genetic problems. Their solution involves some very special mechanisms of gene expression. For example, immunoglobulins turned out to be the first known exception to the "one gene, one polypeptide" rule.

Each light chain and heavy chain consists of two major regions, variable and constant. These were originally identified by comparing the amino acid sequences of different immunoglobulin molecules. As the names imply, the sequences in the constant regions are similar, whereas the variable region sequences differ considerably from antibody to antibody. These comparisons were made possible by the fact that patients with B cell tumors, called myelomas, make large amounts of a given immunoglobulin molecule. The immunoglobulin that accumulates in the blood of each patient is called a *myeloma protein*. The urine of these patients often contains free immunoglobulin light chains called *Bence Jones proteins*.

For light chains, the carboxy-terminal halves of chains of the same type (κ or λ) have the same sequence, while the amino-terminal parts are different. For heavy chains, a variable region of similar size (about 110 amino acids) is present at the amino terminus, while the rest of the molecule is rather constant. Within the variable regions, differences are clustered into three regions of the light chains and four regions of the heavy chains. These regions, each about 4 to 12 amino acids long, are known as *hypervariable regions*. From x-ray diffraction studies it is now clear that the variable regions of the light and heavy chains are so folded that the hypervariable regions form an antigen-binding pocket that can accommodate antigenic determinant the size of about five to six sugars or about 10 amino acids. Thus, the amino-terminal variable parts of the light and heavy chains form the antigen-binding site. Their amino acid differences provide the structural basis for the diversity of antigen binding function.

The interaction of antigen with antibody is a reversible bimolecular reaction. Unlike enzyme-substrate reactions neither of the reactants is permanently altered. The binding of antigen to the antigen-combining site is mediated by the sum of many noncovalent forces such as hydrophobic and hydrogen bonds, Van der Waals forces, and ionic interactions. Since these forces are effective at short distances, a tight fit takes place when the surfaces are complementary, that is, if the size and shape of the antigen fits to the combining site on the antibody. The goodness of the fit is referred to as *affinity*, which can be determined experimentally by quantitating the affinity constant of the antigen-antibody interaction. *Avidity* of the antigen-antibody interaction is the total binding strength of all the sites together; the multivalency of IgM, for example, increases the avidity.

Antibody Specificity and Quantitation

Specificity is defined as the ability of antibodies produced in response to an antigen to react with that antigen and not with others. Antibodies can be incredibly specific. They can discriminate atomic differences between simple chemicals and single amino acid substitutions in proteins. There are exceptions, and specificity may be imperfect, leading to cross reactions. For example, antibody

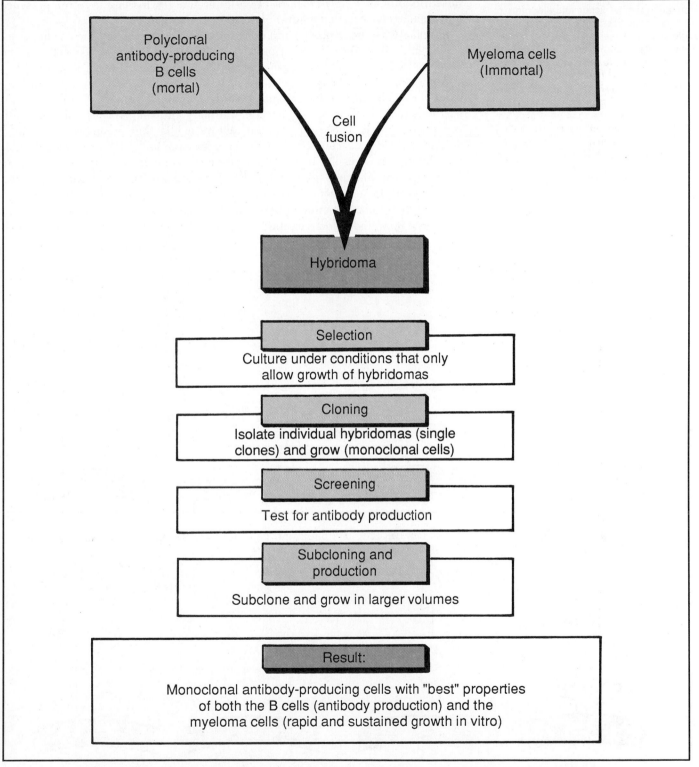

Figure 5.8. Production of monoclonal antibodies. Sequential steps in the procedure used to generate monoclonal antibodies are illustrated.

Figure 5.9. The immunoglobulin supergene family. Schematic diagrams of some of the members of the immunoglobulin supergene family are shown. Immunoglobulin, β_2-microglobulin and class I MHC have been studied by x-ray diffraction and the three-dimensional structure is known. Other structures are predicted from the amino acid sequence inferred from the nucleotide sequences of cloned genes. Homology units (or domains) are depicted by intrachain disulfide–bonded loops. These loops represent globular domains, each with the polypeptide chain folded into a β-pleated sheet configuration. Irregular loops represent imperfect folding into such a configuration.

raised to antigen X may cross react with antigen Y. This is due to the presence of a similar molecular configuration on the two antigens.

Specificity can be improved and cross reactions minimized by the use of monoclonal antibodies. By an elegant procedure illustrated in Figure 5.8, cells can be generated which secrete homogeneous antibody molecules with a single kind of binding site. An antibody-forming B cell is fused with a myeloma cell resulting in a hybrid cell (called a hybridoma) with the combined properties of both fusion partners: the ability to secrete specific antibody and the capacity for rapid and sustained growth. The use of special culture media that permit the growth of only the hybrid cells, coupled with methods for isolation of the progeny of individual hybridomas, results in the propagation of monoclonal antibody–producing cells. This procedure has revolutionized biology and medicine by making unlimited quantities of homogeneous antibodies available for a variety of applications.

The methods for detecting antibody and antigens are numerous. Some rely on the ability of antibody to precipitate antigen that can be visualized or quantitated:

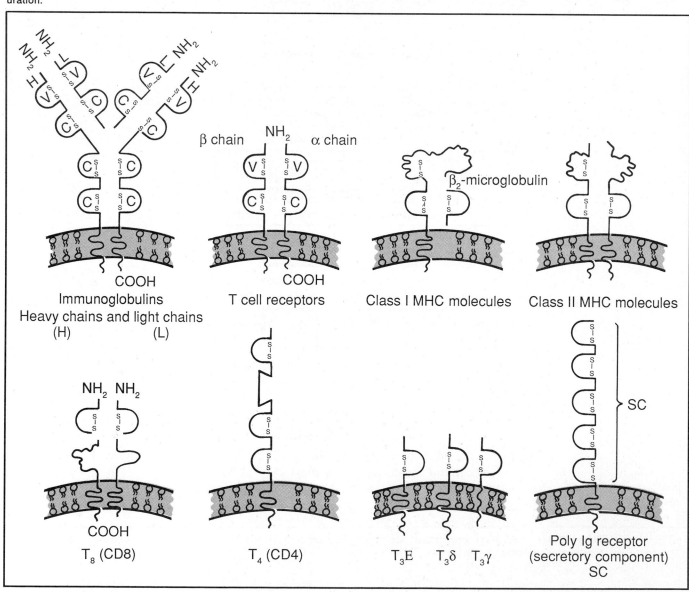

These include quantitative immunoprecipitation; immuno double diffusion, or the Ouchterlony test; single radial immunodiffusion (SRID), or the Mancini test; immunoelectrophoresis (IEP); etc. Other tests rely on antigen-antibody interactions that are detected by coupling antibody or antigen with a radioactive tracer (radioimmunoassay, or RIA), an enzyme (enzyme-linked immunosorbent assay, or ELISA), or a fluorescent compound (immunofluorescence, or fluorescence immunoassays or FIA). These tests are described in Chapter 59. Still other assays make use of the ability of antibody to cross link and agglutinate antigen-bearing cells (e.g, antibodies to red cells can be detected by hemagglutination) or activate complement when bound to antigen (complement fixation test).

Evolution of the Immunoglobulin Supergene Family

As previously discussed, the heavy and light chains are made of homologous domains and each domain has a characteristic three- dimensional structure called the immunoglobulin fold. The homology among the domains suggests that the immunoglobulin chains arose in evolution by a series of gene duplications of the basic 110-amino-acid unit. It is now clear that the immunoglobulin fold is a fundamental structural unit that defines a whole family of homologous proteins, called the immunoglobulin supergene family (Fig. 5.9). Members of the family include immunoglobulin, secretory component (poly Ig receptor) and as we shall see below, the T cell receptor, molecules of the major histocompatibility complex (MHC), and other lymphocyte surface proteins such as T_4, T_8, and the T_3 complex. By 1987 there were 27 known members of the family expressed by cells of the immune system and the nervous system.

It is possible that the supergene family evolved to supply a common function to the family members. It is clear that the functions of the domains of immunoglobulin heavy and light chains are to interact, stabilize the immunoglobulin molecule, and form the antigen-binding site. Similarly, the family may have evolved to mediate cell-cell interactions via significant binding affinity among family members, as discussed below.

Generation of Diversity

One major challenge to the immune system is to provide millions, perhaps billions, of antibodies specific for almost any antigenic determinant. The issue at hand is how to do this without requiring an unreasonably large amount of genetic material.

Immunoglobulins are produced from three gene pools (groups of similar genes) on separate chromosomes, corresponding to the κ light, λ light, and heavy chains. Each pool contains many variable region genes (and subdivisions of variable gene segments), located a very long distance upstream of the constant region genes. During B cell development, variable genes are *translocated* to a position closer to a particular constant gene. By this arrangement, the chains (composed of variable and constant regions) can be transcribed and translated. The first translocation that occurs in B cell development brings a particular variable region gene segment into proximity of the μ constant gene and thus leads to the expression of heavy chains for IgM. Other translocations occur during this differentiation, so that a particular variable gene is connected more closely to other heavy chain constant genes, allowing the expression of other isotypes of antibody (Fig. 5.10). This phenomenon is called *class switching*. These events occur by a process known as *site-specific recombination*, which depends on specific recombination sequences flanking each gene segment. These translocations account

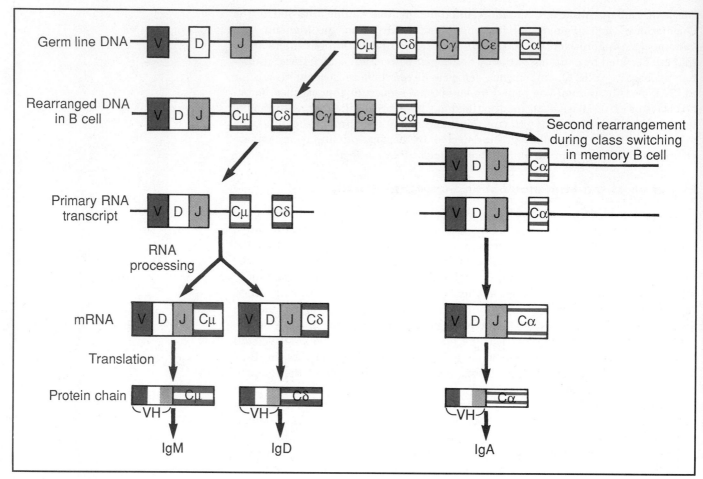

Figure 5.10. Organization and expression of immunoglobulin heavy chain genes. The gene rearrangements that occur during B cell development and the response to antigen are depicted. DNA segments that encode for individual portions of the mature protein are carried separately in the germ line DNA. These gene segments must rearrange as indicated in order for expression to occur. The joining of a given variable gene to different constant region genes permits the production of different isotypes (classes) of antibody with identical antigen-binding characteristics. (The genes are not drawn to scale and many details are omitted.)

for the fact that different classes of antibody may have the same antigen-binding specificity.

Variable-region genes are actually made up of two or three separate variable *gene segments*. A segment is defined as a contiguous stretch of DNA that is ultimately translated into a portion of the mature polypeptide. Two segments code for the variable region of each light chain: they are called V, for variable, and J, for joining, segments. Three segments are involved for heavy chains: V, D (diversity), and J segments (Figs. 5.10 and 5.11). During assembly of a complete variable-region gene, these segments are brought into proximity to permit transcription. Since there are several different V, J, and D segments, many unique combinations can be created by somatic recombination, thereby increasing antibody diversity. For example, in the mouse, variable-heavy-chain genes are made up of about 200 V segments, 10 D segments, and four J segments. Random combination could produce 8000 ($200 \times 10 \times 4 = 8000$) unique variable heavy chains. Similarly, if the 200 or so variable light chain kappa gene segments were to recombine with the four J segments, about 800 unique variable genes would be generated. Also, since the antigen-binding site is generated by both heavy and light chains, the random association of heavy (H) and light (L) chains could yield about 6.4 million ($8000 \times 800 = 6,400,000$) different antibody molecules. (This process is like creating a large number of different meals in a Chinese restaurant by choosing one from column A, one from column B, and so on. See Fig. 5.11.)

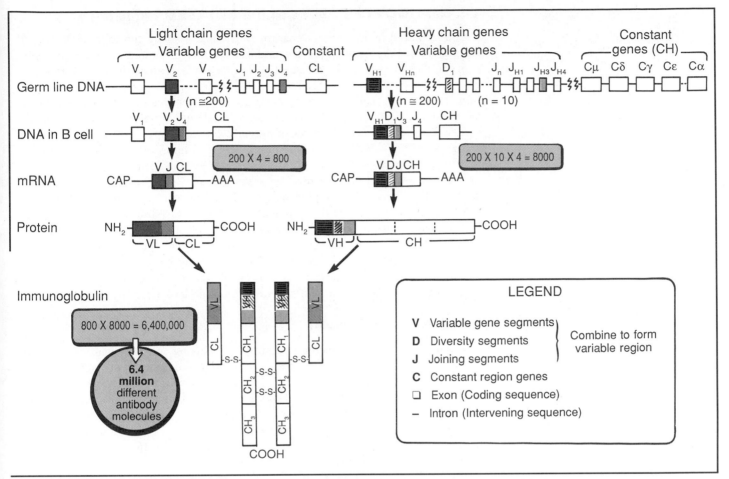

Light chain genes — Variable genes — Constant

Heavy chain genes — Variable genes —

Constant genes (CH)

200 X 4 = 800

200 X 10 X 4 = 8000

800 X 8000 = 6,400,000

6.4 million different antibody molecules

LEGEND

V   Variable gene segments ⎫
D   Diversity segments   ⎬ Combine to form variable region
J   Joining segments   ⎭

C   Constant region genes

☐   Exon (Coding sequence)

—   Intron (Intervening sequence)

Figure 5.11. Generation of diversity. Depicted is the mechanism by which a large number of unique immunoglobulin molecules is created. The number of unique variable regions and antigen combining sites created at each step is calculated. For example, with heavy chains the 200 V segments can combine with any of the 10 D segments and four J segments to create 8000 different variable regions. The number of V, D, and J segments present is, in some cases, a minimal estimate and the actual number of segments varies among different species. A similar mechanism occurs for the generation of diversity in T cell receptors (not shown).

Additional diversity can be created by the inaccuracy during the cutting and joining of the V, D, and J segments, known as *junctional diversity*. Also, point mutations in and around the V region genes can occur. This is called *somatic mutation*. These mechanisms probably increase antibody diversity by a factor of 10 to 100. Somatic mutation may play an important role in antibody production during secondary responses to antigen. Such mutations may serve as a mechanism to "fine-tune" the affinity of a particular antibody. Additionally, somatic mutations may reflect the immune system's attempt to "anticipate" changes in antigens. For example, the genes of an invading microorganism are subject to mutations that can potentially change antigens to a form unrecognizable by a particular antibody and thus evade the immune response. The antibody genes may also "play this game" and "gamble" that somatic mutations in variable genes produce changes in the binding site that complement changes in the antigen, thus permitting successful recognition and destruction of the invader.

Thus, somatic recombination of segments, junctional diversity, somatic mutation, and combinatorial joining of light and heavy chains, all act to increase antibody diversity for a total of possibly 10^8 different antibody molecules. This huge repertoire is apparently sufficient to deal with the antigenic universe. But, this is only half of the story. The other arm of immune defense, the T lymphocytes, can likely generate, by similar mechanisms, a repertoire of 10 million or more antigen-binding molecules.

T LYMPHOCYTES AND CELL-MEDIATED IMMUNITY

Cell-mediated immune reactions are those mediated by the thymus-derived T lymphocytes. Like B lymphocytes and the antibody responses, T lymphocytes can specifically recognize and react to highly diverse structures. Both types of lymphocytes respond to antigen and mediate memory responses by clonal selection. However, T cell antigen recognition and function differ from B cells in several important aspects. (a) There are several functionally distinct categories of T cells: cytotoxic cells, inducer or helper cells, and suppressor cells. (b) T cells recognize antigen when it is associated with proteins of the major histocompatibility complex (MHC). In general, cytotoxic T cells "see" antigen in association with class I MHC molecules, whereas helper T cells recognize a molecular configuration formed by the physical association of processed antigen with class II MHC molecules. (c) The developmental pathways are different: T cells depend on the thymus for important differentiation and selection events. (d) A number of lymphocyte accessory molecules, important for T cell activation, are not expressed by B cells. (e) The receptor for antigen used by T cells is related to immunoglobulin, but is structurally and genetically distinct. In general the T cell receptor is not designed to be a secretory product—like antibody.

T Cell Receptor Complex

T cells recognize and respond to antigen by using integral membrane glycoproteins called the T cell receptors. The major receptor is a disulfide-linked heterodimer of two polypeptide chains, designated α and β, each having a molecular weight of about 40,000 to 50,000. Each chain contains N-terminal variable regions unique to particular clones of T cells and carboxy-terminal constant regions shared among T cells. This basic structure has been identified on both helper T cells and cytotoxic T cells. The receptor(s) for antigen on suppressor T cells have not been identified.

The T cell receptor appears to have a domain structure homologous to immunoglobulin, which would place it in the Ig supergene family (Fig. 5.9). Like immunoglobulin, T cell receptors are constructed by somatic recombination of genes carried separately in the genome. α-Chain genes include a single constant region, 50 or more J segments, and probably an equal or greater number of V segments. Upstream of β constant region genes there are about six J segments, one D segment, and 20 to 100 V segments. With both chains, junctional diversity can increase the repertoire, but somatic mutation may not play a major role in increasing diversity. Like diversity created with the construction of an immunoglobulin gene, many different unique α and β chains can be constructed by the random combinations of V, J, and D segments. By combinatorial associations of different α and β chains a very large repertoire of T cell receptors can be potentially generated. Depending on the inferred contributions of the various mechanisms for diversity and bias of the estimators, the repertoire number is about 10^7 to more than 10^9. It is certainly comparable to the range of antibody diversity and big enough to deal with the antigenic universe.

How does the triggering of these receptors translate into the expression of function? We know that other membrane proteins of T cells are involved in as yet poorly understand but well-established accessory roles. One of these is designated the T_3 complex. This is a group of three major proteins (designated γ, δ, and ϵ) noncovalently linked to the T cell receptor. The T_3 complex must be present for proper T cell function but does not bind directly to antigen. It may be involved in stabilizing the T cell receptor and/or transmitting the signals to the cell interior.

Functional T Cell Subpopulations

T lymphocytes are divided into three main functional groups: cytotoxic T cells, helper or inducer T cells, and suppressor T cells. The latter two are also known as regulatory T cells since they modulate the activity of other cells.

Cytotoxic T Cells

Cytotoxic T lymphocytes can specifically recognize and destroy antigen-bearing cells. They defend us against certain viral diseases (and possibly bacterial diseases caused by intracellular pathogens) by reacting with antigens expressed on the surface of infected cells. Prevention of viral replication results from their ability to recognize very low levels of antigen and to kill such target cells before production of virus progeny. Intimate effector cell-target cell interaction is required for killing. This cellular adhesion is aided in an undefined way by lymphocyte-function-associated molecules such as LFA-1. Following binding to the target cell, the T_8 molecule and the T_3 complex are involved in expression of lytic function.

The mechanism of killing is not certain, but the most attractive hypothesis is termed the *granule exocytosis model*. Evidence exists that the T cell secretes a protein termed *granule cytolysin* or *perforin* from intracellular granules onto the target cell membrane. This protein then assembles into amphipathic channel-forming structures—which are analogous to the membrane attack complex of complement—that cause permeability changes in the target cell and eventual osmotic lysis. *Cytotoxic T lymphocytes* may also induce a nuclease activity in the target cell so that both cellular and viral DNA are destroyed. It is clear that the effector T cell is not damaged in this process and can kill multiple target cells.

Helper T Cells

Helper or inducer T lymphocytes are essential for optimal proliferation and differentiation of B cells and cytotoxic T cell precursors. They are also important for increasing the ability of macrophages to ingest and destroy microbial pathogens and to kill tumor cells. They display characteristic surface markers including T_3 and T_4. T_3 is involved in signal transduction and T_4 acts by stabilizing cellular interactions by binding to portions of the class II MHC molecules present on B cells and macrophages.

When activated, T helper cells release a variety of lymphokines. These include several interleukins (IL) such as IL-2, IL-3, and IL-4 (also known as BSF-1); macrophage activating factors (MAF) such as γ interferon; B cell stimulatory factors (BSF) such as BSF_1 (IL-4) and BSF-2; B cell differentiation factors such as BCDF; B cell maturation factor (BMF); and T cell–replacing factor (TRF). These and others are summarized in Table 5.3.

Because of this secretory function, many if not all of the activities of helper T cells can be duplicated by the appropriate mix of active lymphokines. However, the most efficient delivery of helper T cell–derived lymphokines to B cells and macrophages is accomplished by the direct physical interaction between the cells. This occurs when antigen is presented by B cells so that helper T cells interact with it on the B cell's surface. Likewise, macrophage activation via helper T cell–derived MAF is aided by macrophage-mediated antigen presentation.

Table 5.3
Lymphokines and monokines

Current Name	Other Names	Cell Source	Activity
Interleukin-1 (IL-1)	LAF, BAF Endogenous pyrogen (EP)	Macrophages and others	Promotes T cell proliferation; increases body temperature
Interleukin-2 (IL-2)	TCGF	Predominantly T_{4+} cells	Causes proliferation of activated T cells and B cells
Interleukin-3 (IL-3)	PSH	T cells	Promotes proliferation of a variety of hemopoietic cells
Interleukin-4 (IL-4)	BSF_1	T cells	Promotes B and T cell growth
γ Interferon	Immune interferon, MAF	T cells	Activates macrophages; promotes B cell differentiation
B cell stimulatory factor-2 (BSF-2)	BCDF	T cells and others	Promotes B cell function
Tumor necrosis factor-α (TNFα)	Cachectin	Macrophages	Multiple activities: Causes death of certain cells; promotes growth and differentiation; causes wasting
Tumor necrosis factor-β (TNFβ)	Lymphotoxin	T cells	Causes death of certain cells; multiple activities
Macrophage-activating factor (MAF)	γ Interferon and others	T cells	Causes macrophage activation
Migration inhibitory factor (MIF)		T cells	Decreases macrophage motility
$BCGF_2$		T cells	Promotes growth of activated B cells
α/β Interferon	Leukocyte/ fibroblast interferon	Neutrophils, macrophages, fibroblasts	Antiviral activity; macrophage activation; growth inhibition
T cell–replacing factor (TRF)	Many molecules, e.g., IL-2	T cells	Replaces T helper cells in antibody production

Suppressor T Cells

Suppressor T cells downregulate the response of B cells or other T cells to antigens. They remain the most enigmatic regulatory T cell. One thing that is clear is that they regulate responses in an antigen-specific manner. They certainly do not use the same receptor for antigen employed by T helper cells. Suppression can be mediated by soluble factors from suppressor T cells. The current confusion about suppressor T cells will be mitigated as their antigen receptors are identified and characterized, and the mechanisms involved in complex cellular interactions are elucidated.

Null Cells ("Third Population Cells")

In addition to B and T lymphocytes there are yet other functionally important cells that lack the classical surface markers and functions of T cells, B cells, and macrophages. As the name implies these cells lack the readily detectable markers and functions of macrophages, B cells, and T lymphocytes. While their lineage remains unclear, they are generally considered to be lymphocyte-like. This group includes two types of cells: *natural killer* (NK) *cells* and the *killer* (K) *cells* responsible for antibody-dependent cell-mediated cytotoxicity (ADCC). NK cells can efficiently kill certain types of tumor and virus-infected cells with some selectivity, but not with the precise specificity displayed by cytotoxic T lymphocytes. While NK cells do not require the thymus for development, some evidence indicates that they may be lineally related to T cells. NK cells have prominent cytoplasmic granules and have been called large granular lymphocytes (LGL). These granules contain a protein with several names such as granule cytolysin, perforin, or NK cell cytotoxic factor. Granule exocytosis as described for the cytotoxic T cell is the likely mechanism of killing by NK and K cells.

K cells express high-affinity Fc receptors that are employed to recognize and destroy antibody coated cells. IgG is the predominant class responsible for directing the specificity of cytotoxic activity. These cells can kill certain bacteria and mammalian cells. K cell and NK cells are either the same population of cells or part of largely overlapping subsets.

The activity of both NK and K cells is increased in response to lymphokines such as interferon and they can proliferate in response to IL-2. NK cells themselves can also produce lymphokines such as γ interferon, IL-1, IL-2, CSF, and BCGF.

NK and K cells just do not fit into the standard cellular categories. Perhaps they are "all purpose" cells with some of the properties of both lymphocytes and macrophages.

Macrophages

A discussion of cell-mediated immunity would not be complete without discussion of the mononuclear phagocyte, or macrophage. Macrophages develop from myeloid stem cells in the bone marrow. There, as promonocytes, they are capable of intense proliferation (driven by colony stimulating factor, CSF-1). These cells then enter the blood, where they are called *monocytes*. After several days in the blood they seed various tissues, at which time they are considered mature macrophages. They have several names and specialized functions depending on their anatomical location. For example, in the lung they are called alveolar macrophages; in the brain, microglial cells; in the liver, Kupffer cells; and in the skin, Langerhans cells. (Some believe that Langerhans cells are distinct from macrophages, since Langerhans cells lack the ability for rapid phagocytosis.)

In general, mature macrophages have a limited capacity for proliferation. Thus, the increase in number of monocytes in the blood (monocytosis) or at inflammatory sites is not due to local proliferation but rather to greater influx from the bone marrow. Macrophages are readily distinguished from lymphocytes by function, morphology, and surface markers. Unlike lymphocytes, macrophages have horseshoe-shaped nuclei, prominent cytoplasmic granules, and the ability to ingest particles and to adhere to surfaces.

While macrophages play crucial roles in constitutive defense reactions (as described in Chapter 4) their most important roles may be related to their symbiotic relationship with lymphocytes. Macrophages help lymphocytes by processing and presenting antigen and by elaborating molecules such as IL-1. Conversely, lymphocytes help macrophages through the elaboration of lymphokines.

One such group of lymphokines is known as macrophage-activating factors (MAF), the most well defined of which is interferon. This lymphokine augments a variety of macrophage functions, such as antigen presentation, phagocytic functions involving complement component C3b and antibody fragment Fc, and destruction of intracellular microbial pathogens and extracellular tumor cells.

Macrophages probably have several mechanisms for expression of cytocidal function. In addition to those discussed in Chapter 4, activated macrophages secrete tumor necrosis factor (TNF), or cachectin. TNF has several biological activities, including tumor killing and antiviral effects. Macrophages also release other antiviral substances: α and β interferons. The expression of macrophage-mediated cytotoxicity is dramatically modulated by a number of bacterial products such as lipopolysaccharide (LPS) from Gram-negative bacteria (Chapters 2 and 7). LPS dramatically increases macrophage cytolytic activity and other defensive activities.

The growth and differentiation of macrophages from bone marrow-derived stem cells is mediated by the colony stimulating factors, working in synergy with lymphocyte-derived IL-3. Other T cell-derived lymphokines are thought to be important for the accumulation of macrophages at certain inflammatory sites; macrophages are attracted to the sites of elaboration by macrophage chemotactic factor (MCF) and prevented from leaving by migration inhibitory factor (MIF). Both MIF and MAF are molecularly heterogeneous and require further definition.

Antigen-Presenting and Dendritic Cells

Cells with the ability to present antigens to lymphocytes are functionally classified as antigen-presenting cells. They include macrophages, B cells, and dendritic cells, all of which appear to have the following required functions: antigen binding, antigen processing, expression of class II MHC gene products (see "Major Histocompatibility Complex"), and elaboration of IL-1.

Dendritic cells get their name from their long slender processes and irregularly shaped nuclei. They are effective antigen-presenting cells and are thought to be important in cooperative interactions with lymphocytes. They are found in small numbers in lymphoid tissue, and their lineage is unclear. They have little or no phagocytic activity and carry neither B nor T cell receptors. They do have Fc receptors, C3 receptors, and express class II MHC proteins. (There are at least four kinds of these cells, with somewhat different locations and functional properties: lymphoid, follicular, interdigitating dentritic cells, and Langerhans cells.)

The various cells involved in immune responses are shown in Table 5.4. In summary, the relationships among lymphocytes and their products is so intricate and interdependent that it is difficult to speak of an individual cell without reference to other members of the partnership. Like the nervous system, it is difficult to appreciate the function of an individual neuron without understanding

Table 5.4
Cells of the immune system

Cell	Surface Components	Function
T lymphoctyes	T_3	Involved in cell-mediated immunity
Helper T cells (T_H)	T_4	Recognizes antigen with class II MHC; promotes differentiation of B cells and cytotoxic T cells; activates macrophages
	T cell receptor complex: α, β dimer associated with T_3	
Cytotoxic T cells (CTL)	T_8	Recognizes antigen with class I MHC; kills antigen-expressing cells.
Suppressor T cells	T_8 Receptor for antigen unknown	Downregulates the activities of other lymphocytes
B lymphocytes	Surface immunoglobulin, Fc receptors, class II MHC	Recognizes antigen directly; differentiates into antibody-producing plasma cells, antigen presentation
Large granular lymphocytes (LGL) K cells	Fc receptor	Kills antibody-coated cells (ADCC)
NK cells	Receptor for target "antigen" unknown	Kills cells with some selectivity
Macrophages	Fc receptor, C_3 receptor Some have class II MHC; can bind to wide variety of substance via surface "receptors"	Antigen presentation; phagocytosis killing of microbes and tumor cells; secretion of IL-1.
Dendritic cells	Fc receptor, C_3 receptor, class II MHC	Antigen presentation.
Mast cells (tissues) and basophils (blood)	High affinity receptors for IgE	Allergic responses; histamine release
Neutrophils	Fc receptor, C_3 receptor, C_{5a} receptor and FMLP receptor	Phagocytosis and killing of bacteria, yeast, and fungi
Eosinophils		Phagocytosis and elimination of parasites

the collective activities of networks of functioning cells and molecules. Thus, a major challenge for the future is to define the rate-limiting steps of the various cellular and molecular interactions and to understand the regulation of immune physiology.

MAJOR HISTOCOMPATIBILITY COMPLEX

The MHC consists of proteins originally discovered as being responsible for the rejection of tissue or organ grafts. Only later did it became clear that they perform a far more crucial role, that of helping T cells recognize foreign antigens. The MHC has played several tricks on immunologists. One trick was that the MHC made us focus first on issues concerning graft rejection and tissue transplantation between members of a species. While such strong transplantation antigens are indeed encoded by the MHC (thus the name), the importance of hindering organ transplantation makes no immediate sense for survival value and for the normal protective immune responses against pathogenic microbes. Another trick that immunologists are still struggling with is the association of disease susceptibility with certain alleles of MHC genes. For example, it remains a mystery why Japanese people with a particular MHC allele (HLA B27) are at a 300-fold greater risk of developing the degenerative disease ankylosing spondylitis. Other ongoing tricks include the control of mating behavior (sex) by the MHC. Mating is disfavored among mice with similar MHC genes and this may serve to increase genetic polymorphism. Interestingly, mice can smell minor differences (three amino acids) in the MHC expressed by other mice. Strange but true.

The Straight Dope on MHC

Unless we are being tricked again, we now believe that the main role of the MHC is in mediating cell-cell communication. MHC-encoded cell-surface proteins "hold" foreign antigens in the "proper" configuration for recognition by T cells and serve to "guide" the appropriate subpopulation of T cells to the appropriate antigen-expressing surface. Thus, T cells recognize foreign antigens in association with self-MHC molecules.

Chemistry and Cellular Location of MHC

There are two structurally and functionally different classes of MHC molecules, conveniently termed class I and class II. As summarized in Figure 5.12 and Table 5.5, these classes differ in genetic loci, chain structure, cell distribution, and function with different T cell subsets. In general, class I molecules direct the activity of cytotoxic T lymphocytes. Class II guide the function of helper T cells.

Mature class I molecules are composed of two subunits, a single 345-amino-acid polypeptide encoded by the MHC and a smaller protein called β_2-microglobulin. The class I chains are integral membrane proteins. Like with other members of the immunoglobulin-supergene family, their homologous three-dimensional domain structure can be inferred from sequence data. β_2-microglobulin is also homologous to immunoglobulin constant regions. Class II molecules (also called Ia molecules or Ia antigens) are structured from two noncovalently linked glycoproteins, an α chain (mol wt about 33,000) and a β chain (mol wt about 28,000). Each chain is a transmembrane protein with two external domains, again homologous to immunoglobulin (another family member; see Fig. 5.9).

Table 5.5
Properties of class I and class II MHC proteins

	Class I	Class II
Genetic loci	HLA-A, HLA-B, HLA-C	HLA-D (DP,DQ,DR)
Chain structure	45,000 mol wt glycoprotein $+ \beta_2$-microglobulin	α-chain (33,000 mol wt) β-chain (28,000 mol wt)
Cell distribution	Almost all nucleated somatic cells	B cells, some macrophages, dendritic cells, thymus epithelial cells, and activated T cells
Functions in presenting antigen to	Cytotoxic T cells	Helper T cells

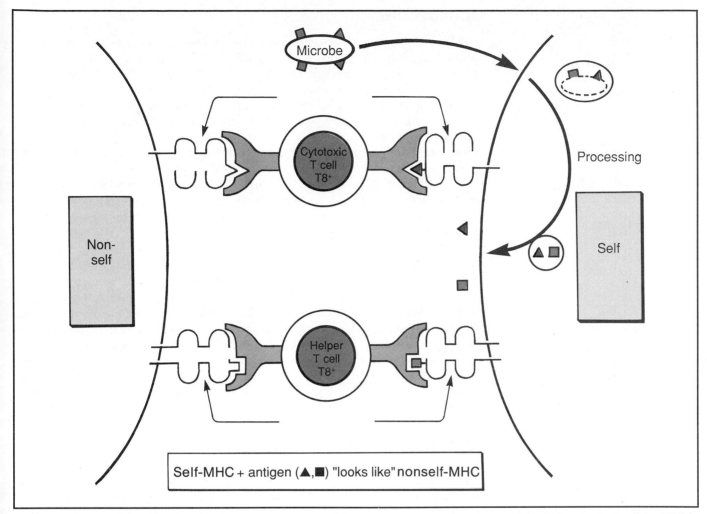

Self-MHC + antigen (▲,■) "looks like" nonself-MHC

Figure 5.12. The role of the MHC in antigen recognition by T cells. Microbial antigens are processed by cells of the self immune system and are expressed on the antigen-presenting cell surface in association with self-MHC molecules. These antigen-MHC complexes are then recognized by T cells. The powerful reaction to nonself MHC, as with transplantation reactions, is thought to be due to the molecular mimicry of [self-MHC + antigen] with nonself MHC. Thus, T cells "sense" alterations of the self-MHC, which can occur in two ways: by the binding of processed antigen or by changes due to different allelic forms of MHC molecules.

Class I gene products are expressed on almost all nucleated somatic cells. Up to 1% of total membrane proteins are class I molecules. In contrast, class II molecules normally display a more restricted cell distribution. All B cells and some macrophages, dendritic cells, thymus epithelial cells and activated T cells express class II molecules. Many cell types (including epithelial, endodermal, and parenchymal cells) can express class II under certain abnormal clinical situations such as graft rejection and autoimmune diseases.

The cellular distribution of class I and II molecules is thought to reflect differences in their function. Cytotoxic T cells patrol the tissues "looking for" abnormal cells such as potentially dangerous cancer cells or virus infected cells. The advantage of recognizing both class I and foreign antigen is that the cytotoxic T cell can focus its function on the source of the potential trouble. This cellular surveillance by cytotoxic T cells requires the global expression of class I molecules. In contrast, the more restricted expression of class II molecules directs the function of helper T cells to the cells requiring the help: B cells and macrophages. Thus, during evolution, T helper cells "learned" to recognize antigens associated with B cells and macrophages, while cytotoxic T cells "learned" to pay attention to all somatic cells expressing suspicious structures—alterations of self.

MHC Genetics

Class I molecules are encoded in humans by gene loci called HLA-A, HLA-B, and HLA-C. Class II proteins are encoded by genes in the HLA-D region, subdivided into the HLA-D region and include the DP, DQ, and DR subregions. Each subregion can encode for one or more polypeptide chains.

The MHC is the most polymorphic group of genes known in higher vertebrates. Within a species, there is a very large number of different alleles (alternate forms of the same gene). For example, hundreds of different class I glycoproteins can be expressed by a species as a whole. However, the diversity of MHC proteins is different than that of antibody molecules. MHC genes do not undergo somatic rearrangements like immunoglobulin and T cell receptor genes. Each of us can make millions of different antibody molecules, but we inherit only a single MHC allele at each locus from each parent. Thus, MHC polymorphism must have to do with survival of the species, not of the individual.

Immune response genes (Ir genes) are the class II MHC genes that control responses of helper T cells (similar control of cytotoxic T lymphocytes by class I MHC genes also occurs). Certain MHC alleles are associated with low responsiveness, while others determine high responsiveness to a particular antigenic determinant. These effects are antigen specific, such that a given individual or group of inbred animals can be a low responder to antigen X but a higher responder to antigen Y. While high responsiveness is dominant, under certain circumstances a cross between two allelic dissimilar low responders can produce a high responder. This results from the creation of a unique class II molecule by combinatorial association of an α chain from one parent with a β chain from the other (or vice versa).

How Do MHC Molecules Work?

Class II molecules can physically interact with antigen. This binding is required for effective immune responses and likely serves as the basis for immune response gene control. Class II molecules for high responders can bind processed antigen, while low-responder class II cannot bind the antigenic determinant in question.

The interaction among the T cell receptor, the MHC molecules, and the foreign processed antigen may be thought of as a ternary complex in which each component of the complex interacts with the other two proteins. The sum of the separate affinities creates a trimolecular interaction of high avidity. The interactive ability of the T cell receptor and the MHC, both members of the immunoglobulin supergene family, may be due to the common three-dimensional structure. Just as the domains of heavy and light chains of immunoglobulin interact to stabilize structure and to form a binding site for antigen, MHC molecules and the T cell receptor may interact to form a binding site for processed antigen. Similarly, the familial structure of accessory molecules such as T_4 and T_8 may contribute to cell-cell interaction through associations with class II and class I MHC molecules, respectively. Family members like to stick together (Fig. 5.9).

Additionally, the T cell receptor may be conceptualized as specific for any "new" molecular configurations created by the binding of foreign antigen to the MHC protein. As such, T cells recognize "alterations of self". Armed with this concept, the obsession of T cells with foreign MHC molecules (as in the powerful transplantation reactions) can be understood. An individual T cell clone (with presumably one type of receptor) can react with both foreign antigen in the context of self-MHC molecules and with certain foreign MHC molecules alone. As such, the T cell is "seeing" nonself in two forms: an allelic form of self—the foreign MHC, and an "altered self" caused by the bound antigenic determinant. Thus, self-MHC + antigen X "looks like" nonself-MHC (Fig. 5.12). Because of this molecular mimicry and the fact that microbial antigens make for a huge number of antigenic experiences, the strong responses to foreign MHC molecules, as with transplantation reactions, is likely due to the many clones of T cells that react with microbial antigens in the context of self-MHC molecules. This unfortunate cross reaction makes transplantation of organs impossible without carefully matching the MHC of the donor and recipient and/or using immunosuppressive treatments.

Similar considerations may also explain why increased risk of certain autoimmune diseases is associated with certain MHC alleles. Since tolerance to self-antigens is controlled by the MHC (just like responses to foreign antigens) it is possible that cross reactions between microbial antigens and self-antigens occur with certain combinations of self-MHC and foreign antigen experience. As such, the defensive reaction to microbes may result in the side effect of autoimmune disease (see "Autoimmune Diseases").

Since the MHC controls immune responsiveness, does MHC polymorphism have survival value? Consider an epidemic within a species caused by a highly pathogenic microorganism that is weakly immunogenic. This hypothetical microbe may have antigenic determinants that bind poorly to most kinds of MHC molecules. In this "Andromeda Strain" scenario, MHC polymorphism may increase the chances that at least certain members of the species would have the "right" MHC molecules (high responders) and make a protective response to the pathogen. At least some members of a species would survive.

In summary, the MHC is crucial to the understanding of T cell specificity and function. Our current understanding of these molecules is that they bind antigenic determinants and guide the activities of T cell subsets. It is possible that they are important carrier proteins that transport the antigenic determinant from the inside of the antigen-presenting cell, where processing occurs, to the cell surface, where recognition can occur. MHC molecules may also protect portions of antigens from complete degradation. Additional roles for the MHC may be as unambiguous markers for self so that the critical process of tolerance to self-tissue can be maintained. The MHC may even be a "leftover" recognition system from the days when we were swimming about in primordial ooze trying to reject the dissimilar and bind to the similar. Their possible role as cell interaction molecules in developmental processes has also not been overlooked. Clearly, all the answers about these crucial molecules are not in. Are we being tricked again? Let's hope not.

REGULATION OF THE IMMUNE RESPONSE (IMMUNOREGULATION)

The immune response to foreign antigen must be regulated. Otherwise, once it were initiated, our body would fill up with lymphocytes and antibody. There are five major ways by which the immune response is downregulated: The limited life span of effector cells, antigen removal, antibody feedback, suppressor cells, and the idiotypic network.

1. The immune response is self-limiting in that the functional life span of effector cells is short. For example, plasma cells can live only a few days.

2. Since continuous production of effector cells requires antigen, another way to downregulate the response is to remove the antigen. This is, in fact, the primary goal of the protective immune responses. The elicited antibody combines with antigen and the resulting immune complexes are more rapidly removed by the garbage collectors of the body, the cells of the reticuloendothelial system. For example, proteins are rendered nonantigenic by complete digestion to amino acids in the lysosomes of macrophages. Such antigen degradation is more efficiently performed by the activated macrophages.

3. Another fundamental mechanism is feedback regulation by antibody. Soluble antibody can cover antigenic determinants and prevent binding to B cell receptors. Also, the Fc parts of the antigen-bound antibody can cross-link Fc receptors on the B cell and thereby send an "off signal" for B cell proliferation and differentiation.

4. Suppressor cells regulate immune responses via complex regulatory cell circuits. Suppressor T cells are generated in response to increased numbers of helper T cells. Thus, helper T cells activate suppressor T cells that can ·in turn downregulate the helper T cells. This feedback pathway allows the activity of both cells to be self-regulating. The action of suppressor cells can be mediated by soluble suppressor factors that are molecularly heterogeneous.

5. The fifth and most intriguing way the immune response is regulated involves the so-called *idiotypic network* as proposed by Niels Jerne. He proposed that the antigen-combining sites of the lymphocytes' antigen receptors are themselves antigenic. He called the antigens associated with the combining sites *idiotypic determinants* (also called *idiotopes*). Because an individual idiotope is present in very small concentrations in the body, immunological tolerance to self-idiotopes is not established. Thus, immune responses can be generated to self-idiotypic determinants. Antibodies raised against these determinants can prevent the binding of antigen to the antibody. Consequently, antigen can block the interaction of the anti-idiotypic antibody with idiotypic determinants on the target antibody. These facts suggested to Jerne the network theory (Fig. 5.13).

The network theory is based on two functions of the antibody molecule: its traditional role in binding antigen and its ability to be an antigen. When animals are immunized with antigen X, the concentration of anti-X antibody is greatly increased. This increase in anti-X antibody is then perceived by the immune system, and antibody reactive to the idiotypic determinants of anti-X antibody is generated. The anti-idiotypic antibody can then elicit the production of another wave of antibody. Thus, antigen X stimulates anti-X antibody (Ab 1) that stimulate anti-(anti-X antibody) antibody (Ab 2) that stimulates anti-[anti-(anti-X antibody) antibody] antibody (Ab 3), and so on. Each response wave, however, is dampened by regulatory mechanisms.

The network theory gives the immune system the ability to regulate itself using only itself. Idiotypic determinants may be thought of as the "internal images" of the external antigens. In other words antibody against an antigen-binding site "looks like" the antigen. Since some antibodies are made even in the absence of foreign antigen a vast number of immune responses are always going on. These internal reflections, a web of opposing immune responses, are in a dynamic equilibrium (a kind of immunological "muscle tone"). What we perceive as an immune response when foreign antigen is introduced is simply the perturbation of the preexisting network and the establishment of a new position of equilibrium.

Anti-idiotypic antibody can regulate immune responses in both positive and negative ways. Anti-idiotypic antibody can be used instead of antigen to immunize

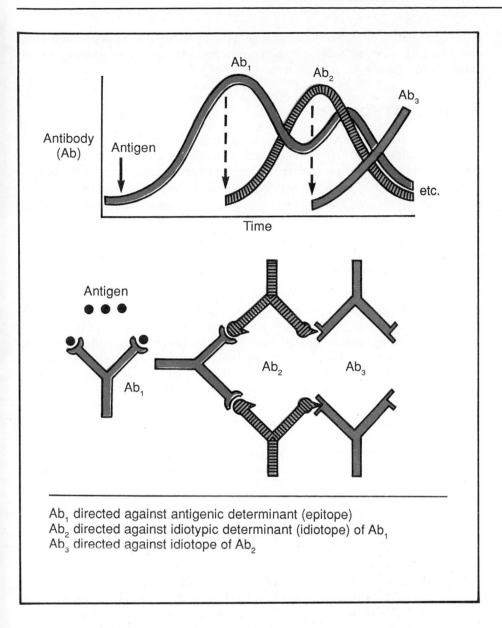

Ab₁ directed against antigenic determinant (epitope)
Ab₂ directed against idiotypic determinant (idiotope) of Ab₁
Ab₃ directed against idiotope of Ab₂

Figure 5.13. The idiotypic network. The amount of antibody produced is plotted as a function of time after injection of foreign antigen. When antibody 1 (directed against the epitope of the antigen) reaches a high concentration, it is sensed by the immune system and antibody 2 is made against the idiotope (or variable region) of antibody 1. A similar reaction then occurs with antibody 3, and so forth.

animals; its potential utility as a vaccine has been well demonstrated in mice and rats. Inhibition, rather than activation, is noted when the anti-idiotypic antibody is of a class that can bind complement and Fc receptors. In this case it is likely that the anti-idiotypic antibody suppresses responses by elimination of the clones of lymphocytes that express the idiotypic determinant.

Using the ability of anti-idiotypic antibody to mimic antigen, it is also possible to generate antibody to a cell constituent that is difficult to purify. For example, it is possible to make antibodies to a hormone receptor (e.g., the acetylcholine receptor) without ever using the receptor as antigen. Because both hormone receptor and the antihormone antibody can bind to the hormone, antibody raised against the antihormone antibody can bind the hormone receptor. These observations illustrate the useful tricks that can be used to identify structures by knowing only their biological activity.

It's all a matter of molecular complementarity. "Nature the idiotypic network, she shows us only surfaces, but she's a million fathoms receptors deep," said Ralph Waldo Emerson.

IMMUNOPATHOLOGY

Immunopathology refers to disease caused by inappropriate immune responses. Immune responses that fail to distinguish self from nonself may result in auto-immune diseases, responses that are exaggerated or inappropriate for protective function are called hypersensitivity reactions, and defects in defense reactions manifested by recurring infections are known as immunodeficiency diseases. Thus, immune responses that are misdirected, too strong, or too weak can result in pathology.

Autoimmune Diseases

Autoimmune reactions are those directed against the body's own tissues, cells, or molecules. These occur when the regulatory events involved in immunological tolerance are subverted or otherwise malfunction. Self-antigens or autoantigens, the targets of autoimmune reactions, may be intracellular components, receptors, cell membrane components, extracellular components, plasma proteins, or hormones. Depending on the autoantigen, the disease may be organ specific (e.g., Graves' disease with the primary site in the thyroid gland) or non-organ-specific (e.g., systemic lupus erythematosus with symptoms affecting many systems). Both antibody and T cell responses to self-antigens may cause disease. Such diseases are catalogued in Table 5.6.

Tissue damage by the immune response may be caused by the sharing of antigenic determinants between host and parasite. Given the biological relationships of hosts and parasites it is not surprising that microorganisms and vertebrates sometimes share antigenic determinants. However, it is not known how such determinants elicit immune response, since they should be recognized by the body as self and tolerance to such antigens should be established.

Autoimmune reactions have been implicated in two puzzling disorders that follow infections by certain streptococci. Rheumatic fever and glomerulonephritis are uncommon but severe sequels of otherwise mundane "strep throats". We know that antigens in the cell walls of the infecting streptococci cross react with components of heart muscle or kidney glomeruli and that antibodies reactive with self-tissues are present in such patients. However, the precise role of autoimmune reactions in these diseases is still unclear.

Since immunological tolerance to self-components hidden from the immune system cannot be established, immune responses to self-antigens occur when such sequestered antigens are released or abnormally expressed. Tissue and cellular damage may result in the release of antigenic intracellular molecules. The resulting immune reactions may cause continued cellular trauma, the further release of sequestered antigens, and perpetuation of the inflammatory process. Self-components present in organs such as the central nervous system (which lack conventional lymphatics and thus, frequent contact with lymphocytes) may elicit strong immune responses in an unusual context. For example, in experimental animals, injection of self-CNS tissue mixed with an adjuvant may cause a demyelinating encephalitis that resembles the human disease multiple sclerosis. It is also thought that the abnormal expression of class II MHC gene products on cells

Table 5.6
Antigens in autoimmune diseases[a]

Disease	Antigen Type[b]					
	A	B	C	D	E	F
Systemic lupus erythematosus	+		+		+	
Sjögren's syndrome	+				+	
Scleroderma	+					
Polymyositis	+		+			
Chronic active hepatitis	+				+	
Mixed connective tissue disease	+					
Insulin-dependent diabetes	+	+				+
Primary biliary cirrhosis	+					
Pernicious anemia	+					+
Autoimmune thyroiditis	+	+				+
Idiopathic Addison's disease	+					
Vitiligo	+					
Gluten-sensitive enteropathy	+					
Chronic active hepatitis	+					
Graves' disease	+	+				
Myasthenia gravis		+				
Autoimmune hemolytic anemia			+			
Autoimmune neutropenia			+			
Idiopathic thrombocytopenia purpura			+			
Rheumatoid arthritis			+		+	
Cirrhosis			+			
Multiple sclerosis			+			
Pemphigus vulgaris			+	+		
Autoimmune infertility			+			
Goodpasture's disease				+		
Bullous pemphigoid				+		
Discoid lupus				+		
Dense deposit disease					+	

[a] Modified from Smith HPR, Steinberg AD. Autoimmunity—a perspective. *Annu Rev Immunol* 1: 175–210, 1982.
[b] A, intracellular. B, receptors. C, cell membrane components. D, extracellular. E, plasma proteins. F, hormones.

other than the antigen-presenting B cells and macrophages may permit effective local immune reactions to self-antigens on these cells.

Autoimmune disease may also result from alterations of self-components by environmental agents. For example, there is a class of autoimmune hemolytic anemias that are known to be drug induced. The drug may bind to red cells and permit immune responses to the drug-associated self-components. Conceivably,

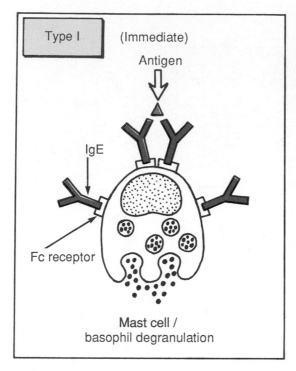

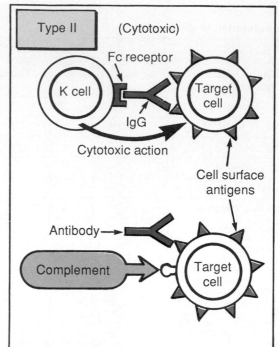

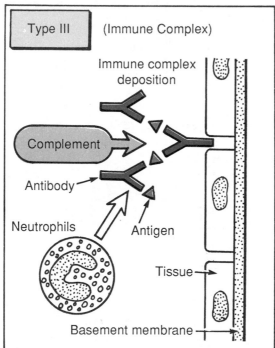

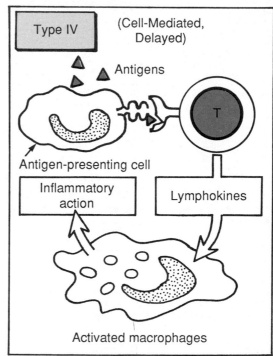

Figure 5.14. Hypersensitivity reactions. Hypersensitivity reactions are secondary responses to antigen that occur in an exaggerated or inappropriate form. These have been classified by Gell and Coombs into four major types: Types I, II, and III are antibody mediated, while type IV is cell mediated. Serious pathology can result from these reactions.

alterations of self-components by interactions with microbial products may also contribute to autoimmune reactions. Additionally, there are many microbial agents that are able to polyclonally activate lymphocytes and thus possibly bypass the normal regulatory pathways that maintain tolerance to self.

Finally, it is important to note that self-reactivity may occur in the absence of pathology. The idiotypic network, for example, is a web of responses to self-idiotopes. Also, the association of a particular disease with autoimmune reactions does not necessarily imply a direct cause-and-effect relationship. An autoreaction may be secondary to the pathological changes caused by another mechanism.

Hypersensitivity Reactions

The term hypersensitivity is used for immune responses that occur in an exaggerated or inappropriate manner. These reactions are also called *allergic reactions* and the antigens involved are called *allergens*. None of the many clinical manifestations of hypersensitivity are pleasant.

As the name implies, hypersensitivity reactions occur in individuals who have been previously sensitized to the antigen; they are secondary responses. They have been classified by Gell and Coombs into four major types according to the speed of the reaction and the nature of the immunological reactions involved. While they are grouped separately, in reality they rarely, if ever, occur in complete isolation from each other. Nonetheless, they are useful conceptual frameworks for review of immune reactions (Fig. 5.14). Types I, II, and III are all antibody mediated; type IV is cell mediated.

Type I (Immediate Hypersensitivity)

These occur within minutes of exposure to antigen. The cross linking of mast cell–bound IgE by the allergen triggers the release of vasoactive amines which produce inflammation. It is not known why some antigens elicit IgE production and cause such responses. While it is not entirely clear why only certain individuals suffer from these reactions, genetic control by class II MHC genes plays a significant role. Examples include allergic asthma, hay fever, urticaria, and anaphylactic reactions to insect venom.

Type II (Cytotoxic Hypersensitivity)

Antibody binding to cell surface antigens is followed by antibody-dependent cell-mediated cytotoxicity by K cells, or complement-mediated lysis. Examples of type II diseases include transfusion reactions, hemolytic disease of the newborn, and certain drug allergies resulting in hemolytic anemia. Tissues can also be damaged by cytotoxic T lymphocytes, but these will be discussed below as a form of cell-mediated hypersensitivity.

Type III (Immune Complex-Mediated Hypersensitivity)

This kind of immunopathological damage is caused by the activation of complement by immune complexes (via the classical pathway) and the mobilization of white blood cells, especially neutrophilis. Antigens may be soluble or associated with small particles such as viruses. The antigen-antibody complex activates the complement pathway and the resulting complement fragments (C3a,

C5a; see Chapter 4) causes an inflammatory response. The resulting vascular permeability changes and the influx of neutrophils (and later macrophages) elicits symptoms such as fever, skin rash, and arthritis. Thus, the deposition of antigen-antibody complexes in certain tissues can elicit inflammatory reactions that result in damage and disruption of normal organ function. The site of deposition of immune complexes dictates the pathology observed. Why complexes show affinity for particular tissues (kidney, joints, etc.) is not clear, but certain hemodynamic factors as well as the size of the immune complexes are thought to be critical. A relatively high or persistent antigen load characterizes these conditions. Hypersensitivity reactions may result from persistent infection with certain bacteria (streptococcal infections), viruses (hepatitis B), parasites (the *Plasmodium* agents of malaria), or worms (filariae, the agents of elephantiasis). Examples of type III reactions include glomerulonephritis, alveolitis, and certain antoimmune diseases.

Type IV (Cell-Mediated Reaction or Delayed Type Hypersensitivity)

This is so named because symptoms appear at least 24 to 48 hours after antigen exposure. It is caused by the activation of T cells, the release of lymphokines and the subsequent influx of macrophages to the site. Allergic contact dermatitis (e.g., poison ivy) and the skin test for exposure to tubercle bacilli, called the tuberculin test, are examples of DTH reactions.

Cell-mediated hypersensitivity is often characteristic of infections by intracellular slow growing pathogens, typified by the tubercle bacilli and fungi by *Histoplasma capsulatum*, the agent of histoplasmosis. Circulating antibodies here play a minor role because the organisms are shielded from them in their intracellular location. Chronic inflammations are usually manifestations of cell-mediated immune reactions. The activation of T cells, the release of lymphokines and the subsequent influx of macrophages to the site of antigen may result in a lesion called the *granuloma*. This is a densely packed collection of macrophages that fuses to produce characteristic giant cells, surrounded by epithelioid cells and lymphocytes. This is usually a slow progressing but nonetheless active lesion, since the host attempts to contain the infection but the microorganisms continue to grow intracellularly at slow rates. Whether the lesion progresses or resolves depends on many factors, principally the rate of release of antigens from the organism.

A prototype of this kind of immunological industry is the disease leprosy. It is caused by an organism called *Mycobacterium leprae*, a relative of the tubercle bacillus. These organisms survive inside monocytes, probably by virtue of possessing a thick layer of wax (see Chapters 2 and 22). In one form of the disease, lepromatous leprosy, the organisms elicit the production of granulomas that damage sensory nerves. This results in anesthesia of fingers or whole limbs. Because the patient has little feeling in the affected areas, these become subject to repeated trauma and secondary infection by bacteria. This cycle of injury and repair leads to some of the deformities characteristic of untreated cases of the disease.

While T_4-expressing T cells are most noted for their release of lymphokines and elicitation of DTH reactions, T_8-bearing T cells can also release lymphokines and participate in cell-mediated immunity. The mouse analogues of T_8 (CD8)$^+$ cells have been shown to play a protective role in cutaneous leishmaniasis (leishmanias are protozoan parasites) and in immunity to certain intracellular bacteria. Whether

Table 5.7
Classification of congenital immunodeficiency disorders according to function affected[a]

Classification	Diseases
Antibody (B cell) immunodeficiency diseases	X-linked (congenital) hypogammaglobulinemia Transient hypogammaglobulinemia of infancy Common, variable, unclassifiable immunodeficiency (acquired hypogammaglobulinemia) Immunodeficiency with hyper-IgM Selective IgA deficiency Selective IgM deficiency Selective deficiency of IgG subclasses Secondary B cell immunodeficiency associated with drugs, protein-losing states B cell immunodeficiency associated with 5'-nucleotidase deficiency
Cellular (T cell) immunodeficiency diseases	Congenital thymic aplasia (DiGeorge syndrome) Chronic mucocutaneous candidiasis (with or without endocrinopathy) T cell deficiency associated with purine nucleoside phosphorylase deficiency
Combined antibody-mediated (B cell) and cell-mediated (T cell) diseases	Severe combined immunodeficiency disease (autosomal recessive, X-linked, sporadic) Cellular immunodeficiency with abnormal immunoglobulin synthesis (Nezelof's syndrome) Immunodeficiency with ataxia-telangiectasia Immunodeficiency with eczema and thrombocytopenia (Wiskott-Aldrich syndrome) Immunodeficiency with thymoma Immunodeficiency with short-limbed dwarfism Immunodeficiency with adenosine deaminase deficiency Episodic lymphopenia with lymphotoxin GVH disease
Phagocytic dysfunction	Chronic granulomatous disease Glucose-6-phosphate dehydrogenase deficiency Myeloperoxidase deficiency Chédiak-Higashi syndrome Job's syndrome Tuftsin deficiency "Lazy leukocyte syndrome" Elevated IgE, defective chemotaxis, eczema, and recurrent infections
Complement abnormalities and immunodeficiency diseases	C1q, C1r, and C1s deficiency C2 deficiency C3 deficiency (type I, type II) C4 deficiency C5 dysfunction, C5 deficiency C6 deficiency C7 deficiency C8 deficiency C9 deficiency

[a] From Amman AJ, Fudenberg HH: Immunodeficiency diseases. In Stites DP et al. (eds): *Basic and Clinical Immunology*, ed 4. Los Altos, CA, Lange Medical Publications, 1982, pp. 395–429.

these effects are due to lymphokine elaboration or by the direct cytotoxic effector function of such cells is unclear.

The tissue-damaging effects of cytotoxic T lymphocytes have been noted in the immunopathology of persistent viral infection. Infection of mice with lymphocytic choriomeningitis virus (LCMV) is a good example. LCMV is an arenavirus that is relatively noncytopathic. When injected into neonatal mice a persistent infection is produced and the mice, even as adults, remain healthy. In contrast, the injection of adult mice with the virus causes a rapid death from meningochoroidoencephalitis. However, death is prevented in adult mice by immunosuppression with x-irradiation, thymectomy, or pharmacological means. Thus, it is the immune response to the virus (cytotoxic T lymphocytes) rather than the virus itself that causes death. Neonatal mice are not killed by the virus because they are immunoincompetent and presumably develop tolerance to viral antigens as in the process of tolerance to self antigens. Similar mechanisms may be involved in the chronic infection of humans with measles virus, which can cause a severe degenerative disease and death due to subacute sclerosing panencephalitis (SSPE). It is believed that the immunopathology associated with a variety of persistent virus infections may be due at least in part to the action of cytotoxic T lymphocytes and other immunological mechanisms (see Chapters 29 and 32).

It is clear that persistent immune responses by both antibody and T lymphocytes may have severe immunopathological results.

Immunodeficiencies

Perhaps the most serious forms of pathology involving the immune system result from the loss of immune function. Immunodeficiency diseases may be acquired or congenital. Congenital immunodeficiencies are tragic "experiments of nature" that have proven to be important tools for defining the differentiation pathways of lymphocytes described above. The functions influenced by these defects are tabulated in Table 5.7. Of the acquired immunodeficiencies, the most worrisome example is, of course, the acquired immunodeficiency syndrome, or AIDS. In AIDS, the virus binds to the T_4 protein of helper T cells and destroys them. The reduction in the number of T_{4+} helper cells produces a profound immunosuppression that leads to severe infections with commensal and normally avirulent microorganisms. *Pneumocystis carinii* pneumonia, herpes simplex infections, candidiasis, and disseminated Kaposi's sarcoma are some of the more common manifestation of AIDS. (See Chapter 33 for further discussion of AIDS and its opportunistic diseases.) Thus, the AIDS virus has developed an ingenious and nefarious strategy for survival: infection and destruction of the very cells that could help fight back. AIDS patients succumb not to HIV infection itself, but rather to overwhelming opportunistic infections. A better understanding of the immune system and of the invading AIDS virus offers hope for the future.

SUMMARY

Our immune system faces three major challenges in maintaining our health: (a) How to distinguish an apparently infinite array of foreign antigens and ensure that a specific response is made even when antigen is present in small concentrations; (b) how to ensure that the response is appropriate to the foreign agent so that the foreign agent is eliminated; and (c) how to avoid responding to self-antigens and damaging self. The immune system meets these challenges with specific acquired immune responses. Such responses have been described as a "microcosm of evolution operating on somatic cells".

The first challenge is met by generating millions of different antigen receptors. These receptors are distributed among millions of different lymphocyte clones. The diversity created by genetic recombination and mutation are not unlike the mechanisms that generated diversity during the evolution of various species. A kind of survival-of-the-fittest process operates with lymphocytes in that those lymphocytes fit for protective defense reactions are encouraged to survive. Lymphocytes respond to antigens in the individual's environment and are stimulated to proliferate and differentiate into long-lived memory cells by a process of clonal selection. The symbiotic relationships among lymphocytes and macrophages ensure that efficient responses are made to even small amounts of antigen.

The second problem of how to ensure that the response is appropriate to the invading foreign agent is solved, at least in part, by the division of labor among the lymphocytes, and may be mediated by the guiding function of the MHC glycoproteins. B cells make various classes of antibody, and cell-mediated responses are mediated by separate subclasses of T lymphocytes. It is thought, but is far from proven, that the MHC channels antigens into pathways for recognition by either helper or cytotoxic T cells. Also, the various antibody isotypes may help to ensure that appropriate responses are made in the proper places and sequences. The amplification of constitutive defense reactions by products of the specific acquired immune responses, (e.g., opsonization with antibody and macrophage activation by lymphokines) makes for efficient elimination of the foreign agent.

The third challenge of preventing damage to self is met by a precise discrimination between self and nonself through the processes of immunological tolerance and immunoregulation. During development lymphocytes with receptors specific for self-components are downregulated, and, perhaps akin to evolutionary pressures, T lymphocytes reactive to self may be eliminated in the thymus. Responses to foreign agents must also be delicately controlled by feedback mechanisms to prevent damage to our tissues. When this immunoregulation is imprecise we have autoimmune disease and hypersensitivity reactions with disastrous consequences to our health.

Thus, the double-edged sword of immune defense is delicately balanced to fight the foreign and protect the self by remarkable abilities for specific recognition and precise regulation.

CODA—THE INTEGRATION OF DEFENSE MECHANISMS

As previously discussed (in Chapter 4 and this one) higher animals have a multitude of means to discriminate self from nonself and to maintain the integrity and health of the individual. Nature has provided a system with many layers of defensive fail-safe mechanisms. The advantages of this should be obvious: Failure at any one level can often be compensated by success at another. These "layered" defense reactions differ in terms of speed, specificity, and strength, but they are interactive and cooperative.

More primitive defense reactions, such as the toxins and enzymes of procaryotic organisms or the phagocytic cells of invertebrates, were not discarded during the development of the more sophisticated specific acquired immune responses of mammals. Instead, the new mechanisms of defense were layered on top of the older ones. And, most important, the specific induced defenses evolved to interact bidirectionally with the more primitive innate or constitutive defense reactions, so that both types of reactions would work best in concert. To prevent infectious disease, humans may avoid contact with microbes, prevent their entry (keep them on the epithelial side), or destroy them if they breach the defensive barriers. We will review briefly the defense reactions against a microbe once it has gained entry. Multiple defense reactions will be emphasized.

The Gauntlet of the Body's Defenses

Consider a microbe running the gauntlet of immune defenses in a human being. There are three phases in these defenses. In the first stage, the microbe is sensed by the host as foreign and innate defense reactions are expressed. In the second stage, the foreign entity is processed by cells and the specific immune response is initiated. In the third phase, the innate defense reactions interact with the induced defense reactions, resulting in the efficient elimination of the invading microbe. The importance of each of these stages in host defense varies with the invading organisms and their principal pathogenic mechanisms (Table 5.8).

Stage I. Innate (Constitutive) Sensing

Important reactions in the first or "sensing" stage involve the functions of complement, interleukins, interferons, phagocytes, killer cells, and other elements of the inflammatory response. Through random collisions and ill-defined attachment

Table 5.8
The relative importance of mediators of antimicrobial defense to various pathogens

immunity, Monocytes/ Macrophages	Neutrophils	Complement	Antibody	Cell-Mediated immunity, Monocytes/ Macrophages
BACTERIA Gram-positive cocci	+++	++		+++
Enterobacteriaceae	+++	+	+	
Pseudomonas	+++	+	+	
Haemophilus influenzae	+	+	+++	
Salmonella (systemic infections)				+++
Listeria monocytogenes				+++
Mycobacterium tuberculosis				+++
FUNGI Candida sp.				
Systemic	++			
Mucocutaneous				+++
Aspergillus sp.	+++			
Cryptococcus neoformans			+++	
Histoplasma capsulatum			+++	
VIRUSES		+	+++	

mechanisms, phagocytes have the intrinsic ability to ingest and destroy microbes. These are amplified by activation of complement and by white blood cell chemotaxis. Important events include the recruitment of phagocytes, especially the faster neutrophils, in response to microbial products such as the bacterial chemotaxin formyl-met-leu-phe (Chapter 4). If the alternative pathway of complement is activated, the movement of phagocytes toward the microbe is aided by C5a. Complement activation may also generate the opsonin C3b, which promotes phagocytosis of the microbe as well as the membrane attack complex, which can directly lyse certain bacteria and viruses.

The concerted action of these cells and molecules may result in death and digestion of microbes. If a microbe fails to negotiate this first level of the gauntlet, no further action is required by the immune system. In fact, specific lymphocyte responses are not even elicited. However, if destruction is incomplete, the short-lived neutrophils begin to disintegrate and the later-arriving macrophages must come into play. Macrophages play important roles as garbage collectors and domestic engineers, as they arrive to digest debris and remaining microbes. Macrophages also play perhaps an even more important role as liaison between phagocytes and lymphocytes in initiating the next stage of immune defense.

Stage II. Specific Immune Responses

The second stage of defense is the generation of specific immune responses (this stage is also called the afferent immune response). Macrophages process microbial antigens and express them on their cell surface in association with class II MHC gene products. In this form, antigens may be recognized by helper or inducer T lymphocytes (T_4/CD4$^+$). Virus infected cells that have escaped innate defenses express viral antigens on the surface in association with class I MHC gene products. These antigen-MHC complexes are recognizable by the precursors of cytotoxic T lymphocytes (T_8/CD8$^+$). Still other microbial antigens may be relatively intact and able to interact directly with the receptors on B lymphocytes.

The engagement of antigen specific receptors and the subsequent cellular and molecular interactions lead to proliferation and differentiation of lymphocytes. This process of clonal selection and memory cell production accounts for specific acquired immunity. Effector cells (e.g., plasma cells and cytotoxic T cells) are also generated in this process. Such cells and/or their products may then mediate several important functions in the third and final stage of immune defenses; the specific, amplified, efferent phase.

Stage III. The Specific and Amplified Efferent Phase

The third stage involves the concerted action and cooperation of both innate and specific acquired immune responses. In this stage, the host uses every means available to eliminate the invader: the ultimate and bloodiest battle in the war. Thus, this stage is not just a simple addition or layering of the specific induced defenses over the innate defenses, but also the synergistic effect of both. For example, antibody helps activate complement more efficiently via the classical pathway. In turn, complement activation makes for more efficient killing of microbes and accelerates chemotaxis and opsonization by phagocytes. Antibodies neutralize toxins that impair the function of leukocytes and prevent the invasion of new microbes. Antibodies also enhance and direct the function of the large granular lymphocytes (NK cells and the K cells) to perform antibody-dependent cell-mediated cytotoxicity (ADCC).

In this stage, functions and products of T lymphocytes also play key roles in amplifying innate defense reactions. Notably, macrophage activating factors elaborated by T cells dramatically improve the phagocytic killing mechanisms. For example, lymphokines increase the expression of macrophage Fc receptors, which in turn promotes the function of antibody as an opsonin. Macrophage activation by T lymphocyte lymphokines is especially important in the elimination of intracellular pathogens that have managed to escape initial destruction and live inside macrophages. Lymphokines released by T cells (e.g., γ-interferon) also increase the expression of MHC molecules on macrophages and other cells and thus augment antigen presentation.

These are just a few of the examples by which products of induced defenses interact with innate defense mechanisms during the elimination of invading microbes. If this array of cooperative defenses was not impressive enough, there is an even more intelligent strategy for defense. Even after the successful resolution of the infection, the immune system quietly waits, anticipating the next encounter with the microbe. Immunological memory ensures that the next response to the microbe will be even stronger and faster and more interactive with innate defense reactions.

SUGGESTED READINGS

Clark WR: *The Experimental Foundations of Modern Immunology.* New York, John Wiley & Sons, 1980.
Golub ES: *Immunology. A Synthesis.* Sunderland, MA, Sinauer Assoc., 1977.
Klein J: *Immunology. The Science of Self-Nonself Discrimination.* New York, John Wiley & Sons, 1982.
Roitt I, Brostaff J, Male D: *Immunology.* St. Louis, C.V. Mosby, 1985.
Williams AE: A year in the life of the immunoglobulin superfamily. *Immunol Today* 8:296–303, 1987

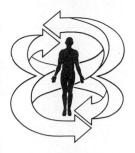

Microbial Subversion of Host Defenses

6

A. Plaut

When a microorganism causes an infectious disease it creates a hostile environment for itself. The host responds by mobilizing defenses that impair the organism's growth and threaten its existence. In most cases the host prevails, but the existence of infectious diseases demonstrates that this is not always true and that microorganisms can thwart or evade the host defenses. The microbial countermeasures involved should be considered to be virulence factors, even though they do not contribute directly to tissue damage. Generally speaking, each species of infectious agents develops an individual spectrum of survival strategies. For every successful infection by a microorganism we must ask, How does it survive in its particular location of the body? We know some of the answers, but by no means all.

Host defenses do not operate in isolation but are interrelated. The strategies that microorganisms use to subvert them are correspondingly complex and difficult to classify. We will divide these strategies into those directed against constitutive defenses, *complement* and *phagocytosis*, and against induced defenses, *humoral* and *cellular immunity*. Microorganisms invading a host that has not encountered them previously will meet these defenses in this order.

Many microbial countermeasures are known from in vitro experimental situations and it is not always possible to determine if they also operate in human disease. This is a subject of intensive research that has clear therapeutic and prophylactic implications. Experimental approaches used in such investigations are presented in Chapter 8.

Table 6.1
Some bacterial anticomplement strategies

Mask activating substances
   Coating with capsule (e.g., staphylococci)
   Coating with IgA antibodies (e.g., meningococci)
Appropriate inhibitor of activation to their surface (component H) (e.g., *E. coli*, group B streptococci)
Cover up target of membrane attack complex (e.g., *E. coli*, salmonellae)
Inactivate complement chemotaxin C5a (e.g., *Pseudomonas aeruginosa*)

DEFENDING AGAINST COMPLEMENT

The most effective way to protect against the antimicrobial components of complement is to prevent their activation. Bacteria do this in several ways (Table 6.1). One is by masking surface components that activate by the alternative pathway. For example, the cell wall murein of *Staphylococcus aureus* is a good complement activator, but is overlaid by a capsule that prevents this activity. Group B streptococci and strains of *Escherichia coli* that possess capsules rich in sialic acid also inhibit activation by the alternative pathway.

Meningococci have another mechanism to avoid activation of complement. When these organisms enter the blood they become coated with *circulating IgA antibodies*, a class of immunoglobulins that do not activate the complement cascade. Furthermore, this binding prevents other kinds of antibodies (capable of setting off complement activation by the classical pathway) from reaching the surface of the organisms. Although this seemingly protective role of IgA sounds superficially like host stupidity, it more likely reveals our ignorance of the role of the IgA class of immunoglobulins.

Some Gram negatives, such as *Salmonella* or *E. coli*, resist the action of complement by yet another mechanism. They do not prevent formation of the complement membrane attack complex, but rather, hinder access to its target, the bacterial outer membrane. "Smooth" strains, which have a long O antigen polysaccharide chain, do not allow access of the membrane attack complex to their cell surface, while "rough" mutants, which have little or no O antigen are readily killed by it. This correlates well with pathogenicity, since smooth strains tend to be virulent, whereas rough strains are not.

There is a price to pay for having capsules and other protective surface structures: Most of them are highly antigenic and in time elicit the production of anticapsular antibodies that enable the activation of complement by the classical pathway. Notice that these organisms defend themselves better against the more immediate host defense, activation of complement by the alternative pathway, than against later events, the formation of antibodies.

SUBVERTING PHAGOCYTOSIS

The very large number of ways microorganisms avoid being killed by phagocytes highlights the central role of phagocytosis in the evolution of parasitism and infection. The host attempts to overcome these microbial countermeasures, and these efforts are answered by yet other microbial tactics. A point must be made at the outset: Being taken up by a cell is not necessarily a bad thing from the microbe's point of view. A powerful counterdefensive strategy is for microor-

Table 6.2
Microbial strategies to evade phagocyte function[a]

Antiphagocyte Activity	Mechanism	Examples
Murder	Membrane lysis	Streptococci (streptolysin O) *Pseudomonas* (exotoxin A) *Staphylococcus aureus* (α-toxin)
Diversion (to nonproductive use)	Activate complement C5a, leucoaggregation, pulmonary sequestration	Streptococci Gram-negative enterics
Humiliation	Release of adenylate cyclase leading to high cAMP levels. All functions depressed	*Bordetella pertussis* (toxin)
Paralysis	Make cells unresponsive to chemotactic factors; induce inhibitors of migration; inactivate chemotaxins (C5a)	Capnocytophaga Tubercle bacilli Leprosy bacilli Leprosy bacilli *Pseudomonas* (elastase)
"Playing hard to get"	Slimy capsule on organisms	*Pneumococcus* *Meningococcus* *Haemophilus influenzae* *Bacteroides fragilis* Many others
	M protein Pili	Group A streptococci Gonococci
Inhibit phagosome-lysosome fusion	Sulfatides?	Tubercle bacilli Toxoplasma
Indifference (resist lysosomal enzymes)	?	*Salmonella typhimurium* *Mycobacteria* sp. *Leishmania* sp.
Escape from phagosomes	Phospholipase? ?	Rickettsiae Influenza viruses
Inhibit oxidative killing	Inhibit respiratory burst Catalase breaks down H_2O_2	Virulent salmonellae *Legionella pneumophila* *Listeria monocytogenes* *Staphylococcus aureus*

[a] From Dr. M. Klempner, unpublished data.

ganisms to grow within nonphagocytic host cells, where they are shielded from antibodies or certain antimicrobial drugs.

Here we will discuss a few examples of strategies used by microorganisms to withstand the killing power of phagocytic cells. Various aspects of phagocytosis are affected, from the arrival of the phagocytes at the scene to the killing powers of phagocytic cells (Table 6.2.).

Inhibiting Phagocyte Recruitment

We have already seen that some microorganisms avoid the activation of complement; in so doing, they prevent the secondary release of chemotaxins for neutrophils, thus reducing the chance of encountering these cells. Other organisms directly inhibit neutrophil motility and chemotaxis, which are essential elements for a successful phagocytic response. An example is the agent of whooping cough, *Bordetella pertussis*, which produces a toxin that increases the neutrophil level of cyclic AMP (Chapter 20). This leads to paralysis instead of chemotaxis of these highly motile cells towards bacteria. Another pertussis toxin impairs the migration of monocytes.

Microbial Killing of Phagocytes

Many pathogenic bacteria produce exotoxins called *leukocidins* that kill neutrophils and macrophages. These soluble products work at a distance and thus may protect bacteria before the phagocytes come near them. In many cases, however, microbes kill after they are ingested—which means that the phagocyte commits suicide by carrying out phagocytosis. Examples of leukocidins are discussed in detail in the chapter on bacterial toxins (Chapter 7). For now, you should know that typical leukocidin producers are highly invasive bacteria, such as pseudomonas, staphylococci, group A streptococci, and the clostridia that cause gas gangrene.

Escaping Ingestion

The preeminent microbial counterdefense to phagocytosis is its capsule. One of the more captivating visual experiences in microbiology is to watch a preparation of live neutrophils and encapsulated pneumococci under the microscope: Every time a neutrophil attempts to embrace a pneumococcus, the slimy bacterium squeezes away with what looks like total indifference. Repeated attempts are no more successful; eventually it becomes difficult not to share the frustration of the neutrophil.

The picture changes when a small amount of specific antiserum is added: Now the neutrophils have no trouble engulfing the opsonized pneumococci. Anticapsular antibodies thus provide protective immunity against infection by encapsulated bacteria. However, bacteria have evolved measures to counter opsonization by either complement components or by specific antibodies. Any mechanism that inhibits activation of complement (see "Inhibiting Phagocyte Recruitment"), or synthesis or activity of antibodies will reduce the probability of opsonization.

Staphylococci, streptococci, and probably other bacteria have evolved a mechanism to reduce opsonization even when antibodies are present: They make a surface component, *protein A*, that binds to IgG molecules by the "wrong" end, the Fc portion. These antibodies cannot act as opsonins because they cannot bind to the Fc receptors on phagocytic cells, not to mention that their Fab region is "waving in the breeze". It is not known to what extent this antiphagocytic mechanism plays a role in actual infections.

How Microorganisms Survive Inside Phagocytes

Microorganisms have many ways to survive once they are taken up by host cells. These include entry into the cytoplasm (a privileged site), inhibiting fusion of lysosomes with the phagosomes, and resisting the oxidative or nonoxidative killing mechanisms of white blood cells. These mechanisms are discussed in detail below.

Escaping into the Cytoplasm

The trypanosomes of Chagas' disease or the rickettsiae of Rocky Mountain spotted fever cross the membrane of the phagocytic vesicle, the *phagosome*, and enter into the cytoplasm itself. Since lysosomes do not release their contents in the cytoplasm, the microorganisms are now protected from lysosomal enzymes. How the organisms exit the phagosome is not known with certainty, although rickettsiae possess a surface-bound phospholipase that may be responsible for weakening the phagosomal membrane.

Inhibiting the Fusion of Lysosomes with Phagosomes

When lysosomes fuse with phagosomes, they release powerful microbicidal enzymes (Chapter 4). Inhibiting this fusion is a clear benefit to intraphagosomal microorganisms. Several examples of this mode of resistance are the bacteria that cause tuberculosis, psittacosis, or Legionnaires' disease. How do they do it? In the case of the tubercle bacilli, this inhibition seems to be induced by complex glycolipids of the organisms called the *sulfatides*, although this point is still under study. Clearly, inhibition of fusion must be due to a modification of the membrane of the phagosome. The microorganisms must contribute to this modification using compounds they secrete or that are present on their surface.

Resisting Lysosomal Enzymes

Some microorganisms are innately resistant to the lysosomal enzymes and survive in the so-called phagolysosome, the vesicle formed by fusion of the lysosomes with the phagosomes. Examples are protozoa called *Leishmania*, which cause several severe tropical diseases. Resistance of leishmanias to lysosomal enzymes may be due to resistant cell surfaces and, in addition, to the excretion of enzyme inhibitors. Note that the pH of the phagolysosome may be as low as 4, which means that *Leishmania* can thrive in what one might regard as an extreme environment.

Inhibiting the Phagocytes' Oxidative Pathway

There are several ways in which microorganisms inhibit the phagocytes' oxidative pathway: The bacillus of Legionnaires' disease inhibits the hexose-monophosphate shunt and oxygen consumption in neutrophils, thus reducing the respiratory burst used by these cells for killing engulfed microorganisms. Staphylococci produce a powerful catalase that breaks down the hydrogen peroxide necessary for oxidative killing.

The Effect of Antibodies

Antibodies against the attacking organisms sometimes help dismantle these survival mechanisms. For instance, rickettsiae that are coated with antibodies lose their capacity to pass through the phagosome membrane; lysosomes will eventually fuse with the phagosomes, leading to the destruction of these organisms. Likewise, antibodies against *Legionella*, the agents of Legionnaires' disease, prevent the organisms from inhibiting the phagolysosomal fusion. Note that in these cases antibodies do not inhibit entry of the microorganisms into cells, but rather interfere with subsequent specific steps.

SUBVERTING THE IMMUNE RESPONSES

Immunosuppression

Some infections result in suppression of the immune responses. What is the outcome of the direct assault on the immunologic apparatus of the host by an invading organism? The host becomes susceptible to other agents and the threat to survival is heightened. Patients may suffer from several infections, which expand considerably the complexities of their clinical problems.

The ability of infectious agents to cause immunodeficiency has reached its known limit with AIDS. Immunodeficiency in this disease is especially profound because the AIDS virus (HIV, human immunodeficiency virus) infects the T_4 (inducer-helper) subset of lymphocytes (see Chapter 5). The process of infection is intimately associated with the immunological role of these cells. Depletion of T_4 cells leads to collapse of the immune system, which topples like a roman arch whose keystone is removed. The result is lymphopenia (reduction in circulating lymphocytes), impaired delayed hypersensitivity, defective responses of T cells to antigens, and reduction in the numbers of T cells cytotoxic for tumor cells and virus infected cells. Even B cell function becomes disordered, with reduced production of specific immunoglobulins and the increased, chaotic production of nonspecific immunoglobulins—paradoxically, AIDS patients may have an abnormally high level of circulating immunoglobulins. All these events lead to the opportunistic infections and tumors that make AIDS a uniformly lethal illness. If evasion of immunity is a biological imperative for HIV, the process clearly reaches grim levels of excess.

The extensive regulatory interactions of the immunocompetent cells may go awry when even minor changes are introduced into the network. For some 85 years, long before AIDS, it has been known that measles is immunosuppressive. There is good evidence, for example, that tuberculosis is more common after widespread measles outbreaks. Since then immunosuppression has been found to follow other viral infections as well, e.g., hepatitis B and influenza. These viruses function more subtly than HIV, impairing the function of lymphoid cells without causing major structural changes. T lymphocytes infected with measles virus in vitro do not die but lose certain functions, e.g., the capacity to mount a delayed hypersensitivity reaction (Chapter 5). B cells infected with measles virus stop synthesizing and releasing immunoglobulins. The effect is intrinsic to B cells and is not secondary to the action of the virus on T cells or macrophages.

In some cases, immune suppression is the result of inhibition of the synthesis of lymphokines. Recent experiments with leishmanias, the protozoa that cause leishmaniasis, showed that when these organisms are growing in macrophages, they suppress the production of interleukin-1. This is significant because interleukin-1 is a critical product of infected macrophages and initiates a series of immunological and inflammatory events that lead to the eradication of the infection (Chapter 4). These findings may explain an old observation, that successful infection in so-called visceral leishmaniasis is associated with T cell unresponsiveness. This parasite seems to go one step further in arranging for immune evasion by suppressing the capacity of macrophages to make the class I and II products of the major histocompatibility complex (MHC), an event that has the potential for marked suppression of cell-mediated immunity.

Infection of lymphocytes is not necessarily an immune suppressive tactic of the microbe. A large number of microorganisms infect the lymphoreticular tissues but do not cause global disturbances to host immunity. For example, the bacteria that cause typhoid fever or brucellosis live in lymph nodes for long periods of time without inducing noticeable immune suppression.

"Masquerading" by Changing Antigenic Coats

Certain bacteria, viruses, and protozoa are unusually adept at frustrating immune recognition by changing their surface antigens. The classical cases are trypanosomes, gonococci, the agents of recurrent fever, and influenza viruses.

The Case of the Trypanosomes

One of the best studied examples of antigenic variation is seen with the protozoan that causes sleeping sickness, *Trypanosoma brucei*. The organism affects humans and domestic animals and infects the blood and interstitial fluids. Thus, trypanosomes are exposed to circulating antibodies. Trypanosomes are covered with a thick protein coat called *variable surface glycoprotein*, which undergoes periodic antigenic changes during the infection. These parasites have several hundred genes that encode for different antigens, but they express only one at a time (Chapters 39 and 40). When antibodies against one type are made, the number of parasites in the blood of an infected host drops, but they are soon replaced by a new antigenic type. There can be many successive waves of antigenically different parasites in a single host. Thus, protective immunity does not function well against this master of disguise.

Gonococcus and Its Adhesin

Like the trypanosome (a eucaryotic cell), some bacteria can also switch their surface antigens. A good example is the gonococcus, which undergoes periodic changes in pilin, the protein that makes up its fimbriae, the apparent means of attachment of host cells. Details of how this occurs are discussed in Chapter 2. In addition to changes in the antigenicity of pilin, the major outer membrane proteins of gonococci also undergo antigenic variation. Thus, the surface of these organisms displays a highly variable antigenic profile to the host immune system.

Influenza and Antigenic Variation Among Influenza Viruses

The tendency of influenza to reappear in a population on a regular basis is due in part to the great ability of influenza viruses to undergo antigenic variation. This is the major obstacle to the development of a truly effective vaccine against this disease. Minor changes are called *antigenic* drift and occur every 2 or 3 years. Major antigenic changes, called *antigenic shifts*, take place every 10 years or so. These changes involve two surface proteins, a *hemagglutinin* that serves to bind to cell surface receptors, and a *neuraminidase* that changes these receptors. How these proteins are involved in attachment and penetration of the virus is discussed in Chapter 30.

Proteolysis of Antibodies

A number of bacteria—gonococci, meningococci, *Haemophilus influenzae*—and some dental pathogenic streptococci make extracellular proteases that specifically inactivate secretory IgA. They cleave it at the hinge region to yield complete but relatively ineffective fragments. IgA is the major immunoglobulin isotype on human mucosal surfaces and consists of subclasses I and II. The relative importance of these subclasses is not known, but only subclass I is cleaved by these proteases. IgA_1 proteases from different bacteria are all highly specific for this substrate but they have biochemical and genetic differences that suggest that this property has evolved independently. The proteases are present in active form in tissues and fluids infected by the bacteria that produce them. Nonpathogenic relatives of these organisms are protease negative. Notice that this suggests, although it does not prove, a role for IgA proteases in pathogenesis.

In some instances it is known that when an organism cleaves IgA, it keeps the Fab fragment attached. This makes the antigens unavailable for binding by intact antibody molecules. This phenomenon has been called *fabulation* (after "Fab") and may serve to protect organisms from antibodies. Fabulation may be more widely used by pathogens than is currently known.

Other Viral Survival Strategies

The more chronic an infection, the more lasting must be the mechanisms for microbial evasion of host defenses. This is well illustrated in herpes infection. To limit access from circulating defenses, herpesvirus do not usually enter the extracellular fluid but pass from cell to cell via cytoplasmic bridges. Also, even intracellular herpes viruses have a major mechanism for evading attack: *latency*, whereby they reside within nerve cells but do not proliferate (Chapter 31). In these circumstances viruses are not affected by antibodies, cell-mediated immunity, or interferon. They can then survive for long periods of time in the presence of well-developed host defense mechanisms. Later—often when the host defenses have subsided—the viruses may reactivate to cause disease and perhaps even cancer. "He who fights and runs away may live to fight another day."

SUGGESTED READINGS

Cox FEG: How parasites evade the immune response. *Immunol Today* 5:29, 1984.
Haywood AM: Patterns of persistent viral infection. *N Engl J Med* 315:939–948, 1986.
Johnston RB, Jr: Recurrent bacterial infections in children. *N Engl J Med* 310:1237–1243, 1984.
Oldstone MBA: Distortion of cell functions by noncytotoxic viruses. *Hosp Pract* July 15:82–92, 1986.
Parsons M, Nelson RG, Agabedian N: Antigenic variation in African trypanosomes: DNA rearrangements program immune evasion. *Immunol Today* 5:43–50, 1984.
Young JD-E, Cohn ZA: Cellmediated killing: a common mechanism? *Cell* 46:641–642, 1986.

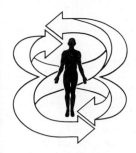

Bacterial Toxins

D. Schlessinger
M. Schaechter

DEFINITIONS

Toxins, like antibiotics, are biological weapons. The analogy is somewhat macabre since antibiotics affect microbes, whereas toxins are directed at us. Bacterial toxins are soluble substances that alter the normal metabolism of host cells with deleterious effects on the host. They are the salient feature of some bacterial diseases and are responsible for their main signs and symptoms. Understanding how they work helps understand the pathophysiology of many infectious diseases and, in some instances, reveals important facts about normal processes. We understand a few toxins in detail and for the rest must await the result of further work. Individual toxins will be treated in detail in the chapters on specific bacterial pathogens. Here we will discuss the basic concept of how bacterial toxins function to cause damage in the host. Traditionally, toxins are associated with bacterial diseases, but this probably reflects our ignorance. It seems quite possible that toxins play important roles in diseases caused by fungi, protozoa, and worms.

A conventional distinction is made between *exotoxins* and *endotoxins*. Exotoxins are proteins produced by bacteria that are usually secreted into the surrounding medium, but are sometimes bound to the bacterial surface and released upon lysis. In contrast, endotoxin is the lipopolysaccharide of the outer membrane of Gram negative bacteria and acts as a toxin under special circumstances only.

Bacterial exotoxins vary in their specificity; some act on certain cell types only, whereas others can affect a wide range of cells and tissues. Some bacteria make a single toxin, others are known to produce 10 or more (Table 7.1 gives some

Table 7.1
Major toxinogenic organisms

Toxin	Effects	Mechanism
Bacillus anthracis		
Protective antigen	Required for others	"B" components
Edema factor	Edema	Internal adenylate cyclase; calmodulin dependent
Lethal factor	Pulmonary edema	Kills certain cells (All three factors together give vascular, permeability, neurotoxicity)
Bordetella pertussis		
Adenylate cyclase	Inhibits, kills white cells	Adenylate cyclase; can be calmodulin independent
Pertussis toxin	Many hormonal effects	ADP-ribosylation of G-binding protein
Tracheal cytotoxin		
(others)	Kills cilia bearing cells	?
Campylobacter jejuni		
Enterotoxin	Diarrhea	Cholera-like
Clostridium botulinum		
Botulinum toxin	Neurotoxins	Blocks neuromuscular junctions presynaptical flaccid paralysis
Clostridium difficile		
Enterotoxin	Hemorrhagic diarrhea	Acts at membranes
Cytotoxin	Cytoplasmic; cells lose filaments	
Clostridia		
α toxin	Necrosis in gas gangrene; cytolytic, lethal	Phospholipase C
β toxin	Necrotic enteritis	?
Enterotoxin (others)	Food poisoning; diarrhea	Cytoxin; damages membranes
Clostridium tetani		
Tetanus toxin	Spastic paralysis	Inhibits GABA and glycine release from nerve terminals at inhibitor synopsis
Corynebacterium diphtheriae		
Diphtheria toxin	Kills cells	ADP-ribosylates elongation factor 2
Escherichia coli		
(and often other enterics)		
Heat-labile enterotoxins	Diarrhea	Identical to cholera toxin
Cytotoxin	Hemorrhagic colitis	Like *Shigella* toxin

examples). Some bacteria, like the pneumococci, make no known toxin and probably cause disease by mechanisms that do not require them. For each pathogen that makes a toxin we would ideally like to know whether the toxin is important in the process of infection. To find out we may ask:

1. Is virulence quantitatively correlated with toxin production?

2. Does the toxin in purified form produce damage? (In experimental animals or cells in culture, of course.)

3. Can a specific antibody (antitoxin) prevent or alleviate the manifestations of the disease?

Table 7.1 *Continued*

Toxin	Effects	Mechanism
Legionella pneumophila Cytotoxin	Lyses cells	?
Listeria monocytogenes Listeriolysin	Membrane damage	Like streptolysin O
Pseudomonas aeruginosa Exotoxin A (others)	Kills cells	Like diphtheria toxin
Shigella dysenteriae *Shigella* toxin	Kills cells	Inactivates 60S ribosomes
Staphylococcus aureus α toxin	Hemolytic, leukocytic, paralysis of smooth muscle	Lytic pores in membranes
β toxin	Cytolytic	Sphingomyelinase
δ lysin	Cytolytic	Detergent-like action
Enterotoxins	Food poisoning (emesis, diarrhea)	
Toxic shock syndrome toxin(s)	Fever, headache, arthalgia, neutropenia, rash	Mediated through IL-1 induction
Exfoliating (others)	Sloughing of skin ("scaled skin syndrome")	?
Streptococcus pneumoniae Pneumolysin	Cytolysin	Similar to streptolysin O
Streptococcus pyogenes Streptolysin O	Cytolysin	Cholesterol target
Erythrogenic toxin (others)	Fever, neutropenia, rash of scarlet fever	Mediated through IL-1
Vibrio cholerae Cholera toxin (others)	Diarrhea	Hormone-independent activation of adenyl cyclase
Yersinia enterocolitica Heat-stable enterotoxin	Diarrhea	Like *E. coli*

4. If toxin production is impaired by a mutation in the pathogen, is the disease process affected?

In cases where a toxin is shown to be important, we want to know how it works:

1. What is its mechanism of action?

2. Why is it specific for certain cells or tissues?

3. Does the pathogen make other toxins? Do they interact with one another?

These questions have been answered in detail only in the few cases where modern research methodology has been fully exploited. The answers come easiest when the action of a single toxin accounts for the symptoms of the disease. This is the case in cholera, diphtheria, tetanus, and botulism. By contrast, many pathogenic bacteria, such as staphylococci and streptococci, make several toxins and their importance becomes difficult to assess.

THE PRODUCTION OF TOXINS

Toxins share with antibiotics an ambivalent position in the life of the organisms that produce them. On one hand they are dispensable, not necessarily required for growth. On the other hand, under some conditions, they may be essential for survival and spread of the bacteria.

In agreement with the dispensability of toxins, their genes are frequently carried by DNA elements that are themselves dispensable: plasmids and temperate bacteriophages. Examples of phage-coded genes are those for the toxins of diphtheria, botulism, and scarlet fever. Plasmids carry genes for the toxins with which *Escherichia coli* causes diarrhea and certain staphylococci cause "scalded skin syndrome". The location of these genes on mobile DNA molecules ensures that the ability to produce toxin may rapidly spread to nontoxigenic bacteria. Conversely, the property may also be lost from the bacteria by "curing" the cells of plasmids or prophages. In experimental studies, this provides a simple way of making nontoxigenic bacteria that are otherwise identical to the toxin-producing ones.

Some toxins are produced continuously by growing bacteria, others are synthesized when the cells enter the stationary phase. Note that this is often true for antibiotics and other "secondary metabolites", which are also made as growth stops or slows down. In some instances there is some teleological sense to this. For example, certain toxins may help bacteria obtain nutrients that have become scarce. High levels of diphtheria toxin are produced only when the diphtheria bacilli run out of iron. Since there is very little free iron in normal tissues, may this be a way for the organisms to obtain it from the cells killed by the toxin?

Sporulating bacteria sometimes release toxins during spore formation. In this process the bacterial cells in which the spores are formed eventually lyse, which leads to the liberation of cytoplasmic proteins including toxins that may have accumulated. Examples are toxins made by the organisms that cause botulism, gas gangrene, or tetanus, all members of the genus *Clostridium*. In a heterogeneous environment, like a contaminated wound, some organisms are growing while others are sporulating. This means that the toxins will be produced continuously and will not be "phased" during the course of the infection.

MECHANISM OF ACTION

Some toxins act locally to help bacteria stay alive by killing nearby white blood cells. Others help the organisms spread in host tissues by degrading the proteins of the connective tissue matrix. Still other toxins disseminate far from the site where they are synthesized. This is the case for diphtheria toxin, which is manufactured in the throat but acts on remote organs, including the heart and the brain. Note that neither the mechanism nor the site of action of a toxin can be predicted. Nor is it always possible to understand the benefit to the bacteria of making toxins, especially those that act at a distance. This only reflects our ignorance, for it must be true that toxins help bacteria grow and survive.

Bacterial toxins work at extraordinarily low levels and include the strongest poisons known. One gram of tetanus, botulinus, or Shiga toxin is enough to kill about 10 million people. One hundred–fold more is required for the action of diphtheria toxin, and 1000-fold more for others (for example *Pseudomonas* A toxin).

Toxins cause damage in various ways (Table 7.1): Some lyse host cells, others stop cell growth, and still others exaggerate normal physiological mechanisms.

By depressing or augmenting particular functions toxins may kill a person without directly damaging any cells. For example, tetanus toxin paralyzes the body without affecting the integrity of the target neurons. Cholera toxin turns up a normal secretory process, using a normal regulatory mechanism of the epithelial cells of the intestine. This results in the huge loss of water characteristic of cholera. No abnormal lesions result—the toxin acts by causing hyperactivity of a normal process.

Toxins That Help Bacteria Spread in Tissues

Toxins that do not target any particular type of cells can nevertheless contribute to causing disease. These include degradative enzymes that function as *spreading factors* by facilitating the dispersal of infecting organisms. For example, some streptococci secrete a *hyaluronidase* that breaks down hyaluronic acid, the ground substance of connective tissue. They also secrete a *DNase*, which thins out pus made viscous by the DNA released from dead white blood cells. A streptococcal protease, *streptokinase*, cleaves a precursor of plasminogen activator to an active form. This converts plasminogen to plasmin, the serum protease that in turn attacks fibrin clots. Streptokinase can thus eliminate fibrin barriers that may be in the way of invading streptococci.

Similar roles have been suggested for the *collagenases* and *elastases* produced by other organisms. Such "meat tenderizers" are unregulated forms of enzymes that also exist in the uninfected host, but whose activity is normally under control.

Toxins That Lyse Cells

A large and common class of toxins kills host cells by destroying their membranes. They usually act as lipases or by inserting themselves in the membrane to form pores.

An example of a lipase toxin is the *lecithinase* formed by the clostridia of gas gangrene. This enzyme lyses cells indiscriminately because its main substrate, phosphatidylcholine (lecithin), is ubiquitous in mammalian membranes. Several toxins of this sort are known as *hemolysins* because they are usually measured by their ability to lyse red blood cells. This does not mean, however, that they only affect these cells only. White blood cells are often targets for these toxins. Organisms thus eliminate potential host defenses and at the same time create a necrotic, nutritionally rich anaerobic milieu in which they thrive.

The other class of membrane-damaging toxins are those that insert themselves in membranes to make *protein pores*. These channels make the membranes more permeable; water pours into the concentrated cytoplasm, and the cells begin to swell. When this process continues beyond a certain point, the cells burst. Even at toxin concentrations too low to cause lysis, cellular functions may be severely damaged because slight perturbations of permeability may cause leakage of the potassium ions needed for protein synthesis and cell viability. Thus, low levels of this kind of toxin effectively inhibit the function of the phagocytes, the first line of host defense. Note that these toxins are not enzymes but act to form nonselective channels for water and ions, "ionophores", much like certain antibiotics (e.g., the antifungal polyenes, which also form "pores").

The pattern of ion leakage and of subsequent damage is similar for many toxins. These nonenzymatic toxins work by a mechanism similar to that of the membrane attack complex of complement (see Chapter 4). The pores formed by this complex contain aggregates of unfolded C9 and other components in a "torus" or tube-like array that is unusually resistant to proteases and detergents. Such a fortified structure is seen with many toxins that make pores. This general resistance very likely contributes to their stability at the cell surface.

α-Toxin of Staphylococci

An example of a toxin that works in this manner is the toxin of *Staphylococcus aureus*. It is an example of a *homogeneous pore former*; i.e., each pore has the same number of protein molecules. Here, a protein with a molecular weight of 34,000 forms hexamers with an external diameter of 8.5 to 10 nm and an internal channel 2 to 3 nm across (Fig. 7.1), more than sufficient to allow free passage of most metabolites.

Offhand, the ability of toxin to insert itself in the membrane would not seem to require specific receptors. However, such receptors apparently exist, since different cells show a 100-fold range in sensitivity to this toxin. Among the specific consequences of the action of this toxin are the aggregation of platelets and narrowing of small blood vessels, leading to tissue necrosis. Toxin, as well as the C9 component of complement, becomes denatured by contact with low-density serum lipoprotein. This effect has suggested that a "nonimmune" neutralization may occur in vivo.

Figure 7.1. Pores formed by membrane-active toxin seen under the electron microscope. **A**, Red blood cells treated with staphylococcus α-toxin. Numerous 10-nm ring-shaped holes are seen. **B**, Isolated α-toxin in detergent aggregate to make a doughnut-shaped structure. **C**, Red blood cell membranes treated with streptolysin O. **D**, Purified streptolysin O incorporated into artificial membranes (liposomes). (From Bhakdi S, Tranum-Jensen J: *Phil Trans Roy Soc London B* 306:311, 1984.) See Figure 4.8 (p. 83) for analogous pores produced by the membrane attack complex of complement.

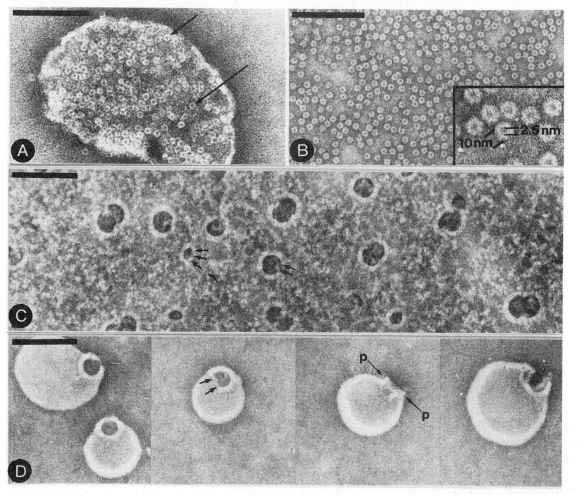

Streptococcal Streptolysin O

The pore-forming toxins of the other major class are heterogeneous, that is, they form pores of various sizes and with different numbers of monomer molecules. The prototype of this class is streptolysin O, one of the toxins produced by certain streptococci. Streptolysin O ("O" for "oxygen labile") binds to cholesterol in the cell membrane. (Again, note the similarity to the action of antifungal polyenes.) The free toxin may be inactivated by cholesterol, but once it is incorporated in the membrane, it becomes impervious to it. The toxin consist of monomers, with a molecular weight of 89,000, which together with cholesterol, form large curved rods. The diameter of the resulting channels is up to 30 nm (Fig. 7.1). The aggregates are large enough to be easily visible in the electron microscope, and the pores are easily demonstrable in both the inner and outer leaflets of the membrane.

For unknown reasons, streptolysin O lyses red blood cells but not neutrophils or macrophages. Still, these white blood cells are killed by low levels of this toxin because it acts preferentially on the membranes of lysosomes, releasing their hydrolytic enzymes. This results in damage to the cytoplasmic contents and leads to cell death. In addition, the lysosomal enzymes released from killed neutrophils damage surrounding tissue. Pores made by toxins need not be large or well defined. A toxin made by *E. coli* binds to the membranes as monomers, yet allows the free passage of ions. Apparently, "minipores" can be very effective.

What happens to pore proteins? At low concentrations pores can be repaired. Since neutrophils can shed membrane-associated components of complement, they probably throw off toxin-mediated channels as well. In general, however, toxin-formed pores resist proteolytic attack and tend to survive for a long time.

Toxins That Block Protein Synthesis

Structure and Mode of Action

In contrast to the toxins that act on the surface of cells, which are highly variable in structure and mode of action, those that act inside cells show a number of similarities: (a) Most have two portions, one involved in binding to the cell membrane, the other responsible for the toxic activity. In some toxins these two activities are carried by a single polypeptide chain, in others by two different chains. They are called A for "active" and B for "binding," and these toxins are known as *A-B toxins*. (b) Binding to the membrane may be followed by receptor-mediated endocytosis and internalization of the toxin, although some investigators propose as an alternative the direct passage through a pore. (c) The A moiety is often still latent after uptake. It may be activated by proteolytic cleavage and reduction of disulfide bridges. For example, diphtheria, cholera, tetanus, and *Shigella* toxins are all synthesized as inactive precursors that must be activated to become toxic. (d) Finally, many of these toxins have a common mode of action: they catalyze the transfer of the adenosine-diphosphate group from the coenzyme NAD to target proteins. These *ADP-ribosyltransferases* are exemplified by diphtheria toxin, cholera toxin, and exotoxin A of *Pseudomonas aeruginosa*.

Diphtheria Toxin

Diphtheria toxin is one of the best understood of all bacterial toxins. Its A and B portions are synthesized as a single polypeptide chain. The hydrophobic B portion binds to a receptor on the membrane that is found on all the cells of susceptible species. By this time, the molecule has been cleaved at a protease sensitive site between the A and B portions, but they are still covalently associated by disulfide linkage. The entire receptor-toxin complex then enters the cell by receptor-mediated endocytosis, just like hormones or certain viruses. Once the toxin enters the cell, reduction of the disulfide bond separates the A and B portions. The acidic conditions prevailing within endosomal vesicles promote insertion of the B chain into the endosomal membrane. Somehow, this facilitates passage of fragment A into the cytosol. Thus, both endocytosis (passage across the cell membrane) and membrane translocation (out of the vesicles into the cytoplasm) are required for fragment A to reach the cytoplasm and begin its toxic action.

The A fragment is resistant to denaturation and is long-lived inside cells. This accounts in part for its potency: a single molecule can kill a cell. Killing takes place by ADP-ribosylation of elongation factor 2, or EF-2, a protein that catalyzes the hydrolysis of guanosine triphosphate, which drives the movement of ribosomes on eucaryotic mRNA. The reaction is

$$\text{EF-2} + \text{NAD}^+ \longrightarrow \text{ADPR-EF2} + \text{H}^+$$

EF-2 is the only known substrate for diphtheria toxin. The reason for the specificity is that EF-2 contains a rare modification in one of its histidine residues and this is the site recognized by diphtheria toxin for ADP-ribosylation. Mutant cells that cannot modify this histidine become resistant to the toxin. The addition of ADP-ribose inactivates EF-2 and kills cells by an irreversible block of protein synthesis. Exotoxin A of *P. aeruginosa* works the same way.

Pharmacological Toxins

Here we will discuss toxins that function by elevating or depressing normal cell functions but which do not result in death of their target cells.

Toxins That Elevate Cyclic AMP: Cholera Toxin

An important class of toxins that do not damage cells work by raising the concentration of cyclic AMP (cAMP). Phagocytic cells are often an important target since an excess of cAMP inhibits chemotaxis and phagocytosis, thus reducing their power to kill microorganisms. The level of cAMP may be increased in several ways. Some pathogens pour out cAMP themselves; others secrete an adenyl cyclase to make more cAMP from adenosine triphosphate; and still others make a toxin that alters the activity of the adenylate cyclase of host cells. One of the best studied is cholera toxin, which acts by modifying the host adenylate cyclase.

The target tissue for cholera toxin is the epithelium of the small intestine. The toxin has separate A and B subunits: The B component has specific affinity for the intestinal epithelial mucosa. As with diphtheria toxin, the A subunit ADP-ribosylates a target protein which, here again, is a GTPase. This target protein is part of a complex that makes cAMP. The synthesis of cAMP becomes unregulated and it is made in large amounts. By an incompletely understood process, this provokes loss of fluids and copious diarrhea characteristic of cholera.

Both the structure of cholera toxin and its mechanism of action are known in detail. The binding component consists of five B subunits that form a doughnut structure visible in the electron microscope. A single enzymatic A subunit sits partly on and partly within the hole of the doughnut. The A subunit is synthesized as a single chain that is cleaved after secretion into two pieces, A_1 and A_2, which are held together by disulfide bridges. The whole toxin (one A_1, one A_2, five B subunits) binds to five ganglioside receptors on the surface of intes-

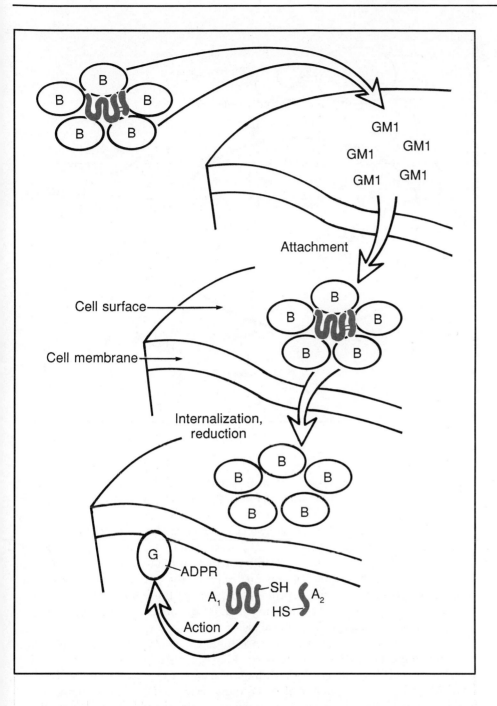

Figure 7.2. Cholera toxin becomes active. The B (binding) component is thought to become incorporated in the membrane and the A (active) component enters the cell.

tinal epithelial cells. The A_1-A_2 portion now enters the cell and is cleaved into the A_1 and A_2 pieces, perhaps by reduction of the disulfide bridges (Fig. 7.2). The A_1 fragment is enzymatically active and can now act on its target protein.

To understand how cholera toxin elevates the cAMP level we must examine how the synthesis of this compound is regulated normally, an intricate business. The adenylate cyclase complex is membrane bound in the intestinal cells and is composed of three proteins: they are known as G_s, R, and the cyclase itself (Fig. 7.3). The key to the working of the cyclase complex is that G_s protein is a GTP-

Figure 7.3. The action of cholera toxin. G, R, and cyclase all interact with the membrane. G protein binds GTP, stimulated by the complex of R protein and its cognate hormone. With GTP bound, G protein activates adenyl cyclase. Cholera toxin ribosylates G protein which now cannot hydrolyze GTP and remains in the stimulatory GTP bound form to keep adenyl cyclase making cAMP.

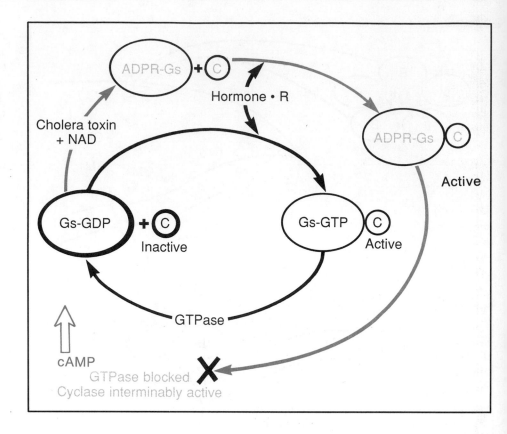

binding protein that has two conformational states: When it binds GTP, it stimulates adenylate cyclase to make cAMP. This effect is normally of short duration, because G_s protein is also a GTPase that cleaves GTP to guanosine diphosphate. The activity of adenyl cyclase is thus determined by the balance of binding and hydrolysis of GTP by G_s proten. What determines this balance? Binding of GTP by G_s protein is stimulated by R protein. This protein, in turn, is a receptor for one of several hormones, such as the adrenergics. We can now paint the whole picture: When R protein binds one of these hormones, it interacts with G_s protein to increase its binding of GTP. G_s protein now remains in the "active" state to stimulate adenyl cyclase.

How does cholera toxin act to increase the level of cAMP? The normal action of R protein is mimicked by cholera toxin. Like R protein, it promotes the "active" state of G_s protein, although by a different mechanism than R protein: Cholera toxin ADP-ribosylates G_s at one of its arginine residues. G_s protein is now locked in the conformation that stimulates adenylate cyclase. As mentioned above, the interminable synthesis of cAMP provokes the movement of massive quantities of fluid across the intestinal membrane and into the lumen of the gut.

Activation of adenylate cyclase by ADP-ribosylation is a strategy adopted by a number of other so-called enterotoxins that produce diarrhea, like the so-called labile toxin, or LT enterotoxin of *E. coli*. Other toxins, like one produced by *Bordetella pertussis*, the agent of whooping cough, raise cAMP in leucocytes. This results in impairment of motility of leucocytes and of their ability to migrate toward invading bacteria.

Toxins That Block Nerve Function

Among the most lethal toxins known are those of tetanus and botulism (Table 7.1). They are produced by members of the anaerobic spore-forming genus *Clostridium*. Both these toxins act on the nervous system: tetanus toxin produces irreversible muscle contraction, botulinum toxin blocks muscle contraction.

Tetanus and botulinum toxins, like diphtheria toxin, consist of single polypeptide chains (molecular weight about 150,000) which contain putative A and B regions. Once again, binding is to ganglioside receptors that, in this case, are those specific to nervous tissue. As are others, these toxins are activated by proteolysis and disulfide reduction, and they function intracellularly. Their potency suggests that they may well act enzymatically, in a manner analogous to diphtheria toxin. This is only speculative at present.

Tetanus Toxin

Tetanus bacilli rarely move from their location in wounds, and their toxin acts at a distance on the central nervous system. This is one of the best examples of a disease that results from the action of a single toxin. Once bound to cell membranes, tetanus toxin is internalized, probably by receptor-mediated endocytosis, and flows via retrograde transport through axonal processes to the spinal cord. There the toxin interferes with synaptic transmission by preferentially inhibiting the *release of inhibitory neurotransmitters* such as glycine from inhibitory interneurons. The excitatory and inhibitory effects of motor neurons become increasingly unbalanced, causing rigid muscle contraction. Thus, while the physiological basis of action is understood, its biochemical basis remains unknown. It is not known why it is more active on the inhibitory synapses.

Botulinum Toxin

Unlike tetanus toxin, botulinum toxin is seldom produced in wounds but is made in contaminated food kept under anaerobic conditions, e.g., improperly sterilized canned beans or sausages. The disease is therefore a true intoxication and does not require the presence of the organisms at all. Botulinum toxin is not destroyed by proteases of the digestive tract, apparently because it is protected by complexing with other proteins. In fact, intestinal proteases activate the toxin, which is a single polypeptide chain with A and B portions.

In contrast to tetanus toxin, botulinum toxin affects peripheral nerve endings. Once across the gut lining, it is carried in the blood to neuromuscular junctions. There it may bind to gangliosides at motor nerve endplates, where it is taken up. The subsequent events are not known, but they result in a *presynaptic block of the release of acetylcholine*. The interruption of nerve stimulation causes an irreversible relaxation of muscles, leading to respiratory arrest.

IMMUNE PROTECTION AGAINST TOXINS

Since toxins are foreign proteins and are antigenic, immune protection of the host is an optimistic possibility. For some diseases, like tetanus, the clinical disease itself does not confer immunity to subsequent infections, probably because only small amounts of toxin are produced, too small to be effective immunogens. On the other hand, vaccination and treatment with antitoxins have been used successfully in tetanus and other diseases. Of course, active immunization cannot be carried out by injecting the toxins themselves. Luckily, many toxins can be modified chemically to retain their immunogenicity while losing their toxicity. Such *toxoids* are commonly used for the prevention of diphtheria and tetanus. Initial doses in the first months of an infant are effective, and boosters every 10 years are sufficient to maintain immunity. As may be anticipated, infection by the organisms can still occur in individuals immune only to the toxin, but serious disease does not ensue.

Active disease in a nonimmune individual may be combated by the administration of antitoxin. However, once toxins are bound to the cells, antitoxins are usually ineffective. Bound toxins are rapidly internalized and become unavailable to the antibody molecules. Therefore, treatment with antitoxins must be very rapid to be useful. Another serious drawback of this "passive immunization" is that the antitoxin is frequently derived from horses or other animals. As a result it can lead to serum sickness, an immune reaction against foreign proteins.

Recombinant DNA technology may refine some of the vaccination procedures and it may be possible to immunize using tailor-made fragments of the toxin. The B fragments seem to be particularly promising candidates since antibodies that prevent binding of a toxin would block the initial steps of toxin action. In the absence of A fragment, the B fragments are innocuous and could be administered with little risk.

Not all toxin-mediated diseases respond to vaccination. In particular, vaccines against cholera administered systemically have been of limited value. Protection here requires the intestinal secretion of IgA antibodies against the toxin (to prevent its action) and against the bacterial adhesins (to prevent their colonization). Vaccines administered by injection give poor or short-lived protection, in part because they do not induce the formation of effective amounts of IgA antibodies. Alternatives are being exploited, based on knowledge of how the toxin works. In one case, a preparation of B subunits is administered orally along with killed cholera bacilli. This procedure produces a secretory IgA response and seems to protect quite well. Another possibility that has been considered is the administration of "protective colonizers", mutants that can only make the B subunit of the toxin but that may colonize by virtue of their adhesins.

Bacterial toxins are being used in attempts to make them useful delivery systems for drugs, for example, coupling a specific antibody to an A subunit of a toxin. The antibody would then seek out the specific cell, and the toxin fragment would kill it. The results of these attempts have thus far been equivocal and have often been colored by side reactions. Nonetheless, the idea of turning toxins to advantage remains appealing.

ENDOTOXIN: SOMETIMES A TOXIN, USUALLY AN IMMUNOSTIMULANT

Endotoxin is the lipopolysaccharide (LPS) of the outer membrane of Gram-negative bacteria. It plays an important role in the diseases caused by these organisms. In small amounts, endotoxin elicits a series of alarm reactions: fever, activation of complement by the alternative pathway, activation of macrophages, and stimulation of B lymphocytes. In large amounts it produces shock and even death. The term endotoxin is misleading on two counts—it is not "endo" (internal), and only in large amount is it a toxin. Endotoxin is full of surprises and complications. To quote from Lewis Thomas' *The Medusa and the Snail* (New York, Viking Press, 1979):

The most spectacular examples of host goverance of disease mechanisms are the array of responses elicited in various animals by the lipopolysaccharide endotoxins of Gram-negative bacteria. Here the microbial toxin does not even seem to be, in itself, toxic. Although the material has powerful effects on various cell and tissue, including polymorphonuclear leucocytes, platelets, lymphocytes, macrophages, arteriolar smooth muscle, and on complement and the coagulation mechanism, all of these effects represent perfectly normal responses, things done every day in the course of normal living. What makes it a disaster is that they are turned on all at once by the host, as though in response to an alarm signal, and the outcome is widespread tissue destruction, as in the generalized Shwartzman reaction, or outright failure of the circulation of blood, as in endotoxin shock.

Endotoxin and exotoxins are different in most important ways. Endotoxin is not a protein, like the exotoxins, but rather a complex molecule with some exotic chemical constituents not found elsewhere in nature. Most exotoxins have a single mode of action. Endotoxin, on the other hand, induces many and different pharmacological and immunological changes at low and at high concentrations. Our knowledge of endotoxin is still fragmentary and at times its study stirs up considerable controversy. Welcome, then, to the immunopharmacologists' Explorers' Club.

Chemistry of Endotoxin

The complex chemistry of endotoxin does not, as yet, cast a light on how it works. As discussed in Chapter 2, bacterial lipopolysaccharide is composed of three parts: a glycophospholipid, called *lipid A*; a core of sugars, ethanolamine and phosphate; and the *O antigen*, a long side chain of species-specific, often unusual sugars (Fig. 2.6). Of these parts of the molecule, the active one is the lipid A, whereas the others serve as carriers. Lipid A alone is water insoluble (because it is hydrophobic) and inert, but its activity is restored when complexed even with artificial large-molecular-weight carriers, like proteins. The structure of lipid A is unusual (Fig. 2.6): it contains uniquely short fatty acids (12, 14, and 16 carbons in length), some with hydroxyl groups.

Major Effects of Endotoxin

In low and high amounts, endotoxin does two major things in the body (Fig. 7.4): At the low range of concentrations it sets off a series of alarm reactions and at high range it induces shock. The extent to which these complex events overlap depends not only on the amount of endotoxin, but also on the route of injection and the previous exposure of the host to this substance.

Four types of cells are the *primary target cells* for endotoxin: the mononuclear phagocytes (peripheral blood monocytes, macrophages of the spleen, bone marrow, lung alveoli, peritoneal cavity, Kupffer cells), neutrophils, platelets, and B lymphocytes. These cells probably have specific endotoxin receptors, although at present this is still an unsettled question.

Alarm Reactions to Endotoxin

Fever

Endotoxin acts as a *pyrogen*, i.e., causes fever, when Gram-negative bacteria accumulate in tissue in sufficient amounts to come in contact with the circulation. In the words of Lewis Thomas elsewhere in his essay, "endotoxin becomes propaganda", information that bacteria are present. Fever is elicited by extremely small amounts of endotoxin. About 100 ng (0.1 μg) injected intravenously in an

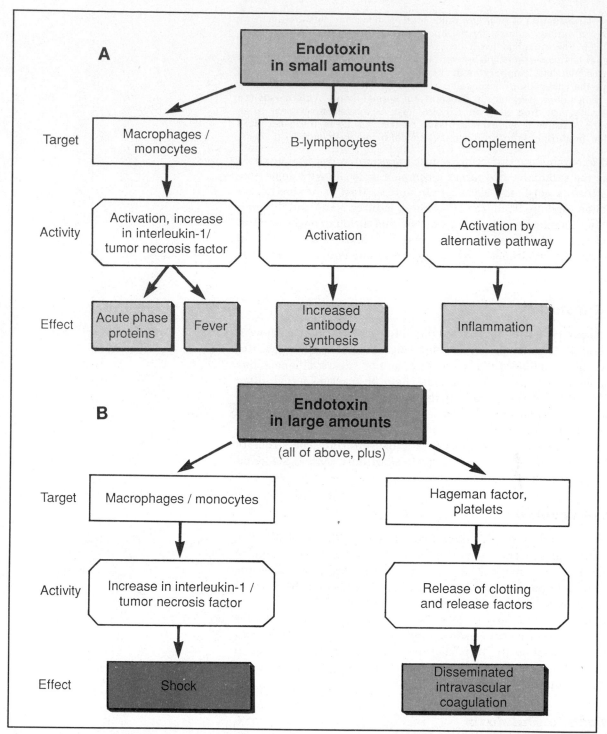

Figure 7.4. The action of endotoxin at low and high concentrations. See text for details.

adult human volunteer produce a measurable pyrogenic response, or fever. Note that this amount comes from about 10 million typical enteric bacteria, not a particularly large amount of microbial mass. The normal intestinal flora contains perhaps one million times more bacteria than that. If all the endotoxin in the bowel were to enter the bloodstream and if fever followed an absurdly linear response, we would have a temperature of about one million degrees! Obviously neither is true and the amount of endotoxin that spills over from the gut into the portal circulation, although not known, is probably quite small. Nonetheless, it serves in healthy people as constant low-level stimulation of the immune response without pathological manifestations. Low titers of antibodies to endotoxin are found in most healthy persons.

Fever is produced by endotoxin inducing the release of proteins known as *endogenous pyrogens* from mononuclear phagocytes. The best known of these proteins are interleukin-1 and tumor necrosis factor, which set off a complex series of events known as the *acute phase response* (Chapter 4). Gram-positive bacteria also induce fever but, lacking endotoxin, they elicit it through their cell wall components, which also causes the release of interleukin-1 and tumor necrosis factor.

Activation of Complement

Endotoxin activates complement directly by the alternative pathway (see Chapter 4). At low endotoxin concentrations, the events most likely to be of consequence to the bacteria are the production of the membrane attack complex, plus phagocyte chemotaxis and opsonization. Neutrophils are called up, especially by C5a, and, because of the opsonizing effect of C3b, become available for phagocytosis. Complement activation also leads to the production of anaphylatoxins (C3a, C5a), which lead to increased capillary permeability and release of lysosomal enzymes from neutrophils (degranulation). Together, these effects produce an inflammatory response.

Activation of Macrophages

Endotoxin activates macrophages; that is, it stimulates them to increase their production of lysosomal enzymes, to speed up their rate of phagocytosis, and to secrete some of their hydrolases into the medium. Once activated, macrophages become supreme scavengers and are able to handle larger numbers of invading microorganisms. Their exuberance extends itself to killing certain cancer cells, partly by direct attachment, partly by releasing proteins such as tumor necrosis factor. The ability of endotoxin—via macrophages—to limit the growth of certain tumors has been recognized for some time and is the subject of continued investigation. Endotoxin derivatives belong to a class of potential anticancer agents known as *biological response modifiers*, which are being evaluated for use in clinical work.

Stimulation of B Lymphocytes

By inducing the release of interleukin-1, endotoxin induces B lymphocytes (but not T lymphocytes) to divide. B lymphocytes mature into antibody-producing cells, thus adding to resistance to infection by increasing the level of antibodies. In this capacity endotoxin is an immunological adjuvant.

Effects of High Amounts of Endotoxin: Shock

The full panoply of the activities of endotoxin is displayed when it is administered in large amounts. This is seen, fortunately rarely, in a condition known as *bacterial sepsis*, when the body is overwhelmed, often by Gram-negative bacteria like *E. coli*, *P. aeruginosa*, or meningococci (see Chapters 19 and 51). The result is a frequently lethal condition known as *endotoxic shock*, which is manifested by a serious drop in blood pressure, *hypotension*, and by *disseminated intravascular coagulation*.

Hypotension is due to a complex series of reactions elicited by endotoxin. It has recently been proposed that the key mediators in endotoxin-induced hypotension are tumor necrosis factor and interleukin-1. Thus, the extent of hypotension is considerably reduced by the administration of antisera against tumor necrosis factor or interleukin-1 prior to the injection of endotoxin. An earlier view is that decreased resistance of peripheral vessels is due to a build up of vasoactive amines (histamine and kinins). Considerable work is being carried out to clarify the situation and to understand the molecular basis for endotoxin shock.

Disseminated intravascular coagulation (DIC) is the name given to the deposition of thrombi in small vessels, with consequent damage to the areas deprived of blood supply. The effect is most severe in the kidneys, where it leads to cortical necrosis. Other organs also affected are the brain, the lungs and the adrenals. In some cases of meningococcal infection, adrenal insufficiency due to infarction leads to rapid death, a condition known as the Waterhouse-Friderichsen syndrome. Endotoxin contributes to coagulation of blood in three ways: (*a*) It activates blood factor XII (the so-called Hageman factor), to set off the intrinsic clotting cascade. (*b*) It causes platelets to release the contents of their granules, which are involved in clotting. (*c*) It makes neutrophils give off basic proteins that are known to stabilize fibrin clots.

Summary

Endotoxin is the visiting card of Gram negative bacteria. When it is noticed, the body sets off a series of alarm reactions that rapidly help it fend off the invaders. These include the mobilization of neutrophils, the activation of macrophages, and the stimulation of B lymphocytes. In large amounts, endotoxin becomes deserving of its name and induces shock and widespread coagulation. This suggests that we have evolved successful defense mechanisms against Gram negative bacteria but have not developed ways of regulating them in every instance.

SELF-ASSESSMENT QUESTIONS

1. Discuss how certain toxins lyse host cells.

2. Why do many toxins have an A-B structure?

3. Which group of toxins has no obvious B portion?

4. What is the basis for believing that diphtheria toxin is the critical feature of the disease?

5. Cholera toxin acts by making adenylate cyclase hyperactive. What other types of diseases are due to excess activity of a normal process? (Hint: Consider effects of the immune response.)

6. Contrast the mode of action of tetanus and botulinum toxins.

7. Discuss the ideal properties of a toxoid to be used for vaccination.

8. List the main differences between exotoxins and endotoxins.

9. Contrast the local and systemic activities of low amounts of endotoxin.

10. Discuss the effects of high amounts of endotoxin.

SUGGESTED READINGS

Bhakdi S, Tranum-Jensen J: Damage to mammalian cells by proteins that form transmembrane pores. *Rev Physiol Biochem Pharmacol* 107:147–223, 1987.

Lewis T: *The Medusa and the Snail.* New York, Viking Press, 1979.

Middlebrook JL, Dorland RB: Bacterial toxins: cellular mechanisms of action. *Microbiol Rev* 48:199–221, 1984.

Stephen J. Pietrowski RA: *Bacterial toxins. Aspects of Microbiology 2.* Washington, DC, American Society for Microbiology, 1984.

Taussig MJ: *Processes in Pathology and Microbiology.* London, Blackwell Scientific Publication, 1984.

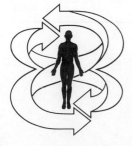

Strategies to Study Microbial Pathogenesis

8

M. Schaechter
D. Schlessinger

The purpose of this chapter is to acquaint you with ways new knowledge is acquired in the field of microbial pathogenesis. This area of very active research relies on methodology derived from molecular biology, immunology, microbiology, and biochemistry.

Microorganisms cause disease because they have special properties, so called *virulence factors*, or, more broadly, *determinants of disease*. The host also has attributes that contribute to the disease state. More often than not, properties of the parasite and the host interact in a complex, multifactorial fashion. To follow the nuances of such interactions we must attempt to dissect them into the component parts. Often, this requires a critical awareness of the difficulties involved in the interpretation of seemingly simple results. This chapter assumes that the agent of a particular disease has already been identified. An example of the strategies used to identify a new etiologic agent is found in the chapter on epidemiological principles (Chapter 60).

CORRELATIONS

Since the earliest days of microbiology, researchers have sought to correlate the ability of microorganisms to cause disease with some of their specific properties. If a certain trait is commonly found among the isolates of a certain pathogen, but only rarely among its nonpathogenic relatives, it is then likely that this property plays a role in the disease. The simplest examples are bacteria that make strong exotoxins. For instance, essentially all diphtheria bacilli isolated from patients with this disease make diphtheria toxin. Furthermore, injection of this toxin in animals closely mimics the major symptoms of the disease in humans, and prophylactic administration of a specific antitoxin prevents it. It seems reasonable,therefore, to believe that diphtheria toxin is a major virulence factor.

In the chapters on individual infectious agents you will find that most of what has been learned about microbial pathogenicity is based on this kind of correlation. However, the need for cautious interpretation should be apparent. Natural isolates may differ in properties other than the ones the investigator has chosen to study. For this reason, this approach is increasingly used in connection with genetic or immunological studies.

THE GENETIC APPROACH AND ITS HIDDEN TRAPS

The need for caution may be seen in an apparently straightforward example. When mice are injected in their peritoneal cavity with virulent pneumococci, they die of a fulminating infection, often within 18 hours. This occurs only if the organisms are surrounded by a capsule that permits them to elude phagocytes. Can it be concluded unequivocally that the capsule of the pneumococcus plays an essential role in the disease process? Let us analyze the situation critically. If the encapsulated and the unencapsulated strains represent separate isolates, they might differ in properties other than just the capsule. Suppose, for example, that the unencapsulated strain contains an additional mutation that makes it dependent on a high concentration of iron for growth. In the test tube this might not be noticed since iron is abundant in the usual culture media, but in the mouse it could make a big difference. This second mutation could be the real reason for the lesser virulence of the strain. To avoid such problems, the appropriate strategy is to construct *isogenic strains*, that is, organisms that are identical except for the mutation to be studied. Genetic techniques allow the exchange of a "good" gene with one that has been knowingly mutated, while keeping the rest of the genome the same. If a strain that carries such a mutated gene becomes avirulent, that gene is very likely to be involved in virulence.

Genetic experiments are relatively easy to carry out with *Escherichia coli* and a few other organisms, but are still quite demanding with most pathogens. With most other bacteria this richness of opportunities is not available, although relevant studies may still be carried out, usually with a greater expense of effort. Table 8.1 shows genetic systems that have been developed with some important bacterial pathogens.

Cloning techniques allow definitive studies of genes suspected of playing a role in pathogenesis. A gene may be purified by cloning in a surrogate organism, mutated, and reintroduced into the original host. This is the basis of one of the experiments described in detail below. An important use for this cloning technology is the study of organisms that cannot be grown in the laboratory, like the leprosy bacillus or the syphilis treponeme. It is possible to purify these agents from infected tissue in sufficient quantity to isolate their DNA. This can then be spliced into a suitable plasmid vector and introduced by transformation into *E. coli* or some other suitable genetic host.

This technique has also been used to make large amounts of gene products that are difficult to obtain by other methods. For example, thanks to cloning, it has been possible to make antigens of the hepatitis B virus, an agent that cannot easily be grown in the laboratory. This has been useful not only for experimental studies but also for the manufacture of a vaccine against the virus.

Table 8.1
Some bacteria used as recipients in genetic exchange experiments

Organisms	Systems of Exchange
Gram-positive cocci	
Staphylococcus aureus	Transduction
Streptococcus pyogenes	Transformation, transduction
Streptococcus pneumoniae	Transformation
Gram-negative cocci	
Neisseria gonorrhoeae	
Neisseria meningitidis	Transformation
Gram-positive rods	
Bacillus subtilis	Transformation, transduction
Corynebacterium diphtheriae	Transduction
Gram-negative rods	
E. coli and other enterics	Conjugation, transformation, transduction
Pseudomonas aeruginosa	Transduction, conjugation
Bacteroides fragilis	Conjugation
Haemophilus influenzae	Transformation

ANIMAL MODELS

Although well-controlled experiments may be carried out with isogenic strains, they are often limited in scope. For example, in the case of pneumococcus, the ultimate question is, how does the organism cause disease in humans? The reaction of the peritoneal cavity of mice is not necessarily relevant to that of the human lung. It would be preferable to induce pneumonia in laboratory animals, but it is difficult if not impossible to mimic the human disease in these animals. This is one important limitation of the genetic approach. Useful experiments not only depend on successful genetic manipulations but they also require a suitable animal model. In the ideal situation, the disease in laboratory animals should closely resemble that in people. Given the differences among vertebrates, this is not often the case. However, even if the situation is usually far from perfect, much can be learned from this approach. The careful experimenter is aware of the need for caution in extrapolating from work with animals to humans.

AN IMMUNOLOGICAL APPROACH

Fortunately, there are other approaches. One is to use specific antibodies against, for instance, the capsule of pneumococci. Mice injected with pneumococci in the peritoneal cavity or people with pneumococcal pneumonia could be treated with antibodies against the capsular polysaccharide of the organisms. They could also be "passively vaccinated", that is, they could receive antiserum prophylactically. To use this approach, a highly specific antibody against the virulence attribute to be studied must be available. If the antiserum prevents the effects of the infection, the capsule may be a virulence determinant. Does this result indicate that the capsule is the *main virulence factor*? Obviously not, because antibodies against any surface component may inhibit pathogenesis of the organisms. Nonetheless, in conjunction with the genetic study discussed above, the use of antipneumococcal capsular antibody could be valuable. This is, in fact, a central theme of this kind of research: Usually, several experimental approaches are used in combination.

TWO EXAMPLES OF RECENT EXPERIMENTS

Two examples of modern studies on pathogenesis are presented below. The first example concerns "invasin", a protein that permits avirulent bacteria to invade mammalian cells in culture. The second deals with the ways that viruses affecting the central nervous system reach their target tissue. These are original articles reprinted with permission of the authors. References and technical details have been omitted and a few explanatory statements, which appear in italics, have been added. The originals should be consulted for further details. Each paper is followed by comments and questions you may want to think about.

The Identification of Bacterial "Invasin"

[*From Isberg RR, Voorhis DL, Falkow S: Identification of invasin: A protein that allows enteric bacteria to penetrate cultured mammalian cells. Cell 50:769-778, 1987.*]

Introduction

A wide variety of pathogenic microorganisms are able to enter and survive within the cells of their host. These include many eucaryotic parasites as well as the bacteria that cause tuberculosis, dysentery, and bubonic plague. These species enter either epithelial cells and other nonphagocytic cells of the host or grow within macrophages, avoiding intracellular killing mechanisms. Little is known about how this is accomplished, even though invasive microorganisms cause common and severe diseases. It is therefore of interest to develop simple systems that allow the dissection of these processes.

We are studying the bacterium *Yersinia pseudotuberculosis* as a model invasive pathogen. *This organism is related to the plague bacillus and causes severe diarrhea in people.* In the body, the organism is found within host cells as well as in extracellular spaces. As is true of many yersiniae, it is able to enter nonphagocytic cells, as well as survive within macrophages of certain hosts. Initially, it invades the host by entering intestinal epithelial cells after ingestion of contaminated foodstuff, eventually gaining access to the lamina propria in a step that takes place without significant intracellular replication. Once it gains entry into the lymphatic system, the bacterium is able to survive and replicate within macrophages and becomes distributed in the liver, spleen, and mesenteric lymph nodes.

Two experimental systems allow an examination of the mechanism of cellular penetration by *Y. pseudotuberculosis* and the role invasion plays in the pathogenesis of disease. (a) The bacterium efficiently enters cultured mammalian cells, such as the human HeLa or HEp-2 cell lines. Monolayer cultures internalize as many as 50% of the added bacteria, allowing easy detection of intracellular microorganisms in a variety of assays. This is a useful phenotype, since monolayers of these cell lines do not internalize most bacterial species at a measurable frequency. Once inside the cell, the bacteria are found almost exclusively in membrane-bound vacuoles. (b) Animal models exist that allow one to evaluate the virulence of mutants. Several recent studies, in which mutant bacteria were introduced into live animals, demonstrated that various *Yersinia* gene products are critical for establishing disease. This approach will allow evaluation of mutations defective in cellular penetration as well.

In order to analyze bacterial penetration of mammalian cells, we have cloned segments of the Y. pseudotuberculosis genome into E. coli. We have isolated clones containing 30 kilobases of Y. pseudotuberculosis DNA that convert the normally innocuous E. coli K12 strain into an organism capable of entering cultured mammalian cells. These clones were identified by selecting for E. coli strains that penetrate the monolayer cells in a fashion similar to Y. pseudotuberculosis. The genetic locus necessary to confer invasiveness, called inv, was shown to be confined to a single region of approximately 3.2 kilobases. This locus allows E. coli strains to behave identically to the parental Y. pseudotuberculosis strain, with respect to both their efficiency of entry and their intracellular localization in membrane-bound vacuoles.

By faithfully reproducing the cell entry phenotype in E. coli, we can utilize the standard genetic techniques developed with this organism in order to dissect the penetration process. In this report, E. coli strains harboring the inv locus are analyzed. This has allowed us to transfer mutations to the parental Yersinia strain and to identify the protein necessary for entry into cultured cells.

Results

The inv Locus Is Required For Y. pseudotuberculosis to Enter Cultured Cells Efficiently

We have shown that the presence of the inv gene is sufficient to convert E. coli into an invader (Table 8.2). Y. pseudotuberculosis and E. coli strains harboring the inv locus were tested for their ability to bind to human cultured HEp-2 cells. Binding was measured by adding radioactively labelled bacteria to a standard amount of HEp-2 cells in culture. Nonbound bacteria were removed by washing 10 times with cold buffer. The remaining radioactive counts were a measure of the amount of bacteria bound to HEp-2 cells. As can be seen in Table 8.2, an E. coli inv$^+$ strain and the parental Y. pseudotuberculosis strain bound cells with equal efficiency. In each case, approximately 40% of the labeled bacteria were bound. In contrast, 40-fold fewer radioactive counts were associated with cells incubated with an E. coli strain harboring an insertion mutation in the inv locus. Insertion mutations are created by the incorporation of transposons—"hopping genes"—at random sites on the chromosome. Here, transposon insertion at the inv locus rendered the strains inv$^-$. A large series of mutants prepared by transposon insertion were used to delineate the inv gene (Fig. 8.1). Genetic deletions were also made and used in mapping of this gene.

So far we have demonstrated that the inv gene allows E. coli to bind to mammalian cells. Is inv also necessary for Y. pseudotuberculosis to bind to animal cells? To approach this question, we introduced a mutated version of the inv gene into Y. pseudotuberculosis using a transferable plasmid. We were able to construct two types of Y pseudotuberculosis strains in this fashion: One had a

Table 8.2
The inv locus encodes efficient binding to HEp-2 cells

	% Bound	
Strain	0°C	37°C
Parental Y. pseudotuberculosis	40.1	43.3
E. coli + inv plasmid	38.3	42.5
E. coli + mutant inv plasmid	0.8	1.0

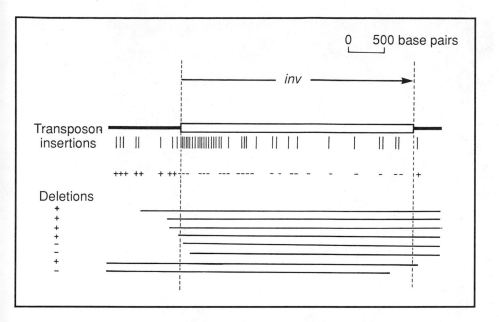

Figure 8.1. Physical and genetic map of inv region encoded on a plasmid that contains a 4.6 kilobase fragment of *Y. pseudotuberculosis* chromosomal DNA. Shown is a restriction map of the chromosomal DNA present on this plasmid, the sites of transposons Tn5 and Tn1000 insertions, deletion mutations, and the phenotypes of these mutations. *Vertical bars* indicate sites of insertion mutations as mapped by digestion with restriction enzymes. *Dashes* indicate insertions or deletions that eliminate the ability of *E. coli* strains harboring this plasmid to enter HEp-2 cells. *Crosses* indicate insertions or deletions that have no effect on the entry phenotype. *Open box* indicates region of DNA encoding *inv* locus, as determined by insertion and deletion mutations. *Horizontal lines* correspond to deletion derivatives present on these plasmids.

genetic duplication and contained both a mutated and an intact copy of the *inv* locus. The other strain was haploid and contained only a single copy of the mutated *inv* locus.

These *Y. pseudotuberculosis* strains were assayed for their ability to bind HEp-2 cells. We found that a *Y. pseudotuberculosis inv⁻* mutant bound with an efficiency of 0.1% that of its parental strain. In contrast, the strain with the genetic duplication that contained one intact copy of *inv* was fully competent to enter HEp-2 cells. Consistent with this was electron microscopic observation of thin sections prepared from these infections. We were unable to find internalized bacteria when HEp-2 cells were incubated with the *Y. pseudotuberculosis inv⁻* mutant (compare panels in Fig. 8.2A–C). The rare bacteria that could be found in these thin sections were always outside the HEp-2 cells (Fig. 8.2B). We conclude, therefore, that the *inv* locus is required by *Y. pseudotuberculosis* for efficient penetration of HEp-2 cells.

Penetration-Defective Mutants Are Defective for Binding Animal Cells

Regardless of the species harboring *inv*, bound bacteria were unable to enter HEp-2 cells at 0°C. Only when the temperature was raised were the externally bound bacteria able to penetrate the cells. Our interpretation of these results is that the presence of the *inv* locus allows binding of the bacteria to a receptor located on the cultured monolayer cells. When the temperature of incubation is raised above 0°C, the HEp-2 cells can internalize the bacteria through some endocytic process. Electron microscopic observation of this process is consistent with this interpretation, since bacteria are seen tightly bound to the surface of the animal cells when incubated on ice, but are internalized only at higher temperatures (Fig. 8.2D, E).

It was of interest to determine whether binding and penetration of animal cells were expressed as two separable functions. For instance, there could be one protein that binds the bacterium to animal cells, and a second protein that facilitates internalization of the bound bacterium. To determine the relationship between these two activities, a series of penetration-defective insertion mutants

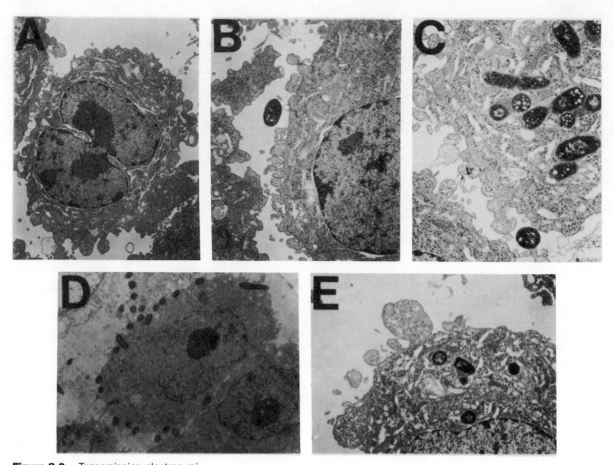

Figure 8.2. Transmission electron microscopy of HEp-2 cells incubated with bacterial strains. HEp-2 cells were infected with bacteria, fixed, and sectioned (as described in the original paper). **A**, **B**, Typical sections of animal cells incubated with *Y. pseudotuberculosis* strain *inv* **B**, Note that the *inv*⁻ strain is never found inside the HEp-2 cells, and that the rare bacterium found in these sections is not in close opposition to the cell. **C** Section showing cytoplasm of cell infected with *Y. pseudotuberculosis* strain *inv*⁺. **D**, **E**, Sections showing HEp-2 cells incubated with *E. coli* strain harboring the *inv* plasmid. Bacteria were incubated with the monolayers on ice for 90 minutes (**D**) and then allowed to enter by raising the temperature to 37°C for one hour (**E**).

were isolated. To determine whether binding and entry are separable activities, we subjected the mutants to the radioactive binding assay. As can be seen in Table 8.3, each of the penetration-defective mutants were also unable to bind the HEp-2 cells. We conclude that the binding activity and the ability to enter cultured cells are inseparable by mutation. Expression of both activities may be due to the presence of a single structure on the bacterial cell surface.

Identification of Invasin, the Protein Encoded by the inv Gene

Several lines of evidence indicated that the *inv* locus is a single gene.

1. We found that all the insertion mutations located within the *inv* locus fell into a single complementation group (data not shown).

2. In experiments in which plasmid-encoded proteins were preferentially synthesized we identified a protein that corresponds in size to the *inv* locus. *These experiments were based on the following: When plasmid-containing bacteria are treated with ultraviolet light, DNA of the chromosome is damaged more rapidly than plasmid DNA (because it is larger). Under these conditions, plasmid-encoded genes are preferentially expressed.* Bacteria containing the *inv* plasmid were treated with ultraviolet light and their proteins labeled with methionine S 35. Extracts of these irradiated cells were fractionated by sodium dodecyl sulfate (SDS) polyacrylamide gel electrophoresis. Three major polypeptide spe-

cies expressed from the *inv* gene migrated at apparent molecular weights between 98,000 and 103,000. In addition, an array of smaller proteins was also seen that might be degradation or premature termination products of the large protein. When *inv*⁻ mutants were analyzed in this fashion, the major peptides encoded by the *inv* locus were all disrupted. It would appear, therefore, that cells harboring the *inv* locus synthesize a 103,000 protein, large enough to encompass the region of *inv* defined by mutation outlined in Figure 8.1. Inasmuch as this protein is the product of the *inv* locus and must be intact for the bacterium to enter mammalian cells, we will call this protein *invasin*.

3. Does the *inv* gene code for a single protein? What is its size? To answer these questions, we determined the sequence of the 3947bp region encompassing *inv*, as well as the sequence endpoints of several deletion mutations described in Figure 8.1. We found a single "open reading" frame corresponding to a 988-amino-acid protein (molecular weight of 102,315). *An "open reading frame" is a stretch of DNA that contains the proper sequences for the initiation and termination of synthesis of a polypeptide chain.* We conclude,therefore, that invasin is the major product of this locus, with a molecular weight of 102,315.

Is Invasin Exposed on the Bacterial Surface?

There are two possible explanations for how invasin could participate in binding and entry into mammalian cells. The simplest model is that invasin is localized on the bacterial cell surface and functions as the ligand that binds the microorganism to a cell receptor. The second model is that invasin acts enzymatically to synthesize the binding structure (such as a carbohydrate) which is in turn placed on the bacterial cell surface. The former model could be discarded if we were to show that invasin is localized in some place other than the outer membrane of the bacterium. The second model, on the other hand, makes no prediction as to the cellular location of invasin.

A protease accessibility experiment was performed to determine if invasin is located on the surface of cells. Methionine S 35 irradiated cells were suspended in buffer containing various amounts of trypsin. After this treatment, the intact cells were washed in soybean trypsin inhibitor, boiled in SDS (*the detergent sodium dodecyl sulfate*), and the labeled protein products were analyzed on SDS polyacrylamide gels. 2.5 μg/ml of trypsin destroyed the 98,000- to 103,000-molecular-weight invasin products, and resulted in the production of two bands of apparent molecular weights 45,000 and 55,000. Since only intact cells were exposed to the trypsin treatment, this implies that invasin was localized on the surface of the bacteria, where the protease could have access to it. Surface exposure of invasin is consistent with the simple notion that this protein is the structure that binds the microorganism to the animal cell, although this result cannot, by itself, eliminate the enzymatic model.

Discussion

We have shown that the *inv* locus is necessary for efficient entry of *Y. pseudotuberculosis* into cultured animal cells. A mutation in this locus eliminates the ability to enter HEp-2 cells. Futhermore, the gene that encodes *inv* is sufficient to allow *E. coli* to bind and to penetrate HEp-2 cells. Bacteria harboring the *inv* locus bind tightly to animal cells at 0°C, and are internalized in a process that appears identical for both *Y. pseudotuberculosis* and *E. coli* strains encoding this locus.

Table 8.3
Entry-defective mutants are also defective for binding cultured mammalian cells

Plasmid Containing	Entry Phenotype[a]	% Bound
inv gene	+	39.0
No *inv* gene	−	0.34
Mutant *inv* gene	−	0.54

[a] Entry was measured by allowing bacteria to bind to HEp-2 cells and, after 200 minutes of incubation, treating the cells with the antibiotic gentamicin. This drug cannot penetrate into HEp-2 cells, thus it kills extracellular but not internalized bacteria. The bacteria that have entered can then be counted by carrying out colony counts ("viable counts") on a suitable agar medium.

The simplest interpretation of these data is that entry-proficient bacterial strains synthesize a structure that is localized on the surface of the bacterium, and are bound by this structure to the cultured cells. The entry process is completed when the mammalian cell internalizes the bound bacteria via an endocytic pathway. This formulation is supported by our data showing that all penetration-defective *inv*⁻ mutants of *E. coli* were also defective for binding animal cells. This is also consistent with a model in which the microorganism plays a relatively passive role in this process. It would appear that the only role of the *inv* locus is to allow binding of the bacterium to a critical site of the animal cell. It is then up to the animal cell to internalize the tightly bound bacteria.

A series of genetic and biochemical experiments indicated that the *inv* locus is a single transcriptional unit that encodes a single gene. This is based on the lack of complementation between *inv* insertion mutations as well as the identification of a 988-amino-acid protein that is large enough to saturate the coding capacity of this region. In vitro synthesis of this protein, which we call *invasin*, also results in a series of degradation and/or premature termination products.

Invasin is localized on the bacterial surface in a conformation that is sensitive to trypsin cleavage. Assuming that live bacteria localize this protein in a similar fashion, this result suggests a simple model for the mechanism of action of invasin. A domain on the surface-exposed region of invasin could act as a ligand that binds the bacterium to receptors on the animal cell. Direct proof of this model, of course, is contingent on determining if invasin itself is able to bind the animal cells. (*Editorial note: This experiment was subsequently carried out. It was found that isolated invasin binds to animal cells.*)

The implication from our data is that invasive bacteria synthesize a class of proteins specialized to interact directly with mammalian cells. The simple ability to encode a protein such as invasin may be a key determinant in differentiating between innocuous intestinal bacteria, and those that are able to penetrate intestinal epithelial cells. This raises the question of whether other enteroinvasive organisms, such as *Shigella* and *Salmonella* species, possess a similar property.

Questions and Comments

The discovery of *Yersinia pseudotuberculosis* invasin relied on a combination of genetics and biochemistry. It first required identifying the invasin gene and then determining which protein it encodes.

1. The identification of the invasin gene depended on two distinct uses of isogenic pairs: The gene was a) introduced into a surrogate organism that lacks it (*E. coli*) or b) it was mutated and then reintroduced in the organism that carries it normally (*Y. pseudotuberculosis*). The comparison was made, respectively, with the identical strain of *E. coli* lacking the gene or with the original strain of *Y. pseudotuberculosis* that carries a normal copy of the gene. Does this prove that *inv* is the only gene required for invasiveness? Does this disprove that invasiveness may be encoded in a "hidden gene"? What about "hidden mutations"? Notice that the gene was introduced into *E. coli* via a 30-kilobase piece of donor *Yersinia* DNA. This much DNA may contain about 20 average-sized genes.

2. The authors went to considerable effort to show that inv codes for a single protein. Why did they do that?

3. Why didn't the authors directly compare the amino acid sequence of the protein with that of nucleotides of the *inv* gene?

4. The authors suggest that bacteria may play a "relatively passive role" in penetration. Can you think of experiments that deal with this question directly? What would you do if you had a preparation of purified invasin available?

5. These results indicate that invasin is involved in penetration into cells in culture. Does this prove that invasin is involved in pathogenesis? What could be done to study this point?

What Genes Determine How a Virus Spreads in the Body?

[*From Tyler KL, McPhee DA, Fields BN: Distinct pathways of viral spread in the host determined by reovirus S1 gene segment. Science 233: 770-774, 1986.*]

For a virus to produce systemic illness, it must first spread from its site of initial entry and primary replication in the host to distant target tissues. This aspect of viral pathogenesis is particularly well exemplified by neurotropic viruses, which, after entering the host through a number of divergent portals (for example, respiratory, gastrointestinal, or venereal), subsequently spread to reach the central nervous system (CNS). Two principal pathways of spread to the CNS have been identified for neurotropic viruses. Most neurotropic viruses (for example, arboviruses, enteroviruses, measles virus, mumps virus, and lymphocytic choriomeningitis virus) spread through the bloodstream to reach the CNS (hematogenous spread), but several viruses, including rabies virus, herpes simplex virus, herpesvirus simiae, and poliovirus can reach the CNS by traveling through nerves. Almost nothing is known about the viral genes and proteins responsible for determining the capacity of viruses to spread through specific pathways within the infected host. Similarly, the precise cellular mechanisms utilized by viruses as they spread have not been identified.

The reoviruses are widespread among many mammalian species and most of the time cause mild or imperceptible diseases. However, in the laboratory these viruses cause infections of the central nervous system that have been useful in identifying genetic and molecular mechanisms of viral pathogenesis. Reovirus type 3 infects neurons and produces a lethal necrotizing encephalitis after intracerebral inoculation into newborn mice. Type 1, in distinction to type 3, does not infect neurons after intracerebral inoculation but instead infects ependymal cells and produces hydrocephalus. These and other differences suggest that type 3 is transported via nerves to the CNS and within it, whereas type 1 utilizes a non-neural pathway to spread to the CNS. Our previous success in studying viral pathogenesis by using reoviruses encouraged us to investigate viral-host interactions involved in viral spread.

To investigate our hypothesis that types 1 and 3 use different pathways of spread to the CNS, we took advantage of the fact that the motor and sensory neurons innervating the hindlimb and forelimb footpads are located in different regions of the spinal cord. If type 3 spreads via nerves, it should appear preferentially in the region of the spinal cord containing the neurons innervating the skin and musculature at the site of viral inoculation. If type 1 spreads through the bloodstream, it should appear in all regions of the spinal cord in equivalent amounts and with similar kinetics. Therefore, we injected type 3 and type 1 into the forelimb and hindlimb footpads of neonatal mice and studied the pattern of spread of these two viruses to the spinal cord. We found that after either hindlimb or forelimb inoculation, type 3 appeared first, and in up to 1000-fold higher titer, in the region of the spinal cord innervating the injected limb (Fig 8.3A, and

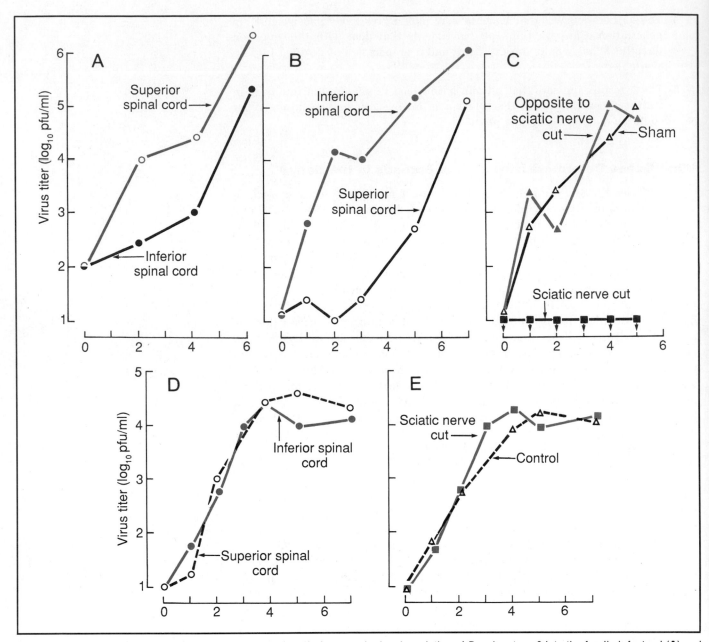

Figure 8.3. Pattern of spread of *Reovirus* to the spinal cord of neonatal mice. Inoculation of *Reovirus* type 3 into the forelimb footpad (**A**) and into the hindlimb footpad (**B**). **C**, The result of sectioning the sciatic nerve at the same side or the opposite side of the inoculation. **D**, Like **A**, with *Reovirus* type 1. **E**, Like **C**, with *Reovirus* type 1. The results of inoculation in the hindlimb are not shown because they were identical to those in the forelimb. The results are expressed as virus titers ($\log_{10}$ plaque-forming units per milliliter) in segments of spinal cord. A plaque-forming unit is the amount of virus needed for the production of a visible focal infection in cell culture monolayers. One-day-old mice were inoculated in the footpad with a 30-gauge needle. Sciatic nerve sections were performed on anesthetized mice by microsurgical techniques. Sham operations were identical except the nerve was not cut.

B). In contrast, type 1, after either hindlimb or forelimb innoculation, appeared at essentially the same time and in equivalent titer in all regions of the spinal cord (Fig 8.3*D,E*). These results support our hypothesis that type 3 spreads through nerves, and type 1 via the bloodstream, to reach the CNS.

To confirm these results, we studied the spread of types 1 and 3 from the hindlimb to the spinal cord in neonatal mice after section of the sciatic nerve. Since the sciatic nerve is the principal neural pathway from the hindlimb to the spinal cord, its section should completely prevent spread of virus from the hindlimb through nerves but should not affect its capacity to spread through bloodstream. As predicted, sciatic nerve section completely inhibited spread of type 3 to the spinal cord. Nerve section contralateral to the injected limb and sham operation had no significant effect on the spread of type 3 (Fig. 8.3C). Section of the sciatic nerve had no significant effect on the spread of type 1 (Fig. 8.3E). Thus, these experiments establish that type 3 spreads to the CNS through nerves and that type 1 uses nonneural, hematogenous pathways.

To identify the role of specific virus dsRNA segments in determining the capacity of type 1 and type 3 to spread by different routes to the CNS, we studied the pattern of spread of 11 reassortant viruses containing various combinations of genes derived from type 1 and type 3. *Reoviruses are unusual because their genome is contained in 10 separate segments of double-stranded (ds) RNA, each encoding different genes. "Reassortant" strains containing segments originating from different viruses can be constructed in the laboratory.* We inoculated each reassortant virus into the hindlimb and forelimb footpads of separate litters of neonatal mice and assayed viral titers in the superior and inferior spinal cord 48 and 72 hours after inoculation (Table 8.4).

A large difference in mean titer (more than 100-fold) between the superior and inferior spinal cord would be indicative of neural spread, whereas a small difference (less than fourfold) would be indicative of hematogenous spread. All reassortant viruses containing a type 3 S1 dsRNA segment showed a neural pattern of spread to the spinal cord, whereas all reassortants containing a type 1 S1 dsRNA segment showed a hematogenous pattern of spread to the spinal cord. The other nine reovirus dsRNA segments are equally represented in the neurally and hematogenously spreading reassortants. If the parental origin (type 1 or type 3) of each gene segment for all the reassortants is analyzed, there is an equal

Table 8.4.
Pattern of spread of type 1 and type 3 reovirus reassortants to the CNS

Origin of Genome Segment[a] Serotype			Differences ($\log_{10}$) in Viral Titer Between Inferior and Superior Spinal Cord After Injection in the Hindlimb Footpad[i]	Pattern of Spread
S1	M2	S4		
1	1	1	0.10	Hematogenous
1	1	3	0.21	Hematogenous
1	3	1	0.48	Hematogenous
1	3	3	0.40	Hematogenous
3	3	3	2.22	Neural
3	1	3	2.82	Neural
3	1	1	2.13	Neural

[a] S1, M2, and S4 are genomic segments of double-stranded RNA. They code for outer capsid proteins. Clearly, the pattern of spread depends on the origin of the S1 segment only. Shown in the original paper, but not here, are the results obtained with reassortment of all other genomic segments from types 1 and 3 viruses. None of these segments influence the results of this experiment and, it is concluded, are not directly involved in the pattern of viral spread.
[b] Mean differences between virus titers in the inferior and superior spinal cord 2 or 3 days after virus inoculation. The original paper shows similar data for the converse experiment, the injection into the forelimb footpad. A difference of 100-fold, or 2.0 on a $\log_{10}$ scale is considered indicative of neural spread, while small differences indicate hematogenous spread.

representation of both parental genotypes, indicating that the genetic mapping was not the result of any preexisting bias favoring the selection of specific genes.

The S1 dsRNA segment of reovirus type 1 and type 3 has been cloned and sequenced previously. The messenger RNA derived from this dsRNA is functionally dicistronic and directs the synthesis of two distinct reovirus proteins. These two proteins are the *viral hemagglutinin* and a small protein that is not part of the virion but is found in infected cells. Although our genetic analysis does not permit a definitive conclusion about which of these two S1 encoded proteins is responsible for determining the pattern of spread of reoviruses, the viral hemagglutinin appears to be the logical candidate. The hemagglutinin is the viral cell attachment protein that determines the tropism of reovirus type 3 for neurons and the tropism of reovirus type 1 for ependymal cells. Passive immunization of mice with monoclonal antibodies (mAbs) directed against the type 3 hemagglutinin, but not with mAbs to type 1 hemagglutinin, inhibits the neural spread of type 3.

In conclusion, our results provide evidence that two serotypes of the same virus use different pathways to spread to the CNS. Reovirus type 3 spreads to the CNS via microtubule-associated fast axonal transport, whereas reovirus type 1 spreads to the CNS via the bloodstream. Using reassortant viruses, we showed that the reovirus S1 dsRNA segment is responsible for determining the capacity of reoviruses to utilize discrete pathways to spread in the infected host, and we suggest that this is mediated via the viral hemagglutinin.

Questions and Comments

This work convincingly demonstrates that two different serotypes of reovirus reach their CNS target by different pathways. Further, it demonstrates that this difference is determined by a specific segment of the viral genome. The original article should be read for interesting details (omitted here) about the transport mechanisms involved.

1. Can you reconstruct the two anatomic experiments that showed the two modes of spread? Do you find the findings sufficient for the conclusions derived?

2. Experiments to identify the genomic segment that determines the mode of spreading relied on the peculiar genomic structure of these viruses. Does this work remind you of classical mendelian genetics, the study of chromosome reassortments?

3. Genetic studies that depend on linkage relationship between genes are difficult to carry out with these viruses. What difficulties are associated with RNA viruses in general? With viruses with segmented genomes in particular?

4. What could be done to study the genetics of these viruses? Could you take advantage of cloning techniques? Could you work directly with the RNA segments, or would you have to convert them into corresponding DNA segments? How would you do that? What would you do with such DNA?

5. How might knowledge of the mode of spread of a virus help design suitable prophylactic or therapeutic strategies? Under what circumstances would a vaccine work better? For which type of virus would the administration of antisera to patients be most indicated?

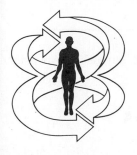

Normal Microbial Flora

M. Schaechter

We live in a microbial world: The human body normally contains thousands of species of bacteria and a smaller number of viruses, fungi, and protozoa. The great majority are commensals, meaning that they eat alongside us without causing harm. We do not carry all of them all the time, but their number at any instant is still formidable. Each of us has a distinct spectrum of microorganisms and, microbiologically speaking, we are highly individualized. In the words of the Romans, *suum quique*, to each his own.

WHAT IS THE NORMAL FLORA?

We define as members of the normal flora those microorganisms that are frequently found on or within the body of healthy persons. Some of these organisms are only found in association with the body of humans or animals, others live freely in the environment.

The line of demarcation of what constitutes the normal flora is often fuzzy. Consider, for instance, the meningococcus or the pneumococcus. Either one is found in the throat of about 10% of healthy people; thus, they can be counted as members of the normal flora in these individuals but not in 90% of the population. In any one of us they may come and go as sporadic denizens of our throat. Therefore, such organisms should be called transient members of the normal flora of some individuals.

The problem with definitions in this field is that they are not absolute. The same problems in defining what constitutes the normal microbial flora pertain to terms such as pathogenicity and virulence. As we will see in subsequent chapters, these terms depend not only on properties of the infectious agent, but also on the state of the defenses of the host.

THE IMPORTANCE OF THE NORMAL FLORA IN HEALTH AND DISEASE

A Common Source of Infection

The normal flora is the source of many opportunistic infections. When our commensal organisms find themselves in unaccustomed sites of the body, they may cause disease. For example, anaerobic bacteria, usually of the genus *Bacteroides*, are carried in the intestine of normal persons and may produce abscesses if they are allowed to penetrate into deeper tissues via traumatic or surgical wounds. Staphylococci from the skin and nose, or streptococci and Gram negative cocci from the throat and mouth, are also responsible for infections of this sort. *In general practice, physicians see more patients with this kind of disease than those afflicted by agents acquired from outside the body.*

These facts point out that the definition of virulence is very elusive and that no microorganism is intrinsically benign or pathogenic. *Under the right circumstances, any microorganism that can grow in our body could cause disease.* This statement needs to be qualified: Members of the normal flora do not all have the same pathogenic potential. Some cause disease more readily than others because they are endowed with special virulence properties. This is readily seen in peritonitis produced after the release of intestinal bacteria from a break in the gut wall. The resulting infection is usually caused by a small number of bacteria, comprising a small fraction of the total number of species in the inoculum.

The definition of virulence is not intrinsic to the microorganisms but depends also on the state of immunocompetency of the host. Members of the normal flora often invade organs and tissues in immunocompromised patients. Thus the yeast *Candida*, a harmless commensal in about one third of normal people, is a common agent of pneumonia in patients undergoing vigorous cancer chemotherapy. *Pneumocystis carinii*, is a common inhabitant of the lungs of healthy persons, but becomes one of the principal causes of death in patients with AIDS.

Immune Stimulation

Our repertoire of immunoglobulins reflects in part the antigenic stimulation by the normal flora. In general, we do not have high antibody titers to the individual bacteria, viruses, or fungi that inhabit our body. Nonetheless, even in low concentrations these antibodies serve as a defense mechanism. Here, then, is a clear benefit from our normal flora. Among the antibodies produced in response to bacterial stimulation are those of the IgA class, which are secreted through mucous membranes. While the role of these immunoglobulins is not well understood, it seems reasonable that they are an important first line of defense and that they interfere, possibly on a daily basis, with the colonization of deeper tissues by commensal organisms.

Antibodies elicited by the antigenic challenge of the normal flora sometimes cross-react with normal tissue components. A good example are antibodies against the ABO blood group substances. You may remember that people that belong to the A group have anti-B antibodies and, conversely, B group individuals make anti-A antibodies. People in the O group make both anti-A and anti-B antibodies.

You may wonder about the source of antigenic stimulation for these antibodies. On reflection, this is not obvious. Why should one make antibodies against a blood group different than one's own? The reason is not that we come in contact with red blood cells of a different type, since obviously very few of us get blood transfusions, especially with the wrong type blood. The answer to this puzzle is that bacteria from the intestinal flora contain antigens that cross-react with both A and B blood substance. These antigens are a source of antigenic stimulation. We make antibodies against these foreign blood group antigens but not against those of our own group because we are immunologically tolerant to the "self" antigens but not to the "foreign" ones.

This type of cross-reactivity does not usually cause disease. It is possible, however, for antibodies cross-reactive to microbial antigens to play an insidious role. For instance, the serious disease lupus erythematosus is associated with the production of antibodies against one's own DNA. There is some evidence that the antigens that set off the production of these antibodies are not nucleic acids but may be cross-reacting bacterial lipopolysaccharides.

Keeping Out Invaders

In some sites of the body the normal flora keeps out pathogens. This happens in two ways. (*a*) Commensal bacteria have the physical advantage of previous occupancy, especially on epithelial surfaces. (*b*) Some commensal bacteria produce substances that are inhibitors to newcomers, such as antibiotics or lethal proteins called bacteriocins. It is not surprising, therefore, that colonization by a new species or a new strain is not a frequent event.

This old fact became relevant once again in the 1970s in connection with experiments done to assess the safety of new bacterial strains engineered by molecular cloning. The most commonly used organism for this purpose was (and probably still is) a particular strain of *Escherichia coli* called K12. This strain was originally isolated from a person's feces, but has had a long residence in the laboratory. When human volunteers were fed this strain in large numbers, they retained it for only 1 day. The conventional interpretation is that in its sojourn in the laboratory the strain had lost its colonizing capacity. In other words, this strain can no longer out compete the resident members of the bacterial flora of the gut.

When the normal flora is nearly wiped out with antibiotics, both exogenous and endogenous microorganisms are given the chance to cause disease. For example, the infecting dose of a *Salmonella* strain decreases almost a millionfold after mice are given streptomycin. Patients treated with certain antibiotics that are particularly effective in the gut may suffer from diarrhea, due to the overgrowth of yeasts or staphylococci. With the administration of some drugs, notably clindamycin, a particular organism, *Clostridium difficile* produces a serious disease called pseudomembranous colitis (see Chapter 21). This organism is a minor member of the normal flora but can grow to a large population density when its neighbors are suppressed.

A Role in Human Nutrition and Metabolism?

The normal flora of the intestine plays a role in human nutrition and metabolism, but little is known about the extent of its influence. Why is it so difficult to figure this out? Obviously, humans cannot be made "germ free" at will; most of the information comes from work with animals and its relevance to human nutrition is uncertain. Nonetheless, it is likely that a biomass as huge and metabolically active as that in the large intestine plays a role in the nutritional balance of the host. It is known, for instance, that several intestinal bacteria, e.g., *E. coli* and *Bacteroides* species, synthesize vitamin K, and this may be an important source of this vitamin for human beings and animals.

The metabolism of several key compounds involves excretion from the liver into the intestine and their return from there to the liver. This enterohepatic circulatory loop is particularly important for sex steroid hormones and bile salts. These substances are excreted through the bile in conjugated form as glucuronides or sulfates but cannot be reabsorbed in this form. Members of the intestinal bacterial flora make glucuronidases and sulfatases that can deconjugate these compounds. The extent to which these activities are physiologically important is not yet known.

A Source of Carcinogens?

The flora of the large intestine may produce carcinogens. The compounds we ingest are chemically transformed by the varied metabolic activities of the gut flora. Many potential carcinogens are active only after being modified. Some of the known modifications are carried out by enzymes of intestinal bacteria. An example is the artificial sweetener cyclamate (cyclohexamine sulfate), which is converted to the active bladder carcinogen cyclohexamine by bacterial sulfatases. The importance of the normal flora in production of carcinogens is difficult to assess but is a subject of considerable scrutiny.

HOW DO WE STUDY WHAT THE NORMAL FLORA DOES?

Much of what we know about the role of the normal flora in nutrition and prevention of disease comes from studying animals reared under sterile conditions, the so-called *germ-free animals*. Rats and mice resemble humans in many physiological properties but differ in important details. Nonetheless, germ-free animal research has produced interesting information.

Small mammals can be reared in the germ-free condition if they are placed in a sterile chamber after a cesarean birth. Chickens can be hatched from eggs whose shell surface has been sterilized. Usually the germ-free chamber is provided with gloves and ports to allow manipulation and the exchange of food and other material without breaking the sterility barrier. Many species of animals breed under these conditions and large colonies can be established. It is even possible to buy germ-free rats and mice from commercial suppliers.

In general, rodents thrive under these conditions as long as their diet is supplemented with vitamins. They even gain weight faster than do conventional animals. As expected, their concentration of immunoglobulins is reduced, especially if the diet is chemically defined and does not contain antigenic compounds. One of the more interesting characteristics of germ-free animals is that the histology of their intestines looks quite different from the usual. The most visible difference is in the lamina propria, which has only a few lymphocytes, plasma cells, and macrophages. By contrast, in conventional animals, the same tissue is heavily infiltrated with these cells. This suggests that the "normal" intestine is in a constant state of chronic inflammation!

WHAT PARTS OF THE BODY ARE INVOLVED?

Let us now consider the parts of the body that are colonized by the normal flora. Those that usually contain large amounts of microorganisms are

• Skin

• Respiratory tract: nose and oropharynx

• Digestive tract: mouth and large intestine

• Urinary tract: anterior parts of the urethra

• Genital system: vagina

Bacteria, and to lesser extent fungi and protozoa, reside and actively proliferate at these sites. Other parts of the body contain small numbers of microorganisms, most often in transit. These sites include the rest of the respiratory and digestive tracts, the bladder and the uterus. Finding pathogenic microorganisms at these sites is highly suggestive of disease, but is not proof. At the other extreme are certain tissues and organs that are usually sterile. The presence of microorganisms at these sites is usually considered of diagnostic significance. Included here are blood, cerebrospinal fluid, synovial fluid, and deep tissues in general.

The number of bacteria in sites which contain thriving microbial communities varies over a wide range. In highly protected areas bacteria are almost as densely packed as is physically possible. For instance, the gingival pockets around teeth contain wall-to-wall bacteria. Normal feces consist of about one third bacteria by weight. It may be worth realizing what that represents in terms of the number of organisms. If the average bacteria are about 1 μm^3 in volume, the densest possible packing would result in a mass of 1×10^{12} ml. Such numbers are actually approached in the "buggiest" parts of the body. In contrast, sites that are not quite as hospitable, such as skin, mouth, and vagina, may have populations that are more of the order of 1 to 10 million bacteria per milliliter of fluid or per gram of scrapings.

THE MEMBERS OF THE NORMAL FLORA

What types of microorganisms constitute the normal flora? The vast majority are bacteria. We also carry viruses, fungi, protozoa, and occasionally worms, but in the healthy person these are present in smaller numbers than the bacteria. In the early days of microbiology, it was thought that most bacteria of the body were aerobes or facultative anaerobes. For a long time *E. coli* was believed to be one of the principal members of the fecal flora. This erroneous conclusion was due to the fact that most of the members of the normal bacteria flora are strict anaerobes. Thus, they do not grow on media incubated in the ordinary manner in air. Only by using special techniques of anaerobic cultivation has it been realized that in the gingival pocket or in feces, strict anaerobes outnumber the others by 1000 to 1 or more. Bacteria do not have to be located far from the air to find themselves under anaerobic conditions, because oxygen has very low solubility in water. Furthermore, the few molecules of oxygen that diffuse into deeper layers are readily used by host cells or by actively metabolizing aerobes and facultative anaerobes. Thus, anaerobic conditions can be found a fraction of a millimeter below the surface.

TABLE 9.1

The normal bacterial flora: examples of frequent types

	Gram Positive		Gram Negative		
	Cocci	Rods	Cocci	Rods	Others
Skin	Staphylococci	*Corynebacteria* *Propionobacterium acnes*		Enteric bacilli (on some sites)	
Oropharynx	α-hemolytic streptococci Gaffkya, micrococcus	Corynebacteria	*Neisseria*	*Haemophilus* *Bacteroides*	Mycoplasma Spirochetes
Large intestine	Streptococci (enterococci)	Lactobacilli Clostridia	Several types	Enteric bacilli *Bacteroides* *Pseudomonas*	Spirochetes Mycoplasma
Vagina	Streptococci	Lactobacilli		*Bacteroides*	Mycoplasma

Table 9.1 shows the distribution and occurrence of the most prominent bacteria in selected parts of the human body. It should be understood that the organisms mentioned, although the most frequently encountered, represent only a minute fraction of the number of genera and species represented. The total number of taxonomic groups is probably well in the thousands. As an example, in a particularly detailed study the intestinal flora of a single person alone yielded about 400 distinct species of bacteria!

Newborn babies become colonized very rapidly by a varied microbial flora, especially in their intestine. In animals and probably in humans, there is a time sequence in the appearance of different organisms. The earliest colonizers are *E. coli*, streptococci, and some clostridia. Within 24 hours or so, lactobacilli appear and are followed within a few days by the major anaerobes that characterize the normal intestinal flora.

Little is known of the complex reasons why different species vary in their colonizing capacity and in their ability to compete with others. It seems likely that specific properties of bacteria, such as their pili, allow them to attach and survive in different microenvironments within the intestine. Thus, the microbial flora is different at the base of the intestinal crypts, in the mucus that covers the villi, or in the lumen of the gut. Normally, the intestinal flora of one individual is remarkably constant. This stability suggests that each successful colonizer is equipped with powerful devices to withstand the challenge from newly ingested microorganisms.

CONCLUSIONS

Our knowledge about the role of the normal flora in health and disease is derived largely from a few circumstances of uncertain significance: studies with germ-free animals, observation of patients on antibiotics, etc. We are left with the impression that from the immunological and microbiological point of view, the normal flora contribute to the maintenance of health mainly by excluding potential invaders and possibly by long-term immunological stimulation. Nutritionally speaking, the microbial biomass within us plays a role in recycling certain important compounds and probably in supplying vitamin K. The negative side is that members of the normal flora are opportunistic pathogens and may cause disease when present in unaccustomed tissues and organs. We do not have the choice of living in a germ-free environment. In a microbe-laden world, it is reasonable to conclude that the normal microbial flora is adapted to do more good than harm.

SELF-ASSESSMENT QUESTIONS

1. Name some infections due to members of the normal flora and the factors that allowed them to cause disease.

2. What is the immunological significance of the normal flora?

3. How does the normal flora ward off colonization by external pathogens?

4. Which portions of the body are usually heavily colonized? Which have a transient microbial flora? Which are usually sterile? What main factors dictate these ecological relationships?

5. Which main groups of bacteria are associated with the heavily colonized parts of the body?

6. What general strategies are available to study the role of the normal flora?

SUGGESTED READINGS

Rosebury T: *Microorganisms Indigenous to Man.* New York, McGraw-Hill, 1962.
Rosebury T: *Life on Man.* New York, Viking Press, 1969 (a delightful popularization).

The Infectious Agents

Bacteria

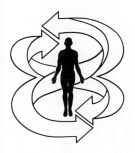

Introduction to the Pathogenic Bacteria

M. Schaechter

Thousands of species of bacteria, both commensal and pathogenic, are found in association with the human body. You will need to know only the principal ones, but even that makes a long list. Before venturing into the thicket of bacterial taxonomy, you may consider a few guide posts. It is useful, for instance, to learn the names of the organisms in relation to where they fit in the microbial scheme of things. For example, it is helpful to know that staphylococci and streptococci both belong to a group called the *Gram-positive cocci*, that *Escherichia coli* is classified among the *Gram-negative enteric bacteria*, that the tubercle bacillus belongs to the *acid-fast bacteria*, and so forth. This chapter is intended as a study aid. We recommend that you do not try to assimilate all this material at once, but that you refer to this chapter later when studying individual types of bacteria.

We will use a practical scheme to divide the main pathogenic bacteria rather than ones used in the science of bacterial taxonomy (Fig. 10.1). In broad terms, medically interesting bacteria belong to one of two large categories:

- The "typical" bacteria, rods and spheres without many morphological embellishments; these "garden variety" bacteria include both Gram positive and Gram negative rods and cocci.
- Those that do not fall in this group.

Like all other forms of life, bacteria are named by their genus, as in *Escherichia*, and species, as in *coli*. Conventionally, after its first use in a text, the genus name is shortened to the first letter, e.g. *E. coli*. Many bacteria also have common names, usually related to the main disease they cause, e.g., the "cholera bacillus",

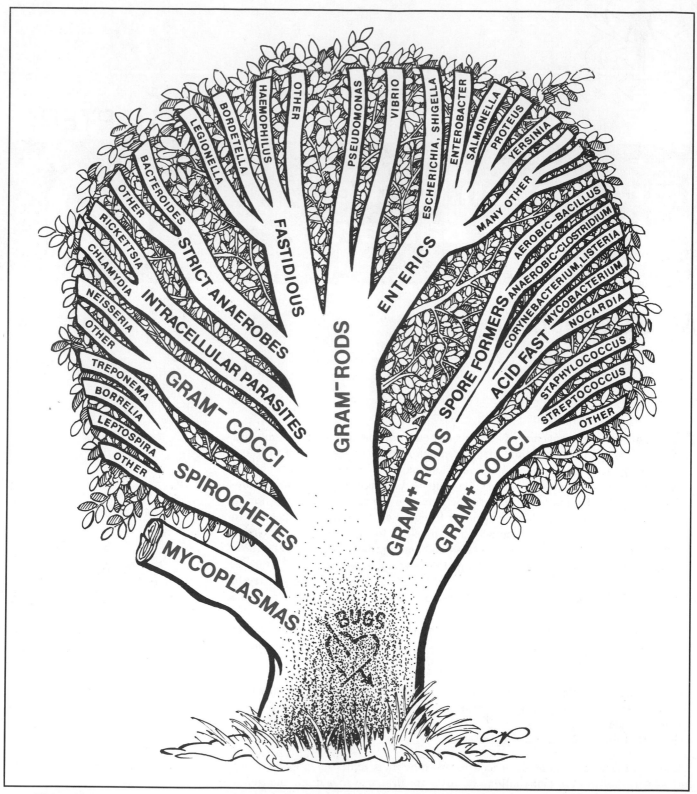

Figure 10.1. The major groups of medically important bacteria. This illustration is a practical representation of the principal groups of pathogenic bacteria. It is meant to be a study aid, and not a taxonomic or phylogenetic tree.

the "tubercle bacillus". Occasionally it may be useful to figure out the derivation of genus and species names. Many of them attempt to honor famous microbiologists (e.g., *Escherichia* is named after Dr. Escherich, *Salmonella* after Dr. Salmon and not after the fish), but some are descriptive. To take examples from other areas of microbiology, "retrovirus" refers to viruses that replicate using reverse transcriptase, "pyogenes" (as in *Streptococcus pyogenes*) indicates that it causes pus, and "nana" (dwarf) means that *Hymenolepis nana* is the "dwarf tapeworm".

A confusing aspect of bacterial taxonomy is that there is usually considerable variety within a species. Thus, a *Staphylococcus aureus* isolated from one patient may be distinctly virulent, whereas another one may not be. We refer to these isolates as *strains*. The point is well illustrated with *Escherichia coli*: This designation includes the common strain of molecular biology, known as K12, as well as less benevolent ones that cause infection of the kidney, the intestine, or the meninges. All are *E. coli*, but each is of a different strain.

"TYPICAL" BACTERIA

Please recall that the *Gram stain* property reflects fundamental differences among bacteria. These differences are mainly in their permeability properties and surface components. The chief differences are the presence of an outer membrane in the Gram negatives and of a thick murein layer in the Gram positives (Chapter 2). These organisms can also be divided into rods and cocci, giving us four boxes in which to place them (Fig. 10.2).

Keep in mind that Gram positives differ more from Gram negatives than cocci do from rods. For instance, the streptococci, which are Gram positive, are closely related to certain Gram positive rods, the lactobacilli, but quite distant from Gram negative cocci such as the gonococci.

In the laboratory, the Gram stain makes the positives look dark violet; the negatives look red (see Chapter 2 for details). If you have never done a Gram stain or if you have forgotten how, it is performed by first treating a smear with a stain called crystal violet, which is taken up by most bacteria. Second, after washing with water, the slide is exposed to a solution of iodine. This modifies the violet dye to make a dye-iodine complex. Third, the preparation is treated with alcohol or acetone for a brief time, a few seconds. At this point, Gram positives retain the violet dye and Gram negatives are decolorized. This step must be carried out with care since too short a treatment will result in underdecolorization and all the stained bacteria will remain violet. Overdecolorization, on the other hand, will remove the dye from Gram positives. With experience, this step can be done just right. In order to be able to see the now colorless Gram negatives, the fourth step is to counterstain them with a red dye.

The four groups in Figure 10.2 are fairly evenly represented in the normal flora of the bacteria-rich milieu of the body, the mouth, the pharynx, and the large intestine. This is not true for the major pathogenic organisms. The Gram-positive cocci and the Gram-negative rods are the most common agents of infections, followed by the Gram-negative cocci, and last, the Gram-positive rods.

Gram-positive Cocci	Gram-positive Rods
Gram-negative Cocci	Gram-negative Rods

Figure 10.2. The "big four" typical bacteria.

Gram-Positive Cocci

Streptococci

Streptococci grow in chains of round cells—like strings of pearls—and constitute a large and diverse group. They are subdivided according to the changes they produce when grown on agar containing blood. Thus, *β-hemolytic* streptococci (or "beta strep") which cause most streptococcal infections, lyse the red blood cell, causing an area of clearing around the colonies. The *α-hemolytic* streptococci produce a different change, a greening of the hemoglobin. Other streptococci do not change the blood at all. Many streptococci are nonpathogenic and are found in the environment as well as in the normal human intestine. Some are associated with dairy products and contribute to the manufacture of cheese.

Streptococci do not carry out respiration but only fermentation. This is characteristic of anaerobic bacteria, and indeed some streptococci are strict anaerobes. Most of the pathogenic species grow in air, which makes them *oxygen-tolerant anaerobes*. Colonies of streptococci are usually small on agar. Streptococci make a lot of extracellular proteins, some of which are virulence factors involved in spreading the organisms through tissues and damaging host cells.

The main pathogens in this genus are the *β*-hemolytic strains. These are further subclassified into groups by the presence of different so called C antigens, which are cell wall polysaccharides. Of all the groups (A through R) the most important ones in human disease are those of group A. They cause "strep throat", infections of soft tissues elsewhere and other serious infections. These infections may be followed by important complications, such as rheumatic fever or glomerulonephritis. The full taxonomic name of these organisms is *Streptococcus pyogenes*, but you will hear them referred to as "group A strep."

Staphylococci

There are three main species of staphylococci; thus this group is not as diverse as the streptococci. They are called *Staphylococcus aureus*, *S. epidermidis*, and *S. saprophyticus*. Staph cells have no specific arrangement under the microscope but look like arrays of buckshot or bunches of grapes ("staphylo" comes from the Greek word for grapes). They are more robust than streptococci and withstand many chemical and physical agents and are hard to eradicate from the human environment. They make larger colonies on agar and are aerobes.

Staphylococci are found on many sites of the body, especially the skin. They are the most likely organisms to cause pus in wounds and may produce serious infections in deep tissues, such as osteomyelitis (infection of the bone marrow), endocarditis (infection of the heart valves), etc. Like the streptococci, they also secrete a large number of extracellular enzymes and toxins. One of these, *coagulase*, clots plasma and is useful in classification since only the more pathogenic species, *S. aureus*, makes this enzyme.

Gram-Negative Cocci

Gram-negative cocci include several genera of medical importance, but the most important one is the *Neisseria*. This genus includes many organisms found in the normal mouth and pharynx and two important pathogens, the *gonococcus* and the *meningococcus*. Like all Gram negatives, they possess an outer membrane that contains endotoxin (lipopolysaccharide). The gonococcus obviously causes gonorrhea, and the meningococcus meningitis and a severe septicemia.

Gram-Positive Rods

Gram-positive rods are abundant in the environment; this group includes bacteria that only infrequently cause diseases, at least in the developed regions of the world. One, diphtheria, was a deadly disease in children until vaccination nearly eradicated it. The agent of diphtheria is called *Corynebacterium diphtheriae* and has many relatives called *diphtheroids*. These are common inhabitants of the skin and mucous membranes and can cause opportunistic infections. (Note that "diphtheria" is spelled with two "aitches".)

In the human environment, the most common organisms in this group are the *spore-forming rods*. Microscopically, they are the largest of the "typical" bacteria, 5 to 10 times the volume of an average *E. coli*, about 1 μm^3. They are divided into two genera: the aerobic *Bacillus*, whose only important pathogen is *B. anthracis*, which causes anthrax, and the strict anaerobes, members of the genus *Clostridum*. Clostridia are medically important because they include species like *C. botulinum*, which cause botulism, *C. tetani*, the agent of tetanus, and several that produce gas gangrene (most often *C. perfringens*). Symptoms of these diseases are caused by powerful exotoxins.

Another important pathogen among the Gram-positive rods is *Listeria monocytogenes*, which occasionally causes serious infections in infants and in adults who are immunocompromised.

Gram-Negative Rods

Enteric Bacteria

The Gram-negative rods are a large group of bacteria and include many important pathogens. Here the enteric bacteria stand out. Their paradigm is *E. coli*, the "typical" bacterium par excellence. The enteric bacteria (for family *Enterobacteriaceae*) comprise many genera, including the *Salmonella* of typhoid fever and food poisoning and the *Shigella* of bacillary dysentery. The enteric bacteria have in common the ability to grow readily on laboratory media, to make middle sized colonies (usually less than 1 mm across), not to make spores, or have special cell arrangements. Many, but not all, are motile. They are divided among those that ferment lactose (*E. coli* and others), and those that do not (*Salmonella*, *Shigella*). Although many pathogens are nonlactose fermenters, this is not a firm rule and has many exceptions both ways. Included in the enterics are also the organisms that cause plague and certain intestinal infections (*Yersinia*).

Among their more distant cousins are Gram-negative rods that differ in metabolism and somewhat in morphology. These include the genus *Pseudomonas* (agents of "blue pus", so called because of a pigment made by these organisms) and the cholera bacillus, *Vibrio cholerae*. A close relative of *Vibrio* is *Campylobacter jejuni*, a common agent of infectious diarrhea. Pseudomonads, as the members of the *Pseudomonas* are sometimes called, are often found in waters—rivers, lakes, swimming pools, tap water—frequent sources of human infection.

"Fastidious Small Gram-Negative Rods"

Besides the organisms mentioned above, the Gram-negative rods include an important and heterogeneous group of genera. They can be lumped, somewhat arbitrarily, into a group that may be awkwardly described as the "fastidious, small, Gram-negative rods" because they have complex nutritional requirements and tend to be smaller than, for example, *E. coli*. Included in this group are the following genera: *Haemophilus* (pneumonia and meningitis), *Bordetella* (whooping cough), *Brucella* (brucellosis), *Francisella* (tularemia), and others. *Legionella*, the agent of Legionnaires' disease, is also a small Gram-negative rod but varies considerably from the others in its habitat (soil, water) and chemical composition.

Strictly Anaerobic Gram-Negative Rods

Lastly, an important group of Gram-negative rods is distinguished by its strict anaerobic way of life. Clinically, the most noteworthy of these organisms belongs to the genus *Bacteroides*. They are extremely common in the human body, often the most frequent members of the intestinal flora. They are also found in the gingival pockets that surround the teeth. Normally not bothersome, members of this genus may cause serious diseases when deposited in deep tissues. They are associated, for example, with peritonitis, the abdominal infection that results from the outpouring of intestinal content into the peritoneum. These organisms usually do not cause disease alone but are found in association with other bacteria to cause mixed or polymicrobial infections. Obviously, they will not grow if incubated aerobically and require special anaerobic techniques for their growth and detection.

"NOT SO TYPICAL" BACTERIA

The "not so typical bacteria," a taxonomic hodgepodge, includes organisms that have their own special characteristics with regard to shape, size, or staining properties. They do not have much in common, other than being of medical importance. Each group, then, stands alone.

Acid-Fast Bacteria

Acid-fast bacteria are almost synonymous with the genus *Mycobacterium*, which includes the *tubercle bacillus*, *M. tuberculosis*, and the *leprosy bacillus*, *M. leprae*. Acid fastness refers to the fact that these organisms are nearly impervious to many chemicals and must be stained by a special procedure (Chapter 2). They are surrounded by a waxy envelope that can be penetrated by dyes only if the bacteria are heated or treated with detergents. For them the Gram stain is irrelevant since they do not take up regular dyes.

The special staining procedure used is called the *Ziehl-Neelsen* technique. Its most frequently used modification consists of treating smears with a solution of a red dye (fuchsin) that contains detergents. After washing, the smear is treated with a solution of 3% hydrochloric acid that removes the dye from all bacteria except the acid-fast ones. The preparation is then exposed to a blue dye, which counterstains other bacteria, white blood cells, etc. Tubercle or leprosy bacilli, the "red bugs", are clearly visible against the blue background.

Several species of mycobacteria found free living in the environment may cause opportunistic infections, especially in immunocompromised patients. These environmental species are sometimes called *atypical acid-fast bacilli*, AFBs. All mycobacteria grow slowly and are quite resistant to chemical agents but not to heat.

The name of this genus contains the root word for fungus (*myco-*). The reason is that these organisms sometimes form branches that vaguely suggest the fungi. Even more akin to fungi in morphology are relatives of the mycobacteria, the *Actinomycetes*. These organisms take up the Gram stain and are Gram positive.

Some are also weakly acid fast. They make true branches and long filaments with complex structures, which places them among the most highly differentiated of the procaryotes. There are two pathogenic genera: *Nocardia*, which are aerobic, and *Actinomyces*, which are strict anaerobes. They cause certain forms of pneumonia and soft tissue infections. A generally nonpathogenic genus, *Streptomyces*, includes organisms that make important antibiotics (streptomycin, tetracycline, etc.).

Spirochetes

Spirochete bacteria are helical, in the shape of a spring (not a screw.) They include the agent of syphilis, *Treponema pallidum*, whose species name ("pale") refers to the fact that these organisms are so thin that they do not take up enough dye to be readily seen under the microscope. Unstained, they can be seen with a phase contrast or a dark-field microscope. The spirochetes of syphilis have the distinction of not being readily cultivated in the laboratory.

Other spirochetes include the genus *Leptospira*, which cause a disease called icterohemorrhagic fever, and *Borrelia recurrentis*, the agent of relapsing fever. A recently described disease known as Lyme disease (after the town in Connecticut) is also caused by a spirochete, *Borrelia burgdorferi*. Lyme disease may become one of the most important spirochetoses in the eastern and western United States. All the organisms of this group stand out because of their distinct helical morphology.

Chlamydiae

Chlamydiae are small strict intracellular little bacteria that cannot be grown in artificial media. They are among the smallest cellular forms of life but have a fairly complex life cycle. They possess a different morphological form when they are growing inside cells or when they are in transit between them. They are the most common cause of sexually transmitted diseases (chlamydial urethritis) and other more unusual infections. They set up housekeeping in phagocytic vesicles of their host cells and obtain their energy from them.

Rickettsiae

Rickettsiae are also small, intracellular bacteria and cause epidemic typhus, Rocky Mountain spotted fever, and other diseases. Each species is transmitted by the bite of a different kind of arthropod (lice, fleas, ticks, etc.), with the exception of *Coxiella burnetii*, the agent of Q fever, which may also be acquired by inhalation. Rickettsiae are small rod-shaped bacteria without distinctive stages in their growth cycle.

Mycoplasma

Perhaps most evolutionarily distant from all other bacteria, Mycoplasmas are organisms that lack a rigid cell wall. They are quite plastic in structure, grow slowly on laboratory media, and have special nutritional requirements. The most unique of these is the need for sterols, which are not required by any other group of bacteria. Mycoplasmas lack murein and, consequently, are resistant to penicillin and other cell wall antibiotics. Only one human pathogen is known with assurance, *Mycoplasma pneumoniae*, which causes a form of pneumonia, but others have been implicated in different diseases.

Mycoplasmas resemble wall-less forms that can be produced in the laboratory, the so-called L forms. Regular bacteria take on the same amorphous appearance as the mycoplasma when their cell wall is removed with lysozyme or when murein synthesis is inhibited with penicillin. This usually leads to cell lysis, but if they are placed in a hypertonic medium they can be grown as colonies that resemble those of the mycoplasma. However, the similarity is only superficial. L forms can usually revert to the regular bacterial form when they are removed from lysozyme or penicillin. Mycoplasmas, on the other hand, do not. Mycoplasmas also differ from all other bacteria in terms of the degree of relatedness as measured by DNA hybridization.

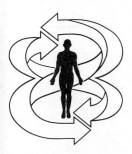

Staphylococci: Abscesses and Other Diseases

F.P. Tally

S taphylococci (Gram-positive cocci) are among the most common of the *pyogenic* or pus-producing bacteria. They produce local abscesses in almost any place in the body, from the skin (pimples) to the bone marrow (osteomyelitis). Occasionally they cause more specific diseases such as endocarditis.

Staphylococci make a large number of toxins and enzymes that act locally, chiefly to help them withstand phagocytosis by neutrophils. They are among the most resistant of the pathogenic bacteria and are hard to eliminate from the human environment. Thus, they are responsible for many hospital-acquired infections. Special strains also produce toxins that cause different types of disease, namely food poisoning, *toxic shock syndrome*, and a disease of children called *scalded skin syndrome*.

CASE

Mr. S., a 45-year-old pastry chef, cut his left forearm with a knife during the course of his work. Over the next week, he noticed swelling, redness, and warmth at the site. He thought it was just a reaction to the cut, but after 4 more days he developed fever with shaking chills and came to the emergency department, with severe low back pain. On physical examination he had a fever of 39.4°C, his left forearm was swollen with an area of central softness, indicating an abscess. He had tenderness to pressure over his lower spine.

The laboratory reported that he had a high white cell count. A Gram stain of pus aspirated from the forearm showed Gram-positive cocci in clusters (Fig. 11.1). Staphylococcus aureus was cultured from the pus. Blood cultures were

Figure 11.1. Gram stain of *Staphylo-coccus aureus* in pus.

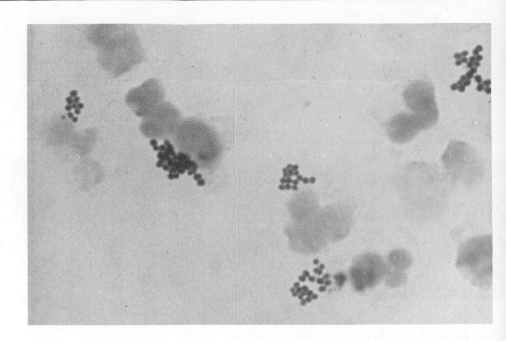

Figure 11.2. X-ray of vertebrae show-ing infection of the intervertebral disk space. Compare the sharp edge of the normal vertebral plates (above and below) with the ragged eroded edges of the involved vertebral plates (*arrows*).

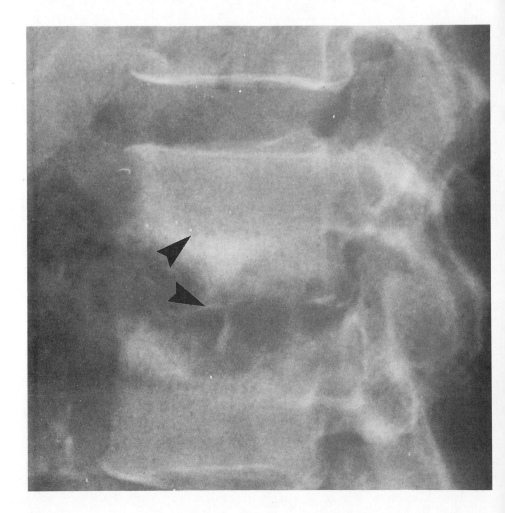

positive for the same organism. X-rays of the lumbar spine showed erosion of the third lumbar vertebra, suggesting the infection called osteomyelitis (Fig. 11.2). The organism was resistant to penicillin but sensitive to oxacillin, which was used to treat Mr. S. with good results.

The day after Mr. S. was admitted to the hospital, the local public health department was notified that eight persons who had patronized his restaurant had developed severe vomiting and diarrhea 4 to 6 hours after eating there. Cultures of cream pies remaining in the refrigerator were positive for S. aureus. A staphylococcal toxin called enterotoxin B was detected in the cream pies. The organisms from the contaminated food belonged to the same phage type (see "The Organism") as the ones isolated from the patient's abscess and blood, and were therefore likely to be the same.

A number of questions arise:

1. What was the source of the organisms that infected Mr. S.?

2. What contributed to the development of the abscess in the skin?

3. How did *S. aureus* invade his bloodstream?

4. How did *S. aureus* cause infection in the bone?

5. What caused the food poisoning in the patrons of Mr. S.'s restaurant?

6. What are the properties of *S. aureus* that allow it to cause such different types of disease?

The case of Mr. S. illustrates several features typical of staphylococcal infections. The initial lesion was mild and localized. It resulted in a boil, which is the most common manifestation of staphylococcal disease. Most of the time this is self-terminating, although in this case it progressed to involve the bloodstream and eventually led to a metastatic involvement of a vertebra. Mr. S. was relatively fortunate because the infection of the vertebra, while highly worrisome, is not immediately life threatening. Had it occurred in his heart or his brain, he would have been at immediate and serious risk.

S. aureus causes more frequent and more varied diseases than perhaps any other human pathogen. Some of these diseases are unrelated with regard to their symptoms and epidemiology. Our case includes infection of the skin, an abscess in deep tissue, and food poisoning, which is far from the end of the list (Table 11.1). Among the more specialized staphylococcal diseases are the toxic shock syndrome, caused by the use of highly absorbent menstrual tampons, and a serious condition of children called scalded skin syndrome.

THE ORGANISM

Staphylococcus aureus is a large Gram positive coccus that grows in clusters. It is one of the hardiest of the non-spore-forming bacteria and can survive for long periods on dry inanimate objects. It is also relatively heat resistant. For these reasons it is hard to eliminate once it is introduced in the human environment.

The genus *Staphylococcus* includes several species (Table 11.2). The most common one is *S. epidermidis*, which is found on the skin of many people and only occasionally causes disease. *S. aureus* is less common but generally more pathogenic. The species name ("golden") refers to the fact that on agar its colonies are pigmented with a bronze color, while other species make white colonies. A third

Table 11.1
Diseases caused by staphylococci

Skin and soft tissue infections
  Furuncles, carbuncles
  Wound infections (traumatic, surgical)
  Cellulitis
  Impetigo (also caused by streptococci)
Bacteremia (frequently with metastatic abscesses)
Endocarditis
Central nervous system infections
  Brain abscess
  Meningitis—rare
  Epidural abscess
Pulmonary infections
  Embolic
  Aspiration
Musculoskeletal
  Osteomyelitis
  Arthritis
Genitourinary tract
  Renal carbuncle
  Lower urinary tract infection
Unrelated diseases caused by toxins
  Toxic shock syndrome
  Scalded skin syndrome
Food poisoning (gastroenteritis)

Table 11.2
Properties of various species of staphylococci

Species	Frequency of Disease	Coagulase	Color of Colonies	Mannitol Fermentation	Novobiocin Resistance
S. aureus	Common	+	Bronze	+	−
S. epidermidis	Common	−	White	−	−
S. saprophyticus	Occasional	−	White	−	+
Others	Different responses by individual species				

species, *S. saprophyticus* is unique in that it apparently causes urinary tract infections only. The genus *Staphylococcus* contains other species of occasional medical importance, which are described in standard microbiological texts. The three species mentioned suffice for our purposes. It is relatively easy to identify this genus in the laboratory. All its members make large, creamy colonies on nutrient agar and in a Gram stain they look like clusters of grapes. *S. aureus* is best distinguished from other species of the genus using the *coagulase test*. Coagulase, an enzyme that clots plasma, is made by *S. aureus* but not by the others.

Within a species of staphylococci, individual *strains* can be identified by differences in resistance to different antibiotics, or, more commonly by a procedure called *phage typing*. This is performed by determining the sensitivity of a strain to a number of standard bacteriophages. Its usefulness in epidemiology can be seen in our case report: Finding the same pattern of phage sensitivity in the isolates from Mr. S.'s abscess and from the contaminated cream pies served to establish their epidemiological link.

ENCOUNTER

Staphylococci share their environment with that of human beings. They live on people and survive on inanimate surfaces with which they have contact, such as bedding, clothing, door knobs, etc.—the so-called fomites. Humans are the major reservoir for *S. aureus*. The organisms frequently colonize the external nares and are found in about 30% of normal individuals. They can also be found transiently on the skin, oropharynx and in feces. Staphylococci are well equipped to colonize the skin since they grow at the high salt and lipid concentrations. In the laboratory they can grow in media containing upward of 10% NaCl, which is unusual among the bacteria associated with humans. The growth of staphylococci and other skin organisms is favored by poor hygiene and the accumulation of dirt and sloughed skin. Moist conditions, as are found in skin folds of obese persons or under occlusive bandages, also favor their growth.

Staphylococci spread from person to person, usually via hand contact. They can also spread by aerosols produced by patients with pneumonia. Babies are colonized shortly after birth, a present from people in their immediate surroundings. Some will become carriers for prolonged periods of time while others will harbor the organisms only intermittently. For unknown reasons, people in certain occupations are more prone to colonization, including physicians, nurses, and other hospital workers. Also, certain patient groups, including diabetics, patients on hemodialysis, and chronic intravenous drug abusers, have a higher carriage rate than the general population.

ENTRY

Staphylococci and most other bacteria do not usually penetrate into deep tissue unless the skin or the mucous membranes are damaged or actually cut. This may come about by burns, accidental wounds, lacerations, insect bites, surgical intervention, or associated skin diseases. In the case of Mr. S., the organisms penetrated via a cut. If present in very large numbers, some bacteria are able to enter spontaneously and cause disease. This happens with staphylococci in cases of poor hygiene or prolonged moisture of the skin, which permit their growth in large numbers. Skin infections can also be caused by immersion into swimming pools that contain large numbers of *Pseudomonas* (Chapter 19). It is not known if these instances are really due to spontaneous penetration or if the organisms enter through unseen cuts and abrasions.

SPREAD AND MULTIPLICATION

Once they have entered tissues, survival of staphylococci depends on several factors: the number of entering organisms, the site involved, the speed with which the body mounts an inflammatory response, and the immunological history of the person. When the inoculum is small and the host is immunologically competent, infections by these and other organisms are usually aborted. Nonetheless staphylococci possess a particularly complex but effective pathogenic strategy and even healthy persons find it difficult to combat *S. aureus*. Luckily, the area of inflammation most often remains localized and the organisms are contained.

DAMAGE

Local staphylococcal infections lead to the formation of a collection of pus called an *abscess*. Abscesses in the skin are called boils, or, in medical parlance, furuncles. Multiple interconnected abscesses are called carbuncles. Alternatively, staphylococci may spread in the subcutaneous or submucosal tissue and cause a diffuse inflammation called *cellulitis*. In most cases, these infections are caused by *S. aureus* and not by the other staphylococcal species.

The development of an abscess is a complex process that involves both bacterial and host factors (Fig. 11.3). The early events are characteristic of an *acute inflammatory* reaction, with the rapid and extensive participation of neutrophils. Chemotactic factors, derived both from bacteria and complement, are made in large amounts. A proportion of the bacteria not only survive this onslaught but are even capable of killing and lysing many of the neutrophils that have ingested them. This results in the outpouring of large amounts of lysosomal enzymes, which damage surrounding tissue.

The inflammatory area rapidly gets surrounded by a thick-walled fibrin capsule. It is tempting to attribute this in part to the coagulase made by the organisms. The center of the abscess is usually necrotic and consists of the debris of dead neutrophils, dead and live bacteria, and edematous fluid. This, then, is an abscess: a well-defined area containing pus. From the point of view of the host it represents a containment of invading organisms in one site. There is, however, an associated cost: Abscesses may cause serious symptoms if they are located in vital parts of the body.

From this picture it becomes apparent that staphylococcal infection represents a titanic struggle between the white blood cells and the invading organisms (Fig.

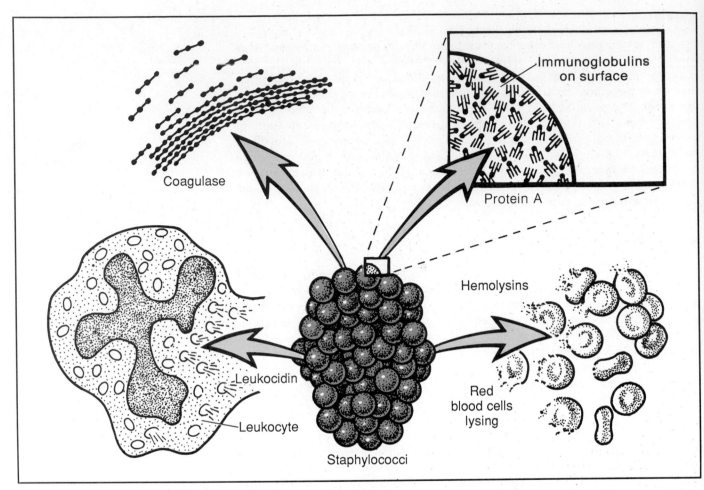

Figure 11.3. Virulence properties of *Staphylococcus aureus* in pus and abscess formation.

11.3). Many of the virulence factors of *S. aureus* are designed either to avoid their being phagocytized or to survive in the phagocytes once taken up. They will be discussed in detail below. Despite their impressive strategy, *S. aureus* do not always win, and neutrophils usually gain the upper hand. The importance of neutrophils in this fight is highlighted in children with a hereditary defect in phagocyte function called *chronic granulomatous disease* (Chapters 4 and 54). This is a fatal disease characterized by frequent and serious infections with *S. aureus*. Neutrophils of these patients are defective in their ability to make sufficient hydrogen peroxide to set off the oxidative killing pathway. In these children the balance between staphylococci and phagocytes is clearly shifted toward the microorganisms.

The interaction between staphylococci and neutrophils is an example of how complex the struggle between them can be. The organisms produce an unusually large number of relevant substances: soluble enzymes, toxins, and constituents of the cell envelopes (Table 11.3). This formidable list invites speculation: Why has it been necessary for these successful organisms to develop such a varied strategy? With other organisms, a capsule suffices to resist phagocytosis. Perhaps different factors predominate in different loci of the infection. The staphylococcal situation is not easy to analyze, and much remains to be learned. The genetic methods outlined in Chapter 8 have been developed in the past few years for

Table 11.3

Soluble virulence factors of *Staphylococcus aureus*

Leukocidin	—Damages white blood cells
Catalase	—Probably reduces killing by phagocytes
Coagulase	—Causes plasma to clot
Hemolysins	—Lyse red blood cells and others (five kinds known)
Hyaluronidase	—May help spread by destroying connective tissue ground substance
β-Lactamase	—Inactivates penicillins
Exfoliatin	—Causes sloughing of skin in scalded skin syndrome
Toxic shock toxin	—Involved in toxic shock syndrome
Enterotoxins	—Cause food poisoning (seven kinds known)

these organisms, and studies of staphylococcal pathogenesis using this approach are under way.

What are the main factors that are thought to allow survival vis-a-vis the neutrophils? To begin with the cell surface: *S. aureus* are sometimes surrounded by a *capsule* that prevents phagocytosis, but probably not to the extent seen with pneumococci or meningococci. The cell wall *murein* of *S. aureus* activates complement by the alternate pathway, thus contributing to the inflammatory response. Note that in this regard staphylococcal murein resembles the endotoxin of Gram negatives. Another important wall constituent is *teichoic acid* (a polymer of ribitol and glycerophosphates; see Chapter 2), which also appears to be involved in complement activation and possibly in the adherence of these organisms to mucosal cells.

A fourth wall component, *protein A*, has a most unexpected property: it binds nonspecifically to the Fc terminus of immunoglobulin G of almost all subclasses (Fig. 11.3). This incapacitates these molecules in their function as antibodies since their business end, the Fab portion, is now dangling away from the surface of the organisms. This interferes with opsonization by reducing the amount of Fc residues available for opsonization. Although the protein A-Fc combination is nonspecific, it acts like an antigen-antibody complex in that it activates complement through the classical pathway.

In addition to these components, *S. aureus* secretes several enzymes and toxins that are almost certainly directed towards the struggle with phagocytes (Fig. 11.3). *Leukocidin* makes pores in the membrane of neutrophils and is probably responsible for their killing. *Catalase* converts hydrogen peroxide to water and may help counteract the neutrophil's ability to kill via the production of oxygen free radicals. *Coagulase* converts fibrinogen to fibrin and probably helps prevent the organisms from getting phagocytized since white cells penetrate fibrin clots poorly. The role of coagulase sounds plausible because coagulase negative mutants have recently been shown to be less virulent in animal models.

As if this weaponry were insufficient, *S. aureus* elaborates other enzymes that probably participate in its pathogenesis. Among them are several *hemolysins* (α through ε) that may contribute to the availability of iron for the organisms by lysing red blood cells. Many strains make a *hyaluronidase* which hydrolyzes the matrix of connective tissue and perhaps facilitates the spread along tissue planes. Clearer is the role of *β-lactamase*, a powerful enzyme that hydrolyzes the classical penicillins. It is found in about 90% of *S. aureus* strains and is responsible for the infamous penicillin resistance of this organism. The gene for this enzyme is born on plasmids that can be readily transferred, probably accounting for the rapid spread of penicillin resistance among the staphylococci.

In the case of Mr. S., the organisms escaped from the abscess in the skin and found themselves in the bloodstream. This is not the usual outcome since most local staphylococcal diseases are self-limiting and do not result in metastatic infections. In healthy individuals the organisms that escape from the local abscess are usually destroyed by the clearance mechanisms of the blood and the lymph. In the case of Mr. S. there was no reason to think that his defenses were impaired, although this could have been true temporarily. On the other hand, the "shower" of organisms from the skin lesion could have been so great that it overwhelmed the capacity of the body to destroy them. When staphylococci become implanted in deep tissues they colonize best areas that have been previously traumatized by previous diseases or by surgical intervention. Otherwise the choice of the site seems random and is probably dictated by the clearing capacity of the organ and the amount of blood flowing through it. The main sites of metastatic abscesses are highly vascularized organs: bones, lungs, and kidneys. Immunocompromised patients frequently have multiple staphylococcal metastases, which can lead to serious and often fatal diseases.

Once implanted in deep tissue and able to survive, staphylococci elicit an inflammatory reaction similar to that of skin abscess. In the words of Pasteur, "Osteomyelitis is a boil of the bone marrow". The consequences of abscess formation in deep sites depends on their location. Nowhere is it more devastating than in the heart or the brain. On the other hand, if the function of the organ is not directly compromised, staphylococcal abscesses can endure for considerable time and give relatively mild symptoms. At times, these tax the diagnostic acumen of the physician.

This is not the end of the story. *S. epidermidis*, the common inhabitant of the normal skin, rarely causes disease. However, infections with *S. epidermidis* are found with increasing frequency in patients with implanted artificial devices such as prosthetic joints or intravenous catheters. When defense mechanisms are impaired they can cause serious infections, such as septicemia and endocarditis. A potential virulence factor of these organisms is a slime layer that has been found in upwards of 80% of disease-causing isolates. It is thought that this slime layer allows the organisms to stick to the surface of plastics used in various devices.

S. saprophyticus may be the most highly specialized staphylococcus in terms of pathogenicity because it is almost entirely associated with urinary tract infections. The reason for this is not yet known, but seems likely that this organism has unique binding properties to the epithelium of the urethra or the bladder.

In contrast with these classical complicated infections, three staphylococcal diseases are relatively straightforward. The symptoms of each of these diseases are caused by a different toxin. The first is called scalded skin syndrome and is a life-threatening disease of children that results in extensive sloughing of the skin. A toxin, known as exfoliatin, causes these symptoms in laboratory animals. Its role has been clearly established because the administration of specific antitoxin prevents the skin lesions in humans or mice.

A second disease caused by a toxin, called toxic shock syndrome, is characterized by fever, skin rash, hypotension, and the dysfunction of several systems. The disease is associated with the use of highly absorbent menstrual tampons, which apparently foster the growth of the organisms. The toxin involved cannot be studied as readily as exfoliatin because it does not cause all the symptoms of the disease in laboratory animals. It does cause fever by the same mechanism as the endotoxin of enteric bacteria, namely by stimulating the formation of interleukin-1, the endogenous pyrogen. It can be clearly implicated in staphylococcal toxic shock because it has been found in all strains isolated from patients with this disease and only rarely in other isolates.

Finally, there is a group of staphylococcal *enterotoxins*, which are a major cause of food poisoning, as in our case report. They cause intensive intestinal peristalsis, apparently by working directly on the vomit center of the brain. They are very heat stable and are not necessarily destroyed by cooking. These toxins mimic the disease when administered to laboratory animals. Note that the same strain of *S. aureus* can cause several of the diseases mentioned. In the case described here, a single strain was responsible for Mr. S.'s bone and soft tissue infection as well as for food poisoning in the unfortunate people who ate the pastries prepared by him.

DIAGNOSIS

Recognizing staphylococcal infections is not usually a difficult diagnostic problem. They are among the most frequent infections seen both in the community and in the hospital. However, they must be quickly recognized so that appropriate therapy can be initiated.

A localized abscess in a seriously ill patient should be aspirated and the contents examined by the Gram stain and by culture. Clusters of large Gram-positive cocci point to staphylococcal infection. The patient's blood should also be cultured to determine if the organisms have invaded the bloodstream. A common problem with blood cultures is to distinguish between *S. aureus* and *S. epidermidis*, since the latter is a common contaminant and is considered pathogenic only under special circumstances. The coagulase test serves to separate these two species.

THERAPY

A staphylococcal abscess like the one seen in Mr. S. should be drained and an appropriate antibiotic should be administered. The early and widespread arrival of penicillin-resistant strains in the 1960s caused grave therapeutic problems and sent a shock wave through the medical community. It seems entirely in character that the earliest organism to accommodate to these powerful drugs should have been the adaptable staphylococcus.

The human response was to develop penicillins and cephalosporins that are resistant to β-lactamase, the hydrolytic enzyme responsible for penicillin resistance. In most cases, antibiotic resistance is coded for by genes carried on plasmids, which probably accounts for the rapid spread of resistant organisms. There appears to be a race between the synthetic chemists and the organisms, because no sooner are new drugs introduced than reports of staphylococcal resistance begin to appear. More recently, there has been a disturbing increase in numbers of infections caused by staphylococci resistant to the newer β-lactamase-resistant penicillins and cephalosporins. Both *S. aureus* and *S. epidermidis* fall within this group and infections by these organisms require treatment with vancomycin.

Other classes of antibiotics (e.g., aminoglycosides, macrolides) may be useful second line agents in the treatment of certain kinds of staphylococcal infections (particularly in penicillin allergic patients), although some strains are resistant to them as well. The choice of drugs should be based on the antibiotic sensitivity of the infecting strain and the special characteristics of the patient. Therapy should also be sufficiently prolonged to ensure elimination of the organisms.

Over the years vaccines have been developed for the treatment of recurrent, recalcitrant staphylococcal infections and to prevent the carrier state. Success has been limited, probably because circulating antibodies play a relatively minor role in these infections.

CONCLUSION

Staphylococci are potent pathogens, widely found in the human environment and able to cause a number of infections. They are hardy organisms that can survive under adverse conditions. They possess a large number of virulence determinants that allow them to cause serious diseases by different mechanisms. The most common diseases caused by these versatile pathogens are pyogenic infections, sometimes leading to the formation of abscesses in deep tissues. They can also cause distinct disease entities by making specific toxins.

Staphylococci have learned to adapt to new environments by acquiring antimicrobial resistance and even new virulence factors, as witnessed recently by the emergence of a new disease, the toxic shock syndrome. These organisms have been around for a long time and will probably employ new mechanisms to cause serious diseases. It behooves the physician to respect them and to be aware of their presence.

SELF-ASSESSMENT QUESTIONS

1. What general types of diseases are due to staphylococci? Which are the most frequent and serious?

2. What are the structural, physiological, and ecological characteristics of the staphylococci? Which are the main types?

3. Regarding different staphylococcal diseases, how do we encounter these organisms?

4. How do staphylococci enter deep tissues? How do they set up residence? How do they cause disease? Why is this question particularly difficult for some staph infections but not for others?

5. How does the body respond to different staphylococcal infections?

6. What are the therapeutic problems encountered in different staphylococcal infections? How has this changed through recent history?

SUGGESTED READINGS

Chesney PJ, Bergdoll MS, Davis JP, Vergeront JM: The disease spectrum, epidemiology, and etiology of toxic shock syndrome. *Annu Rev Microbial* 38:315, 1984.

Easmon CSF, Adlam C: *Staphylococci and Staphylococcal Infections.* New York, Academic Press, 1983.

Radetsky P: The rise and (maybe not the) fall of toxic shock syndrome. *Science* 85:72, 1985.

Sheagren, J.N. *Staphylococcus aureus:* the persistent pathogen. Parts 1 and 2. *N Engl J Med,* 310:1368–1373, 1437–1442; 1984.

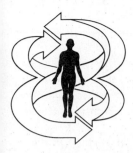

The Streptococci

12

D.T. Durack

The genus *Streptococcus* includes a large number of Gram positive cocci. Some cause disease in humans and animals, others live on the human body as commensals, and yet others are found freely in the environment. The pathogens among them also comprise a heterogeneous group that is responsible for a wide spectrum of diseases.

The best known of these bacteria is *Streptococcus pyogenes*, also called "group A strep", which causes *pyogenic infections* in many organs and tissues, ranging from "strep throat" to deep tissue infections. Other streptococci cause specific infections in newborns, elderly persons, or immunocompromised patients.

CASE

Stephanie, a healthy 10-year-old, complained of a sore throat as she left for school one morning in March. Later that day she became feverish, with nausea and vomiting. Her mother picked her up from school and took her to a pediatrician who found her to be flushed and distressed, with a temperature of 39.9°C. Her tonsilar lymph nodes were enlarged, firm and tender, with several swollen lymph nodes nearby. Her pharynx was diffusely reddened, with enlarged tonsils that showed several small patches of gray-white exudate on their surface.

The pediatrician swabbed Stephanie's throat with a sterile swab, which was used to make a streak plate on blood agar. After an 18-hour incubation, scattered among other colonies representing the normal throat flora, were many small grayish colonies surrounded by areas of clearing (β-hemolysis). After this report from the laboratory, Stephanie's mother was given a prescription for 10 days treatment with oral penicillin with firm instructions to finish the treatment no matter how Stephanie felt. Within 2 days of treatment Stephanie's sore throat had resolved and she felt so well that she forgot to take most of her remaining tablets. When this was discovered at a later visit, the pediatrician expressed her displeasure in a forceful tone.

Stephanie had many of the typical features of "strep throat", which is the acute pharyngitis caused by Streptococcus pyogenes. At her age, these features include occurrence in early spring, high fever, nausea and vomiting, striking pharyngitis and tonsillitis with exudate, and rapid resolution within 2 to 3 days. The pediatrician took a culture because she knew that only about a quarter of cases of acute sore throat are caused by these organisms in children of Stephanie's age. Even in this group, most cases are produced by viruses, including those of the common cold, influenza and parainfluenza. Some cases are caused by mycoplasma, gonococci, and even diphtheria bacilli. The proportion of sore throats caused by agents other than streptococci rises to about 90% in adults.

The following questions arise in the case of Stephanie:

1. Despite their frequency, are "strep throats" the casual diseases they are often thought to be? Why was the physician concerned about Stephanie not continuing her treatment for 10 days when Stephanie felt perfectly well?

2. Streptococci can cause many other diseases. Are they the same species or strains as those that caused Stephanie's sore throat?

3. How do people "catch" streptococci? Are these organisms part of the normal bacterial flora?

4. Stephanie's throat showed purulent inflammation. Is pus typical of streptococcal diseases? Do streptococci cause pus by the same mechanisms as, say, the staphylococci?

Answers to these questions must take into account the great variety of disease caused by members of the genus Streptococcus (Table 12.1). These include the most common infection of humans, dental caries, as well as diseases of the skin (impetigo, erysipelas) and mucous membranes (pharyngitis, tonsillitis), of the blood (septicemia), and infections of wounds or of the damaged heart valves (bacterial endocarditis). In addition, streptococcal infections lead to serious nonsuppurative sequelae: rheumatic fever and poststreptococcal glomerulonephritis. This

Table 12.1
Some of the medically important streptococci

Organisms	Hemolysis	Lancefield Group	Main Diseases
"Group A β-strep" (S. pyogenes)	β-	A	Pyogenic infections, erysipelas, scarlet fever, rheumatic fever, glomerulonephritis
Group B strep (S. agalactiae)	β-	B	Neonatal sepsis, meningitis, other pyogenic infections
Enterococci (S. faecalis and other)	variable	D	Urinary tract infections
"α-hemolytic strep" (S. salivarius and others)	α-		Caries, endocarditis
Pneumococcus	α-		Pneumonia, meningitis, other pyogenic infections

is not a complete list. Physicians have many opportunities to become acquainted with these organisms because streptococci cause such a broad spectrum of disease.

THE STREPTOCOCCI

Streptococci comprise a large and heterogeneous group of bacteria. Unlike the staphylococci, there are dozens of species of streptococci. Nonetheless, all streptococci share a few characteristics: They are Gram positive cocci in chains, have a fermentative metabolism only, and need rich media for cultivation. Beyond that, the genus includes species that are associated with humans and animals, often in a commensal relationship, but also capable of causing serious diseases. Other species are found in the environment, especially in dairy products.

Why the Chains?

The reason streptococci make chains is twofold: They keep dividing along the same plane as in the previous division, and they do not separate readily after they divide. Apparently divisions are along one plane because streptococcal cells are not perfectly spherical but are ovoid. As in rod shaped bacteria, division takes place across the long axis (Fig. 12.1). The length of the chains varies with the species and the conditions of growth, from a few cells to hundreds linked together.

In some strains the individual cocci are variable in size and shape, sometimes within the same chain (Fig. 12.2). Thus, Gram stains from older cultures or purulent exudates may show large, swollen, football-shaped cells that sometimes lose their Gram positiveness. This may be due to damage to the cell walls due to autolysis or the action of antibiotics. Thus, recognition of streptococci under the microscope is straightforward when their morphology is typical, but sometimes can be difficult.

How Do Streptococci Obtain Energy?

A word about the energy metabolism of streptococci: They do not respire, they obtain their energy entirely by fermentation of sugars. As discussed in Chapter 2, fermentations are incomplete oxidation of sugars, whereas in respiration sugars

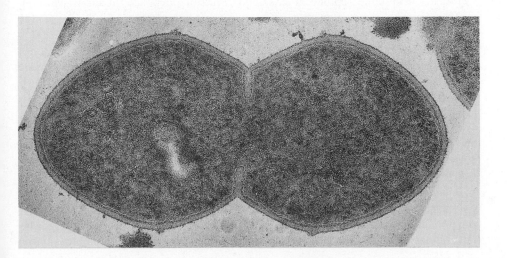

Figure 12.1. An ultrathin section of *Streptococcus faecalis*, showing short chain, ovoid cells under the electron microscope. (Courtesy of Dr. Michael Higgins.)

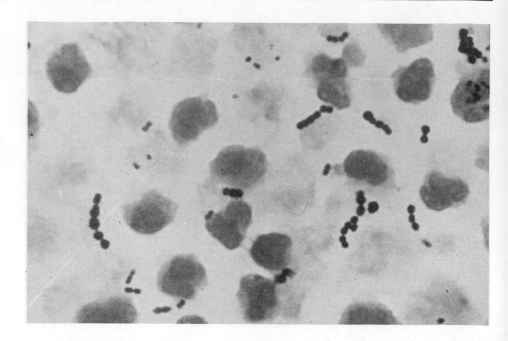

are oxidized to CO_2. Most strictly fermentative organisms are obligate anaerobes. However, many streptococci can grow in oxygen as well as in its absence. These organisms can be said to be *oxygen indifferent* and to be able to carry out the same metabolism in its presence or absence.

In some species fermentation of glucose produces lactic acid only; while in others this is mixed, with several end products. Without exception, growth of streptococci leads to marked reduction in pH. This strong acid production has several consequences: It contributes to dental caries in humans and to clotting of milk, and it may slow down the growth of the streptococci themselves. We depend on special strains of streptococci for the first steps of cheese making (for instance cheddar or Swiss).

What Kinds of Streptococci Are There?

How are different streptococci classified? For our purposes the main grouping is by the hemolytic reaction that surrounds their colonies on blood agar (Table 12.1). Thus, we call those that produce a characteristic greening of the blood α-hemolytic. This group includes some of the most common bacteria in our mouth and pharynx as well as the pneumococci. β-hemolysis is due to the rapid lysis of red blood cells, and is produced by some of the main pathogens of the genus. Many species of streptococci cause no hemolysis at all.

The β-hemolytic (and some nonhemolytic) streptococci are further divided into about 20 groups by the serological differences of a major cell wall polysaccharide, the so called C-carbohydrates. They are known as the *Lancefield groups*, after Rebecca Lancefield, who devised this classification in 1933. We speak of "group A, B, or C, streptococci", and so on. The main human pathogens belong to groups A, B, and D; occasional infections are caused by other groups. The organisms within each group have regular taxonomic names, such as *pyogenes*, the most common human pathogen. It belongs to group A. The specific C-carbohydrate that defines Group A strains of *S. pyogenes* is a dimer of N-acetylglucosamine and rhamnose; it contributes 30% to 50% to the dry weight of the cell wall. Cell walls of group A streptococci also contain protein antigens, known as R and T, which have been used for classification purposes.

Surface Components of *Streptococcus pyogenes* Are Important in Pathogenesis

The surface structures of S. *pyogenes* have been intensively studied, partly because this is such an important pathogen for humans and partly in an attempt to find components responsible for pathogenesis. Virulent strains usually possess the following surface structures outside their cytoplasmic membrane (Fig. 12.3):

• An outer capsule;

• A complex cell wall;

• Surface fibrils composed of protruding macromolecules.

The *capsule* is composed of *hyaluronic acid* and forms a slimy outer coat that retards phagocytosis by leukocytes. Hyaluronic acid is also an important component of connective tissue and is therefore nonantigenic, so that opsonizing antibodies cannot form against the capsule. Paradoxically, some streptococci also excrete the enzyme hyaluronidase, which breaks down both host-derived and streptococcal hyaluronic acid.

The cell wall has several major components. The rigid skeleton is provided by a thick layer of murein, fleshed out by other major cell wall components, polysaccharides, and proteins. Among the polysaccharides are teichoic and teichuronic acids, whose precise role and ultrastructural location are unknown.

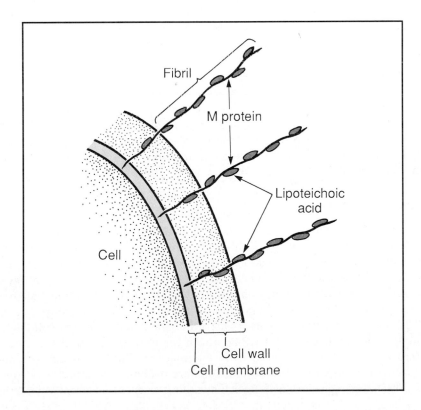

Figure 12.3. Surface structures of *Streptococcus pyogenes*. Extruding from the cell membrane are fibrils of M protein "decorated" with molecules of lipoteichoic acid.

The surface *fibrils* are also known as the "fuzzy layer" because of their appearance in the electron microscope. These fibrils protrude through the cell wall and consist of two macromolecules, known as M protein and lipoteichoic acid. Fibrils play important roles in the pathogenesis of *pyogenes* by inhibiting phagocytosis and by promoting adherence of the organisms to host cells.

M proteins make up 30% to 50% of the dry weight of the cell and occur in about 80 antigenic types. They are probably anchored in the cytoplasmic membrane by a hydrophobic amino acid sequence at their carboxy end (Fig. 12.3). M proteins are a major streptococcal virulence factor because they are strongly antiphagocytic; strains of group A streptococci lacking M proteins are avirulent. The antigenicity of these proteins elicits the formation of IgG antibodies, which act as opsonins, promoting phagocytosis. These antibodies provide a means to serotype strains of *pyogenes*, which has proven useful for following epidemics of streptococcal infection and for identifying strains associated with rheumatic fever and glomerulonephritis (see "Nonsuppurative Sequelae of Streptococcal Infection").

Lipoteichoic acid (LTA) is a polymer consisting of repeating units of glycerophosphate and a terminal glycolipid. LTA molecules interact with M proteins to form the extracellular fibrils (Fig. 12.3). The combination of the two promotes adherence to cell surfaces, such as pharyngeal epithelium. This attachment may be blocked *in vitro* either by antibody to LTA, or by pretreatment of the cells by exogenous LTA.

ENCOUNTER

Many streptococcal infections are caused by members of the patient's own flora, while others are acquired from other persons. It is not easy to tell the origin of organisms in a given patient because *pyogenes* is carried asymptomatically by a substantial number of people. However, the frequency of carriers in the population is not constant; it increases with crowded living conditions, cold and humid climate, and probably other factors. Under the usual conditions, about one in six healthy young people, such as medical students, is likely to carry these organisms in the throat. In the case of Stephanie, a careful epidemiological history may reveal that others in her surroundings, school or home, may have symptoms of streptococcal disease. In other words, streptococcal pharyngitis is one of the many conditions that are described as "What's going around". Where are these organisms when they are not "going around"?

Hygiene and History

The recognition that streptococci may be transmitted from person to person has played a seminal role in the history of infectious diseases. In the 1840s, antedating the modern era of microbiology, the Hungarian Ignaz Philipp Semmelweis and the American Oliver Wendell Holmes proposed that puerperal fever, a lethal sepsis of women following childbirth, was due to transmission from obstetricians to patients. It turned out later that this disease is due to group A streptococci. This infection, once a frequent and often fatal consequence of childbirth in hospitals, has now been almost wiped out in the developed countries.

Improvement in hygienic practices in the home and in the hospital is a major reason why certain streptococcal infections are declining in importance. For example, these organisms are no longer the leading cause of nosocomial infections, especially in surgical patients. On the other hand, the reason why other types of streptococcal infections, such as scarlet fever and erysipelas, have lost their pre-eminence is not clear, although improvements in hygiene may be a contributory factor. Thus, Stephanie's pharyngitis is now a mild disease: In the past it was more often associated with high fever and prostration and, frequently, with a generalized skin rash, in which case it was called scarlet fever. The rash is caused by one of the exotoxins produced by group A streptococci, erythrogenic toxin. Scarlet fever is seldom seen nowadays even though sore throats are still commonly caused by strains that make erythrogenic toxin. The reason for the waning of scarlet fever is unknown.

SPREAD AND MULTIPLICATION

S. pyogenes is highly adapted to spread through tissues. Not only is it able to resist phagocytosis, but it also makes a number of extracellular enzymes that liquefy tissue components and allow it to escape from the confines of an area of inflammation (Fig. 12.4). Among these are *streptokinase*, a protein that activates

Figure 12.4. Some of the pathogenic properties of *Streptococcus pyogenes*: lysis of neutrophils and release of their lysosomes, hydrolysis of fibrin, hyaluronic acid, and DNA.

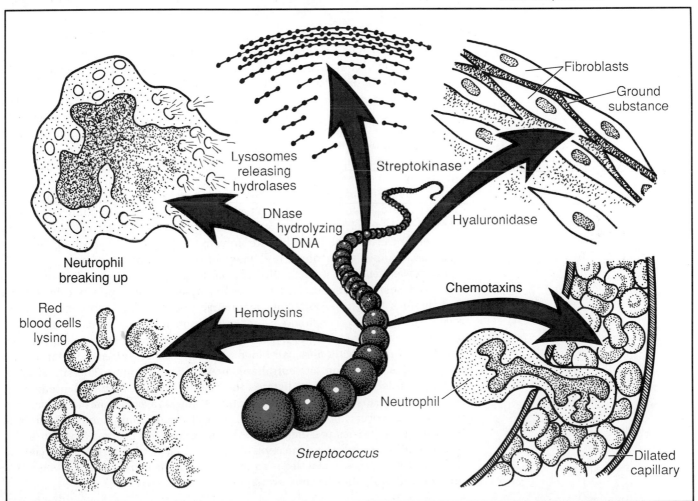

a plasma enzyme (*plasminogen*) to become an active protease (*plasmin*) which digests fibrin clots. This hinders the buildup of fibrin barriers that may contain the organisms. *Hyaluronidase*, another typical streptococcal enzyme, digests the ground substance of connective tissue and aids the movement of organisms through tissues. Similarly, streptococcal *deoxyribonucleases* thin out the viscous deposits of DNA (resulting from the lysis of white blood cells) that would also contain the organisms to restricted sites. Antibody to one of these, DNase B, is a useful serologic marker for recent group A streptococcal infection. Other streptococcal enzymes that presumably function in attacking host-derived substrates are lipoproteinase, proteinase, amylase, esterase, and NADase.

This unique ability to spread is reflected in some of the clinical manifestations of streptococcal disease. Infections due to these organisms often result in thin, spreading exudates rather than the thick pus of the well-localized abscesses that typify staphylococcal infections.

Despite their apparent wanderlust, *pyogenes* have efficient mechanisms to adhere to the cells of their host. This is not unexpected because these organisms often must penetrate mucous membranes before they may cause disease. Attachment is mediated by the fibrils of lipoteichoic acid and M protein.

DAMAGE

S. pyogenes elicits an inflammatory response in a manner similar to that of other pyogenic bacteria: They cause release of chemotaxins for white blood cells, and they activate the alternate pathway of complement, which also results in the production of strong chemoattractants (Fig. 12.4). Once neutrophils arrive at the scene, they cannot easily ingest the organisms because of the antiphagocytic M protein and the hyaluronic acid capsule. Antibodies against M protein provide strong immunity, probably by inhibiting this antiphagocytic activity.

Not only can group A streptococci evade phagocytosis by neutrophils, but like the staphylococci, they may also kill them via the production of a number of cytotoxins. Thus, *S. pyogenes* makes a toxin called *streptolysin O*, which causes cell lysis by intercalating into the cell membrane at cholesterol-containing sites (see Chapter 7). Lysis of neutrophils results in the release of their lysosomes, which themselves can now be lysed by streptolysin O. The strong hydrolytic enzymes from these granules contribute to damage of the surrounding tissues.

The consequences of inflammation caused by *S. pyogenes* depend on both bacterial and host factors. *Scarlet fever*, for example, is due to infection by strains that, besides the virulence factors mentioned above, make toxins called erythrogenic toxins (type A, B, and C), that are responsible for the rash seen in this disease. The mode of action of these toxins is complex and not completely understood. They act directly on small blood vessels to cause extreme dilatation and leakage. This action can be neutralized by specific antibodies. The site of entry of the organisms sometimes dictates the type of lesions they will produce. *S. pyogenes* may cause many types of infection of the skin, sometimes in association with staphylococci. *Impetigo* is a superficial skin infection, mainly of children. Entry of the organisms presumably is through minute abrasions. *S. pyogenes* also causes a diffuse cellulitis, an infection of superficial layers of the skin and lymphatics called *erysipelas*, which leads to fever and septicemia. Erysipelas was often fatal before antibiotics became available.

Nonsuppurative Sequelae of Streptococcal Infection

We now turn to two serious consequences of infections by *S. pyogenes*, which are the reason why Stephanie's physician worried about the interruption of the treatment. She had prescribed penicillin not only to shorten the course of Stephanie's current disease, which probably would have been self-limiting anyway, but to prevent the continued colonization of Stephanie's throat by these organisms. Acute streptococcal infections have been linked epidemiologically to two serious diseases, *acute rheumatic fever* (ARF) and *poststreptococcal glomerulonephritis* (PSGN). These diseases are known as *nonsuppurative sequelae* because they are not direct infections: Organisms cannot be cultured from the lesions. Table 12.2 compares some of their main characteristics. A thorough coverage of these very important illnesses is beyond the scope of this book. Here we should note the following:

Table 12.2

Comparison of some features of acute rheumatic fever and poststreptococcal glomerulonephritis

Characteristic	Acute Rheumatic Fever	Poststreptococcal Glomerulonephritis
Age	Rare in infancy; old age	Any age
Sex incidence	Equal	Males predominate
Familial factors	Familial tendency	Family contacts
Geographic distribution	Decreasing in northern latitudes	Uniform
Preceding infection	Pharyngeal only	Pharyngeal or skin
Attack rate (epidemic)	1–3% or less; fairly constant	1–28%; variable
Attack rate (sporadic)	Less than 0.1%	Less than 1.0%
Second attacks	Common	Rare; may occur after skin infections
Average latent period between infection and first attack	18 days	Pharyngeal: 10 days, skin: up to 6 weeks
Latent period between infection and exacerbation	Same as latent period in first attack	Shortened as compared with latent period in first attack
Relation of degree of ASO titer increase to incidence of first attacks	Incidence proportional to degree of ASO titer increase	No relationship to ASO titer
Time of ASO increase in relation to onset of relapse	Before	After
Serum complement and C3	Increased	Decreased
M types of initiating group A hemolytic streptococcus	Any pharyngeal type; skin strains not rheumatogenic	Pharyngeal type: 1,4,12,18 Skin type: 2,31,49,52,55,57,60
Main pathologic findings	Pericarditis; arthritis; rheumatic nodules	Proliferative, exudative glomerulonephritis; immunoglobulins and complement present

Rheumatic fever follows infection of the pharynx (strep throat), while glomerulonephritis results from either skin or pharyngeal infection. The two conditions apparently follow infections by different strains of S. pyogenes. Indeed, some strains are closely linked to PSGN and are called *nephritogenic*. A lesser correlation is found with strains that cause ARF and is termed *rheumatogenic*. The reason for the differences between these strains is not yet known.

Much is known about each condition, but after intensive study the essential mechanisms of pathogenesis remain elusive. The main reason is the lack of suitable animal models for laboratory investigation. The most widely held view on the pathogenesis of rheumatic fever is that it is due to immune cross-reactivity between myocardial components and streptococcal antigens. However, it has also been proposed that the disease may be caused by production of a streptococcal rheumatic cardiotoxin.

The cross-reaction hypothesis can be bolstered by a number of arguments: Antibodies that react with heart antigens may be found in patients' sera after infection with S. pyogenes. Rabbits immunized against various streptococcal components (protoplasmic membranes and peptides derived from M protein) develop antibodies which bind to heart sarcolemma and subsarcolemmic sites and to myosin. Immunoglobulins and complement are indeed found bound to heart muscle in children who died of rheumatic fever. An argument against this hypothesis is that autoantibodies against heart muscle are sometimes produced without rheumatic fever and do not always accompany this disease. Notice that none of these pro and con arguments (or many others) are easy to evaluate.

Theories regarding the pathogenesis of poststreptococcal glomerulonephritis are also varied and, so far, equally difficult to prove. The following mechanisms have been proposed:

• Cross-reaction between antigens of the streptococci and the glomeruli,

• Deposition of streptococcal antigens in the glomeruli, followed by an in situ reaction with antibodies from the circulation,

• Formation of circulating immune complexes that deposit in the kidney and initiate an inflammatory response,

• Nephrotoxic effects of streptococcal toxins.

S. pyogenes has a number of other poorly understood immunological properties. For instance, it has surface receptors for the Fc portion of immunoglobulins (reminiscent of protein A of staphylococci). If immunoglobulins were to bind to these receptors, the antigen-combining sites (on the Fab portions) would still be available for further interactions. It is not known if this plays a role in streptococcal pathogenesis (you may wish to speculate about what such a role might be). Murein from these organisms is very stable and is resistant to breakdown by lysozyme and other enzymes. It persists within macrophages for long periods, possibly accounting for late immune-mediated events that contribute to glomerulonephritis or rheumatic fever.

Clearly, many observations favor the idea that pathogenesis for ARF and PSGN is based on immunological mechanisms. However, primary immune events that actually cause disease are difficult to distinguish from secondary immune reactions that are associated with disease, but do not cause it. This big nut remains to be cracked.

OTHER STREPTOCOCCI

The changing pattern of streptococcal infections makes *S. pyogenes* less pre-eminent and requires greater awareness of the diseases that other streptococci inflict on humans. Thus, the group B streptococci, which used to be important mainly in veterinary medicine, are now a common cause of septicemia, meningitis and pneumonia in neonates. These organisms are carried by about one third of pregnant women, either as members of the intestinal or vaginal flora or both. The reasons for the marked tropism of group B streptococci for the meninges is not known. Like other bacteria that reach the central nervous system via the blood, these organisms are encapsulated. Group B streptococci also cause opportunistic infections in adults, especially diabetics and alcoholics. The rise in incidence of infections by these organisms is not due solely to better diagnosis. Again, we do not yet know why.

Most of the streptococci discussed so far are β-hemolytic. α-Hemolytic strepto-cocci are also clinically important. By far the most pathogenic one is the pneu-mococcus, which is discussed in Chapter 13. Other α-hemolytic streptococci are among the most abundant organisms in the human mouth and pharynx. They are known collectively as the "α-hemolytic", "viridans", or "greening" streptococci because they cause α-hemolysis or greening of blood agar. Some of these orga-nisms cause brief, low-grade bacteremias, due to injury to the gums during tooth brushing or chewing of fibrous food, and especially during tooth extractions. They do not possess protective devices against host defense mechanisms and are rapidly cleared from the circulation. However, should they find themselves in a protected niche they may survive and cause serious diseases. The best example is the disease *subacute bacterial endocarditis*, which is due to the growth of viridans streptococci on damaged heart valves. This damage may be caused by post–group A streptococcal rheumatic fever, thus leading to one streptococcal disease on top of another. Despite the low intrinsic virulence of the organisms, this is a serious disease with severe local and systemic manifestations that was uniformly fatal in the preantibiotic era.

To these streptococcal infections we must add those due to other groups, mainly group D. These streptococci are collectively known as the *enterococci* because they are common members of the intestinal flora. They commonly cause endocarditis and urinary tract infections and nosocomial (hospital-acquired) in-fections (Table 12.1 and Chapter 57). The sensitivity of enterococci to penicillins and other antibiotics varies widely. Thus, clinical isolates must be carefully tested for their sensitivity to penicillins, aminoglycosides, and sometimes other anti-biotics.

DIAGNOSIS

The diagnosis of strep throat is of cardinal importance, because it calls for che-moprophylaxis of poststreptococcal sequelae. Fortunately, throat cultures done properly are reasonably sensitive indicators of infection by these organisms. It should be remembered that among the population at greatest risk of rheumatic fever, children between ages 5 and 15, up to 50% of sore throats are due to group A streptococci, at least during the winter and early spring months. In other age groups, the incidence decreases to 5% to 10%, with the majority of cases due to viral infections.

Obtaining a throat culture is done by firmly swabbing the back of the throat and tonsils. The swab is then used to streak a blood agar plate. Physicians often make the streak plate, so medical students should learn this technique. Growth of β-hemolytic colonies suggests but does not prove the presence of group A β-hemolytic streptococci because other denizens of the throat also carry out this kind of hemolysis. Fortunately, some simple tests allow us to tell them apart. Group A streptococci are almost invariably sensitive to the antibiotic bacitracin, while almost all the other β-hemolytic bacteria are resistant to it. The test is easy to perform: A suspected colony is restreaked on a blood agar plate and a commercially available bacitracin disc, called an "A disc," is placed on the area of the streak. If the organisms are β-hemolytic streptococci, a zone of growth inhibition is seen around the disc after incubation. Group A streptococci can also be identified by easily performed antibody tests. It is fortunate that easily recognizable characteristics, β-hemolysis, sensitivity to bacitracin, and the group A serotype are diagnostic of group A streptococci, because microbiological diagnosis could otherwise be quite complicated in material so laden with other bacteria as a throat swab.

Cultures are easier to interpret when obtained from specimens of tissue fluids that are normally sterile, such as blood or cerebrospinal fluid. The determination of the group to which a streptococcus belongs is done by serological tests that are not always within the capability of a small diagnostic laboratory.

A serological test that is widely useful in detection of S. pyogenes infection depends on the presence of anti–streptolysin O (ASO) antibodies. An increase in the titer of these antibodies in serum warns of the possible development of rheumatic fever (Table 12.2).

TREATMENT AND PREVENTION

S. pyogenes is one of the few major pathogenic bacteria of humans that so far shows few signs of becoming resistant to antibiotics. Penicillin is the drug of choice; erythromycin or a cephalosporin are alternatives for patients who are hypersensitive to it. Treatment should continue for 10 days to prevent nonsuppurative sequelae. Of these, glomerulonephritis is not as easily avoided as rheumatic fever. Long-acting preparations of penicillin can be given by intramuscular injection, thus avoiding the problem, encountered in Stephanie's case, of patients often discontinuing the drug after they begin to feel better.

Antimicrobial prophylaxis should be used before dental procedures in patients with rheumatic heart disease in an attempt to prevent subacute bacterial endocarditis.

CONCLUSIONS

Streptococci are classical causes of human infections. They produce a wide range of different illnesses that vary greatly in severity, from trivial to fatal. In some cases, a rather mild infection such as pharyngitis or impetigo is followed by severe immunological sequelae, rheumatic fever or glomerulonephritis. In view of their ubiquitous nature, streptococci should be recognized as potential agents in many opportunistic infections.

The pattern of streptococcal infections is changing, possibly because of social factors and improvements in sanitation. The diseases that were associated with crowding and poor hygiene are giving way to those that are transmitted more directly, as during birth of a child. Fortunately, streptococci have remained sensitive to antibiotics.

SELF-ASSESSMENT QUESTIONS

1. What morphological and physiological properties distinguish the genus *Streptococcus*? What are the main groups within this genus?

2. What factors contribute to spread in streptococcal lesions?

3. Discuss the role of M protein in streptococcal pathogenesis.

4. What are the main diseases caused by streptococci? How can they be grouped by (*a*) symptoms and (*b*) types of streptococci?

5. Discuss the immunological aftermath of suppurative streptococcal infections.

6. What are the problems in the microbiological diagnosis of streptococcal infections?

SUGGESTED READINGS

Ferretti JJ, Curtiss R III: *Streptococcal Genetics*. Washington, DC, American Society of Microbiology, 1987.

Read SE, Zabriskie JB (eds): *Streptococcal Disease and the Immune Response*. New York, Academic Press, 1980.

Unny SK, Midlebrook BL: Streptococcal rheumatic carditis. *Microbiol Rev* 47:97–120, 1983.

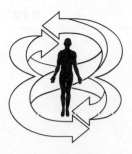

The Pneumococcus and Bacterial Pneumonia

13

G. Storch

The pneumococcus is the most frequent causative agent of acute bacterial pneumonia and one of the classic bacterial pathogens. It yields to antibiotic therapy but remains a serious medical problem, especially in certain risk groups.

The pneumococcus, *Streptococcus pneumoniae*, is a Gram positive coccus that belongs to the group of α-hemolytic streptococci. Its outstanding characteristic is an ample polysaccharide capsule that shields it from phagocytosis and is highly antigenic. The capsule is the main virulence factor of the organism, which does not make important exotoxins but causes disease by eliciting a powerful inflammatory reaction.

CASE

Mr. P., a 58-year-old salesman who is a heavy smoker and an alcoholic, noted that he had nasal congestion and a low-grade fever. Two days later he abruptly developed a shaking chill, cough, and severe pain on the right side of his chest that got worse with breathing. The cough was productive of rust-colored sputum. When he was seen in the emergency room, he appeared acutely ill and had a temperature of 104°F. His respiratory rate was relatively rapid at 40 per minute. His breathing was shallow, with little movement of the right side of the thorax. This pattern of breathing, in which one side of the chest is held immobile by pain, is knows as "splinting".

The laboratory reported that his white blood cell count was 23,000/μl, with 23% "band" forms, indicative of leucocytosis (an increase in the number of

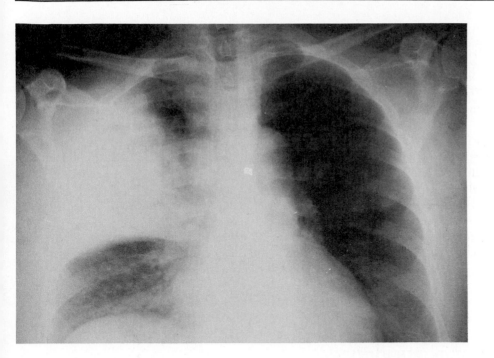

circulating white blood cells). A chest x-ray revealed consolidation of the right upper lobe (Fig. 13.1). A Gram stain of the sputum showed many neutrophils and lancet-shaped Gram positive diplococci (Fig. 13.2). Blood was obtained for culture and treatment was begun with penicillin. Both the blood cultures and sputum cultures were positive for the pneumococcus, S. pneumoniae. Two days later Mr. P. was much improved, and, after two more weeks on penicillin, he recovered completely.

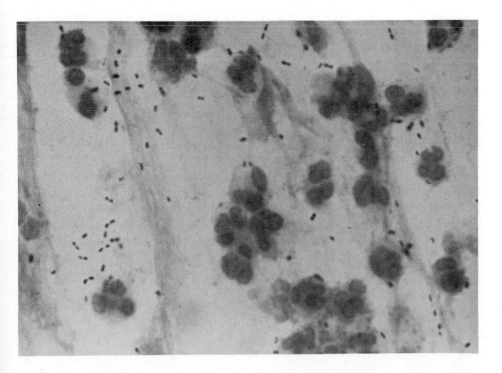

Mr. P.'s case illustrates many of the classical manifestations of pneumococcal pneumonia: abrupt onset of severe symptoms, ill appearance of the patient, rust-colored sputum, involvement of an entire lobe of the lung, leucocytosis, and rapid response to penicillin. This is a dramatic illness, serious enough to threaten the life of an affected patient who may have been well only a few days earlier. It was one of the most important causes of death in the pre–antibiotic era. Today, thanks to penicillin and other antibiotics active against the pneumococcus, it is less often a fatal illness. Nevertheless, it remains the most common form of bacterial pneumonia and may still be extremely serious. Even now, about 5% of all patients die from it; fatality rates are much higher in elderly or debilitated patients, even when they are treated with an appropriate antibiotic.

Many aspects of pneumococcal pneumonia have been carefully studied and merit attention. Perhaps the central motif is that the pneumococcus appears to cause disease in an existential way: As far as is known, its ability to elicit an acute inflammation alone accounts for the major symptoms. It produces no powerful exotoxins. Certain other respiratory pathogens, especially *Haemophilus influenzae* type b and *Klebsiella pneumoniae*, also have a thick polysaccharide capsule and do not produce exotoxins. However, the pneumococcus differs from these Gram negative bacteria in that it does not contain endotoxin.

THE PNEUMOCOCCI

The pneumococcus is classified in the genus *Streptococcus*, based on its morphology and purely fermentative energy metabolism. Like other "aerobic" streptococci, the pneumococcus is anomalous in being able to grow in air, a somewhat unusual feature of strictly fermentative bacteria. The placement of *S. pneumoniae* among the streptococci is supported by the high degree of DNA homology among these organisms.

Pneumococci are Gram positive and commonly grow in pairs (diplococci), but may form short chains. They are surrounded by an ample polysaccharide capsule that imparts a mucoid or "smooth" appearance to colonies on agar. You may recall that the ability of an extract from smooth strains to transform "rough", unencapsulated strains to smooth led Avery, McCarty, and MacLeod in 1944 to the discovery that DNA is the carrier of genetic information.

When a suspension of killed pneumococci is injected into a rabbit, the most prominent antibodies made are ones directed against the capsular polysaccharide. When early workers tested antipneumococcal antisera against different strains of pneumococci, they found a strong reaction with the strains used to produce the antiserum and only weak or no reaction with many other strains (Fig. 13.3). This allowed them to determine that there are some 84 different *serotypes*, each reacting with its specific typing serum. The basis for these antigenic differences lies in the chemical structure of the capsular polysaccharide of each serotype. Since the capsule prevents phagocytosis, nonencapsulated strains rarely if ever cause disease and are rarely found in nature. Antibodies to the capsule play a major role in protection against subsequent infections by pneumococci of the same serotype.

The capsule is not the only pneumococcal component of immunological interest. Also important is the so called *C-substance*, a choline containing teichoic acid that is part of the cell wall. The serum of most people contains a *nonantibody β-globulin*, called *C-reactive protein* because it reacts with the C-substance. When these two components react with one another, the resulting complex activates

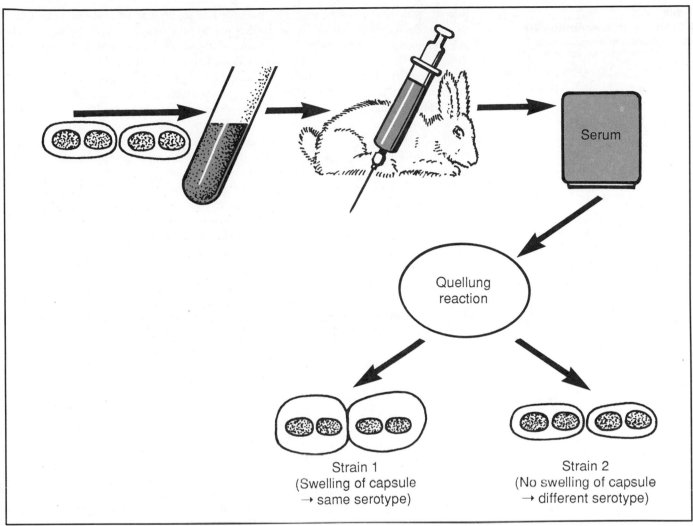

Figure 13.3. The Quellung procedure for serotyping pneumococci. Type-specific antiserum is produced by inoculating a rabbit with a suspension of a pure culture of *Streptococcus pneumoniae* of one capsular type. Typing is performed by mixing a drop of the antiserum with a drop of a suspension of the organism being tested. Swelling of the capsule, visible by light microscopy, denotes that the organism being typed is not of the same serotype as the organism used to produce the antiserum.

the complement cascade, leading to the release of inflammatory mediators. C-reactive protein levels are increased in the sera of patients with many inflammatory diseases, not just pneumococcal infection, and is thus referred to as an *acute phase reactant* (Chapter 5). These characteristics have led to the speculation that C-reactive protein is a primitive, undifferentiated host defense mechanism against infection. The fact that all strains of pneumococci have the same C-substance has led to attempts to use this single component in a vaccine that would elicit protection against all serotypes. Unfortunately, this has not proved successful to date.

ENCOUNTER

Pneumococcal pneumonia is the major form of bacterial pneumonia acquired in the community (as opposed to being hospital-acquired; see Chapter 45). It is estimated that there are about 500,000 cases of this disease per year in the United States. The incidence is higher in certain subgroups, including children younger than 5 years, adults older than 40, blacks, and native Americans. The reason for

Table 13.1

Likelihood of colonization with Streptococcus pneumoniae[a]

Group	% with S. pneumoniae colonization
Preschool children	38–45
Elementary school children	29–35
Junior high school children	9–25
Adults with children at home	18–29
Adults without children at home	6

[a] Adapted from Hendley JO, Sande MA, Stewart PM *et al.*: Spread of *Streptococcus pneumoniae* in families. I. Carriage rates and distribution of types. *J Infect Dis* 132:55–61, 1975.

this distribution is not known, but poverty and a debilitated state of health are risk factors. Certain diseases also predispose to pneumococcal infections, including sickle cell anemia, Hodgkins' disease, multiple myeloma, and the absence of the spleen for any reason. Pneumococcal infections are also distinctly seasonal: the highest incidence is in the winter and early spring. Most cases are sporadic, but outbreaks take place, particularly in residential institutions, army barracks, and work camps, where people are housed under crowded conditions.

The reservoir of *S. pneumoniae* is thought to be humans who harbor the organism, rather than animals or the inanimate environment. Transmission occurs directly from person to person. In this light, it might seem surprising that if the physician had asked Mr. P. whether he had been exposed recently to another person with pneumonia, the answer would probably have been no. The reason is that most people who harbor pneumococci experience no symptoms at all.

Colonization by pneumococci typically occurs in the nasopharynx. The outcome may be (*a*) clearance of the organisms, (*b*) asymptomatic persistence for several months (the carrier state), or (*c*) progression to disease. The outcome of colonization is determined by the intrinsic virulence of the colonizing strain and the efficiency of host defense mechanisms. It turns out that some serotypes of *S. pneumoniae* are more virulent than others. Some cause severe disease, whereas others are commonly isolated from the nasopharynx of asymptomatic persons. The interval between colonization and the onset of disease is variable (and ordinarily undefinable in clinical practice), but there is some evidence that disease is most likely to occur shortly after colonization.

Several aspects of colonization with *S. pneumoniae* have been elucidated by longitudinal studies in which nasopharyngeal cultures were obtained at regular intervals from healthy individuals. Pneumococci were recovered in as many as two-thirds of normal preschool children. In general, colonization is less common in adults, although contact with children increases its frequency. The results of one study that illustrates these findings are shown in Table 13.1. One individual may become colonized many times, usually with different serotypes. The extent to which colonization stimulates the immune response is not known. In one study, 50% of colonized children but only a few adults had antibodies to their homologous strain. It has been suggested that secretory IgA antibodies are important in determining whether or not colonization takes place after exposure.

Transmission from a sick person, or more commonly, from an asymptomatic carrier, is via droplets of respiratory secretions that remain airborne over distance of a few feet. Infecting organisms may also be carried on hands contaminated with secretions. Transmission occurs readily within families and in closed institutions. Since there are many more healthy carriers than sick people, most of the links in the chain of transmission from person to person are invisible. This contrasts with a disease such as measles, which is also transmitted from person to person but where asymptomatic colonization does not take place, so that each link in the chain is evident.

ENTRY

Most of the time, infections of the lung are prevented by elaborate mechanisms, including the tortuous pathway that air and inhaled particles must follow to reach the lungs, the epiglottis that protects the airway from aspiration, the cough reflex, the presence of a layer of sticky mucus that is continuously swept upward by the cilia of the respiratory epithelium, and alveolar macrophages. These mechanisms are ordinarily highly effective in preventing progression from colonization to infection. However, a number of factors can interfere with them, including loss of consciousness, cigarette smoking, alcohol consumption, viral infections, or excess fluid in the lungs.

How do these considerations relate to the case of Mr. P.? The source of the infecting organisms was certainly another individual who may have been entirely healthy. It is possible that Mr. P. had the misfortune to acquire one of the more virulent pneumococcal serotypes. His smoking and alcohol consumption may have depressed his defense mechanisms by weakening his cough reflex and decreasing the activity of alveolar macrophages.

SPREAD, MULTIPLICATION, AND DAMAGE

Pneumococci have a particular predilection for the human respiratory tract, but we do not know the reasons for this marked tropism. Besides the lung, they are also a major cause of infection at two other sites in the respiratory tract: the paranasal sinuses, the middle ear, and the conjunctivae. In addition, they are one of the three most common causes of bacterial meningitis, along with *H. influenzae* type b and the meningococcus. Finally, pneumococci may cause infection at other sites, such as the heart valves, the joints, or the peritoneal cavity.

Much of what is known now about the pathogenesis of pneumococcal pneumonia derives from studies carried out in the 1940s by W. Barry Wood and his colleagues. They produced pneumonia by injecting pneumococci suspended in mucin into the bronchi of anesthetized mice. Animals were sacrificed at various times and histological sections of the lungs were examined. Four zones of the pneumonic process were identified (Fig. 13.4). In the original study all four zones

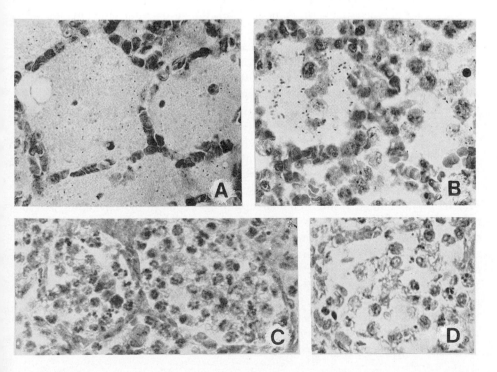

Figure 13.4. Four zones or stages of lung involvement in pneumococcal pneumonia. Pneumonia was induced in rats by intrabronchial installation of live pneumococci suspended in mucin. **A**, Alveoli filled with clear exudate (×430). **B**, Early consolidation. Organisms are plentiful, some engulfed by neutrophils (×430). **C**, Late consolidation. A closely packed cellular infiltrate is present and phagocytosis of organisms has occurred (×530). **D**, Resolution found at center of lesion. Macrophages are present, and the exudate is beginning to clear (×430). (From W.B., Wood, Jr., Studies on the cellular immunology of acute bacterial infections. *Harvey Lectures.* 47:72–98, 1951–52.)

were found simultaneously in different regions of the lung, with the first one located at the expanding edge of the involved area. Thus, it makes sense to think that the four zones correspond to four stages of the inflammatory process.

In the first stage the lung alveoli become filled with serous fluid containing many organisms but few inflammatory cells. In some unknown manner, pneumococci in the alveoli stimulate the outpouring of fluid, which serves as a culture medium for the rapid multiplication of the organisms. The alveolar fluid also provides a rapid means of spread of the infection, both into adjacent alveoli through the pores of Kohn, and to nearby areas of the lung via the bronchioles. Note that the outpouring of fluid could have less severe consequences in many other organs. In the lungs it represents a threat to the basic function of that organ, namely gas exchange.

In the second stage, *early consolidation*, the alveoli are infiltrated by neutrophils and red blood cells. Strong chemotactic signals, produced by the pneumococci and by the alternate pathway of complement, lead to the recruitment of large numbers of neutrophils. The stage is now set for the classic struggle between bacteria and phagocytes. On the one hand, pneumococci resist being taken up by virtue of their capsule; on the other hand, if they are ingested by the neutrophils, they are rapidly killed. Clearly, the extent of successful phagocytosis determines the outcome of the infection. Fortunately, there are mechanisms that make even the heavily encapsulated pneumococci more "digestible" to the neutrophils. If the patient has had previous contact with pneumococci of the invading serotype, he or she will have developed type-specific antibodies that interact with complement to opsonize the organisms and facilitate their uptake. If the individual lacks specific immunity, the organisms may be opsonized by complement components, activated by the alternative pathway and possibly by the interaction of pneumococcal C-substance with C-reactive protein of the serum. Binding of complement components differs among pneumococcal serotypes, which may explain in part why some are more virulent than others.

In the case of our patient, Mr. P., neutrophils failed to contain the pneumococci early on, and the infection progressed to adjacent areas until a whole lobe of his left lung became involved. What accounted for his fever and ill appearance? We do not really know, because while the lung involvement was serious the resulting impairment of gas exchange cannot really explain why the patient is so sick in this disease. It is likely that the systemic manifestations are due either directly to pneumococcal components in the circulation or to products of the inflammatory response induced by the bacteria.

The third stage of pneumococcal pneumonia is called *late consolidation*. Here, the alveoli are packed with victorious neutrophils and only a few remaining pneumococci. On a gross level, the affected areas of the lungs are heavy and resemble the liver in appearance, a state that early pathologists called *hepatization*. In the fourth and final stage, *resolution*, neutrophils are replaced by scavenging macrophages, which clear the debris resulting from the inflammatory process. One of the remarkable aspects of pneumococcal pneumonia is that in most cases the architecture of the lung is eventually restored to its normal condition. This is very different from what takes place in many other forms of pneumonia, where recovery is accompanied by necrosis, with normal lung tissue being replaced by fibrous scar tissue during recovery.

Pneumococcal pneumonia may lead to both local and distant complications. The most common local complication is pleural effusion, the outpouring of fluid in the pleura, present in about one quarter of all cases. Usually, the pleural fluid is a sterile exudate, stimulated by the adjacent inflammation. However, in about 1% of cases, pneumococci can be isolated from this site. Infection of the pleural space is called *empyema*, a condition that must be treated by drainage of the infected fluid and administration of appropriate antibiotics.

Distant complications of pneumococcal pneumonia result from spread of the organisms via the bloodstream. In the early stages of pneumonia, the organisms may enter the lymphatics draining the infected area of the lungs, pass into the thoracic duct, and from there pass into the bloodstream. Pneumococcemia can be documented by positive blood cultures in about 25% of the cases but probably occurs much more often, at least transitorily. When bacteremia is present, the organisms may cause infection at secondary sites, such as the meninges, heart valves, joints, or peritoneal cavity. Had Mr. P. not responded quickly to penicillin therapy, the physician caring for him would have been on guard for such complications.

Host defenses against pneumococcal bacteremia depend largely on the reticuloendothelial system to remove circulating bacteria from the bloodstream. Humoral factors, including antibodies, complement, and perhaps C-reactive protein, assist macrophages in the spleen, liver, and lymph nodes in carrying out their filtering function. The critical role of the spleen is demonstrated by the overwhelming bacteremia that sometimes strikes individuals whose spleen has been removed surgically, or whose splenic function is compromised by another disease such as sickle cell anemia. In these people, bacteremia caused by pneumococci or occasionally by other encapsulated bacteria, such as *H. influenzae*, may be so fulminant that death occurs within hours of the first symptoms.

DIAGNOSIS

Pneumococcal pneumonia can often be suspected on clinical grounds. Even though the astute physician may be able to make an educated guess, laboratory confirmation is essential. The first step is to do a Gram stain of a specimen of sputum. If it contains neutrophils and more than 10 lancet-shaped Gram positive diplococci per oil immersion field, the diagnosis of pneumococcal pneumonia is likely. In the case of Mr. P., the results of the Gram stain of sputum confirmed the clinical suspicion and justified the use of penicillin as initial therapy.

In Mr. P.'s case, final identification was made by culturing the sputum. The culture was performed by streaking the specimen on blood agar and chocolate agar (so called because of its appearance, due to its content of boiled blood). Pneumococcal colonies are surrounded by an area of α-hemolysis, familiar to those who have seen it. Since most streptococci normally present in the body are also α-hemolytic, pneumococci must be differentiated by other properties, their lancet shape and their sensitivity to a compound called *optochin*.

Unfortunately, the interpretation of a positive sputum culture is not always straightforward. It may indicate the cause of the patient's pneumonia, but it may also be the result of contamination of the sputum specimen as it passes through the mouth of a colonized individual. This is an instance where a laboratory finding must be interpreted with an eye towards the clinical context. In contrast, growth of *S. pneumoniae* from Mr. P.'s blood could be considered definitive proof of the etiology of the disease. In recent years there has been interest in the use of specific antisera to detect the capsular antigen directly in sputum, blood, or urine, thus obviating the need for culture. Unfortunately, these techniques tend to be positive in no more than 50% of the cases of pneumococcal pneumonia. To sum this up, laboratory confirmation is not achieved even now in a substantial proportion of cases of pneumococcal pneumonia.

PREVENTION AND TREATMENT

Penicillin revolutionized the treatment of pneumococcal pneumonia. Before its advent, treatment of this disease consisted of the administration of specific immune horse serum. This was associated with complications, especially serum sickness, but it did reduce the mortality rate. The effectiveness of penicillin became evident from its first use in the 1940s, and it rapidly supplanted serum therapy. Other antibiotics, such as erythromycin, are available for patients who are allergic to penicillin.

Despite the dramatic effectiveness of penicillin, the mortality rate in pneumococcal pneumonia remains unacceptably high. There are two reason for this: First, pneumococcal infections sometimes progress very rapidly and patients are already near death when they seek medical attention. Second, some patients are debilitated by other diseases and succumb from the combined effects of the two conditions. Drug resistance is another problem in the therapy of pneumococcal infections. For many years, penicillin resistance was virtually unknown in the pneumococcus. However, in 1977 an outbreak in South Africa was caused by strains with a high level of resistance to penicillin and other antibiotics. This has not yet been a problem in the United States, although an increasing number of isolates have a low or intermediate level of penicillin resistance. Fortunately, most infections by these strains yield to high levels of the drug. This is not the case in pneumococcal meningitis, where incomplete penetration of penicillin into the central nervous system may make it impossible to achieve therapeutic levels.

What about a vaccine? It would be useful, especially for the members of the population who are at risk. Of course the antigenic diversity of the pneumococcus is a significant barrier to developing a vaccine based on the polysaccharide capsular antigens. Nonetheless, most cases of pneumococcal pneumonia are caused by 12 to 18 serotypes. Accordingly, a vaccine based on these types was approved for use in 1977. It is recommended for the elderly and those with diseases that predispose to pneumococcal infections. Unfortunately, patients with Hodgkins' disease or multiple myeloma, who are especially at risk, often do not respond to the vaccine. Likewise, young children, in whom pneumococcal infections are also important, also respond poorly to polysaccharide vaccines in general, including this one (see Chapter 15 for a discussion of vaccination of children against *H. influenzae*). For these reasons the vaccine has yet to have a dramatic impact on the overall morbidity and mortality caused by this organism. Perhaps when its use becomes more widespread or a more effective vaccine is developed, vaccination may affect the prevalence and severity of pneumococcal infections.

CONCLUSIONS

Pneumococcal pneumonia has evolved from one of the major infectious causes of death to a fairly frequent disease that usually yields to treatment. Certain risk factors can be clearly identified, but it remains obscure why some seemingly healthy people become affected. Pneumococci are frequent colonizers, and it is not obvious what makes them cause disease in some individuals but not others.

Pneumococcal pneumonia begins locally as an acute inflammation that involves mainly the alveoli and spreads laterally to adjacent areas. It exemplifies the classical stages of inflammation: exudate formation, influx of neutrophils, and re-solution via macrophages. The local pathological manifestations do not explain the high fever and other systemic signs of the disease.

The main virulence factor and principal antigen of pneumococci is a capsular polysaccharide. It has many antigenic varieties that subdivide this species into distinct serotypes. A "polyvalent" vaccine composed of the most common serotypes is currently available.

SELF-ASSESSMENT QUESTIONS

1. Discuss the epidemiological features of pneumococcal pneumonia.

2. What properties of pneumococci are thought to be relevant to their pathogenesis? Given that the pneumococcus can be transformed with DNA, what experiments would you suggest that may help elucidate them?

3. Describe the histopathological events in pneumococcal pneumonia.

4. What would be your main concerns in treating an elderly patient with this disease?

5. Discuss the complications in the diagnosis of pneumococcal infections of different organs.

SELECTED READINGS

Heffron R: *Pneumonia, with Special Reference to Pneumococcus Lobar Pneumonia.* New York. The Commonwealth Fund, 1939.
Rein MF, Gwaltney JM, Jr, O'Brien WM, Jennings RH, Mandell GL: Accuracy of Gram's stain in identifying pneumococci in sputum. *JAMA* 239:2671–73, 1978.
Austrian R: Random gleanings from a life with the pneumococcus. *J Infect Dis*; 131:474–484, 1975.
Austrian R, Douglas PM, Schiffman G, Coetzee AM, Koornhof HJ, Hayden-Smith S, Reid RDW: Prevention of pneumococcal pneumonia by vaccination. *Trans Assoc Am Phys* 89:184–194, 1976.

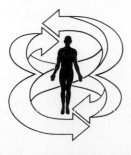

CHAPTER

The Neisseriae: Gonococcus and Meningococcus

14

E.N. Robinson, Jr.
Z. McGee

The genus of Gram-negative cocci, *Neisseria*, has two major pathogenic species, *N. gonorrhoeae*, the agent of gonorrhea, and *N. meningitidis*, the cause of meningococcal septicemia and meningitis. These organisms do not manufacture known exotoxins but have a lipopolysaccharide endotoxin. The gonococcus enters the submucosal connective tissue, usually of the urethra, where it elicits a brisk inflammatory response. Gonorrheal urethritis is characterized by production of pus and pain on urination. The location of the inflammation may lead to important sequelae. For instance, inflammation of the fallopian tubes, pelvic inflammatory disease, may result in scarring and subsequent infertility as well as ectopic pregnancy.

Certain strains of gonococci invade the bloodstream and localize in particular parts of the body, i.e., the skin and the joints. Meningococci have a greater ability to withstand defense mechanisms in the circulation and may grow to high numbers in the blood. This results in the systemic signs of meningococcemia, disseminated intravascular coagulation and shock, probably caused by the large load of endotoxin in the blood, and secondarily by the release of very potent mediators, such as tumor necrosis factor. The meninges and the adrenal glands are often involved.

CASE

The night before coming to the emergency room, Ms. P., a 19-year-old, felt the gradual onset and relentless progression of severe pain in the lower left

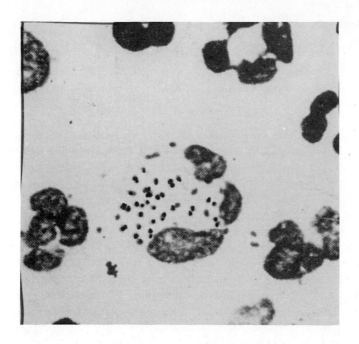

quadrant of her abdomen. She felt nauseated and vomited once without relieving her nausea. She felt feverish, but did not take her temperature. At first, she thought she had appendicitis but then remembered that the appendix is on the right side.

A pelvic examination revealed a green-yellow discharge from the cervical os. Marked tenderness of the left adnexa was elicited both by direct palpation and by moving the cervix back and forth. A cervical swab was placed into the cervical os and left in place for 15 to 30 seconds to absorb secretions. The swab was then rolled on a glass slide and Gram stained. Under the microscope many neutrophils were observed to contain Gram-negative diplococci—two kidney-shaped bacteria abutting one another (Fig. 14.1). This is the characteristic Gram stain appearance of gonococci.

The cervical swab was also streaked directly on plates containing chocolate agar plus antibiotics that inhibit the growth of other bacteria (Thayer-Martin medium). The plates were incubated in a "candle jar" to increase the carbon dioxide concentration to about 5%, which is necessary for the optimal growth of Neisseriae. The next day the laboratory reported that colonies of gonococci were growing on the agar. This confirmed the preliminary diagnosis of gonococcal infection. She was treated with doxycycline and cefoxitin and appeared free of infection on direct examination after completion of therapy. Her cervical cultures at this time were negative. She had previously reported that she had two sexual partners, neither of whom appeared to have symptoms of gonococcal disease during this time.

We can ask the following questions:

1. From whom did Ms. P. acquire the organisms? Could she have gotten them from, say, a toilet seat? Can she infect other people?

2. How extensive is the infection? What organs might be affected?

3. Is Ms. P. at risk of complications?

4. How do gonococci invade deep tissues?

5. How can the disease be prevented? Even though they may be asymptomatic, should the sexual contacts of Ms. P. be notified and treated?

It is most likely that Ms. P. had gonococcal salpingitis (inflammation of the fallopian tubes). Even though she was cured of the active infection, scarring of the fallopian tubes due to inflammation places her at risk of subsequent episodes of *pelvic inflammatory disease* (PID), infertility and ectopic pregnancy. Since her sexual partners were asymptomatic and therefore unlikely to seek treatment on their own, it is particularly important that they be contacted and advised to see a physician for tests and possible therapy.

The gonococcus, *Neisseria gonorrhoeae*, causes several diseases other than simple gonorrhea and PID (Table 14.1). They can be divided into local genital or disseminated infections. About one million new cases are reported every year in the United States. Of the infectious diseases that must legally be reported to the U.S. Public Health Service, gonococcal infections surpass in frequency all other bacterial or viral infections. Note, however, that more frequent diseases, such as upper respiratory or chlamydial infections are not reportable at present. It is estimated that the cost of treating PID and its associated sequelae (ectopic pregnancy and infertility) exceeds 2.6 billion dollars per year in the United States alone. Infertility resulting from gonococcal salpingitis has a devastating impact on the populations of some African countries, threatening the continued existence of some tribes.

Table 14.1
Gonococcal infections

Local infections
Urethritis
Epididymitis
Abscess formation in glands adjacent to the vagina, e.g., Skene's duct or Bartholin abscesses
Cervicitis
Proctitis (rectal gonorrhea)
Pharyngitis
Uterine infection (endometritis)
Infections of the Fallopian tube, the ovary, or adnexal tissues (pelvic inflammatory disease)
Ophthalmia neonatorium (bilateral conjunctivitis in infants born of mothers infected with gonococci)

Disseminated infections
Local extension of the infection to areas contiguous with the pelvis causing peritonitis or perihepatitis (so called Fitz-Hugh-Curtis syndrome)
Direct bloodstream invasion with spread of infection to distant organs
Joint infection (arthritis)
Skin involvement either by immune complexes or whole gonococcal organisms (pustules on a hemorrhagic base)
Rarely, infection involves heart valves (endocarditis) or the central nervous system (meningitis)

THE NEISSERIAE

The gonococcus belongs to the genus *Neisseria*, the main group of Gram-negative cocci associated with the human body. This genus includes one other important pathogen, the meningococcus, or *N. meningitidis*, and a number of non-pathogenic members. One of these, recently renamed *Branhamella catarrhalis*, is emerging as an important cause of upper respiratory tract infections, especially in immuno-compromised patients. The neisseriae are aerobes and require complex media but can grow anaerobically. They have typical Gram negative cell envelopes containing endotoxin.

There are substantial differences in the pathogenic potential of different strains of gonococci. Individual strains differ in the frequency with which they produce uncomplicated urethritis, PID, or disseminated gonococcal infection. In some cases, biochemical and genetic differences among strains can be measured in the laboratory (see "The Survival of Gonococci in the Bloodstream").

The neisseriae die rapidly even under laboratory conditions. This is also true for most agents of sexually transmitted diseases. It is highly unlikely that Ms. P. acquired gonococci from the inanimate environment.

ENCOUNTER AND ENTRY

Gonococci are bacteria of human beings. They do not spontaneously infect other animals, nor do they reside freely in the environment. It follows that humans must serve as the reservoir for these organisms. Both men and women can carry gonococci without demonstrating symptoms. The incidence of such asymptomatic carriers is generally greater among women than men, especially with the more common strains, those that cause uncomplicated gonorrheal urethritis. Asymptomatic carriers of either sex represent the major problem in the control of gonorrhea because they are unlikely to seek treatment. For this reason, it is important to attempt to determine the presence of the organisms among the known contacts of a patient with this disease. In the case of Ms. P., it is possible that she acquired the organism from one of her asymptomatic sexual partners.

Once gonococci are introduced into the vagina or the urethral mucosa of the penis, they attach to the surface of epithelial cells and multiply. Several surface structures of the organisms allow them to anchor to the urethral or vaginal epithelial cells. Gonococci possess pili (Fig. 14.2) that are presumed to mediate attachment to as yet unidentified receptors on the surface of human genital cells and prevent them from being washed away by normal vaginal discharges or by the strong flow of urine. From the point of view of the gonococcus, moving up the male urethra may be likened to swimming up Niagara Falls.

Gonococci that possess pili are also less susceptible to being phagocytized by neutrophils. Although gonococci are sometimes described as "intracellular diplococci" in smears of urethral pus, they may in fact simply be attached to the surface of neutrophils and protected from ingestion by their pili. The outer membrane of gonococci contains another protein, called protein II, which is also thought to function as an adhesin. It is inferred that once the gonococcus comes in close contact with the mucosal cells via its pili, protein II helps anchor the organisms to the surface of the host cells. Thus, gonococci have at least two components that allow them to stick to the slippery mucosal surface.

The primary localization of gonococci in the urogenital tract is due largely to their mode of transmission and not necessarily to a marked tissue tropism. In

Figure 14.2. Transmission electron micrograph of *Neisseria gonorrhoeae.* Note the presence of pili, long thin strands of protein, emanating from the surface of the organisms.

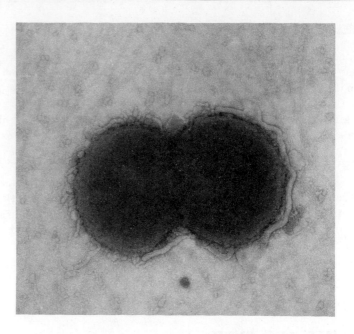

fact, gonococcal pharyngitis and proctitis are common infections in groups that practice oral-genital sex and anal intercourse (i.e., homosexual males).

SPREAD AND MULTIPLICATION

Once they attach to the mucosal cell surface gonococci multiply rapidly and spread upward in the urethra in the male and through the cervix in the female. Gonococci do not have flagella and are not motile, thus their spread must be aided by extrinsic mechanisms. These are the eddy currents in the mucus in which they are entrapped or, more actively, sticking to spermatozoa and hitching a ride on these highly motile cells. Spread is limited by tissue planes and, in the submucosa, takes place along adjacent urethral or genital structures.

Mucosal secretions contain two major types of immunoglobulins, IgA$_1$ and IgA$_2$. Gonococci apparently protect themselves from the action of IgA$_1$ by producing an extracellular protease that specifically cleaves this immunoglobulin at its center. This property is shared with some bacteria that also inhabit mucosal epithelia, such as *Haemophilus influenzae* or certain streptococci. The protease may help the organisms escape phagocytosis by removing the Fc end of the immunoglobulin, the portion that is recognized by phagocytes and that serves as the opsonin.

Invasion

Once gonococci attach to the non-ciliated cells, microvilli extend and embrace the organisms, holding them against the cell surface. Gonococci are then internalized by these "nonprofessional" phagocytes and then transported to the interior via phagocytic vacuoles. These coalesce to form larger vacuoles, within which the gonococci can apparently multiply. Inside the nonciliated cells, gonococci are sheltered from antibodies and professional phagocytes. As Pollock and Harrison wrote in 1912:

When the gonococci have been allowed to penetrate to the interepithelial spaces (or inside epithelial cells) they are protected from the action of any drug applied to the surface of the mucous membrane and to almost equal extent from the action of any substance circulating in the blood. Once firmly established in these spots they are like the garrison of a bomb-proof fort, which, in spite of a fierce attack from all sides, can go quietly existing, ready to sally forth whenever a suitable occasion arrives.

After internalization, the gonococci are transported to the base of the nonciliated cells. The vacuoles that contain them fuse with the basement membrane and discharge their contents into the subepithelial connective tissue. From here the organisms either cause a local damage or they enter blood vessels and cause disseminated disease.

The Survival of Gonococci in the Bloodstream

Normal human serum has the capability to kill a number of Gram-negative organisms, including *N. gonorrhoeae*. The serum factors responsible for this natural protective effect include IgG, IgM, and complement components. The targets for antibodies are the lipopolysaccharide, an outer membrane protein called protein I, and other proteins exposed on the surface of the organisms. Thus, the ability of gonococci to survive in the bloodstream is predicated on the evasion of this defense mechanism. Strains that are usually associated with disseminated infections are serum resistant by virtue of having different surface constituents than their serum sensitive counterparts. Serum-resistant strains are also distinguishable from those that tend to cause uncomplicated urethritis in being more sensitive to penicillin and having specific nutritional requirements. Host factors also affect the outcome of gonococcal infections. For example, individuals unlucky enough to be deficient in the terminal components of the complement cascade (the membrane attack complex) are predisposed to recurrent systemic neisserial infections, both from gonococci and meningococci.

Gonococci need to enter the bloodstream to cause symptoms at distant sites. Frequently, women infected with gonococci present other manifestations, such as hemorrhagic skin lesions, inflammation of the tendons and joints (tenosynovitis) and/or frank infections of the joints (suppurative arthritis). Despite appropriate attempts at cultivation, more times than not, cultures of the blood, joint fluid, or skin lesions are sterile. Several explanations for this phenomenon are possible: (*a*) Gonococci are present but in numbers too low to be viable in culture. (*b*) Immune complexes composed of gonococcal antigens and host antibodies deposit in synovial tissue and evoke local inflammation. (*c*) Gonococcal substances carried into the bloodstream from local sites are directly toxic for joint tissue. The latter possibility is supported by recent experiments in rats which showed that purified gonococcal murein induces arthritis. If this were to apply to humans, the whole gonococcus need not be present at the site of intense inflammation.

DAMAGE

Gonococci do not make exotoxins, thus little is known about how they cause damage. Since they normally only infect humans, not much can be inferred from laboratory animal studies. Most of what we know about how they infect, damage, and invade mucous membranes comes from experiments using human fallopian tubes obtained from surgery and maintained in organ culture media (Fig. 14.3).

Figure 14.3. Scanning electron micrograph of human fallopian tube tissue 20 hours after infection with *Neisseria gonorrhoeae*. Note that gonococci attach almost exclusively to the surface of nonciliated cells. The damage occurs to the ciliated cells. Ciliated cells sloughed from the surface of the mucosa are seen at the *left* and at the *center*, whereas intact ciliated cells are seen at the *top* and *right* of the photomicrograph. (From McGee Z, et al: Pathogenic mechanisms of *Neisseria gonorrhoeae*: Observations on damage to human fallopian tubes in organ culture by gonococci of colony type 1 or type 4. *J Infec Dis* 143: 413–422, 1981.)

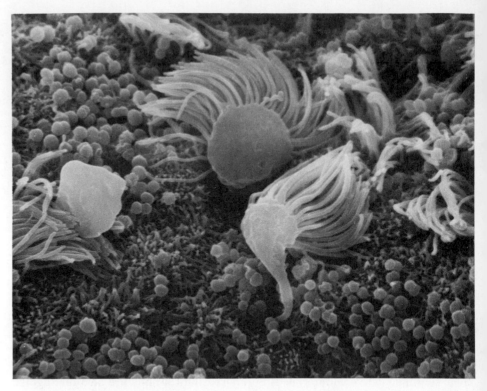

Two types of cells line the mucosal surface of human fallopian tubes: ciliated cells and nonciliated cells. The nonciliated cells have finger-like processes on their surface termed microvilli. When suspensions of live gonococci are added to the organ culture, they attach only to the tips of the microvilli of nonciliated cells. Subsequently there is a rapid decline in the beating of the cilia and the sloughing of the ciliated cells from the mucosal surface (Fig. 14.3). Ciliary activity is thought to be important not only in transporting the egg from the ovary to the uterus but, as in the respiratory tree, in providing a toilet mechanism for clearing bacteria from the mucosal surface. Once this mechanism is lost, the fallopian tube becomes susceptible to infection by organisms that ascend through the cervix and the uterus. This is the likely reason why Ms. P. is at risk; her initial salpingitis may be followed by recurrent pelvic inflammatory disease caused by other bacteria from the vaginal flora.

How gonococci damage the ciliated epithelial cells is surmised by the following observation. Portions of the organisms' outer membranes flare out into blebs, which, when they come in contact with the adjacent ciliated cells of the mucosa, damage them severely. At least two components of the gonococci have been implicated: (a) purified endotoxin extracted from gonococci; and (b) fragments of murein called muramyl monomers (see also Chapter 20 for a similar property of *B. pertussis*).

Damage by the gonococci in the submucosal connective tissue is due to their ability to evoke a brisk inflammatory response. The inflammatory response in the male urethra leads to local symptoms such as pain on urination (dysuria) and a urethral discharge of pus. These symptoms do not distinguish gonococcal urethritis from that caused by other genital pathogens, such as the chlamydiae (Chapter 24), but the urethral discharge in gonorrhea tends to be more copious, thick, and greenish-yellow; and the pain, more intense.

THE OUTCOME OF GONOCOCCAL INFECTION

What is the outcome of gonorrhea? In males symptoms of urethral infection usually subside in several weeks even without treatment. However, repeated infections, if untreated, lead to scarring and stricture of the urethra. Such sequelae of gonococcal infection are relatively unusual, since most males seek medical attention once urethritis becomes apparent. Paradoxically, local urogenital infections in females are frequently asymptomatic and are heralded by the onset of the symptoms of complications of the infection. Sequelae of fallopian tube damage include ectopic pregnancy, recurrent PID by other organisms, chronic pelvic pain, and infertility due to blockage or dysfunction of the tubes. Disseminated gonococcal infections occur predominantly in women. Thus, gonococci may be only a nuisance in a man, but they can potentially lead to death of a woman and her unborn child.

The outcome of gonococcal infection depends not only on the gender of the patient but also on the promptness with which the infected individual seeks medical attention. Prompt treatment increases the chances that the infection remains localized and does not lead to disseminated disease.

SIMILARITIES AND DIFFERENCES BETWEEN GONOCOCCI AND MENINGOCOCCI

It may help to understand the pathobiology of disease caused by gonococci to contrast them with their taxonomic cousins, the meningococci. The two organisms share about 80% of their DNA as measured by hybridization, neither one makes a known exotoxin, and both possess a lipopolysaccharide endotoxin and are relatively good colonizers. Nonetheless, they cause a contrasting spectrum of diseases: Gonorrhea is a localized inflammation and is rarely lethal, whereas meningococcal infection is the herald of a systemic and life-threatening disease. Why do they cause such different illnesses?

The systemic diseases caused by these two organisms are very different. The entry of meningococci into the bloodstream can lead to a devastating disease, *purpura fulminans*, meningitis, disseminated intravascular coagulation, and death. Although gonococcal meningitis and endocarditis have been reported on rare occasion, gonococcal bacteremia is seldom fatal.

In an attempt to explain the differences between these two organisms, we can point to two clues:

1. There are occasional epidemics of meningococcal meningitis when people are exposed to new serotypes of the organisms, but the more usual outcome is colonization with no local symptoms or systemic consequences. The posterior pharynx of approximately 10% of healthy young adults is colonized with these organisms. The reason why some people develop disease and others do not is not easy to fathom because the mechanism of penetration through mucous membranes appears to be similar for the meningococcus in the nasopharynx and the gonococcus in the fallopian tube. The two organisms, however, usually penetrate very different mucous membranes.

2. When the gonococcus reaches the bloodstream, it is usually killed by defense mechanisms. Even the serum-resistant strains do not grow appreciably in the circulation, although they may survive long enough to reach other organs. The meningococcus, on the other hand, grows extremely fast in the bloodstream, reaching blood titers that are among the highest known for any bacteria. It is possible,

for example, to observe the organisms directly on a smear of buffy coat, something that seldom happens with other bacterial septicemias. The reason for this survival is apparently that most strains of meningococcus have a large capsule that helps them resist killing by phagocytes. Some also have outer membrane proteins that contribute to their survival in serum. Thus, meningococci have evolved so that some strains evade human host cellular defenses as well as killing by serum. These are the strains that cause rapidly lethal sepsis with shock and disseminated intravascular coagulation ("purpura fulminans") as well as meningitis.

These differences between gonococci and meningococci may explain the differences in the signs and symptoms of the diseases they cause. The highly invasive gonococci cause symptoms frequently, but the sites affected are usually localized. The highly serum-resistant meningococci, on the other hand, cause a fulminating septicemia with involvement of several organs, especially the central nervous system. Much of the damage is caused by *disseminated intravascular coagulation* (DIC), attributable in part to the large amount of endotoxin in tissues and the circulation. DIC is accompanied by shock, fever, and other responses to endotoxin, as well as to the potent biologic mediators such as tumor necrosis factor, which the endotoxin releases from host cells. Thus, these systemic signs are the direct consequence of the ability of the meningococcus not only to survive but to be able to thrive in the bloodstream. That being so, would a well-encapsulated gonococcus produce manifestations similar to the meningococcus?

DIAGNOSIS

Finding Gram negative intracellular diplococci in vaginal, cervical, or urethral secretions is suggestive evidence of gonococcal infection. It is yet another very good reason why medical students should learn how to do and interpret Gram stains. Positive microscopic findings justify beginning antibiotic therapy before the results of cultures are known, though initial microscopic examination should be followed by culturing.

Culturing clinical specimens is particularly important in the case of gonococcal infections. The reasons are fourfold:

1. Culturing identifies infected individuals and their consorts. Infected consorts can then be treated before symptoms and tissue damage occur. As the social implications of gonorrhea can be as serious as the medical consequences, the physician must be knowledgeable about how the laboratory goes about culturing and identifying these organisms. Misidentifying nonpathogenic neisseriae for *N. gonorrhoeae* can damage personal relationships and lead to lawsuits.

2. For several decades, most strains of gonococci have gradually increased their resistance to antibiotics. The capacity of the human buttocks is the limiting factor for today's penicillin doses. There is, however, considerable variation in the antibiotic susceptibility of individual strains, and the determination of the degree of susceptibility is particularly important for planning proper antimicrobial therapy.

3. Some gonococcal infections will not be eradicated despite the proper administration of currently accepted antimicrobials. Therefore, all individuals should be cultured after therapy as a "test of cure" and to establish that their strains are not drug resistant.

4. Gonococcal infections are often asymptomatic and all persons with multiple sexual partners should be suspected of harboring the organisms and should be

routinely cultured even if asymptomatic. This would greatly aid in diminishing the spread of gonococci.

Gonococci grow on several kinds of media that allow presumptive identification within a day. The most commonly used medium is called "chocolate agar" because it contains boiled blood and has the appearance of milk chocolate. These media are known by such names as "Thayer-Martin medium" and "Martin-Lewis medium", which contain antibiotics to inhibit other bacterial species. Cerebrospinal fluid, blood, or synovial fluid should be cultured on chocolate agar without antibiotics since these fluids are normally sterile. Specimens taken from the vagina and other sites that contain bacteria should always be cultured on chocolate agar with inhibitors of the normal flora (e.g., Thayer-Martin medium). Also, an occasional strain of gonococci is sensitive to the antibiotics used in the Thayer-Martin medium and would be missed otherwise.

All members of the genus *Neisseria* possess an oxidative enzyme that makes the colonies turn purple when flooded with a so-called "oxidase reagent". If a Gram-negative diplococcus is oxidase positive, it is a member of the *Neisseria*. To distinguish *N. gonorrhoeae* from the other species of this genus, the microbiological laboratory determines the pattern of fermentation of various sugars. Unlike other neisseriae, gonococci oxidize glucose but not maltose or sucrose.

PREVENTION

Despite effective antimicrobials and active public health measures, gonococcal infections are extraordinarily frequent in the United States and elsewhere. In the absence of environmental or animal reservoirs, the chain of transmission is tenuous enough to be broken, at least in principle. The best hope at present lies in the development of an effective and safe antigonococcal vaccine. Early versions containing killed whole gonococci failed. The best candidates for antigens to be included in an antigonococcal vaccine should (a) be shared by all strains of these organisms, (b) be exposed to their surface and be bound by antibodies, and (c) play a role in the disease process. At first glance, the most obvious candidate would be the pili. In theory such a vaccine would elicit antibodies that inhibit the attachment of the organisms to urogenital cells. However, gonococcal pili differ from strain to strain, and antibodies against pili from one strain do not bind to the pili from another. A single strain can produce four or more kinds of pili. The ensuing difficulties became disappointingly evident when a vaccine composed of a single antigenic type of purified pili was given to Army personnel in areas of Southwest Asia, where antibiotic-resistant gonococci are frequent. No reduction in gonorrhea was seen.

Why not make a polyvalent pili vaccine? The problem is that the total number of antigenic types of pili is unknown but surely exceeds what can be included in a single vaccine. Are there alternatives? Investigators are studying vaccines made with that portion of the pili protein that is identical among different strains of gonococci. Such vaccines are currently under investigation.

Other surface proteins are also being considered for inclusion in a gonococcal vaccine. Antibodies against the molecules responsible for invasion could theoretically prevent disseminated infection. However, there is a risk that such a vaccine would merely convert invasive gonococci into commensal ones. This may prevent the symptoms that proclaim the disease but would not get rid of the organisms. Since asymptomatic people do not usually seek treatment, the result may be an increase in the number of carriers of gonococci in the community. Such a vaccine would be useful only if everybody received it.

CONCLUSIONS

The mode of transmission as well as the biological properties of the gonococci combine to give the infections by these organisms a unique set of characteristics. Gonococci, by virtue of possessing strong adhesins, are well adapted for their usual portal of entry, the genital tract of humans. They have the unusual ability to traverse epithelial cells and either to cause local inflammation or, infrequently, to disseminate to other parts of the body.

Gonococci are found only in human beings, some of whom act as asymptomatic carriers. In principle, an effective vaccine should prevent new cases and even obliterate gonococcal diseases. It is hoped that such a vaccine will become available soon.

SELF-ASSESSMENT QUESTIONS

1. What are the microbiological distinguishing features of the gonococci? Who are their microbiological kin?

2. Discuss the events that lead to gonococcal urethritis.

3. What are the known virulence factors of gonococci?

4. What problems would be encountered in attempting to eliminate gonorrhea from the face of the earth?

5. Why is it difficult to make an effective vaccine against the gonococcus?

6. Discuss the serious clinical consequences of gonorrhea.

SELECTED READINGS

Brooks GF, Donegan EA: *Gonococcal Infection.* London, Edward Arnold, 1985.

Centers for Disease Control: Guide for the Diagnosis of Gonorrhea Using Culture and Gram Stained Smear. U.S. Department of Health and Human Services Publication, January 1985.

Fleming TJ, Walsmith DE, Rosenthal RS: Arthropathic properties of gonococcal peptidoglycan fragments: implications for the pathogenesis of disseminated gonococcal disease. *Infect Immun* 52: 600–608, 1986.

Holmes KK, Mardh P, Sparling PF, Wiesner PJ, (eds): *Sexually Transmitted Diseases.* New York McGraw-Hill, 1984.

Hook, III EW, Holmes KK: Gonococcal infections. *Ann Intern Med* 102:229–243, 1985.

Schoolnik GK, (ed): *The Pathogenic Neisseria.* Washington, DC American Society for Microbiology, 1985.

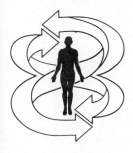

Haemophilus influenzae: An Important Cause of Meningitis

A.L. Smith

Haemophilus influenzae, a nutritionally fastidious small Gram negative rod, causes pneumonia in persons of all ages and meningitis in young children. The reason for this distribution may be immunological: The principal antigen of these bacteria is a polysaccharide that is processed by a T cell independent route, which is not yet developed in these children.

These organisms are not known to produce soluble toxins but have endotoxin. They are usually surrounded by a thick capsule, which allows them to escape phagocytosis and travel to the central nervous system. A vigorous attempt is under way to develop an effective vaccine for children in the risk group.

CASE

Michael, a 9-month-old baby, awoke from his afternoon nap fussy and slightly irritable. His mother thought he had a low-grade fever and gave him some liquids and acetaminophen to reduce his fever. She reported he was fussy throughout the next night and seemed less feverish in the morning. However, he felt warm around noon, refused lunch, vomited, and could not be consoled. His temperature was 103.2°F and he became difficult to arouse. He was then taken to a pediatrician, who interviewed the mother, examined the infant, and performed a lumbar puncture.

A Gram stain of the cerebrospinal fluid showed white cells and many pleomorphic Gram negative rods (Fig. 15.1). A sample was mixed on a slide with specific antisera against the serological types of the capsular antigen of Haemophilus influenzae. The antisera are absorbed on the surface of latex

Figure 15.1. Gram stain of *H. influenzae* in pus. (Reproduced with permission of Schering Corp., Kenilworth, NJ, the copyright owner. All rights reserved.)

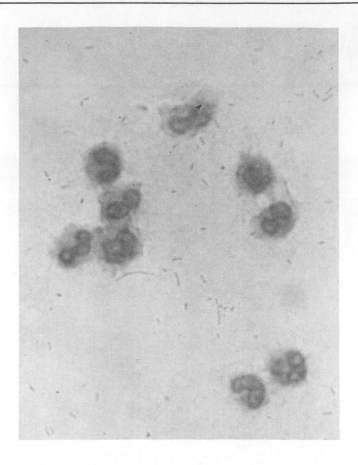

particles, which agglutinate (through lattice formation) in the presence of antigen. This permitted the immediate diagnosis of meningitis due to H. influenzae type b. The diagnosis was later confirmed when the organism grew in culture.

Michael's parents had many questions: What are Michael's chances? Are there complications of the disease? What is the treatment? Could Michael's sister, 3-year-old Ann, acquire the disease?

To answer these questions you should know something about the following:

1. How the disease is acquired and how the organism gets into the central nervous system. How does *H. influenzae* cause disease?

2. What complications may arise?

3. What is the epidemiology of this infection?

4. What are the immune mechanisms operating in this infection?

5. What treatment and preventive measures are available?

Bacterial meningitis is a serious disease, primarily of infants and children. It can be caused by a variety of organisms (Table 15.1), with *H. influenzae* heading the list. The fatality rate has not changed substantially since the introduction of antibiotics and is currently around 10%. In addition, meningitis may cause permanent neurological sequelae, but early treatment minimizes the duration and

Table 15.1
Etiology of bacterial meningitis

Age	Underlying Disease	Bacterial pathogen	
		Most common	Other
Birth to 2 mos	None	*Streptococcus agalactiae* (group B)	*Escherichia coli* *Listeria monocytogenes*
2 to 60 mos	None	*Haemophilus influenzae*	*Neisseria meningitidis* *Streptococcus pneumoniae*
>60 mos	None	*Streptococcus pneumoniae*	*Neisseria meningitidis*[a]
Any age	Cranial surgery	*Staphylococcus aureus*	*Staphylococcus epidermidis*
Any age	Immunosuppression from cancer chemotherapy	*Streptococcus pneumoniae*	*Escherichia coli* *Pseudomonas aeruginosa* Klebsiellae *Listeria monocytogenes*

[a] Occurs in epidemics.

severity of the infection. Meningitis imposes a diagnostic imperative on the physician, and diagnosis must be attempted with great dispatch.

H. influenzae causes infections of the upper and lower respiratory tract in persons of all ages. However, meningitis due to these organisms is confined to a narrow age group, usually between 6 and 60 months of age.

INTRODUCTION TO THE AGENT

Haemophilus are small Gram negative facultative anaerobic rods with complex nutritional requirements. Their name means "blood loving" and was given because members of the genus need either one or both of two compounds found in blood, the so-called X and V factors. X factor is hematin and V factor is NAD or something similar.

The most important human pathogen is *H. influenzae*, known colloquially (in English-speaking countries) as "H. flu". It got its name in a great influenza pandemic during the First World War. And while it was first thought to cause the disease, it took over a dozen years to figure out that influenza is caused by the influenza virus and that H. flu was a common secondary invader.

Many strains of these organisms are surrounded by a capsule that is antiphagocytic. The capsular material comes in six antigenic types that can be distinguished readily by their reaction with specific antibodies. Note that the detection of specific capsular antigen permitted a nearly instantaneous diagnosis in Michael's case. His organism was type b, which accounts for nearly all cases of H. flu meningitis. This capsule is made up of polymers of the pentoses ribose and ribitol linked through phosphodiester bonds. Some other strains of H. flu that cause disease, notably middle ear infections, are nonencapsulated.

ENCOUNTER

H. flu is an organism totally adapted to humans and not naturally found elsewhere. It can frequently be recovered from the nasopharynx of almost anyone except newborn infants. By 3 months of age, virtually all children carry the organism. However, there is a significant difference between these normal commensal strains and those isolated from patients with meningitis. The usual strains are seldom encapsulated, whereas the ones cultured from spinal fluid invariably are. It is not clear what goes on. Are there two totally separate kinds of H. flu? Or can nonencapsulated strains acquire a capsule by induction of latent capsule genes or by a genetic change, and thus become pathogenic? The first possibility, that H. flu is at least two distinct strains, is the favored one but the issue has not been settled. Note that it is not easy to distinguish between the two alternatives. What would you do if you were working on this problem? Keep in mind, among other things, that H. flu infection seems to be preceded by a predisposing viral infection that may well cause local environmental changes.

In experimental studies with infant animals the introduction of *H. influenzae* type b into the nose is all that was necessary for infection to occur. In the same studies it was found that the organisms were readily transmitted to infant animals in close contact. In humans there is a similar type of secondary transmission that is also age dependent. About 4% of children less than 5 years of age in close contact with H. flu patients develop the disease. Thus, Michael's sister Ann is at significant risk.

ENTRY, SPREAD, AND MULTIPLICATION

In many regards, the first steps in the pathogenesis of pneumonia due to H. flu are similar to those of the pneumococcus (Fig. 15.2). Lung infection by both organisms follows colonization of the oropharynx and deposition into the lower reaches of the respiratory tree by inhalation. At these sites both organisms provoke an inflammatory response and resist phagocytosis by virtue of their capsule. However, H. flu is the more invasive of the two and soon reaches the submucosa of the respiratory epithelium. In addition, H. flu has two distinct adherence mechanisms, while the pneumococcus does not appear to have any. H. flu is outfitted with pili and another surface adhesin that has not yet been well characterized.

H. flu meningitis follows the invasion of the bloodstream (Fig. 15.2). How do the organisms enter the circulation? Most likely, this is the consequence of inflammation of the subepithelial tissue, which allows direct penetration of the organisms into lymphatics or small blood vessels. The organisms survive in the blood as long as circulating antibodies are not present in effective amounts. The titer of bactericidal antibodies correlates well with immunity. Anticapsular antibodies are strong opsonins and permit the organisms to be taken up and killed by fixed and circulating phagocytes.

We can now attempt to explain the unusual age dependence of H. flu meningitis. In a classic microbiological study, Fothergill and Wright showed in 1933 that immunity to these organisms is inversely related to the case incidence (Fig. 15.3). The greater the ability of serum to kill H. flu, the fewer the cases of the disease. The change with age has been explained as follows: Children are born with maternal antibodies and are protected as long as these antibodies are present. Hence the low incidence of cases before a few months of age. Much later, after the age of 3, antibody titers rise and the disease becomes less frequent. The puzzling aspect of the curve is, why don't younger children make antibodies if they are colonized with the organisms earlier in life? The answer is twofold: Early colonization is not usually by encapsulated strains, thus the young children may not actually have encountered the capsular antigens. In addition, and more puzzling, is the fact that immunity against capsular antigen type b does not arise before 2 or 3 years of age. The reason for this immunological unresponsiveness

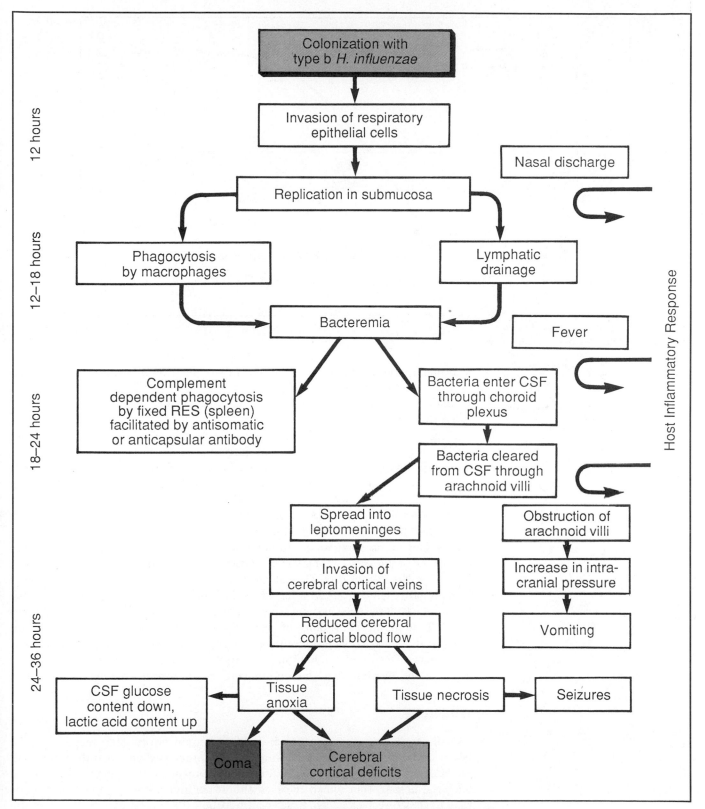

Figure 15.2. The pathogenesis of *H. influenzae* meningitis.

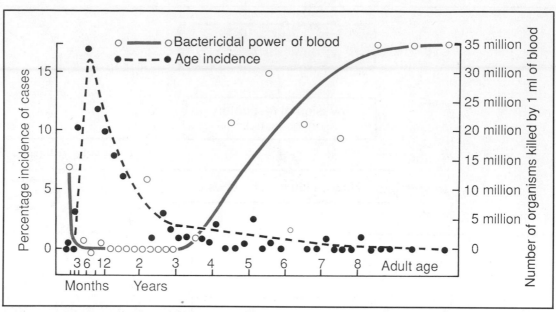

Figure 15.3. Relation of age to the incidence of *H. influenzae* meningitis and the bactericidal titers in blood of the population (From Fothergill LD, Wright J: Influenza meningitis: the relation of age incidence to the bactericidal power of blood against the causal organism. *J. Immunol* 24: 273–284, 1933.)

is probably due to the chemical nature of the polyribophosphate antigen. Polysaccharide antigens like this are not processed via T cells but are T cell independent. This immune response is not yet developed in infants, who rely on T cell antigen processing.

Once in the blood, how do the organisms reach the meninges? From studies with laboratory animals we know that the route of delivery is the cerebral arteries. The very first histological lesion in the brain is an acute inflammation of the choroid plexi. Note that this is the most logical site to cross the blood-brain barrier since it is the site of manufacture of the cerebrospinal fluid (CSF) and is highly vascularized. However, other organisms that cause bacteremias do not have such marked tropism for the meninges. The marked predilection of H. flu for these tissues has not been explained. At any rate, local damage on the plexal capillaries allows the organisms to enter the cerebrospinal fluid. Since the choroid plexi are located in the lateral cerebral ventricles, the organisms enter this compartment first and are then carried into the cisterna magna and over the convexities of the brain. The CSF becomes enriched with inflammatory exudate and is a good place for H. flu to multiply. Blockage of CSF outflow through the arachnoid villi by the inflammation causes the intracranial pressure to increase. This produces the early symptoms of meningitis—vomiting, lethargy, and depressed cortical function. It accounts for the rapidity of the symptoms in the disease, as seen in Michael's case.

DAMAGE

H. flu makes no known exotoxins. Its endotoxin is probably responsible for fever, intravascular coagulation, and perhaps other systemic manifestations. H. flu causes damage by evoking an inflammatory response. Phagocytosis results in bacterial degradation which releases endotoxin and possibly other compounds that have a direct effect on tissues. In addition, the organisms make an extracellular protease that is specific for human secretory immunoglobulin, IgA. They share this property with other bacteria that inhabit mucous membranes, such as the gonococci and certain streptococci (see Chapters 6 and 14). The role of this protease can only be surmised at present, but it may work to inhibit phagocytosis by removing the Fc fragments (which are pointing away from the organisms but are recognized by receptors on phagocytic cells).

Cerebral cortical dysfunction occurs both via impairment of the circulation and of the flow of cerebrospinal fluid. The meninges support part of the vasculature of the brain; cerebral arteries and veins run through this connective tissue to nourish the outer gray matter. Inflammation of the meninges may extend through the wall of the cerebral veins, which then become partially or completely thrombosed. Decreased blood flow leads to various forms of cerebral dysfunction, depending on the site of the cortex that is affected. Inflammation around the arachnoid villi in the dura mater blocks the flow of CSF. Pressure in the subarachnoid space then increases, leading to a rise in intracranial pressure.

This picture is similar in meningitis caused by the other common agents of acute bacterial meningitis, the meningococcus and the pneumococcus. However, the consequences are different. Meningococcal meningitis usually resolves without sequelae, and patients commonly recover without any further signs. H. flu meningitis, on the other hand, leads to further neurological damage in about 1 of 10 infants. This includes blindness, deafness, or obstructive hydrocephalus. Mental retardation is also common, manifested primarily in reading and language skills. One explanation for this difference is the magnitude of the inflammation of the subarachnoid space. It is least with meningococci, moderate with H. flu, and intense with pneumococci. About one third of the survivors of pneumococcal meningitis have severe neurological sequelae.

DIAGNOSIS

In the case of Michael we have already seen how examination of the CSF can yield rapid and accurate diagnosis. When the number of bacteria present is small, direct microscopic examination may not be revealing, and cultures must be performed. *Haemophilus* colonies are small but appear within 24 hours on enriched media. Three of the common meningeal pathogens can be differentiated using the information in Table 15.2.

Other tests on the CSF seek to document the extent of the inflammation and its effects on brain metabolism. These tests include counting the number and type of leukocytes and determining the protein and glucose content. Inflamed capillaries leak proteins into the CSF, increasing their concentration. Decreased glucose content in the CSF is indicative of meningitis because of the decrease in

Table 15.2
Bacteriological identification of common meningeal pathogens

Organism	Commonly Used Media (Agar)	Gram Stain Reaction/Cell Shape	Colonial Morphology
Haemophilus influenzae	Chocolate	Negative, pleomorphic	Iridescent gray, smooth
Streptoccoccus pneumoniae	Blood, chocolate	Positive, lancet-shaped	Gray-white, smooth mucoid
Neisseria meningitidis	Chocolate	Negative, diplococci	Small, bluish gray

cerebrocortical blood flow. Under conditions of partial anoxia, glucose is predominantly metabolized via glycolysis. Since this is an inefficient mode of energy production relative to respiration, more glucose must be utilized than is delivered to the brain. As the glucose concentration decreases, the concentration of lactic acid increases, lowering the pH and leading to other metabolic consequences.

TREATMENT AND PREVENTION

For antibacterial agents to be effective in bacterial meningitis they must be able to enter the CSF and be bactericidal. The reason why bacteriostatic drugs usually do not do well is that the infection takes place in a virtually closed system. Here even nongrowing bacteria can cause significant damage. For two thirds of the cases of H. flu type b meningitis, ampicillin meets these criteria. If administered intravenously it can achieve effective concentration in the CSF. However, one third of the strains of this organism are ampicillin resistant by virtue of making a β-lactamase. For these cases, there are useful antibiotics that are not inactivated by β-lactamases.

A vaccine against H. flu is highly indicated. The greatest preventive challenge with this organism is to protect the children who are at highest risk of getting meningitis from this organism. Note, however, the paradox: The children who are in greatest danger belong to an age group that is immunologically unresponsive to type b capsular antigen. It may seem, then, that a vaccine would stand little chance of working, and, indeed injections of type b antigen do little good in most of the children younger than 2 or 3 years. Recent efforts have been directed towards conjugating the type b antigen to proteins and to render this complex T cell dependent and immunogenic. This has met with some success but is still under investigation.

The antibiotic rifampin can be used as a *chemoprophylactic* for children who have been in contact with patients. Ann, the sister of our sick infant, could well benefit from the administration of this drug. However, this type of prevention should be used in a limited way because of adverse side effects and the rapid emergence of drug resistance among the organisms.

CONCLUSION

H. influenzae is a typical human pathogen that causes respiratory infections as well as a serious form of acute meningitis. This disease seeks out individuals that do not have anticapsular antibodies in their blood, namely young children who are immunologically unresponsive to the principal capsular antigen.

These organisms cause damage mainly by eliciting an inflammatory response. When this takes place in the meninges the consequence is a very severe disease. In an unacceptably large proportion of children, this leads to mental retardation. These are some of the outstanding problems in understanding and controlling these organisms:

1. How are the pathogenic varieties acquired?

2. Why do they have a marked tropism for the meninges?

3. How do they elicit a strong inflammation?

4. Can a truly effective vaccine be produced?

SELF-ASSESSMENT QUESTIONS

1. What are the microbiological characteristics of *H. influenzae*?

2. Explain the age distribution of *H. influenzae* meningitis.

3. What problems are in the way of making an effective vaccine against this disease?

4. What virulence factors of *H. influenzae* can you name?

5. How do you suppose *H. influenzae* enters the CNS? (This requires speculation, not knowledge.)

6. Contrast meningitis caused by *H. influenzae* and by meningococci.

SELECTED READINGS

Sande MA, Smith AL, Root RK: *Bacterial Meningitis.* New York, Churchill-Livingstone, 1985.

Sell SH, Wright PF (eds): *Haemophilus influenzae: Epidemiology, Immunology and Prevention of Disease.* New York, Elsevier, 1982.

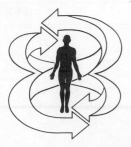

Bacteroides and Abscesses

F.P. Tally

Spillage of microbe-laden materials, such as the contents of the intestine or the oropharynx, into deep tissues often results in infections due to a mixture of bacteria. Examples are peritonitis caused by a ruptured appendix, or a pulmonary abscess due to inhalation of oropharyngeal bacteria. From such sites it is usually possible to isolate many different combinations of infecting bacteria. These infections represent the opposite pole from the "one germ, one disease" concept.

The bacteria involved include strict anaerobes and facultative anaerobes, probably interacting in complex metabolic ways. This chapter will focus on one of the most frequently involved genera, the *Bacteroides*. These strictly anaerobic Gram negative rods are common members of the normal oral and gut flora. However, the main pathogen of the genus, *B. fragilis*, has special pathogenic attributes because it is not one of the major members of this flora. One of these properties is probably its antiphagocytic capsule, but others still remain to be elucidated.

A HISTORICAL VIGNETTE

The famous magician Houdini died of peritonitis. Houdini was known for his astounding feats of escape while enchained and enclosed in containers submerged in water. He possessed amazing physical strength, and, as a point of outside interest, could control many muscles, including, it is said, some that are normally not under voluntary control. His fame was the cause of his demise. Houdini received an unexpected blow to his abdomen from a bystander intent on testing his legendary muscular powers. This resulted in the rupture of the magician's large intestine and his death a few days later.

Had Houdini lived today and been in the hands of a competent physician, he would have had a good chance of surviving as the result of antibiotic therapy. Let us contrast what happened to Houdini with a more recent case of a related problem, a perforated appendix.

CASE

Ms. A., an 18-year-old college freshman, was admitted to the hospital with diffuse abdominal pain, diarrhea, and nausea without vomiting. Her pain was localized to the right side of the abdomen. Physical examination revealed tenderness in the lower quadrant of her abdomen, principally over McBurney's point. She was given a cephalosporin antibiotic and taken to the operating room, where her ruptured appendix was removed. Cultures of the peritoneal cavity in the neighborhood of the appendix grew a mixture of bacteria, typical of those found in stool. On the second day after the operation her temperature spiked to 38.6°C. Blood cultures obtained preoperatively grew Escherichia coli.

Ms. A. improved postoperatively and completed a 7-day course of the cephalosporin. Since she had no further symptoms and her blood cultures were negative, the antibiotic was stopped. However, 36 hours later her temperature was 38.8°C and she felt diffuse pain over the site of the appendectomy. A CAT scan of her abdomen revealed a retroperitoneal abscess. Cultures obtained after drainage of the abscess grew B. fragilis. She was again treated with antibiotics (this time a mixture of gentamicin and clindamycin) for 8 more days and had an uneventful recovery.

Several questions are raised by Ms. A.'s case:

1. How did the two episodes of her disease differ with regard to pathogenesis and to the kind of bacteria involved?

2. How did anaerobic bacteria survive in oxygenated tissue? Why did they survive the first course of antibiotic treatment?

3. How do the organisms involved, specifically *B. fragilis*, cause damage?

4. Was Ms. A. treated properly?

No other place in the body is more prone to becoming contaminated by a large number of endogenous bacteria than the peritoneal cavity. The resulting intra-abdominal sepsis illustrates dramatically what happens when microorganisms are introduced in large numbers into the wrong place. The spillage of a few millimeters of intestinal content in the peritoneal cavity delivers many billions of bacteria to a customarily sterile site. Left untreated, peritonitis is often fatal, as in the case of Houdini. Indeed, in the preantibiotic era, perforation of the colon was a medical catastrophe. Nowadays the mortality rate is still significant, between 1% and 5%, and the diagnosis and management of these cases are far from simple. The physician who is not aware of the proper choice of antibiotics and the need for supportive therapy may well lose a patient to this disease.

Two points will be emphasized. First, intra-abdominal infections typically result in *biphasic diseases*, as in the case of Ms. A. They start with an acute inflammation and progress to the formation of localized abscesses. Second, of the hundreds of species contained in the colonic inoculum a few are most commonly isolated from abscesses. *Bacteroides fragilis* is found in 80% to 90% of all cases and is the single most important of the anaerobic bacteria associated with abscess formation. It is seldom found alone and is typically cocultured with a variety of other bacteria.

The largest number of intra-abdominal infections are caused by the rupture of infected appendices or intestinal diverticula, the abnormal outpouchings of the colon. It has been estimated that in 1983 there were over 250,000 cases of appendicitis and some 350,000 cases of diverticulitis. Of these infections, about 15% perforate and result in peritonitis and many produce abscesses as a late complication. The prevalence of diverticula increases with aging and so does diverticulitis as the cause of intra-abdominal infection.

INTRODUCTION TO THE *BACTEROIDES* AND OTHER STRICTLY ANAEROBIC BACTERIA

Bacteroides are obligate anaerobic, Gram-negative rods, present in large amounts in the large intestine of humans and other vertebrates. They number 10^{11} or more per gram of feces and are the dominant organisms along with anaerobic streptococci. Among *Bacteroides*, *B. fragilis* is a minor component, usually present in concentrations of 10^8 or 10^9 per gram of feces. The reasons why this species becomes dominant in deep tissue infections will be discussed below. Other members of the genus that are implicated in human infections include *B. melaninogenicus*, so called because it produces black-pigmented colonies on blood-containing agar. This organism is often found in the oral cavity as a member of the gingival flora and has been implicated in periodontal disease. Although this organism is also found in other sites, it is most commonly associated with infections of oral origin, including aspiration pneumonia (Chapter 45) and rather serious infections following human bites. Other *Bacteroides* are associated with infections of the peritoneal cavity that originate from the vagina. Table 16.1 includes the major strictly anaerobic bacteria of clinical significance, except the clostridia, which are described in Chapter 21.

Bacteroides are not killed by short exposure to oxygen, although they clearly do not grow in its presence. *B. fragilis* is among the most oxygen-resistant members of the genus. This is because it contains *superoxide dismutase*, which detoxifies

Table 16.1

The major clinically signicifant non-spore-forming anaerobic bacteria

Genus	Typical Species	Typical Diseases
Gram-Negative Rods		
Bacteroides (fragilis group)	fragilis thetaiotaomicron	Intra-abdominal infections
Bacteroides (pigmented group)	melaninogenicus gingivalis	Oral, dental, pleuro-pulmonary infections
Bacteroides	bivius	Pelvic infections
Fusobacterium	nucleatum necrophorum	Oral, dental, pleuro-plumonary infections
Gram-Positive Rods		
Actinomyces	israelii	Actinomycosis (lumpy jaw)
Propionibacterium	acnes	Infections of prosthetic devices
Gram-Positive Cocci		
Peptostreptococcus	magnus asaccharolyticus anaerobius	Intra-abdominal, soft tissue, bone and joint infections

oxygen radicals, and *catalase*, which breaks down hydrogen peroxide. The *Bacteroides* obtain energy by fermentation of carbohydrates. They can use complex polysaccharides such as the mucins present in the colon, which may be why they are present in such large numbers in feces.

The outer membrane of *B. fragilis* contains a *lipopolysaccharide* different from that of the typical endotoxins of the *Enterobacteriaceae* in that it is not toxic. This characteristic is not typical of this group of organisms. For example, the lipopolysaccharide of *Fusobacterium necrophorum*, another common oral Gram negative strict anaerobe, is distinctly endotoxic. An outer polysaccharide capsule protects *B. fragilis* from phagocytosis and is involved in some unknown manner in attachment to mesothelial cells and in abscess formation. These organisms produce many periplasmic enzymes, such as *lipases*, *proteases*, and a *neuraminidase*. Their role in pathogenesis is suggestive but has not been well documented as yet. Most likely, *B. fragilis* has multiple virulence factors, as seen in the staphylococci, streptococci, pseudomonads, and other multifactorial pathogens.

ENTRY, SPREAD, AND MULTIPLICATION

Breaching of the colon wall can result from blunt trauma, a ruptured bowel, a penetrating wound, or from abdominal surgery. In the case of Houdini, a sudden impact caused the colon literally to explode. In Ms. A.'s case, obstruction of outflow from the appendix led to inflammation and eventually to its perforation. Whatever the mechanism, the number of organisms contaminating the peritoneal cavity is enormous. Despite this, phagocytes can be mobilized rapidly in huge amounts to the infected site and, up to a point, dispose of large numbers of bacteria. The minimal infecting dose that results in disease in humans is possibly quite high, perhaps several milliliters of intestinal content, as judged from experiments with laboratory animals.

Organisms that enter the peritoneal cavity find themselves first in a liquid phase that could, in principle, lead to their dissemination throughout the cavity. However, the omentum and the loops of the small intestine drape themselves around areas of inflammation and serve to contain the infection. This takes time, but the abscesses that eventually develop are usually well localized. Lymphatic drainage and the effect of gravity also influence the location of abscesses. These are the likely reasons why Ms. A.'s abscess was found at a retroperitoneal site even though the original bacterial spill took place by her appendix.

Given the diversity of the bacterial inoculum, a large number of factors must be involved in determining which species become dominant in the infection. Many intestinal bacteria can grow in the peritoneal fluid, which is not particularly antibacterial. The first line of defense is most likely the mobilization of phagocytic cells, which happens rapidly. Thus, bacteria that eventually survive and grow must be quite resistant to phagocytosis. In fact, many are encapsulated. This may well be one major reason for the predominance of *B. fragilis*, since it is among the best encapsulated members of the genus *Bacteroides*.

At the moment when the colon contents are spilled, the peritoneal cavity is well oxygenated and highly oxygen-sensitive anaerobes are killed. The first organisms that become numerically dominant are facultative anaerobes, especially *Escherichia coli*. However, many of the less oxygen-sensitive strict anaerobes survive and can be isolated both from the fluid and from the surface of mesothelial cells. Eventually, the site of infection will become increasingly anaerobic, partly because facultative anaerobes metabolize what oxygen is present and partly because the site becomes increasingly avascular. The surviving strict anaerobes can then take over. That synergy between various microorganisms is required for abscess formation is clearly demonstrated in studies with animals. The inoculation of single species of intestinal bacteria seldom leads to infection, while infection with a mixture of facultative and strict anaerobes produces acute inflammation and abscess formation.

In peritoneal abscesses, the dominant *B. fragilis* is often accompanied not only by facultative anaerobes but also by other strict anaerobes, such as members of the genus *Clostridium* or anaerobic streptococci (*Peptococcus, Peptostreptococcus*).

DAMAGE

If the peritoneal defenses are unable to eradicate spilled intestinal contents, an abscess will usually develop. The areas of inflammation become walled in and surrounded by a thick, fibrous collagen-containing capsule. Inside are live and dead white blood cells, bacteria, and cell debris. In general terms, these abscesses resemble those caused by the staphylococci (Chapter 11).

Intra-abdominal abscesses exact a high toll from the host because they can extend to nearby sites, with resultant necrosis of adjacent tissue. In addition, they may enter the bloodstream. The resulting bacteremia may produce septic shock or cause metastatic infections at distant sites. The reasons for shock are not known, but may not be due to the lipopolysaccharide (LPS) of these organisms, since it is nontoxic. Vigorous intervention with antibiotics helped Ms. A. overcome her bacteremia.

OTHER *BACTEROIDES* INFECTIONS

In addition to *B. fragilis*, other species of this genus are also found in abscesses of the female genital tract, usually due to contamination with the vaginal flora. Here the infecting organisms ascend through the cervix, the uterus, and fallopian tubes to reach the neighborhood of the ovaries. The resulting infection is known as *pelvic inflammatory disease* (PID). Predisposing causes are scarring of the fallopian tubes due to previous infections by chlamydiae or gonococci (see Chapter 14). This impairs the downward action of the cilia of epithelial cells in the fallopian tubes. Resulting from the entry of organisms are so-called tubo-ovarian abscesses, which often lead to infertility. The most common agent of this disease is not *B. fragilis*, but *B. bivius*, a common inhabitant of the human vagina.

DIAGNOSIS

Proper chemotherapy of mixed bacterial infections requires the determination of the bacterial species involved and of their antibiotic sensitivity. Specialized techniques are required for growing members of the genus *Bacteroides* and other anaerobes. In general, these call for limiting the exposure of the specimen to oxygen because even oxygen-tolerant strains may eventually be killed. Clinical specimens must be protected from the air using special collecting devices and transported to the laboratory without delay. The most convenient way to handle and culture clinical specimens is by the use of an incubator in the form of a glove box (Fig. 16.1), a device in which the atmosphere can be made anaerobic by flushing with a mixture of inert gases. This equipment is specialized and costly and not all hospital laboratories are equipped with it. It is possible, however, to carry out anaerobic microbiological work with smaller but less convenient glass jars, as in Figure 16.2.

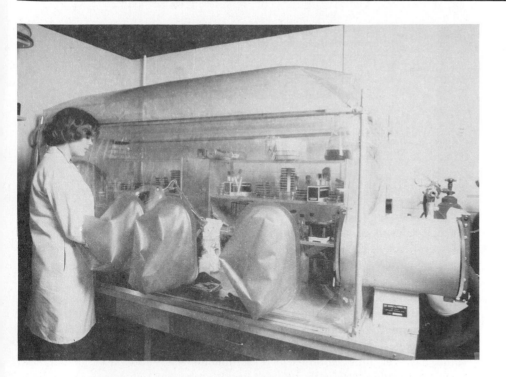

Figure 16.1. An anaerobic glove box used for the culture of strictly anaerobic bacteria. Such a device is used for large-scale work and for experimentation. Note the port on right, which is used to introduce and remove material from the chamber. It has two doors (not visible) and can be independently flushed free of oxygen. (Courtesy of Coy Laboratories, Ann Arbor, MI.)

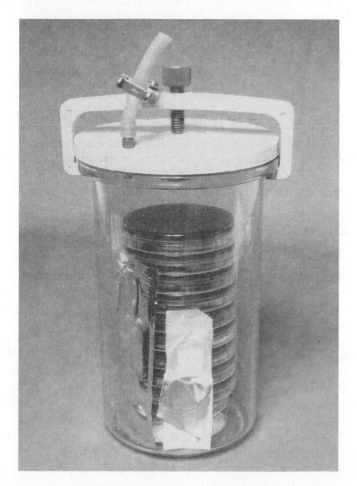

Figure 16.2. An anaerobic jar used for small-scale incubation of petri dishes. The small piece of aluminum visible on the left is a little bag containing a catalyst to rid the atmosphere of oxygen. The strip of paper in the foreground contains an indicator of anaerobiosis. (Courtesy of Baltimore Biological Laboratories, Baltimore, MD.)

Table 16.2
Antimicrobial therapy of experimental peritonitis

Treatment regimen	Acute Mortality, %	Abscess Formation in Survivors, %
Untreated	37	100
Gentamicin alone	4	98
Clindamycin alone	35	5
Gentamicin and clindamycin	7	6

TREATMENT

Localized purulent infections such as abscesses usually require dual therapy, namely drainage of the contents and administration of antibiotics. Additionally, the anatomical defect that allowed spillage from the intestine must be repaired. Thus, a combined medical and surgical approach is often necessary in cases of intra-abdominal infections.

In the past, antibacterial therapy was difficult because *B. fragilis* is resistant to many common antibiotics. Fortunately, a number of new agents have excellent activity against this organism (clindamycin, metronidazole). It must be kept in mind, however, that the target in these infections is seldom a single bacterial species but a mixed flora with different sensitivities. For this reason, a combination of antibiotics is usually given. The need for using more than one drug is seen in a study with experimental animals described in Table 16.2. In the case of Ms. A., it is likely that the cephalosporin first administered was not effective against *B. fragilis*. Her second treatment recognized the need for an appropriate choice, and she also received clindamycin, an effective drug against this organism.

Bacteroides cells possess sophisticated genetic systems to transfer genes for drug resistance. Plasmids and transposons can be transferred between *B. fragilis* and *E. coli*. Although genes from *B. fragilis* are not efficiently expressed in *E. coli* and vice versa, this transfer may be important in the epidemiology of drug resistance. Some of these organisms are undoubtedly the source of resistance genes for others. From a practical point of view, drug resistance has become a significant problem in the treatment of infections by *B. fragilis*.

CONCLUSION

Bacteroides fragilis is a versatile pathogen that colonizes the human large bowel. It possesses special virulence characteristics because it emerges from a numerically inferior position in the normal intestinal flora to become a dominant pathogen in normally sterile tissue. Left for future work is the elucidation of the role of the virulence factors. Among the many questions that may be asked: Is the capsule alone sufficient to resist phagocytosis? Do the various enzymes secreted by the organisms participate in damage? How do they do it? What is the role of the capsule? Two facts bode well for our ability to obtain answers to at least some of these questions. One is the development of a genetic system that allows the manipulation of the corresponding genes and the construction of suitable mutants. The other is the existence of relevant animal models for experimental abscess formation by this organism. Thus, genetically well-characterized mutants can be tested for their virulence.

Although the diseases caused by *B. fragilis* can be cured, the organisms still present challenges to therapy and, above all, to prevention. Unfortunately, there is presently no way to prevent these infections.

SELF-ASSESSMENT QUESTIONS

1. What are the major medical problems caused by this organism? How serious are they? Why was *Bacteroides* not implicated in many of these conditions until recently?

2. What are *Bacteroides*? Describe their major structural, physiological, and ecological properties.

3. What predisposes to infections by these organisms?

4. What do we know about the pathophysiology of *Bacteroides* infections? (Clue: Not much.)

5. What are the special therapeutic and diagnostic problems of these infections?

SELECTED READINGS

Finegold SM: *Anaerobic Bacteria in Human Disease.* New York, Academic Press, 1977.
Gorbach SL, Bartlett JG: Anaerobic infections. *N Engl J Med* 290:1177–1184; 290:1237–1354; 290: 1289–1294, 1974.
Tally FP, JL Ho: Management of patients with intra-abdominal infection due to colonic perforation. In *Current Clinical Topics in Infectious Diseases.* New York, McGraw-Hill, 1987.

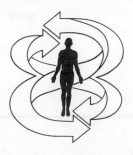

The Enteric Bacteria: Diarrhea and Dysentery

17

G. Keusch

Diarrhea is experienced by all of us at some time in life. It is usually little more than a bothersome watery stool. However, in developing countries it is one of the leading causes of infant mortality, killing over five million children every year at a minimum. In addition, it contributes greatly to malnutrition and to retarded physical and mental development. For these reasons, diarrhea has been singled out for a determined control effort by the World Health Organization.

Diarrhea lies at one end of the spectrum of intestinal infections and consists of *loss of electrolytes and fluids*, often in enormous amounts. In adults, the extreme example of this disease is cholera, with "traveler's disease" a milder form. At the other end of the spectrum are bloody diarrheas and dysentery, diseases caused when certain organisms *invade the intestinal mucosa*, which leads to inflammation and local tissue damage.

These diseases occur when the organisms overcome powerful defenses in the digestive tract. In every case the causative agents must be able to colonize or invade the mucosa of either the small or the large intestine and they may produce powerful toxins. A large variety of different bacteria are involved, collectively known as "enteric pathogens."

CASE

Mr. D., a 33-year-old accountant, his 29-year-old wife, and their 20-month-old son returned from a 2-week trip to Latin America. The next morning the infant seemed listless and his appetite was depressed. By the afternoon his stools became liquid and his temperature was mildly elevated at 38°C. As his diarrhea continued, he refused feeding, became dry, and looked glassy eyed. At the same time his mother developed abdominal cramps and passed several explosive bowel movements, which were followed for several days by semiliquid stools.

The child was brought to a pediatrician who recommended admission to the hospital. Microscopic examination of the stool revealed neither leukocytes nor red blood cells. Over the next 3 days the child was rehydrated by the oral administration of a sugar-salt solution. His fever soon abated and his appetite returned although the diarrhea persisted. The report of stool cultures was "normal fecal flora", with no enteropathogenic Escherichia coli present. He was discharged after 4 days, markedly improved but with mild diarrhea still present. His mother recovered with no specific treatment. The father experienced only a single abnormally loose stool during that period.

This family suffered to different degrees of intensity from traveler's diarrhea. This condition results from the encounter with certain bacteria, viruses or protozoa normally absent from the traveler's usual environment. The most common offenders are special strains of E. coli present in food or water contaminated with human feces. These strains circulate in the local population, usually without symptoms, undoubtedly due to the immunity afforded by previous exposure.

The scope of this disease is vast: The day that the child was admitted to the hospital, some 200 patients arrived at the hospital of the International Center for Diarrhoeal Disease Research in Dhaka, Bangladesh. Indeed, this scenario is repeated every day of the year in Dhaka. All these people have diarrhea, most are under 10 years of age, and about 1 in 10 will be admitted to the hospital wards because they are losing body fluids at such a tremendous rate that unless treated, they will desiccate within 24 hours. Some are already in shock because of the severe dehydration and will die unless replacement fluids are administered right away. Others have different complaints: They have high fever and dysentery, a syndrome marked by cramps and small but bloody and mucoid stools that are very painful to pass. About 1 in 10 of this group of patients is bacteremic, with Gram negative rods in the bloodstream. Half of them are likely to die unless given proper antibiotics.

Most of the patients crowding the outpatient area are not so profoundly ill. They will receive fluid treatment and be sent home, perhaps to return more severely ill in a day or two, or with a new episode within a few months. Pathogenic bacteria will be readily isolated from about one third of these patients' stools, but the predominant isolate is E. coli, indistinguishable by routine laboratory studies from the strains isolated from healthy individuals. As many as 40% of the younger patients suffer from rotaviruses (see Chapter 46) and protozoa such as Giardia lamblia (see Chapter 41).

The following questions suggest themselves:

1. Are all enteric bacteria capable of causing disease or are some more frequently pathogenic than others?

2. Where do the organisms come from?

3. What are the main types of intestinal diseases due to enteric bacteria? Why do the organisms cause different intensity of symptoms in individual people?

4. What virulence factors are involved in colonization? What virulence factors are involved in causing symptoms?

5. What is the proper therapy for different kinds of diseases of the intestinal tract?

6. Can these diseases be prevented?

INTRODUCTION TO THE AGENTS

Most of the bacteria that cause diarrheal disease belong to a large family of Gram negative rods, the Enterobacteriaceae. This family includes members of the normal flora of the colon that are only occasionally pathogenic. In spite of their name, the group also includes organisms that cause diseases in other systems of the body, especially the urinary and respiratory tracts. The Enterobacteriaceae comprise a large number of species that are differentiated on the bases of serological and metabolic details (Table 17.1).

E. coli is a typical member of this group and the enormous amount we know about its structure and function applies in general to the rest of the group. They are facultative anaerobic Gram negative rods, and many, but not all, have flagellar motility. When living or killed enterics are injected into animals or humans, the antibody response is usually to the *O antigens* (the long polysaccharide chains of their lipopolysaccharide) and, for those that are motile, to the flagellar proteins (*H antigens*).

E. coli is the most abundant facultative anaerobe in normal human feces, commonly present in concentrations of 10 to 100 million/g. It should be remembered that in the colon strict anaerobes outnumber facultative anaerobes by 100-fold or more. Most of the *E. coli* isolates seldom cause disease. Some human strains have been cultivated in the laboratory for so long that they have lost the ability to colonize humans. These include the famous K12 strain, which occupies center stage in molecular biology and has the distinction of being the best known of all cellular forms of life.

Individual serotypes of *E. coli* cause different characteristic diseases, which helps us to correlate specific bacterial properties with particular forms of intestinal infections. Many of these *E. coli*–associated diseases resemble those caused by other organisms. Thus, the watery diarrhea of Mr. and Mrs. D.'s infant is similar to that seen in mild cases of cholera. Other strains of *E. coli* cause a febrile

Table 17.1

The main genera of Pathogenic Enterobacteriaceae

Genus	Main Reservoirs	Principal Diseases
Escherichia	Colon of vertebrates	Diarrhea, dysentery; urinary tract infections; meningitis in children
Shigella	?[a]	Dysentery
Salmonella	Gastrointestinal tract of animals and humans	Diarrhea, septicemia; enteric fevers (including typhoid fever); focal infections
Proteus	?Colon of vertebrates, ?water, ?soil	Urinary tract infections
Klebsiella *Enterobacter* *Serratia* *Citrobacter* Others	?Colon of vertebrates, water, sewage	Pneumonia; septicemia, infections of compromised patients
Yersinia	Rodents, pigs, water	Plague, dysentery; lymphadenitis

[a] "?" denotes uncertainty

Table 17.2
Examples of serotypes of pathogenic *E. coli*

Enteropathogenic (EPEC)	Enterotoxigenic (ETEC)	Enteroinvasive (EIEC)	Enterohemorrhagic (EHEC)
O26:H11	O6:H⁻	O29:H⁻	O157:H7
O44:H18	O78:H11,12	O32:H⁻	
Many more	A few more	Many more	No or few others

O refers to "somatic" antigens, part of the bacterial lipopolysaccharide, and their numbers to different antigenic serotypes. H refers to "flagellar" antigens, and the numbers to different antigenic serotypes. H antigens are missing in nonmotile strains.

dysentery not unlike that due to the classic agents of bacillary dysentery, the *Shigella*. Some others cause a newly described condition, hemorrhagic colitis.

All strains of *E. coli* share the taxonomic characteristics of the species, even though they may have different virulence factors. Thus, *E. coli* is a taxonomic lumper's dream, but this is not without problems. The microbiological laboratory does not usually distinguish among the different strains of this species. Indeed, for Mr. and Mrs. D.'s infant, the report did not state which *E. coli* was isolated from his feces, but only excluded a group of a dozen serotypes known as EPEC, enteropathogenic *E. coli* (see "Other Infections Caused by *E. coli*"). Whereas one *E. coli* may superficially resemble another, the clinician and the epidemiologist know that this is far from being the case. The patient may know this even more intimately!

How then can one tell these strains apart? This is can be done by determining their antigenic differences. There are about 170 different serological types of O antigens. In addition, the motile strains have different kinds of H antigens, the flagellar protein. Some strains of *E. coli* also have a *capsular polysaccharide* antigen called K. The various assortments of these antigens help subclassify a strain of *E. coli*. Similar serologic typing is especially useful for the *Salmonella*, which comprise approximately 2000 serotypes. As suggested above, serological differences have practical significance, for certain serotypes of *E. coli* are associated with distinct clinical syndromes and with both intestinal and nonintestinal diseases (Table 17.2). A number of virulence traits are associated with these surface components and account for different effects on the host.

ENCOUNTER

Some enteric pathogens are *well adapted to the external environment* and only incidentally cause disease. The best example are the cholera bacilli, which live in brackish rivers and tidal estuaries. Such bodies of water serve as the source of the organisms without having to be reseeded with the feces of cholera patients. Instead, transmission to humans may be considered the abnormal event. Other enteric pathogens, on the other hand, are *host adapted* and are found mainly in association with the body of humans and of certain animals, usually in the colon. Although these organisms survive in the environment for a short time only, water supplies or foodstuff become a steady source of the pathogens if they are constantly contaminated with feces from carriers or diseased individuals.

Enteric pathogens vary considerably with regard to their host specificity. Some infect a limited number of host species while others have a broad host range. Some strains of *E. coli* are quite human specific; most of the infections they cause are by organisms derived from other humans. In contrast, many strains of *Salmonella* colonize or infect animals as well and are transmitted as zoonoses from animals to people (see Chapter 55).

When the number of organisms needed to cause infection is small, for example less than 100,000, they may be acquired by contact with contaminated objects, for it is surprising how many times individuals, especially children, put fingers, toys, or other inanimate objects in the mouth during ordinary daily activities. Flies may transmit virulent organisms by picking them up on their feet or proboscis and depositing them on foodstuffs. Here the organisms may multiply further.

The number of organisms required to cause disease is probably better known for enteric bacteria than for most other organisms. Experimental human infections have been induced in volunteers who agreed to drink buffered solutions containing a known number of living bacteria. These studies showed that a few hundred *Shigella dysenteriae* strain 1 are sufficient to cause disease in half the volunteers. In contrast, 1,000 to 10,000 *Shigella flexneri* 2a and more than 100 million enterotoxigenic *E. coli* are required to cause the same attack rate. A direct consequence of a small infective dose is that under the same conditions, *Shigella* are generally transmitted from person to person, since small inocula are readily passed by fingers or objects after contact with stool or soiled diapers. It is unlikely, however, that the large required amount of *E. coli* is transferred directly. It would take about a visible pea-sized lump of feces! It is much more likely that large numbers of organisms enter by the ingestion of contaminated food or water.

Despite the high standards of modern hygiene, we are nonetheless in constant touch with enteric bacteria. Our earth can be described as a globe coated with a veneer of feces, the difference between one place and another being the thickness of the veneer. This means that each day we all ingest feces to a greater or lesser extent, depending on our age (which determines behavior) and the state of environmental sanitation. Since potential pathogens are so common, we might ask why don't we get diarrhea every day? The answer to this question requires an understanding of the mechanisms of pathogenesis of these diseases.

ENTRY

Having arrived at the mouth, microorganisms face a watery, long, and perilous journey along the alimentary canal. The gastrointestinal tract is an open tube lined with differentiated epithelial cells that keep bacteria outside the body and deliver them to the exterior through the anus. The journey is perilous, because the microorganisms face host defenses designed to kill them or get rid of them. They are subjected to wide variation in pH, from about 1 in the stomach to 9 or higher near the ampulla of Vater, where the bicarbonate buffered pancreatic juice enters the lumen of the gut. Moving into the small intestine, they will be submerged in the 9 or so liters of fluid that enter the gut each day, partly from food and drink but primarily from endogenous secretions. They will be kneaded and squeezed and swept distally unless they find a way to hold on. They will also be smothered in mucus, rolled up in sticky polysaccharide balls, and propelled toward the anus by peristaltic motions of the bowel. On their way they will be accosted by soluble proteins such as lysozyme, proteases, and lipases, as well as bile salts, secretory immunoglobulins of the IgA class, and phagocytic and lymphoid cells. When they pause on their journey in the large intestine, they meet the populous normal flora that resists implantation by new species, in part by previous occupancy of adhesion sites on the gut wall, in part by producing inhibitory substances.

The efficiency of these host defenses is the reason why the infectious dose of most enteric pathogens is high and disease is not the norm. Still, sometimes bacteria get an advantage. When they arrive in the stomach mixed with food, they are protected from stomach acid, and their infectious dose is lowered considerably. In some patients, gastric acidity and secretory capacity are seriously diminished. Whether this is due to intrinsic disease (chronic gastritis or pernicious anemia), prior surgery (gastric resection, diversions, or transections of the vagus), or anti-ulcer drugs that inhibit gastric acid secretion, these patients are at risk of infection with bacteria that are acid sensitive, such as the cholera bacillus and *Salmonella*.

SPREAD AND MULTIPLICATION

The kind of *E. coli* that cause the uncomplicated diarrhea seen in the D. family are called *enterotoxigenic*, or ETEC. These strains colonize the upper small intestine and are noninvasive. They recognize preferred hosts and tissues by means of surface adhesins specific for receptors on the intestinal brush border membranes. This allows them to attach to the intestinal epithelium and avoid being swept away. At the level of the jejunum and ileum they have little competition because the resident flora is scant or nonexistent.

Adherence is not a simple feat since the surface of both microbe and host is negatively charged and should be mutually repulsive. However, the surface charges are not evenly distributed in either, and patches of greater or lesser negativity permit electrostatic attractions, aided by weaker attractive forces, such as hydrogen bonding, Van der Waals forces, and hydrophobic interactions. If such contact were via long, thin appendages the attachment would be stronger than by the apposition of large flat surfaces. This is indeed what nature has chosen to do. Adhesins (or colonization factors) are frequently found in pili, long thin structures that fulfill the above criteria.

DAMAGE

The diarrhea of the D. family was due to the action of two exotoxins that act on the epithelial cells of the small intestine. These *enterotoxins* are called LT and ST because one is heat labile, the other heat stable. Both act by changing the net fluid transport in the gut from absorption to secretion. Their biochemical mode of action is described in Chapter 7. The two differ in that LT, like cholera toxin, activates the adenylate cyclase-cyclic AMP system, while ST works on the guanylate cyclase-cyclic GMP system. Thus, traveler's diarrhea resembles cholera in the mode of action of one of its toxins; however, cholera is a much more serious disease because it leads to the secretion of much greater amounts of liquid. In neither disease is the intestinal mucosa visibly damaged, and the watery stool does not contain white or red blood cells. Accordingly, after recovery these diseases leave no pathological traces.

It is not easy to figure out why the members of the D. family had symptoms of such different intensity, although this is a common experience. Do the greater symptoms in the infant reflect lack of immunity from previous exposure or a higher inoculum? Did these factors matter in the two adults?

The ability to carry out genetic experiments with *E. coli* has allowed us to evaluate systematically the role of the two main virulence attributes of ETEC strains, *colonization* and *toxigenicity*. Strains with various combinations of these properties were engineered (Table 17.3). The experiments show that efficient

Table 17.3
Virulence determinants in pig strains of *E. coli*

Strains with Plasmidborne Genes for	Colonization of Jejunum	Animals with Diarrhea
None	No	0
K88 pili	Yes	3/11 tested (mild)
Enterotoxin	No	0
Both K88 pili and enterotoxin	Yes	12/16 tested

colonization requires the pilial adhesin but that the symptoms of the disease are full blown only when both adhesin and toxins are made.

OTHER INFECTIONS CAUSED BY *E. COLI*

ETEC strains of *E. coli* represent one end of the enteropathogenic spectrum of this species. The repertoire is quite large and includes a veritable alphabet soup of pathogenic groups: EIEC, EHEC, EPEC, and possibly more awaiting in the wings. Each is associated with a limited number of serotypes (Table 17.2) and causes distinctive conditions.

At the other end of the spectrum from ETEC are the *enteroinvasive*, or EIEC strains. They cause dysentery and resemble the classical agents of this disease, the *Shigella*. These strains are taken up into the epithelial cells of the colon within membrane vesicles by a phagocytosis-like mechanism. These cells are considered nonprofessional phagocytes but can be enticed to respond to proper stimuli. They are, however, quite selective, or else they would spend their lives ingesting the abundant bacteria in the colonic lumen. Some of the specificity resides in outer membrane proteins of the organism. These proteins are coded by plasmid genes, and curing the bacteria of the plasmids renders them noninvasive and nonvirulent (Chapter 9).

After invading the epithelial cells, shigellas or EIEC *E. coli* strains divide within the cytoplasm and produce intracellular colonies that spread to adjacent cells. Like shigellae, they make a toxin that inhibits protein synthesis and kills cells. When the infected epithelial cells die and slough, a microulcer is produced. This leads to a marked inflammatory response in the lamina propria, with outpouring of neutrophils, erythrocytes, exudate, and cell debris into the lumen. The discharge from goblet cells fills the lumen with mucus. Along with the pus and blood from the damaged epithelium, this results in the typical dysenteric stool, a small bloody viscous glob that is passed with great pain (Fig. 17.1). It is not clear if death of the epithelial cells triggers the inflammatory response, or vice versa. Either way, the intense inflammation disrupts normal peristaltic movement and pro-

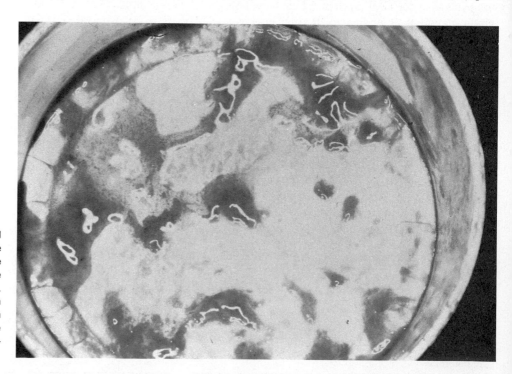

Figure 17.1. Typical dysenteric stool consisting of blood and mucus. Under the microscope, many white blood cells are seen. Such stools are small in volume and passed as often as 40 times a day. They are associated with intense pain upon straining to defecate and with abdominal cramps. Together with the characteristic stool, these symptoms constitute the dysenteric syndrome.

Table 17.4
Gram negative rods that cause diarrhea and dysentery

	Diarrhea	Dysentery	
		Ileitis	Colitis
Enterobacteriaceae			
Escherichia coli ETEC	+		
Escherichia coli EIEC			+
Escherichia coli EHEC			+
Escherichia coli EPEC		+	
Shigella			+
Salmonella (not *typhi*)	+		
Salmonella typhi		+	
Yersinia enterocolitica			+
Vibrionaceae			
Vibrio cholerae	+		
Campylobacter jejuni	+		
Other vibrios	+		

duces the severe cramps characteristic of dysentery. Inflammatory lesions are directly visible by endoscopy of the colon or by microscopic examinations of a biopsy.

A different group is the *enterohemorrhagic* (EHEC) *E. coli*. These strains cause a hemorrhagic colitis, but without invading the cells of the colon. They also produce large amounts of a toxin similar to that of *Shigella*, which may be the factor that damages the intestinal cells and leads to their necrosis and sloughing. Infection by these strains results in a bloody diarrhea in one-third to two-thirds of patients. In these instances the diarrhea is described as "all blood, no stool". Other serotypes, called *enteropathogenic*, or EPEC, cause a watery diarrhea, particularly in infants under 1 year of age, but are localized in the ileum instead of colon. They may also produce a *Shigella*-type toxin, but in lesser amounts. They are noninvasive but cause distinctive histopathology of the microvillus membranes (Table 17.4).

This is not the end of the list of diseases caused by *E. coli*. For example, these organisms are the most common cause of urinary tract infections (Chapter 48). Many of the *E. coli* strains that cause pyelonephritis possess pili that bind to a glycolipid constituent of kidney tissue. This does in part explain the tropism of these organisms. Other strains, which possess a capsular polysaccharide called K1 antigen, are invasive in young infants and cause bacteremia and systemic diseases such as meningitis (Chapter 47). In every case, specific virulence factors are critical in determining the nature of the resulting disease. Many of these are known, others are being investigated. Still others remain to be discovered.

DIAGNOSIS

Let us consider how the stool from baby D. was handled. It was inoculated into various media designed for both *selection* and *differentiation* of possible pathogens. Just by incubating cultures in air, the numerically dominant strict anaerobes were unable to grow. The media were chosen to permit the growth of enteric bacteria and not others. Media of this sort contain dyes (e.g., eosin and methylene blue, as in the so-called EMB agar) or bile salts, which inhibit growth of Gram positives. These media are not especially rich and do not allow the growth of the fastidious Gram negatives. In the case of the more delicate shigellas, the sample must be delivered to the laboratory promptly or the organisms may die in transit.

All the pathogenic strains of *E. coli* described look alike, both on agar plates and under the microscope. Most enteric Gram negative rods are also similar under the microscope and on nutrient agar. They are further classified on the basis of biochemical and nutritional properties, such as differences in the sugars they ferment. Some of the classical intestinal pathogens, *Salmonella* and *Shigella*, do not ferment lactose, and for this reason this sugar is usually included in the medium, together with a colored pH indicator. Lactose-fermenting colonies turn a distinctive color due to the production of acid. The lactose negatives are picked for further determinative work. But other pathogens cannot be selected by this method and must be sought by other techniques.

With the help of this ingenious array of differential and selective media it is usually simple to isolate *E. coli* even from samples that contain many different bacteria. These media and other special tests permit the laboratory to narrow down the identification to the main groups of Enterobacteriaceae (Table 17.1). Classifying *E. coli* into serological subgroups is not a task that most clinical laboratories are prepared to carry out. Indeed, the only serological reagents currently available commercially are antisera directed against some of the EPEC strains. Development of specific gene probes using DNA hybridization assays will no doubt simplify the task in the future. They are currently under development.

THERAPY AND PROPHYLAXIS

The therapeutic needs in the case of the D. family are to restore fluid losses, correct metabolic imbalances, and improve their physiological function. Luckily, the "secretory" diarrheas are usually self-limiting and terminate without specific antibiotics, as long as the patient can be kept well hydrated and prevented from going into shock. Baby D. was given a salt-sugar solution, and that was sufficient to achieve the necessary rehydration.

This simple form of therapy, if universally applied, could save the lives of millions of children every year throughout the developing world. Unfortunately it is not an easy task to ensure that such a simple solution becomes available in every household. Considerable experience has taught us that there are practical problems in making sure the salt-and-sugar solution is made correctly and that adequate amounts are given at the right time. Much effort is now being devoted to determining how to teach this methodology, but the problem has not been solved.

The dysenteries present different challenges: the eradication of the organisms, the modification of the inflammatory response, or both. Successful antimicrobial therapy requires that the drug reach the site occupied by the organisms and remain active under local conditions. Invasive organisms such as *Shigella* or EIEC strains of *E. coli* are located both in the lumen and within the intestinal mucosa, and respond only to drugs that reach therapeutic levels in both compartments. Unfortunately, the enteric bacteria can rapidly acquire plasmidborne multidrug resistance, and this is a constant challenge. Some intestinal infections, such as salmonella gastroenteritis, do not respond clinically even if the organisms are sensitive to antibiotics. Sometimes drug therapy even worsens the clinical condition of the patient. For example, the use of anti-intestinal motility agents, by decreasing intestinal transit time, may provide invasive pathogens a greater opportunity to breach the mucosal barriers.

Considerable efforts have been devoted to vaccine development. The challenge has been twofold: to identify and prepare protective antigens, and to find a way to present the antigen that leads to a local immune response in the intestine. So far, partial success has been achieved with a live oral vaccine with attenuated strains. It is important to note that no vaccines for enteric pathogens have become available for routine use. Molecular techniques are being used to develop a new generation of vaccines, which should result in significant progress in the near future and may allow the use of purified nonviable antigen preparations.

CONCLUSIONS

Diarrhea is not only the trivial bother that besets all of us occasionally. It is a major cause of infant death in the developing world. Symptomatic treatment by fluid replacement requires widespread educational effort.

Intestinal infections encompass a wide spectrum of manifestations, from the characteristic fluid loss seen in cholera and "traveler's disease" to the tissue invasion that characterizes dysentery. These diseases are caused by specific agents, such as the cholera or dysentery bacilli, or by distinct strains of *E. coli*. Exotoxins are involved in the pathobiology of many of these diseases and may account for all of the main symptoms. In addition, each of these organisms has a special ability to attach to certain cells in the intestinal tract and in some cases, invade them.

In every instance, local defenses of the gastrointestinal tract must be overcome. The efficacy of these defense mechanisms is best demonstrated by the fact that in developed countries we seldom succumb to intestinal infections, despite the fact that the gut is a tube open to the exterior. Disease is seen when the load of pathogens in the environment and their opportunity for transmittal are high. Predisposing causes such as malnutrition also play a role.

SELF-ASSESSMENT QUESTIONS

1. What are the main defenses of each segment of the gastrointestinal tract against microorganisms?

2. Which are the main types of bacteria that cause intestinal infections? What distinguishes them in the laboratory?

3. Explain the main virulence factors of each group of intestinal pathogens.

4. How many types of disease do different strains of *E. coli* produce?

5. How would drugs effective against bacterial diarrhea and dysentery differ?

6. What issues should be considered in the prevention of intestinal bacterial infections?

SUGGESTED READING

CIBA Foundation: *Microbial Toxins and Diarrhoeal Diseases.* London, Pitman, 1985, Ciba Foundation Symposium No. 112.

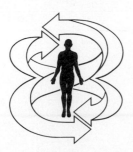

CHAPTER

The Salmonellae: Typhoid Fever and Gastroenteritis

18

G. Keusch
D.M. Thea

almonellae are closely related to other enteric pathogens, such as *Escherichia* and *Shigella*, and cause specific diseases: typhoid fever, gastroenteritis, and septicemia. Typhoid fever is still one of the severe epidemic diseases in certain developing countries but is found only sporadically in the more developed ones. On the other hand, salmonella gastroenteritis is among the most frequent of the foodborne diseases in many countries. It is a mild disease of short duration, but in rare cases it may lead to serious complications.

The pathogenic properties of *Salmonella* are not well understood. The organisms do not produce powerful exotoxins. Salmonellae do resist phagocytosis by macrophages and grow within these cells. Thus, they may become distributed to various organs through the circulation and produce local lesions in important sites.

CASE

Mr. J., a Southeast Asian exchange student, returned home for a 3-month visit. While there he was well, until he cared for an adult family member with fever and diarrhea of 3 days' duration. Two weeks later, Mr. J. had a shaking chill, fever to 38.5°C, headache, muscle aches, a sore throat, and abdominal pain. His symptoms resolved spontaneously after a few days. He returned to the United States 3 weeks later. Several days after his return he had an abrupt onset of chilis, fever of 40.0°C, and a watery diarrhea. These symptoms also abated *without specific treatment, but 10 days later he felt sicker and went to the emergency room of the student health service.*

On examination, his temperature was 40.8°C and he appeared ill and confused. His abdomen was diffusely tender and his liver and spleen were enlarged. He was admitted to the hospital and blood cultures were drawn. The next day the laboratory reported a Gram-negative rod that was identified 1 day later as Salmonella typhi, *the agent of typhoid fever. Mr. J. was treated for 2 weeks with trimethoprim/sulfamethoxazole and eventually made an uneventful recovery.*

The following questions arise:

1. What is the likely source of the typhoid bacilli that infected Mr. J.?

2. Why did Mr. J.'s illness wax and wane?

3. What was the cause of his fever, diarrhea, and mental confusion?

4. How can the disease be diagnosed with assurance?

5. Is Mr. J. at risk of coming down with typhoid fever again on a return visit to his country? May he become a source of the organisms?

To answer these questions you should have an understanding of the epidemiology and the pathobiology of typhoid fever.

In the United States, several hundred cases of typhoid fever are reported each year, some from local outbreaks, some from travelers returning from developing countries where the disease is more prevalent. However, in recent years a few cases have been seen among visitors to the most highly developed countries, such as Switzerland. Typhoid fever has been one of the important epidemic diseases in human history and we still have not seen the end of it. It figured prominently as the first chapter in Osler's 1897 textbook, in which he estimated that there were some 500,000 cases a year in the United States, with about 40,000 deaths. Fully 20% of the U.S. troops in the Spanish-American war had this disease, with over 1500 deaths. Typhoid fever is thought to be a major and increasing problem in some developing countries, where it may have a disproportionate social and economic impact because it often affects young and healthy individuals.

The name of the disease is derived from typhus, a very different disease with which it shares only a few clinical manifestations (see Chapter 25 for typhus). Typhoid fever is a foodborne or waterborne systemic disease still prevalent in regions with poor sanitation, where without therapy it causes death of 10% to 30% of those affected. The disease yields to the administration of appropriate antibiotics.

Typhoid fever is caused by a member of the genus *Salmonella, S. typhi.* Clinically, similar, usually milder forms known as *paratyphoid fever* are caused by two related salmonellae. Two other clinical presentations, *gastroenteritis* and *septicemia*, are caused by still other salmonellae. Typhoid fever is a highly complex disease, with several unique pathobiological features: It is at times a systemic, and at others, a localized infection.

THE SALMONELLAE

The genus *Salmonella* is a large group of enteric bacteria, closely related to the *Escherichia*. The salmonellae are highly motile and as a rule do not ferment

Table 18.1
The species of *Salmonella*

Name	Usual Host	Antigens
Salmonella typhi	Humans	O, H, Vi
Salmonella enteritidis	Animals	Many different O, H
Salmonella cholerae-suis	Animals	Many different O, H

lactose. According to current taxonomy, the genus contains three species only (Table 18.1), *S. typhi*, *S. choleraesuis and S. enteritidis*, which is an umbrella designation for what were previously nearly 2000 different species. The reason for this earlier taxonomic orgy of "splitters" is that investigators were focusing primarily on antigenic differences rather than on the unifying features.

Salmonellae have two major kinds of antigens on their surface: the *polysaccharide O antigen* of the outer membrane lipopolysaccharide, and the *flagellar protein*, known as the *H antigen*. The value of the antigenic classification, known as the Kauffman-White scheme, is that it allows one to fingerprint agents of specific outbreaks. This becomes an invaluable tool in the epidemiology of salmonellosis. Individual serotypes often contain more than one of each of these antigen types, which allows for an endless number of combinations. In the past each serotype was given a species name that is likely to persist in common usage. The names often refer to the location where the organism was isolated, hence *S. newport*, *S. dar-es-salaam*, or *S. montevideo*. A few are called after the animals with whom they are associated, e.g., *S. gallinarum* (chickens), *S. anatum* (ducks).

The three species of salmonellae cause different diseases and have *distinct host ranges* (Table 18.1) *S. typhi* is adapted only to humans; *S. cholerae-suis* and many strains of *S. enteritidis* are not so strict and attack many different animals. Others (e.g., *S. pullorum*) are so well adapted to animals that they only rarely cause disease in humans. Another distinguishing feature of *S. typhi* is that, in addition to the O and H antigens, it contains a so-called *Vi antigen*, a capsular polysaccharide that is associated with virulence in laboratory animals and perhaps in humans.

ENCOUNTER

Salmonellae are ingested with food or water contaminated with feces of infected hosts. *S. typhi* is exclusively a human pathogen, and its source is a human patient or a carrier of the organisms. The timing of Mr. J.'s disease in relation to his care of a relative with diarrhea suggests that this could have been the source of the organisms. *S. typhi* contrasts with largely waterborne organisms, the cholera bacilli, which are naturally found in bodies of water, or other salmonellae that infect domestic and other animals. Because of its limited host range, typhoid fever is a candidate for eradication, while cholera and other salmonelloses almost certainly are not.

Under experimental conditions, the infecting dose of typhoid bacilli is quite high, around 10^5 to 10^6. It becomes smaller if the organisms are ingested with a meal, with bicarbonate to neutralize stomach acid, or if the individual lacks the capacity to make normal amounts of stomach acid (achlrohydria). The relatively large inoculum size required to produce salmonella infection contrasts sharply with the smaller number of *Shigella* needed to cause disease.

ENTRY, SPREAD, AND MULTIPLICATION

S. typhi is not primarily an opportunistic organism: Typhoid fever readily affects healthy nonimmune persons such as Mr. J., not just debilitated people. This attests to the intrinsic invasiveness of the organism and to its ability to overcome constitutive host defenses. Typhoid bacilli display unusual ecological relationships within the body and, as a consequence, typhoid fever is a complex and unique disease. It consists of a series of definable steps, which are not always so sharply delineated (Fig. 18.1):

• Typhoid bacilli that survive passage through the stomach cross the wall of the small intestine. They penetrate the epithelial cells and cross them without apparent damage. They are then rapidly taken up by macrophages, in which they

Figure 18.1. Pathogenesis of typhoid fever. From Taussig MJ: *Processes in Pathology and Microbiology*, 2nd ed. Oxford, UK, Blackwell Scientific Publications, 1984.

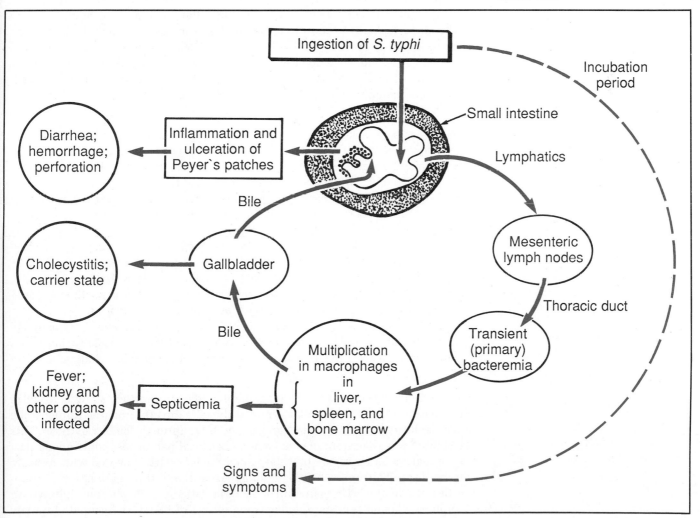

not only survive but actively multiply. *Prolonged intracellular residence* is the hallmark of these organisms and is probably due to intrinsic resistance to lysosomal enzymes. This has been demonstrated in different salmonellae, some other bacteria (e.g., the plague bacilli), and protozoa (e.g., *Leishmania*, Chapter 40).

• The organisms are soon carried inside macrophages to the mesenteric lymph nodes, where they continue to multiply. Eventually, they are released into the thoracic duct and enter the bloodstream.

• The number of bacteria that initially reach the blood is not very large, not enough to cause noticeable symptoms. They are rapidly filtered by the fixed macrophages of the reticuloendothelial system, especially in the liver, spleen, and bone marrow. They continue to multiply within these cells.

• When the intracellular population reaches a critical level, the organisms emerge and invade the bloodstream. This marks the end of the incubation period and the start of the clinical illness, with the beginning of a sustained period of high fever. These events take time, which is why the incubation period of typhoid is relatively long, 1 or 2 weeks from ingestion of the organisms to onset of symptoms.

The brief initial appearance of typhoid bacilli in the bloodstream may explain why killed typhoid vaccines have had limited success. Although the organisms are sensitive to lysis by antibody and complement, the bacteremic period is very brief and humoral defense mechanisms have only a fleeting opportunity to operate. The defense mechanism that ultimately controls the infection is cell-mediated immunity, which takes longer to develop and is only weakly elicited by the vaccine.

• Secondary bacteremia leads to the localization of the now abundant organisms at many sites of the body, accounting in part for the numerous clinical manifestations of enteric fever. Many of these manifestations can be better understood if one thinks of typhoid fever as a disease of the reticuloendothelial system (RES) and a disorder of the areas of the body where there are localized collections of cells of this system, especially macrophages (e.g., spleen, bone marrow, liver, Peyer's patches of the gut). Aggregates of infected mononuclear cells form the basic pathological lesion, the *typhoid nodule*. Such nodules are commonly found in the intestine, mesenteric nodes, liver, spleen, and bone marrow, but may be found in any tissue. These granulomatous lesions may necrotize from the occlusion of small vessels. If the nodules are located in the gut, this results in ulceration of the intestinal wall and diarrhea, as seen in the case of Mr. J.

Hyperplasia and necrosis of lymphoid tissue account for much of the symptomatology of typhoid fever but do not explain all of them, especially the mental confusion seen with Mr. J., and other neuropsychiatric manifestations seen in about half the cases of this disease.

• Typhoid bacilli eventually reach the gallbladder, where they grow actively in the bile. It is not known if they arrive at this site directly from the Kupffer cells via the bile canaliculi or if they are carried there through the bloodstream. This localization is somewhat unusual among bacterial pathogens and is due in part to the particular resistance of the organisms to bile salts. Note that what appears to be a specific tropism for the gallbladder is due to the combination of properties not shared with many other bacteria, i.e., the ability to multiply within Kupffer cells and to resist the damaging effects of bile. It is fortunate that few other bacteria have evolved these characteristics.

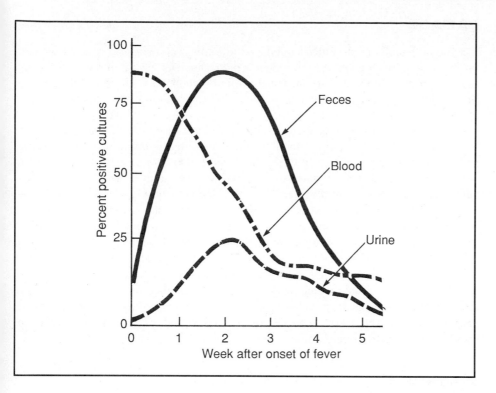

Figure 18.2. The isolation of typhoid bacilli from various sources in the course of untreated typhoid fever. The late rise in positive stool cultures is because of secondary invasion of the gut by organisms from the gallbladder.

• Contaminated bile infects the intestine for the second time, leading to the enteric manifestation of the disease. The inoculum size is now much larger than in the initial encounter and leads to a localized disease. It has two major manifestations. (*a*) The organisms localize in the lymphatic Peyer's patches of the lower ileum. They probably penetrate via the so called M cells, specialized epithelial uptake cells that overlay the lymphatic patches. At these sites, the organisms cause a strong inflammatory response. The process leads to ulceration and sometimes massive bleeding. (*b*) The intestine may perforate, resulting in peritonitis, a common cause of death in typhoid patients. This stage of the disease takes place when cell-mediated immunity has already begun to appear. Thus, while macrophages have become activated and are capable of killing the intracellular typhoid bacilli, the brisk inflammatory response may also result in tissue damage from the release of large amounts of inflammatory mediators.

The usual course of typhoid fever is 4 to 6 weeks in uncomplicated untreated cases. As seen in Figure 18.2, the sequence of events described above reflects the observed sequence of positive blood, feces, and urine cultures. In about 1% to 2% of patients the organisms persist in the gallbladder, causing an indolent chronic infection. Typhoid bacilli may also take advantage of the presence of gallstones and can be found in their interior. Infected gallstones dipped in antibiotic solutions for some time still grow the organisms when cut open. Since these persons continue to shed the organisms through their feces, they become carriers and may contribute to the spread of the organisms in the community. The paradigm in history was "Typhoid Mary", a cook in New York City who early in this century was the unwitting instrument of an estimated 10 outbreaks of the disease.

DAMAGE

Typhoid bacilli are not known to make exotoxins. Their endotoxin is almost certainly responsible for some of the systemic signs, such as fever and the debilitating wasting of muscle tissue seen in some patients (cachexia). These are manifestations of the *acute phase response* mediated by interleukin-1 and other mediators of inflammation (Chapter 4).

As we have seen above, typhoid bacilli may also cause local damage indirectly: When enough time has passed to elicit a cell-mediated immune response, macrophages become capable of killing the bacteria, but in the process they set off a strong mononuclear cell inflammatory response. The result is necrosis of the tissues. The mesenteric lymph system, and to a lesser extent other elements of the RES, contain areas of necrosis that progressively coalesce, leading to disruption of the vascular channels and other damage. This is different from the granulomatous pattern of inflammation seen with many other chronic type diseases, such as tuberculosis, brucellosis, and systemic fungal infections. In these diseases, granulomas are more distinct and necrosis is less prominent. The picture in typhoid fever more closely resembles certain parasitic diseases, such as toxoplasmosis or leishmaniasis. It is not known why S. *typhi* does not produce well-defined granulomas, but the secret is likely to be what signals it possesses to turn on specific inflammatory mediators.

DIAGNOSIS

Typhoid fever cannot be diagnosed clinically or microbiologically during the asymptomatic incubation period when blood cultures are negative. As seen in Figure 18.2, blood cultures usually become positive early in the disease. Blood cultures are easy to perform and do not require special techniques—only one kind of bacteria is likely to be present in the sample. Urine samples become positive later in infection, after the secondary bacteremia has seeded bacteria in the kidneys. Stool cultures are useful after secondary infection of the intestine.

For the detection of salmonellae in feces, selective media must be used to allow their preferential growth. These media contain bile salts at a concentration that inhibits the normal Gram positive and Gram negative fecal flora (Chapter 17). Notice that all fecal organisms have some intrinsic resistance to bile salts; however, because these compounds are reabsorbed in the ileum, their concentration is considerably lower in the large intestine (where most of the organisms live) than in the gallbladder, where typhoid bacilli thrive.

The detection of circulating antibodies against typhoid is useful in diagnosis, especially if several blood samples are taken over time. A stable, moderate antibody titer could be found in people who have been vaccinated, have recovered from the disease, or are carriers. Serological diagnosis relies on finding a rising antibody titer, or, if only a single sample is available, a titer that is unusually high. The test for antibodies is usually carried out by mixing dilutions of the patient's serum with suspensions of killed typhoid bacilli and, after incubation, observing a characteristic *agglutination*, that is, the formation of visible clumps of bacteria. The highest serum dilution that shows agglutination is referred to as the *antibody titer*. Other tests measure typhi Vi antibodies; however, they are not routinely done because other organisms also carry the Vi antigen and elicit the formation of anti-Vi antibodies.

TREATMENT

Several antibacterial drugs, e.g., chloramphenicol or ampicillin, or, as with Mr. J., trimethoprim/sulfamethoxazole, are effective in treating cases of typhoid fever. As stated already, patients must be treated for prolonged times, lest the organisms that remain sheltered in an intracellular location cause relapses. Interestingly, early antibiotic treatment is more frequently associated with relapses than if delayed somewhat in the course of the disease. This strongly suggests that cell-mediated immunity plays a role in preventing relapses.

PREVENTION

On a large scale, sanitation measures that prevent waterborne or foodborne transmission have proved effective and are the reason for the waning of typhoid fever in developed countries. Vaccination with a vaccine consisting of killed organisms is of limited efficacy in preventing typhoid fever but is still used for travelers to endemic areas. It produces pain at the site of the injection, headaches, and fever, all of which are preferable to typhoid fever. New, live oral vaccines are being tested in order to produce a greater degree of immunity, possibly including cell-mediated responses.

Typhoid carriers are a public health concern because they often are shedders: They not only carry the organisms but actively spread them via their feces. Treatment of typhoid carriers, though difficult, is a social imperative but must take into account the rights of the carrier as well. Since there was no successful treatment in her day, Typhoid Mary was put in jail! Today the recommended course of action is long-term antibiotic therapy. If that fails, removal of the gallbladder should be considered.

SALMONELLA GASTROENTERITIS ("SALMONELLA FOOD POISONING")

Many salmonellae other than those that cause typhoid fever are involved in human disease. The most common salmonella disease by far is an *acute gastroenteritis*. It is often referred to as "food poisoning," but this is a misnomer because the condition is not caused by a bacterial toxin present in the food but is a true infection. Salmonellae are the most common cause of gastroenteritis in the United States, with about two million documented cases a year. Staphylococci (Chapter 11) and other bacteria cause food poisoning by producing toxins in the food (Chapter 58).

Salmonella gastroenteritis is possibly the most common zoonosis or animal-derived disease in this country (Chapter 55), with *Campylobacter jejuni* closing in on the leader. Chicken, turkeys, and cattle may acquire the organisms from contaminated feed and either become asymptomatic carriers or acquire infection ("shipping fever") during transport to market. Their meat may also become contaminated in the slaughterhouse or at the food market. Thus the organisms are not host adapted but are more or less pathogenic for all their animal hosts. The most common *Salmonella* isolated in the United States, *S. typhimurium*, causes a typhoid fever syndrome in mice and other rodents that befoul animal fodder. The meat sold in markets, especially poultry, often contains salmonellae picked up from fecal material during the dressing of carcasses. Eggs, dried or frozen, are also common sources of the organisms. Salmonellae are killed by thorough cooking but survive in "rare" meat. Is it advisable to place the meat cooked on an outdoor grill on the same platter used to take it out from the kitchen?

The symptoms of salmonella food poisoning are noticed 24 to 36 hours after eating contaminated food, much later than the time after ingesting food containing, say, preformed staphylococcal enterotoxin. This relatively long incubation time is due to the need for the organisms to multiply to a sufficient concentration in the small intestine. The main symptom, familiar to most readers, is a watery diarrhea, sometimes bloody, and accompanied by low-grade fever. These symptoms may be due to the production of a cholera-like toxin (though this is still a controversial matter) and the initiation of an inflammatory reaction in the intestinal mucosa.

Food poisoning usually does not require treatment, except in children or debilitated adults who may experience heavy loss of liquids. An unusual sequela of salmonella gastroenteritis is a sterile inflammation of the joints, probably caused by an immunological cross-reaction. For unknown reasons, it is found in persons who carry the HLA-B27 histocompatibility marker, in common with other invasive enteric pathogens, such as *Shigella flexneri* and *Campylobacter jejuni*.

THE INFECTIVE COMPLICATIONS OF SALMONELLA GASTROENTERITIS

Although the disease is almost always self-limiting and mild, it has serious consequences in a small percentage of those affected. Salmonella may cause a variety of more serious diseases such as septicemia, osteomyelitis, or meningitis. Attesting to the central importance of the macrophage in determining the outcome of salmonellosis, conditions that result in the overloading of the RES enhance susceptibility to salmonella bacteremia. For example, patients with sickle cell anemia, in which chronic hemolysis may nearly saturate the body's scavenging system, have a 10-fold higher frequency of salmonellosis. Other arms of the immune system are also involved in fighting the infection, and salmonellosis is more frequent in patients with AIDS, leukemia, lymphoma, or chronic granulomatous disease.

The various species of *Salmonella* differ with regard to their ability to adhere to endovascular surface and cause endocarditis. Interestingly, despite its predilection for the bloodstream, *S. typhi* only rarely adheres to vascular epithelia, in contrast to *S. choleraesuis* and *S. enteritidis*, which have a great ability to attach to these surfaces. The resulting cardiovascular infection is more tenacious and difficult to treat than that caused by most other bacteria and often requires valve replacement.

CONCLUSIONS

Salmonella causes three main types of diseases: typhoid or enteric fever, gastroenteritis, and septicemia followed at times by localized infections. Typhoid fever is caused by a specific organism, *S. typhi*, whereas the other illnesses are produced by one of many serotypes of the other *Salmonella*. The pathophysiology of typhoid follows a unique series of systemic and localized events, resulting in a complex clinical picture. The most relevant properties of the organism are its ability to withstand phagocytosis by macrophages, its resistance to bile, and its endotoxin.

Salmonella gastroenteritis is a common disease, usually mild and self-limiting. However, in rare instances, infection by the causative organisms may result in serious systemic infections, especially in immunocompromised patients.

SELF-ASSESSMENT QUESTIONS

1. Describe the steps in the pathogenesis of typhoid fever. Relate the events to the emergence of symptoms.

2. Which symptoms of typhoid fever are systemic? Which ones are due to local damage?

3. Describe the properties of typhoid bacilli that help explain the complex cycle of typhoid fever.

4. What factors contribute to the persistence of typhoid bacilli within and outside the body?

5. Why does salmonella food poisoning take 24 hours or longer to manifest itself?

6. Did you know that raw food is often contaminated with salmonellae? What precautions will you consider in the future to avoid salmonella food poisoning?

SELECTED READINGS

Cohen JI, Bartlett JA: Extraintestinal manifestations of Salmonella infections. *Medicine* 66:349–388, 1987.

Hornick RB: Typhoid fever and other *Salmonella* infections. In Warren KS, Mahmoud AAF (eds): *Tropical and Geographic Medicine.* New York, McGraw-Hill, 1984, pp 710–722.

Rubin RH, Weinstein L: *Salmonellosis: Microbiological, Pathologic and Clinical Features.* New York, Stratton Intercontinental Med. Book Corp., 1977.

Taylor DN, Pollard RA, Blake PA. Typhoid in the United States and the risk to the international traveller. *J Infect Dis* 148:599–603, 1983.

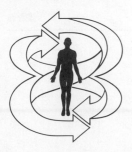

Pseudomonas aeruginosa: A Ubiquitous Pathogen

19

D.T. Durack

Pseudomonads are among the most common bacteria found in water, so we encounter them frequently. They are opportunistic pathogens that cause a variety of infections, usually in immunocompromised hosts such as burn victims, children with cystic fibrosis, and cancer patients. These Gram negative rods produce pigments that may make pus look blue or green. They also make a variety of important toxins, some of which may cause shock, while others kill tissue cells or hydrolyze structural tissue proteins such as elastin.

CASES

The multiplicity of factors that predispose to *Pseudomonas* infection is best illustrated with several clinical cases.

Case 1. *Ms. P., a 53-year-old schoolteacher, received chemotherapy for breast cancer. She became neutropenic; that is, her peripheral blood neutrophil count fell far below normal. One week later a small painful area of inflammation with a black center developed under her left breast (see Fig. 49.6 for a similar lesion), followed within a few hours by high fever and shaking chills. She was taken to the emergency room, where her temperature was high, at 40.5°C, and her blood pressure low, at 80/45 mm Hg. Her total white blood cell count was 400/mm³ (normal, 4500 to 10,500/mm³), with only 25% neutrophils (normal, 50% or more). Two blood cultures taken on admission and one the next day were positive for Pseudomonas aeruginosa. The clinical picture and the*

*laboratory reports permitted the diagnosis of septicemia induced by
P. aeruginosa.*

*Case 2. Mr. B., a healthy 30-year-old rigger, suffered third-degree burns over
40% of his body in an oil rig fire. After 3 weeks of intensive supportive care
in a burn unit, he suddenly became anxious and confused. His temperature fell
to 35.5°C, his blood pressure fell to 70/30 mm Hg, and his total peripheral white
blood cell count, which had been elevated, fell to 1900/mm³. Three blood
cultures grew P. aeruginosa.*

*Case 3. Mr. D., an unemployed drug addict, came to an emergency room
complaining of "feeling bad all over". Numerous needle tracks were found on
his arms and legs, some with superficial infection and associated phlebitis. His
temperature was 39.9°C; white blood cell count was 31,000/mm³, with more than
90% neutrophils. Chest x-ray showed multiple small patches of pneumonitis;
cardiac examination showed signs of tricuspid valve incompetence. Six blood
cultures were positive for P. aeruginosa.*

For each case, these questions are important:

- What was the main predisposing factor?

- How did the *Pseudomonas* gain entry? From what source did the organisms
  enter the bloodstream?

- How did the organisms make these patients so ill?

- What is an appropriate treatment and likely outcome?

- What other infections are caused by *Pseudomonas*?

These three cases have a common feature, namely finding *Pseudomonas* in the
bloodstream. The term *septicemia*, also known as *bacterial sepsis*, denotes proliferation of bacteria in the blood with the production of signs and symptoms. It
differs from *bacteremia*, which means solely that bacteria are present in the blood,
with or without clinical effects. Septicemias are infrequent in healthy persons
but are common in compromised patients, such as those described above. This
underscores the role of the normal defense mechanisms. To make matters worse,
Pseudomonas are among the most antibiotic resistant of the clinically important
bacteria, although some drugs are effective against them. The physician treating
a diabetic or a burn victim with *Pseudomonas* septicemia gets some sense of the
practice of medicine in the preantibiotic era.

Septicemia causes more than 100,000 deaths a year in the United States alone.
It is most often caused by Gram-negative rods, staphylococci, and streptococci.
The most common causative agents are *Escherichia coli* and other enterics, but
P. aeruginosa is responsible for 10% to 20% of the cases. This is not the only
disease caused by *P. aeruginosa*: These organisms are also responsible for many
other serious infections, such as pneumonia in children with cystic fibrosis. In all
the infections caused by these organisms the theme is the same: In nearly every
case there is a discernible predisposing cause.

THE PSEUDOMONADS

The members of the genus *Pseudomonas*, colloquially called the pseudomonads,
belong to a large group of aerobic nonfermenting Gram negative rods with polar
flagella. They are actively motile. About one third of clinical isolates are pigmented,
producing characteristic green or blue-green colonies colored by the water-soluble

pigment pyocyanin. Occasionally, other pigments are produced. Nonpigmented strains of *Pseudomonas* form colonies that are pale gray in color. Colonies on agar plates have a characteristic fruity or grape-like odor, which is sometimes noticed near wounds or other sites that are heavily colonized with these organisms. Some strains make a polysaccharide capsule, resulting in mucoid colonies. This is especially typical of stains isolated from patients with cystic fibrosis, whose lungs are nearly always colonized with this organism.

Pseudomonads are rapidly growing, robust organisms that can persist in marginal environments. Consequently, they are difficult to eradicate from contaminated areas such as hospital rooms, clinics, operating rooms, and medical equipment such as respiratory support devices. They may even survive in some antiseptic solutions used to disinfect instruments and endoscopes. They do not carry out fermentations, obtaining their energy from the oxidation of sugars; thus they are obligate aerobes. Pseudomonads have minimal nutritional requirements, needing only acetate and ammonia as sources of carbon and nitrogen. These simple needs are met by any of the large number of organic compounds, so they grow well on simple media, including nutrient agar and the media used for enteric bacteria. Being nearly omnivorous makes them popular candidates for industrial and environmental uses, such as cleaning up toxic wastes. The first patent awarded for a genetically engineered bacterium was for a pseudomonad designed to clean up petroleum spills by oxidizing hydrocarbons.

Most pseudomonads (except *P. mallei*) are motile, with one or several polar flagella. In this they differ from *E. coli* and other Enterobacteriaceae, which have flagella all around the cell. In fact, pseudomonads are taxonomically quite distant from the enteric bacteria. Most pseudomonads produce indophenol oxidase, the enzyme that renders them positive in the oxidase test frequently used in diagnostic microbiology. They share this characteristic with the neisseriae; few other clinically important bacteria are oxidase positive.

Pseudomonads are resistant to many commonly used antibiotics, including first- and second-generation penicillins and cephalosporins, tetracyclines, chloramphenicol, and vancomycin. The aminoglycosides and some newer ß-lactams are usually effective. Because the resistance pattern among pseudomonas strains varies from hospital to hospital and changes from year to year, proper choice of antibiotics must be based upon continuous surveillance of drug sensitivity.

ENCOUNTER AND ENTRY

Pseudomonas aeruginosa, the most important species for medicine, is commonly present in our everyday environment. It is typically a water organism that thrives in ponds, rivers, drains and sewerage. In homes and hospitals it is usually present in kitchens and bathrooms, especially around taps and sink drains, on damp surfaces and in moist, dirty corners. Outdoors, it is found in the slime layer on the banks and bottoms of pools and streams.

Because of their distribution, *Pseudomonas* inevitably are ingested into the human alimentary tract at frequent intervals. Nevertheless it usually does not become a permanent colonizer; they are found in the fecal flora in only about 1 in every 10 normal people. Although not commonly present in the oral flora of normal humans, it and other aerobic Gram negative bacilli proliferate in the oropharynx of elderly, debilitated, or hospitalized patients, especially if they are receiving antibiotics. *Pseudomonas* strains commonly colonize wounds and ulcers, in which case the pus may be colored green or blue.

Table 19.1

Relationship between selected predisposing factors and varieties of *Pseudomonas* infection

Predisposing Factor	Type of Infection
Early age—premature infants and neonates	Septicemia, meningitis, enteritis
Diabetes	Malignant otitis externa
Burns	Burn wound infection, septicemia
Trauma	Osteomyelitis
Intravenous drug abuse	Endocarditis, septic arthritis osteomyelitis
Cystic fibrosis	Pneumonia, chronic or recurrent
Neutropenia	Septicemia, pneumonia, abscesses
Neurosurgical operations	Meningitis
Surgical operations	Pneumonia
Tracheostomy	Pneumonia
Intravenous lines	Cellulitis, suppurative thrombophlebitis
Corneal injury	Panophthalmitis
Kidney stones	Urinary tract infection
Catheterization	Urinary tract colonization and urinary tract infection

P. aeruginosa is an opportunistic human pathogen par excellence. One or more major predisposing factors can usually be found. These include surgical operations, urinary catheters and the presence of other foreign bodies, neutropenia and others (Table 19.1). *Pseudomonas* cause 10% to 15% of all nosocomial infections. Because it is resistant to many common antibiotics, and has the capacity to develop high levels of resistance to other antibiotics during treatment, it poses serious problems for the affected patient and the physician. Although *P. aeruginosa* is the most important species for human infection; many other species in this genus—among them *P. cepacia, P. mallei, P. pseudomallei, P. putida,* and *P. stutzeri*—occasionally cause disease.

The portal of entry is different for each of the three illustrative cases above. In the neutropenic patient (Case 1, Mrs. P.), the precise portal of entry cannot be determined, but the organisms probably entered the bloodstream from the gastrointestinal tract. In normal people, neutrophils and other defenses in the bowel wall usually contain the organisms that cross the mucosal barrier. In neutropenic patients this critical element of the normal defenses against *Pseudomonas* is deficient, allowing the organisms to multiply unchecked in the tissues. This results in septicemia. Other potential portals of entry in a neutropenic patient are intravenous cannulas, central venous lines, and urinary catheters. These can provide direct access for environmental organisms to the bloodstream.

In the burned patient (Case 2, Mr. B.), the surface of the burn wound became colonized with *P. aeruginosa* from the environment, despite the use of topical antiseptics to which these organisms are often resistant. In one or more sites in the burnt skin, colonizing organisms invaded deeper layers and began to multiply in the damaged tissue below the burn. Normal host defenses, especially neutrophils, do not function normally in burned tissue that is deprived of normal blood flow. Once the organisms mutliply to a count of 10^5 or more per gram of tissue they are likely to spill over into the bloodstream, resulting in septicemia.

Another important potential entry site is the urinary tract. If a patient is catheterized in the course of intensive care, the urinary tract may become colonized or infected with enteric bacteria or *Pseudomonas*. Colonization with associated recurrent infection will usually persist as long as the catheter remains in place, even for life.

In the drug addict (Case 3.), the portal of entry was provided by one of his injection sites. Addicts often draw unsterile water from sinks or toilet bowls to mix and dilute their drugs. Alternatively, the drugs themselves might be contaminated with *Pseudomonas*. Contamination from either source results in direct intravenous injection of *Pseudomonas*. These organisms may also cause local cellulitis or suppurative thrombophlebitis at an injection site, which in turn can give rise to secondary bacteremia. Bacteria passing through the heart from any of these origins may colonize the heart valves, causing endocarditis. The tricuspid valve is commonly infected in this way, but primary or secondary infection of left-sided heart valves also is common in drug addicts.

If present in large enough numbers, pseudomonads may enter the skin, possibly through insignificant abrasions. This happens when people take baths in contaminated hot tubs, which may result in furuncles (boils) all over the body. The favorable conditions of temperature in hot tubs allow for spectacular blooms of *Pseudomonas* that reach up to 100 million organisms per milliliter!

SPREAD, MULTIPLICATION, AND DAMAGE

Pseudomonads are typical extracellular pathogens. Their growth in tissue depends largely on their ability to resist ingestion by neutrophils. Many strains possess an antiphagocytic polysaccharide slime layer and make cytolytic exotoxins. Nonetheless, the low frequency of pseudomonad infections in healthy persons shows that the phagocytes usually have the upper hand. Patients like Mrs. P., with reduced numbers of circulating neutrophils, are at high risk.

What accounts for the striking symptoms and signs in these three cases? *Pseudomonas* damage the host in a variety of ways. Like other Gram negatives, they can cause hypotension and shock, most likely because their cell walls contain lipopolysaccharides that act as endotoxins (see Chapter 7). The organisms also elaborate a wide variety of exotoxins (Table 19.2). These can cause local inflammation, tissue destruction, and abscess formation. For example, during the course of endocarditis *Pseudomonas* frequently destroy part of the affected valve, causing heart murmurs as in Case 3, Mr. D.

Circulating *Pseudomonas* have a special tendency to infect vascular endothelium. They can invade the wall of small arteries or arterioles where they multiply rapidly to reach vast numbers. The resulting endothelial damage promotes thrombosis, so that affected segments become obstructed by an infected clot. In turn this leads to necrosis of the overlying skin, producing a characteristic lesion termed *ecthyma gangrenosum*. This is the lesion described above in the neutropenic patient (Case 1). It is virtually pathognomonic (specifically distinctive) for

Table 19.2
Some of the toxins produced by *Pseudomonas aeruginosa*

Name	Activity
Elastase	Breakdown of elastin
Proteases	Breakdown of proteins
Phospholipase C	Hemolysis; breakdown of surfactant
Exotoxin A	Dermonecrosis; cell necrosis
Lipid A component of lipopolysaccharide	Endotoxin

the *Pseudomonas* infection, although other Gram negative rods occasionally cause the same lesion.

Once in the bloodstream, these bacteria may set up secondary or metastatic infections in other anatomic sites. These include bone (causing, for example, vertebral osteomyelitis), the central nervous system (meningitis), or the lung (Gram negative pneumonia). However, these localized metastatic infections are less likely to occur with *Pseudomonas* bacteremia than with some other organisms, especially *Staphylococcus aureus*. *Pseudomonas* osteomyelitis and meningitis are caused more often by direct introduction of organisms from local trauma than from hematogenous seeding.

In summary, the likelihood that *Pseudomonas* infection will develop is highly dependent on host factors. The normal host is usually unharmed by this common inhabitant of our environment, but local damage to tissues or neutropenia may render the patient highly susceptible. If a high enough inoculum is present, even normal host defenses may be overwhelmed, as in parenteral drug addicts or in normal people bathing in highly contaminated water. The outcome of *Pseudomonas* infection depends on the nature and severity of the infection, the state of host defenses, and treatment. A high-grade bacteremia in a neutropenic patient carries a high mortality, 50% to 70%. Pseudomonas endocarditis likewise carries a high mortality, up to 50%.

PREVENTION AND TREATMENT

By far the most important and most effective prophylactic strategy is the maintenance of normal host defenses. After these have been breached, several strategies may help reduce the risk of *Pseudomonas* infection. First, the environment should be kept relatively free of these organisms. Rooms and hospital equipment should be cleaned and sterilized. Leafy salads and fruits should be omitted from the patient's diet because they often carry pseudomonads. Unnecessary broad-spectrum antibiotic prophylaxis or therapy should be minimized to avoid overgrowth of Gram negative organisms in the oropharynx and increasing antibiotic resistance in the host's flora. The number of intravenous or intra-arterial lines should be kept to an absolute minimum.

Passive immunization has been attempted with antisera against an antigenic determinant common to most Gram negative organisms including pseudomonads. A strain of *E. coli*, J5, carries an antigenic determinant common to most enteric Gram negative aerobes including *Pseudomonas*. Polyclonal antibodies raised against this strain have been used to treat neutropenic patients with fever. The results indicate significant therapeutic benefit, but the lack of a standard preparation so far has kept this promising form of therapy from general use. Active immunization is not available.

Supportive treatment includes intensive monitoring and care for patients with hypotension or shock. Local treatment is necessary to reduce colonization and infection of wounds and intravenous sites. Choice of specific therapy may present a challenge because the pseudomonads are relatively drug resistant. Treatment options include fourth-generation penicillins, third-generation cephalosporins, aminoglycosides, or quinolones. Combination therapy with two, or even three, antibiotics is frequently chosen for serious infections. The regimen selected should be given parenterally and at full doses.

Leukocyte therapy has been tested rather extensively in neutropenic and other patients. It has been marginally successful, but only when large and repeated infusions of neutrophils are used. Most reviewers conclude that leukocyte transfusions are likely to be useful only in carefully selected cases when an ample supply of leukocytes is available.

CONCLUSIONS

P. aeruginosa are a paradigm of an opportunistic environmental pathogen. They are abundant in our environment, causing diseases mainly in patients who have impaired body defenses. Occasionally they overcome the defenses of healthy persons, but this is likely only if the inoculum size is very large. Prevention and treatment of *Pseudomonas* infection in patients debilitated by major underlying diseases are important goals in modern medicine.

SELF-ASSESSMENT QUESTIONS

1. Describe the microbiological characteristics of the pseudomonads.

2. What are the main clinical syndromes caused by *P. aeruginosa*?

3. What types of patients are most often infected?

4. Describe some of the virulence factors of these organisms.

5. List some of the therapeutic problems encountered in pseudomonad infections.

SUGGESTED READINGS

Baltch AL, Griffin PE: *Pseudomonas aeruginosa* bacteremia: a clinical study of 75 patients. *Am J Med Sc* 274:119–129, 1977.
Bodey GP: Infections caused by *Pseudomonas aeruginosa*. *Rev Infect Dis* 5:279, 1983.
Cross A, Allen JR, Burke J, et al: Nosocomial infections due to *Pseudomonas aeruginosa*: review of recent trends. *Rev Infect Dis* 5 (Suppl):S837–S845, 1983.
Olson B, Weinstein RTA, Nathan C, et al: Epidemiology of endemic *Pseudomonas aeruginosa*: why infection control efforts have failed. *J Infect Dis* 150:808–816, 1984.
Pollack M: *Pseudomonas aeruginosa*. In Mandell GL, Douglas RG, Bennett JE, (eds): *Principles and Practice of Infectious Diseases*, 1985, pp 1236–1250.

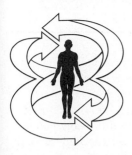

Bordetella pertussis and Whooping Cough

20

A. Smith

In patients with whooping cough the agent, *Bordetella pertussis*, is found on epithelial cells of the bronchioles. These Gram negative rods make powerful toxins that penetrate tissues and kill cells. These toxins immobilize the ciliary elevator and cause the accumulation of thick mucus. The characteristic whooping cough may be due to sensitization of "cough receptors" in the trachea by a toxin. These organisms are incorporated in killed form in the DPT vaccine given to infants. The pertussis component of the vaccine is responsible for some of its rare side effects.

CASE

Eight weeks after her birth, Peggy was taken to her family doctor for a checkup and her first baby shot. The immunization was postponed for a month because she had a slight cold and a runny nose. This may have been acquired from one of her three siblings or her grandfather who lived with the family, all of whom had colds recently. Subsequently, Peggy began sneezing and coughing. It seemed as if any loud noise would bring on a coughing spell. Peggy's mother became concerned when Peggy turned blue after a series of coughing spells that ended with vomiting. Later, during an examination of the infant by a physician, Peggy had a series of "barky" coughs, after which she vomited and could not catch her breath. Her mother was told that Peggy had whooping cough and needed to be hospitalized.

The laboratory report showed an elevated white blood cell count, chiefly due to a large increase in the number of lymphocytes. A nasopharyngeal specimen grew Bordetella pertussis, the causative agent of whooping cough.

Peggy's mother wanted to know the following: How dangerous is whooping cough? Why was the physician sure of the diagnosis? Where did Peggy catch the "bug"? Will antibiotics make her better? When can she get her baby shots?

If you had to answer these questions, you would have to know something about the following:

1. The epidemiology of *B. pertussis.*

2. How the infection causes disease.

3. The pros and cons of vaccination.

4. How whooping cough is diagnosed.

Whooping cough, or pertussis, is a severe childhood disease that has been nearly eradicated due to vaccination. Baby shots contain killed *B. pertussis*, the "P" in DPT, which is very effective in preventing the disease. However, DPT vaccination often causes mild adverse reactions and, rarely, serious complications. In recent years the number of infants who have not received the vaccine has increased. The result is that the number of cases of whooping cough in the United States has risen sharply in recent years. In 1981 the childhood incidence of whooping cough was 0.5 cases per 100,000 population. This increased threefold, to 1.5 cases per 100,000 children by 1985.

Whooping cough is an important disease for three reasons:

• It is highly communicable among susceptible infants less than 1 year of age.

• It is life threatening in infants with underlying cardiac or pulmonary disease.

• It can lead to neurological sequelae.

The *local manifestations* of whooping cough are those of bronchitis, with accumulation of mucus, inflammatory debris, and bacteria. The mucociliary elevator is impaired by damage to the ciliary epithelial cells. As a result, the only clearance mechanism available is the violent cough that gives the disease its name. In addition, patients with whooping cough have systemic symptoms, such as low grade fever, lymphocytosis, and heightened sensitivity to histamine and serotonin.

THE BORDETELLA

Bordetella are small Gram negative, strictly aerobic rods that belong to the group of *nutritionally fastidious* organisms that includes the genus *Haemophilus*. *Bordetella* are grown in complex media that fulfill their nutritional requirements and also contain blood or other additives to neutralize inhibitory compounds, such as fatty acids. *Bordetella* are also very sensitive to chemical and physical agents in the environment and do not survive outside the body for appreciable periods of time.

B. pertussis cause disease without penetrating through epithelial membranes (Fig. 20.1). They have specific adhesins that permit them to attach to epithelial cells of the respiratory tract. They also manufacture exotoxins, which penetrate

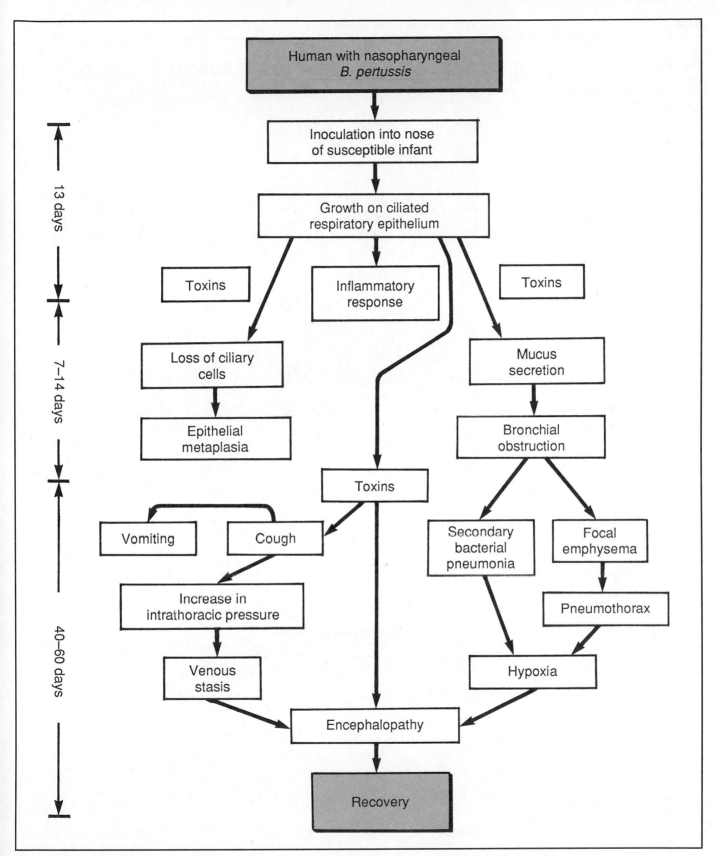

Figure 20.1. Pathogenesis of *B. pertussis*.

Figure 20.2. *Bordetella pertussis* adhering to ciliated respiratory epithelial cells seen in the scanning electron microscope. Note the clump of bacteria attached to the partially extruded epithelial cell (*arrow*). From Muse KE et al: Scanning electron microscopic study of hamster tracheal organ cultures infected with *Bordetella pertussis. J Infect Dis* 136:771–777, 1977.

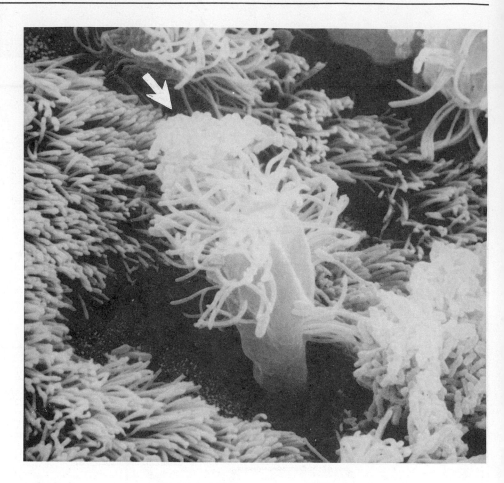

into host cells and contribute to the signs and symptoms of the disease. As with other Gram negatives, *B. pertussis* possess endotoxin, which is probably responsible for the fever and perhaps for some of the other signs of the disease as well (Table 20.1)

Table 20.1
Major toxins of *Bordetella pertussis*

Name	Chemical Nature	Site of Action	Biochemical Activities	Physiological Effects
Pertussis toxin	Protein	Local and systemic	ADP-ribosylates protein	Impairs neutrophil chemotaxis, phagocytosis, and bactericidal activity; encephalopathy; lymphocytosis
Adenylate cyclase	Protein	Local	Converts ATP to cAMP	Histamine sensitization mimics pertussis toxin activity on neutrophils. Increases capillary permeability leading to edema
Tracheal cytotoxin	Murein	Local	?	Kills ciliated respiratory epithelial cells; adjuvant
Endotoxin	Lipopolysaccharide	Systemic	?	Fever; adjuvant

ENCOUNTER

These delicate bacteria are thought to be exclusively human pathogens since they neither survive in the environment nor are known to infect other animal species. Their reservoir is not really known, and they are rarely found in the nasopharynx of healthy persons. The organisms are exceptionally contagious and may affect upward of 90% of the members of a nonimmune family that becomes exposed. Not all people will recognize that they have been infected because the classical symptoms of whooping cough are dependent on the state of immunity. Young infants typically have whooping, paroxysmal cough with vomiting and respiratory distress.

In people older than 15 years the disease may be indistinguishable from a mild "viral" upper respiratory tract disease without cough. This milder manifestation of B. pertussis disease may be attributed to host resistance due to immunization or previous infection. It becomes important, then, for the physician who is treating a baby like Peggy to take a complete history of all family members and to alert them to the possibility that they may contract whooping cough. It should be pointed out that the epidemiology of this disease is not always clear: Vaccination records for childhood diseases are often poorly kept.

ENTRY

B. pertussis enters the trachea and bronchi by inhalation. The organisms attach to the cilia of epithelial cells of the large airways and are seldom found anywhere else (Figs. 20.1, 20.2). Whooping cough is entirely a superficial infection, which means that the organisms rarely enter deep tissue; other important bacterial diseases with this characteristic include diphtheria and cholera. B. pertussis shows a strong tissue tropism for the ciliated epithelium of the respiratory tract. The reason for this phenomenon is not clearly understood, but it may be due to the specific interaction between pertussis adhesins (which are as yet poorly characterized) and receptors on the cells of this tissue. The cell receptors to which B. pertussis binds are probably glycoproteins. Table 20.2 describes an experiment that suggests that the ligand on the bacteria is a protein (trypsin sensitive) and the receptors on the cells contain carbohydrate (binding can be prevented by competition with added carbohydrates or by oxidation with periodate).

SPREAD, MULTIPLICATION, AND DAMAGE

The first stages of whooping cough result in a mild inflammatory response in the submucosa that is manifested clinically by infrequent coughing, a runny nose, and a low-grade fever. Administration of the vaccine at this stage is not indicated

Table 20.2
Effect of pretreatment of bacteria or ciliated cells on cell binding of _Bordetella pertussis_

Treatment	Bacteria	Cells
Trypsin	Decrease	No effect
Antibodies to _B. pertussis_ adhesins	Decrease	No effect
Specific carbohydrates	No effect	Decrease adherence
Periodate	No effect	Decrease adherence

(which is one of the reasons why the physician postponed Peggy's baby shots). At this so-called *catarrhal stage*, the organisms multiply rapidly and spread to contiguous areas. Within a few days there are masses of bacteria entrapped in the cilia and thick mucus (Fig. 20.2). The epithelium remains intact, but the submucosa beneath it becomes increasingly inflamed and the peribronchial lymph nodes become enlarged. Deeper tissue involvement strongly suggests that bacterial products are transported from their superficial origin in the bronchial lumen. There is also evidence to suggest that destruction of ciliated epithelial cells may occur in prolonged infections.

Approximately 3 weeks after entry of the organisms, the cough becomes intense and uncontrollable. At the end of a series of coughs there is a forced inspiration, the "whoops". This cough persists with varying severity for another 2 months. It results from attempts by the body to clear the airways of the large amount of material that accumulates on the epithelium when the ciliary epithelium is impaired (Chapter 45). The organisms thus act locally on at least two levels: They induce an inflammatory response, and they specifically destroy the ciliated epithelial cells.

Whooping cough is a toxin-mediated disease. *B. pertussis* make a complex set of toxins responsible for their pathogenic activities (Table 20.1). They may be classified for convenience into two groups:

• Toxins that are relevant to the inflammatory processes.

• Toxins that damage the ciliary epithelium.

Among the former, the best studied one is *pertussis toxin*. This toxin increases the level of cyclic AMP, which results in impairment of both chemotaxis and bacterial killing power of phagocytes (see Chapter 7). Pertussis toxin has, in addition, a large repertoire of pharmacological activities (Table 20.1). The expression of many of the genes for these virulence factors is regulated by a "master gene", called *vir*. Thus, all the virulence genes may be turned on or off together. The reason for such regulation remains elusive. Would you speculate about how it may be related to the life style of the organisms?

Pertussis toxin resembles cholera toxin in affecting cyclic AMP metabolism. It is also an *A-B* toxin, consisting of an A (active) subunit and a B (binding) subunit. After attaching to host cells via the B subunit, the A fragment enters and acts in the cytoplasm. Like cholera toxin, diphtheria toxin, and *Pseudomonas* exotoxin A, pertussis toxin is also a *ADP-ribosyl-transferase*: It splits the nicotinamide portion from NAD and attaches the remaining ADP-ribose (adenosine-diphosphoribose) to host cell proteins. As with cholera toxin, one of these is involved in the regulation of adenylate cyclase and ADP-ribosylation of this enzyme results in an increase in cyclic AMP. In its preoccupation to make a lot of cyclic AMP, *B. pertussis* also secretes an *extracellular adenylate cyclase* that can enter the host cells and increase their content of cyclic AMP.

Local damage is probably caused by a tracheal cytotoxin, which kills ciliated cells specifically and leads to their extrusion from the epithelium. Curiously, this exotoxin is not a protein but consists of a portion of the cell wall murein (Fig. 20.3). Its biochemical origin is not known, but it may originate from murein biosynthesis or processing. A similar compound made by gonococci (Chapter 14) acts in an analogous fashion by killing ciliated epithelial cells in the fallopian tubes. It is likely that tracheal cytotoxin is not the only one involved in local damage, but that other substances elaborated by these organisms also contribute to it.

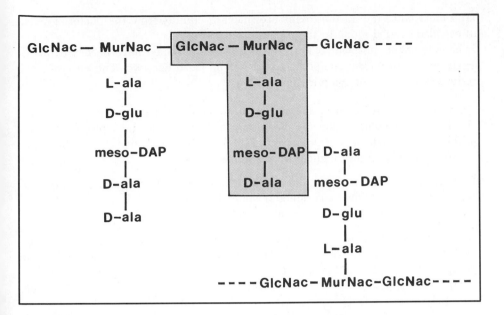

Figure 20.3. Portion of cell wall murein that corresponds to the structure of tracheal cytotoxin. GlcNac, *N*-acetylglucosamine; MurNac, *N*-acetylmuramic acid; meso-DAP, meso-diaminopimelic acid; ala, alanine; glu, glutamic acid. (Courtesy of Dr. WE Goldman.)

Given the nature of the local damage, is it likely that antibodies will have a significant effect on the course of the disease? Preexisting antibodies produced by previous infections or by vaccination prevent the disease, especially if they are of the IgA type. However, once the disease is established, antibodies may play a lesser role. When the exotoxins have reached their target cells, they become impervious to antibodies. On the other hand, local antibodies may prevent the spread of the disease.

DIAGNOSIS

Whooping cough is an uncommon disease in countries where the DPT vaccine is widely used. For this reason, neither clinicians nor the laboratory are always alert to this particular diagnosis. This is true even though the clinical symptoms are usually quite distinctive. It is important to remember that laboratory diagnosis of *B. pertussis* is difficult because the organisms are not resistant outside the optimal growth conditions in the lungs. Thus, as a clinician you will find that *B. pertussis* can be cultivated from a small number of patients only.

Specimens for culture must be taken with care to minimize potential contamination from commensals in the throat. A small swab is placed in the posterior wall of the pharynx and the patient is allowed to cough. The swab is treated with a drop of penicillin solution to kill other normally occurring bacteria that are sensitive to penicillin (to which *B. pertussis* is resistant). The swab is then applied to the surface of a plate containing a medium called Bordet-Gengou, which is incubated for 2 to 3 days. Positive identification of the organisms may then be carried out using specific antisera.

PREVENTION AND TREATMENT

The vaccine against pertussis consists of a killed suspension of *B. pertussis* cells mixed with purified diphtheria and tetanus toxoid proteins. Such a suspension contains significant amounts of the various pertussis toxins, some less than others since not all the toxins are released equally from the bacterial cells. Pili are also carried along in the preparation.

The side effects associated with the use of DPT vaccine have been attributed largely to the pertussis component and not to the other two. The vaccine can produce three types of complications:

• Fever, malaise, and pain at the site of the injection are seen in about 20% of the infants inoculated. This is commonly seen with vaccines prepared from whole bacteria, which contain murein, LPS from Gram negatives, and other substances that elicit an inflammatory response.

• Convulsions occur in about one in 2000 children vaccinated. This may not represent the true incidence since a small number of children, about one in 30,000, suffer from spontaneous convulsions called idiopathic seizures.

• More serious central nervous system reactions occur rarely, at an estimated rate of 1 in every 110,000 children vaccinated. What would the number of these complications be in similar populations that do not receive the vaccine? Such a comparable population does not presently exist in countries where the vaccine is widely used.

In assessing the risks of using the DPT vaccine, one must weigh the potential for severe complications against the undisputed benefits of the vaccine in nearly eradicating whooping cough. Many epidemiologists are convinced that vaccination should be widespread. In fact, all states in the United States have laws requiring children to be immunized against pertussis. Vaccination is required prior to enrollment in school or, in some areas, in day-care centers. In special cases, most states allow exemptions for certain medical reasons. For example, the vaccine should not be given to children with minor illnesses, or those receiving antihistamines or certain other types of medication. The vaccine is usually administered by three injections over a period of 2 months. If the first of these gives an adverse reaction, the treatment should be discontinued.

Meanwhile, there is considerable effort to make the vaccine risk free. If specific immunogens could be identified, whole bacterial cells would not have to be used. Presumably, some of the side effects are due to bacterial constituents other than those required to stimulate a protective response. These "impurities" would be left out of a more purified vaccine preparation. It may turn out, however, that purified pertussis toxin is itself responsible for some of the side effects of the vaccine. In addition, this protein is an immunological adjuvant, and it may contribute to the immunogenicity of the other components of the DPT vaccine. Thus, pertussis vaccination is not a simple matter.

CONCLUSIONS

Until a safer vaccine become available, whooping cough will continue to be a serious medical concern. Meanwhile, there is much to be learned from the specific aspects of the pathogenesis of the causative agent. *Bordetella pertussis* is a superficial pathogen, rarely penetrating into deep tissues. It produces a series of powerful toxins, most of which function to counteract the defense mechanisms of the lower respiratory tract.

SELF-ASSESSMENT QUESTIONS

1. Discuss the aspects of whooping cough that can be directly attributed to the location of the organisms in the body.

2. How does *B. pertussis* cause systemic symptoms, given its superficial location?

3. Describe the activity of the main toxins of *B. pertussis*.

4. Discuss the pros and cons of the pertussis component of the DPT vaccine.

5. Why is it unlikely that whooping cough will be completely eradicated from the planet?

SUGGESTED READINGS

Goldman WE: *Bordetella pertussis* tracheal cytotoxin: damage to the respiratory epithelium. In Leive L (ed): *Microbiology—1986*. Washington, DC, American Society for Microbiology, 1986, pp 70–74.

Hewlett EL, Weiss AA: Conclusions. In Leive L (ed): *Microbiology—1986*. Washington, DC, American Society for Microbiology, 1986, pp 79.

Hewlett EL, Weiss AA: Pertussis toxin: mechanisms of action, biological effects, and roles in clinical pertussis. In Leive L (ed): *Microbiology—1986*. Washington, DC, American Society for Microbiology, 1986, pp 75–78.

Tuomanen E: Adherence of *Bordetella pertussis* to human cilia: implications for disease prevention and therapy. In Leive L (ed): *Microbiology—1986*. Washington, DC, American Society for Microbiology, 1986, pp 59–64.

Weiss AA, Hewlett EL: Virulence factors of *Bordetella pertussis*. *Ann Rev Microbiol* 40:661–686, 1986.

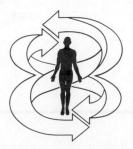

CHAPTER

21

The Clostridia

E. Rubin

Clostridia are strict anaerobic Gram positive rods that cause several unrelated diseases with different clinical manifestations. These include *botulism*, *tetanus*, soft tissue infections including muscle invasion (*cellulitis*—an infection of subcutaneous connective tissue—and *gas gangrene*), *food poisoning* and *pseudomembranous colitis* (an inflammatory disease of the colon). Many of these diseases are very dangerous and all are caused by *exotoxins* secreted by the causative clostridial species. In the case of botulism, the disease is caused by eating toxin-containing food; this disease then is an intoxication rather than an infectious disease. The other diseases are caused by organisms from the environment and are rarely contagious.

The genus *Clostridium* contains a large number of distinctive species (Table 21.1). The clostridia make up the only medically important group of bacteria that are Gram positive rods, spore formers, and strict anaerobes (Fig. 21.1). They are large rods, although usually not as wide as their spores, which gives them a tennis racket appearance during sporogenesis. The likely reason for their strict anaerobiosis is that they lack superoxide dismutase and catalase, enzymes that inactivate toxic products of oxygen metabolism (hydrogen peroxide and superoxide radicals; Chapters 2 and 16). However, they are not killed by the presence of oxygen, especially in the spore state.

Clostridia are very common in the environment, especially in soil; they are also found in the large bowel of humans and other animals. If you were to heat a sample of soil or feces to the boiling point, you would invariably isolate one or more species of these organisms from their spores, thus illustrating both their frequency and their heat resistance. As will be discussed below, both spore

Table 21.1
The principal pathogenic *Clostridia*

Name of Organism	Principal Diseases	Type of toxin	Site of Action of Toxin
C. botulinum	Botulinal food poisoning	Neurotoxin (seven antigenic types)	Neuromuscular junction
	Infant botulism		Neuromuscular junction
	Wound botulism		Neuromuscular junction
C.tetani	Tetanus	Neurotoxin	CNS
C.perfringens (mainly) many others	Gas gangrene (myonecrosis) Anaerobic cellulitis	Lecithinase and others	Cell membranes
	Food poisoning	Enterotoxin	GI tract
C. difficile	Pseudomembranous colitis	Cytotoxin, enterotoxin	Colon

formation and anaerobiosis are necessary for the pathogenesis of clostridial diseases.

The ability of clostridia to cause disease depends on another characteristic of the genus: efficient extracellular secretion of large numbers of proteins. These include two of the most powerful toxins known, botulinum and tetanus neurotoxins (Chapter 7). The genes for many clostridial toxins are encoded by transferable elements, such as plasmids and temperate phages. Therefore, it is not surprising to find different species of clostridia that cause the same disease (e.g., gas gangrene) and synthesize the same toxins.

Clostridia are metabolically highly active and thus have important industrial uses: Clostridial fermentation of crude substrates produces useful chemicals (e.g., alcohols and acetone). The clostridia used for these purposes, like most members of the genus, are not ordinarily pathogenic.

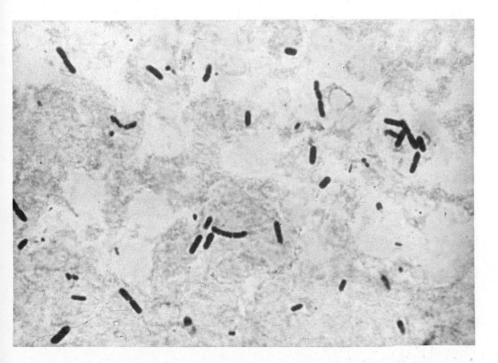

Figure 21.1. Gram stain of *Clostridium perfringens* in exudate from gas gangrene. Note the absence of neutrophils. (Reproduced with permission of Schering Corp. Kenilworth, NJ, copyright owner. All rights reserved.)

BOTULISM

Case

Over the objections of Mrs. B., Mr. B. purchased a can of vichyssoise (a cold potato and leek soup). Mr. B. ate heartily, while Mrs. B. adventurously tried some but resorted to peanut butter and jelly. The next day Mr. B. experienced some nausea, which he ascribed to food poisoning. By that night, Mr. B. began "seeing double" and having difficulty swallowing. Mrs. B. brought him to a physician, who, on strictly clinical grounds, diagnosed the disease as botulism and immediately admitted Mr. B. to the hospital. A team of public health workers searched through Mrs. B.'s trash and carefully removed the nearly empty can of vichyssoise. Examination of the remaining vichyssoise revealed spores of Clostridium botulinum. Other cans of the same brand of vichyssoise were recalled by public health authorities and later found to be contaminated with this organism.

Mr. B.'s condition progressively worsened. By the following day he could no longer raise his head and had difficulty breathing. Within a couple of days Mr. B. was joined in the hospital by his wife, who was experiencing similar but less severe symptoms. By now Mr. B. was breathing with the aid of a respirator and could only weakly contract any of his muscles. Mrs. B. felt weak but remained capable of breathing on her own. Over the course of the next few months both slowly regained their strength, and a year later had no residual symptoms.

The following questions arose:

1. Why was the canned soup such a good vehicle for botulism?

2. What caused the paralysis?

3. Why did Mrs. B. get sick when she only tasted the soup?

The answer to these questions requires knowledge of the clostridia, their life style, and the toxins they produce. While botulism is a rare disease (affecting fewer than 100 patients each year in the United States), it is the most deadly of the foodborne diseases and as such is widely known among the public. Since therapy is difficult and immunization not practical, the mainstay of botulism control is public awareness of how to prevent exposure.

Encounter

Spores of *C. botulinum*, like those of the other clostridia, are widespread in soils and are thus on the surface of many vegetables used for canning. They survive boiling and are killed only after heating to the high temperatures used in proper canning techniques. The presence of spores alone does not present a risk because only actively metabolizing bacteria can form and secrete the toxin. Spores of *C. botulinum* must be able to germinate and grow in an anaerobic environment before they produce the toxin. Germination of the spores may actually be helped by inadequate heating because they need to be *activated* in order to germinate. Heating is an effective stimulus for this. Heating also kills other bacteria that may otherwise compete for growth with *C. botulinum*. Improperly canned food then may provide the right conditions for botulinum toxin production:

Temperature too low to kill the spores but high enough to activate them, and anaerobiosis for the growth of vegetative cells.

Damage

The diseases caused by *C. botulinum* are caused entirely by its neurotoxin. Actually, *C. botulinum* produces seven antigenically distinct toxins (designated A, B, C_1, D, E, F, and G). Most of these are thought to be encoded on the chromosome, whereas C_1 and D are known to be carried by bacteriophages and thus can be transmitted to nontoxigenic species of clostridia, making them pathogenic. Almost all cases of human disease result from types A, B, and E. While these types can be distinguished by antisera, they have similar structures and seem to be equally toxic. All are proteins with a molecular weight of about 150,000. It is likely that all these serotypes of botulinum toxin act by identical mechanisms.

Botulinum toxin has an unusual property: It forms aggregates with other clostridial proteins. These complexes are highly resistant to gastric acidity and the digestive enzymes of the intestine. Thus, when the toxin is eaten in food it survives long enough to get to an area of the gut where it can cross into the bloodstream. Botulinum toxin is absorbed in the gut and transferred into the bloodstream by unknown mechanisms. This makes it the most deadly of the bacterial toxins. One microgram is more than sufficient to kill 10 people; about 0.25 kg could kill all the people on earth. The only other known toxin with similar toxicity is tetanus toxin, but it is not easily taken up from the intestine. As Mrs. B. could tell you, it is not surprising that many victims become ill and may even die after tasting a small amount of contaminated food (less than a teaspoonful). Thus, tasting to see if food is spoiled is not a smart thing to do.

Botulinum toxin is a neurotoxin that does not act by killing cells (Chapter 7). Instead, it acts at the neuromuscular junction, preventing the release of acetylcholine from the α-motor neuron. The muscle cannot then receive signals from the nerve telling it to contract. This results in *flaccid paralysis* of the muscle. As seen in Mr. B.'s case, this paralysis is long-lasting and its reversal probably requires the sprouting of new nerve terminals.

Clinically, botulism is characterized by descending paralysis of muscle groups. Initially the cranial nerves are affected. Most commonly, patients suffer from ocular disturbances. They become unable to control fine movements of their eyes. The first symptoms are often double vision (diplopia), which results from their inability to move their eyes conjugately. Their vision often blurs because the iris and ciliary muscles become paralyzed and the pupils remain widely dilated even in bright light. Other patients first complain of pharyngeal symptoms such as pain and difficulty on swallowing (dysphagia) or difficulty speaking. As the disease progresses it affects muscle groups farther down the body. The toxin causes weakness and then paralysis of the large muscle groups of the trunk and limbs. Eventually patients begin to have difficulty breathing because the respiratory muscles lose their strength. Many patients require mechanical ventilatory support.

C. botulinum causes two other syndromes besides botulinal food poisoning: *infant botulism* and *wound botulism*. Infant botulism, which is usually a mild infection, is caused by *C. botulinum* residing in the gut of infants. There is evidence that many babies are colonized with *C. botulinum* but few suffer ill effects. Alternatively, spores may be ingested with many foods (honey has often been implicated) and resist the acidity of the stomach. They germinate in the infant's large bowel and then produce their toxins. Infant botulism is usually mild and affected infants have lower levels of circulating toxin than do adults with botulinal food poisoning. In the case of food poisoning, toxin is absorbed in the small intestine, whereas in infant botulism it is synthesized and absorbed in the colon. This provides a possible explanation for the differences in clinical presentation: The toxin is not absorbed as efficiently in the large, as in the small, intestine. Despite its usual mild symptoms, infant botulism can be threatening to some children and has been implicated as the cause of some cases of sudden infant death syndrome.

Wound botulism is a rare disease caused by contamination of deep wounds by spores. The spores must enter a poorly perfused anaerobic area in order to germinate. Wound botulism shows a different clinical picture than does botulinal food poisoning. Paralysis starts at the site of the wound and usually extends from the initial area to become generalized.

Treatment and Prevention

Botulism is difficult to treat. Most patients are given antitoxin to bind any toxin remaining in the circulation. It is likely, however, that by the time symptoms occur, most of the toxin is already fixed in tissue. Thus, treatment is primarily supportive: Respiration and blood pressure are maintained, the patient is well nourished, and care is taken to ensure that the patient does not suffer muscle contractions and bed sores while paralyzed. Such care is often very long in duration since recovery may take many months.

Botulinal food poisoning can be readily prevented by proper canning methods. The toxin itself is heat sensitive and is easily destroyed by boiling. Thus, if canned food is boiled for 5 minutes, there is no risk of intoxication (Mr. and Mrs. B. ate a cold meal and therefore did not destroy the toxin that had been synthesized after inadequate canning). As the result of research by K.F. Meyer and others, controls were instituted by the canning industry in California early in this century (upgrading of sterilization methods, quality controls for autoclaving). Since then botulism resulting from commercially canned food has been rare. As a matter of fact a 1963 outbreak of botulism in the United States from contaminated cans of tuna fish was the first one in 40 years caused by a commercially canned food. However, sporadic cases (one involving canned vichyssoise) have been reported since then. Nevertheless, it is likely that home canning remains the more frequent source of the disease.

TETANUS

You will get tetanus, I told myself, and you will die of lockjaw. It was a Deptford belief that in this disease you bent backward until at last your head touched your heels and you had to be buried in a round coffin.

(Robertson Davies, Fifth Business)

While the people of Deptford were not quite accurate in their belief, they did realize the danger of tetanus to wounded World War I soldiers, such as the narrator. Tetanus has been dreaded for centuries, particularly in times of war. The tetanus vaccine, which has made the disease very rare in the developed world, is one of the triumphs of preventive medicine. Tetanus, however, remains a serious public health problem in some developing countries. The number of cases in the United States is around 100 per year. There are over 50,000 fatalities yearly worldwide.

Encounter

The spores of *C. tetani*, like those of the other clostridia, are found frequently in soil and excreta of various animals. *C. tetani* is found in the intestine of many people without causing symptoms, but is usually only a transient member of the intestinal flora. Tetanus toxin lacks the ability of its cousin, botulinum toxin, to cross the intestinal epithelium.

Entry, Spread, and Multiplication

Wounds contaminated with feces or soil may become infected with *C. tetani* spores. In some developing countries, the umbilical stump of newborn children is packed with mud or dung to soothe the infant. Why does such a procedure not invariably lead to tetanus? One reason is that *C. tetani* spores require an anaerobic environment to germinate and cause disease. This condition is found in wounds where the blood supply to the area is compromised, usually when tissue becomes necrotic. In the United States it is usual to treat tetanus patients with penicillin as soon as they are diagnosed. It seems likely, however, that debriding a wound will keep the organisms from growing.

Damage

C. tetani produces tetanus toxin, which is responsible for all of the symptoms of the disease. The toxin, a protein, with a molecular weight of 150,000, is encoded by a plasmid carried by all toxigenic *C. tetani*. On a cellular level, tetanus toxin has an action similar to botulinum toxin, although they are not antigenically similar. Both block neurotransmitter release at the synapse. However, tetanus toxin acts on the central nervous system and botulinum toxin affects peripheral nerves. Thus they produce completely different clinical syndromes. Both toxins bind to the α-motor neuron, which supplies motor impulses to the muscle. Unlike botulinum toxin, which exerts its action on this neuron, tetanus toxin is

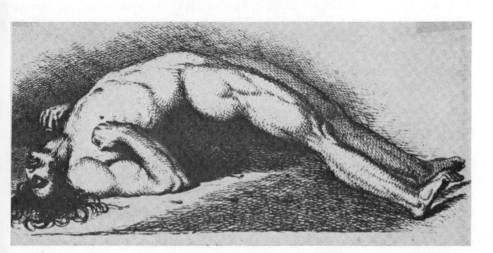

Figure 21.2. Advanced tetanus may lead to *opisthotonos*, the bending backwards of the body caused by spastic paralysis of the strong extensor muscles of the back. This classical illustration of a British soldier wounded in 1809 in the Napoleonic Wars, portrays this condition, as well as "sardonic smile" and lockjaw, caused by spasms of facial muscles.

taken up and travels back up the nerve axon into the central nervous system. There it apparently blocks the release of several types of transmitters, including glycine and γ-aminobutyric acid. Many of the impulses reaching the α-motor neuron are inhibitory; i.e., they reduce the likelihood that a stimulatory impulse will be transmitted to the muscle. The net effect of tetanus toxin is to block these inhibitory neurons. Thus, stimulatory signals remain unopposed and muscles are constantly stimulated.

Clinically, this is manifested as *spastic paralysis*. Muscles contract uncontrollably. Most commonly, the first symptoms are caused by contraction of the powerful masseter muscles resulting in *trismus* (lockjaw). Next, the muscles of the face contract, resulting in a characteristic expression of a "sardonic smile" (*risus sardonicus*). As the disease progresses, opposing groups of muscles contract, with the strongest predominating and forcing the joints into rigid positions. Contractions are painful and come in spasms, often induced by stimuli such as light and sound. Severe contraction of the muscles of the back causes the patient's back to arch and may be so severe as to crush the spinal processes (Fig. 21.2). Mortality rates are high, particularly in developing countries. Death often results from respiratory failure caused by the paralysis of respiratory muscles.

Treatment and Prevention

Like botulism, tetanus is very difficult to treat. We do not know how to reverse the action of the toxin and thus can only provide patients with supportive care. Wounds should be carefully debrided and cleaned. Giving antitoxin to patients after they develop symptoms is probably of limited value, as with botulism. It is important to keep patients in quiet, dark rooms to prevent stimuli that can trigger waves of muscle spasms. In severe cases, patients must be given ventilatory support.

Immunization is the mainstay of the control of tetanus. Since the disease is entirely due to the toxin, antibody to the toxin effectively prevents the disease. The antigen used is *tetanus toxoid*, toxin that has been inactivated with formalin but that retains its antigenicity. It is given in the first few months of life, and is the "T" of the DPT vaccine. The disease itself does not immunize patients, and those who recover from tetanus are still susceptible to it. The apparent reason is that the amount of toxin produced in a patient is sufficient to cause the disease but too small to induce an effective antibody response. Tetanus immunizations should be kept current (every 5 to 10 years) and patients should be reimmunized when they have incurred a so called "tetanus prone wound" (necrotic tissue, contamination with soil). Tetanus antitoxin is given to nonimmune patients who have suffered such wounds.

WOUND INFECTIONS AND GAS GANGRENE

Wounds may become infected by a variety of other clostridia that cause necrotizing lesions, usually beginning at the site of entry. They range from a relatively localized and manageable cellulitis to life-threatening gas gangrene (see Chapter 49). Like tetanus, clostridial wound infections have been a major cause of death and disfigurement during times of war. With better wound management, the incidence of these diseases in soldiers has decreased dramatically. Gas gangrene, however, remains a serious threat to the postoperative patient.

Encounter

Many species of clostridia can cause these infections, but about 90% are caused by a single species, *C. perfringens*. The clostridia that cause wound infections are commonly found in soil, like most other clostridia. Many of the agents of wound infections, including *C. perfringens*, are also normal members of the colonic flora of many individuals.

Entry, Spread, and Multiplication

Any wound exposed to soil may contain clostridial spores, which as mentioned above, only germinate under anaerobic conditions. In addition, after abdominal surgery, wounds are commonly contaminated with clostridia from the gastrointestinal tract. These may also cause disease if they lodge in a poorly perfused area. Unlike *C. tetani* and *C. botulinum*, clostridia that cause wound infections are capable of maintaining their own anaerobic environment.

Damage

The danger of clostridial wound infections depends on their location. Often the infection is confined to the subcutaneous tissues, producing a slowly developing process that classically produces inflammation without serious pain. The gas trapped in tissue may be palpated, creating a sign known as "crepitance". This infection, known as *clostridial anaerobic cellulitis* is not very dangerous by itself; it must be carefully differentiated from the potentially deadly gas gangrene.

Gas gangrene results from a deeper infection of the muscle. As toxins are secreted into the muscle, they quickly cause necrosis, or myonecrosis. This results in acute pain and rapid progression of the symptoms. The muscle first becomes pale and fails to respond to stimulation. Within hours, it turns beefy red, and then turns black as gangrene sets in. The overlying skin appears tense and acquires a bronze discoloration. Blisters filled with dark fluid develop, and the skin eventually turns black. It is often difficult to detect crepitance through the massively inflamed tissue.

How do the invading clostridia cause gas gangrene? After germination, the organisms produce a lecithinase (termed α-toxin in the case of *C. perfringens*). This powerful enzyme hydrolyzes lipids of tissue cell membranes, resulting in lysis. As cells die, the blood supply to the area is cut off, creating an even larger anaerobic area. The clostridia multiply and secrete more α-toxin, which results in an even larger area of necrosis and anaerobiosis. As the bacteria multiply they produce gas as a product of their fermentation. This gas becomes trapped in the area, producing one of the characteristic signs of the disease. In a spatially confined area, such as within a muscle, the gas itself extends the anaerobic area by compressing the tissue and blocking blood flow.

The threat of death in gas gangrene patients is severe. Some α-toxin eventually escapes the affected area and finds its way into the circulation. Here it causes massive hemolysis and renal failure. Death may result only hours after the initial presentation of the disease.

Treatment and Prevention

Gas gangrene is a medical emergency. Whenever a clostridial infection is suspected, it is important to bring the patient to surgery immediately and to examine the affected underlying tissue. The wound should be extensively debrided and affected tissue removed. Amputation is often necessary to prevent further spread of the disease. Some patients are also treated with antitoxin, but it is probably useful only if administered immediately. More recently, patients with gas gangrene have been treated by placing them under high oxygen tension in a hyperbaric chamber. This is thought to decrease the extent of surgery needed. Why do you think this is so?

As with most clostridial diseases, prevention is the key to the control of gas gangrene. Once again, this requires good wound management. Gas gangrene has always thrived in times of war, often claiming a large percentage of seriously wounded soldiers. In recent times, however, physicians have paid greater attention to the risks; for example, in the Vietnam War gas gangrene was extremely rare among wounded American servicemen. A reason for this success was the prompt evacuation of the wounded to hospitals, so that wounds could be debrided and treated rapidly.

Clostridial Food Poisoning

Unlike botulinal food poisoning, which is caused by the ingestion of toxin, clostridial food poisoning is a true infection of the gastrointestinal tract. Food, especially meat, is often contaminated with *C. perfringens* and other species of clostridia. These organisms may infect the large intestine and produce enterotoxins that induce a diarrhea which most frequently is mild and self-limited. Patients with this infection have abnormally high numbers of clostridia in their stool (see Chapter 58 for detailed comparison with other forms of food poisoning). Rarely, *C. perfringens* may also cause a more serious disease known as *necrotizing enteritis*.

PSEUDOMEMBRANOUS COLITIS AND *C. DIFFICILE* DIARRHEA

Soon after the antibiotic clindamycin was introduced into therapeutic usage it was found to cause diarrhea in some patients. The colonic mucosa of these patients had an unusual appearance: It was covered with a fibrinous pseudomembrane. At first, this was thought to be a direct effect of the antibiotic, but later this was also observed in patients who were being treated with other antibiotics. Eventually, it was shown that the disease was associated with still another species of clostridium in the patient's stool, *Clostridium difficile*.

Encounter, Entry, and Multiplication

C. difficile is normally present in the colon of most infants and some adults. The organism is not an abundant member of the intestinal flora. Even though *C. difficile* may be present, pseudomembranous colitis develops only after a stimulus of some kind that promotes germination of spores. In the preantibiotic era, the disease was seen primarily after intestinal surgery. Since then, it has become associated most commonly with antibiotic treatment, particularly with clindamycin and lincomycin. The clinical symptoms of the disease usually develop several days after the initiation of antibiotic therapy.

Does pseudomembranous colitis result because members of the normal intestinal flora are killed by antibiotic therapy? Is *C. difficile* an opportunistic organism that, when this happens, may multiply and cause disease? This is probably not a complete explanation because some strains of *C. difficile* are themselves sensitive to clindamycin. Possibly *C. difficile* exists in the gut in the form of resistant spores, but this has not yet been definitely demonstrated. *C. difficile* has earned its species name!

Damage

As in other clostridial diseases, toxins are responsible for the manifestations of pseudomembranous colitis. All clinical isolates of *C. difficile* produce two toxins: a *cytotoxin*, which causes characteristic changes in the morphology of cultured cells, and an *enterotoxin*, which induces secretory diarrhea in experimental animals. Both of these toxins appear to play a role in pathogenesis. The pseudomembranes can be seen with a colonoscope as adherent gray patches that cover the colonic walls. They are formed from necrotic tissue, inflammatory cells, and fibrin released during this inflammation. The pseudomembranes are reminiscent of the structures seen in the throat of patients with diphtheria, another toxin-induced disease.

Treatment

Patients who have diarrhea from antibiotic therapy should be treated by discontinuing the antibiotic and prescribing one of several others that are effective against *C. difficile*. It is not clear whether patients with this disease are infectious; occasionally cases occur in clusters. Also, the incidence varies from one hospital to another. Some experts have advocated isolating patients with this disease.

CONCLUSION

There are two reasons why the major pathogenic species of clostridia cause different, very characteristic diseases: They or their toxins enter the body by different routes, and different toxins have distinct modes of action. In botulinal food poisoning, the organisms do not invade the body at all, in tetanus they barely set up household in tissues, and in clostridial gangrene they have considerable invasive capacity. The infectious diseases caused by these organisms (other than botulism) are generally of the opportunistic type and require their breaching the defense mechanisms of the body in order to become established.

The toxins of tetanus and botulism have a common site of action in the nervous system and both are extraordinarily potent. They differ, however, in the way they enter the body and in the details of their mode of action. These toxins cause serious disease without killing their target cells, whereas those involved in wound infection and pseudomembranous colitis are generally cytolytic.

SELF-ASSESSMENT QUESTIONS

1. Discuss the properties of clostridia that help explain their ecology.

2. Why is ingesting botulinum toxin more dangerous than ingesting tetanus toxin? Why is infant botulism usually a mild disease?

3. Contrast the mode of action of tetanus and botulinum toxins on the nervous system.

4. What elicits pseudomembranous colitis? Which people are at risk from this disease?

5. We are usually immunized against tetanus early in life. Why don't we get immunized against the other clostridial infections?

SUGGESTED READINGS

Bizzini B: Tetanus toxin. *Microbiol Rev* 43:224–240, 1979.
Simpson LL: The action of botulinum toxin. *Rev Infect Dis* 1:656, 1979.

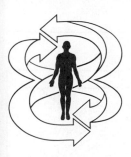

CHAPTER 22

Mycobacteria: Tuberculosis and Leprosy

J. Spitznagel

The captain of all the men of death that came against him to take him away, was the Consumption, for it was that that brought him down to his grave.

John Bunyan (1628–1688)

Tuberculosis conjures up the image of a contagious, chronic, severe disease of the lungs that is often fatal. Actually, that is only one of the manifestations of infection by tubercle bacilli. Tuberculosis is not a single disease but varies in severity depending on the history of previous exposure to the organisms. The infection of a previously unexposed person is usually mild and self-limiting. In rare instances it can proceed directly to a severe generalized disease. Much more often though, the infected person heals and never manifests full-blown tuberculosis.

A few individuals come down with a secondary disease, often many years after the primary exposure. They become ill because the bacteria that caused the primary disease persist in the body by escaping host defense mechanisms. The secondary illness more often fits the classical description of tuberculosis. Many of the symptoms of this form of the disease are not caused by the tubercle bacilli themselves, but result from immunological hypersensitivity reactions of the host to products of the bacteria. If uncontrolled, these can be destructive to tissues.

Thus, tuberculosis is a complex of microbiological and immunological events that escapes simple definition. It serves as a paradigm of chronic infectious diseases, most of which share with it the persistence of the agent in the body and the prominent role of the host responses in the manifestations of the disease.

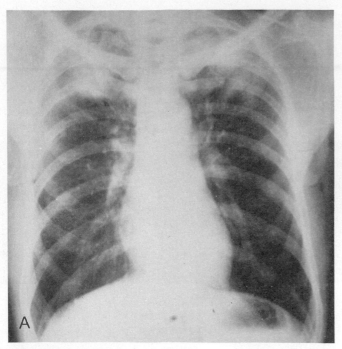

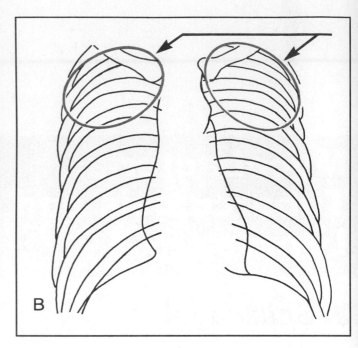

Figure 22.1. Pulmonary tuberculosis. **A**, Posteroanterior radiograph of chest of young adult with recent cough and loss of weight showing bilateral upper lobe shadowing. The x-ray is of a different person from the one described in the text, but the abnormalities are comparable to those seen in the x-rays of that patient. **B**, The areas most affected are circled in the drawing.

CASE

Ms. C., a 24-year-old black schoolteacher and housewife, had recently lost more than 10% of her weight, had night sweats, and felt feverish. She had a cough that produced greenish sputum flecked with blood. Her physician suspected that she might be suffering from pulmonary tuberculosis and administered a tuberculin skin test. Forty-eight hours later, Ms. C. showed a strong positive skin test (redness and thickening at the injection site). The physician referred her to the local health department, where the diagnosis of tuberculosis was confirmed by a chest x-ray (Fig. 22.1) and the presence of "acid-fast bacilli" in a stained smear of her sputum. A careful history revealed that between the ages of 10 and 12 she had lived with an aunt, now deceased, who was said to have had tuberculosis. Given the symptoms, the tuberculin test, plus the radiological and laboratory findings, Ms. C. undoubtedly suffered from tuberculosis.

Ms. C. became worried about her health and wondered about her ability to continue working in school. She and her husband had planned to have a baby soon, but she thought that "pregnancy and new babies do not mix well with tuberculosis". Her physician reassured her that she stood a good chance of being cured. Effective antibiotics could be taken by mouth, although she had to take them for many months. Once treatment was initiated, she could resume her teaching and, in time, plan a pregnancy.

The following are relevant questions:

1. How could Ms. C. have contracted tuberculosis in today's world? Did she get it from her aunt?

2. Did she later develop clinical signs and symptoms from this possible early contact with tubercle bacilli?

3. Why did it take so long for Ms. C. to show signs of an active tubercular infection?

4. What pathobiological events account for her current signs and symptoms? Why did she have fevers, weight loss, cough, bloody sputum, a "positive" skin reaction, and an abnormal chest x-ray?

5. What is the chance that Ms. C. may pass the disease to her husband, her students, or others?

Tuberculosis, or "consumption" (as it used to be called), has been one of the great afflictions of mankind. It has, however, yielded dramatically to improvement in the living standard and is generally responsive to chemotherapy. Still, tuberculosis ranks among the most serious diseases in the developing countries of the world, or wherever poverty, malnutrition, and poor sanitation prevail. In fact, it remains a major problem in the United States, with about 22,000 cases reported every year (Figs. 22.2, 22.3). Although it can affect apparently healthy persons, it is more dangerous to immunocompromised patients. Typical and atypical forms of tuberculosis have made a recent resurgence among the victims of AIDS.

In the last century tuberculosis was a puzzling topic of myths; it was even

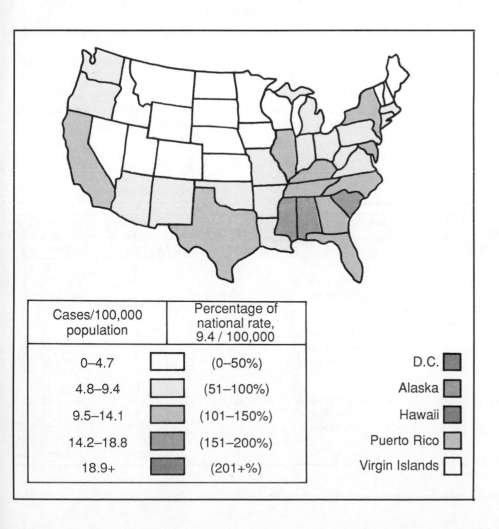

Cases/100,000 population		Percentage of national rate, 9.4 / 100,000
0–4.7		(0–50%)
4.8–9.4		(51–100%)
9.5–14.1		(101–150%)
14.2–18.8		(151–200%)
18.9+		(201+%)

D.C.

Alaska

Hawaii

Puerto Rico

Virgin Islands

Figure 22.2. Rates of tuberculosis by state in the United States in 1984. (From Centers for Disease Control. MMWR, 33:67, 1986.)

Figure 22.3. The incidence of tuberculosis by age, race, and sex in the United States in 1984. (From Centers for Disease Control. MMWR, 33:68, 1986.)

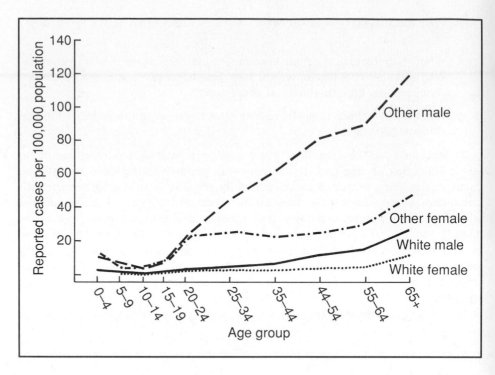

referred to as the "consumptive passion". The disease was thought to afflict sensitive, passionate people, and to endow them with a pale, languid look that was celebrated in literature and opera (e.g., Shelley's *The Sensitive Plant*, Verdi's *La Traviata*, Puccini's *La Boheme*). It was not until the end of the last century, when the cause of the disease was made known by Robert Koch, that the myth was dispelled.

Table 22.1
Characteristics of mycobacteria of major clinical importance[a]

Species	Reservoir	Virulence for Humans	Disease Caused	Case-to-Case transmission	In Vitro Growth Rate	Optimum Growth Temp. (°C)
M. tuberculosis	Human	+++	Tuberculosis	Yes	S	37
M. bovis	Animals	+++	Tuberculosis	Rare	S	37
Bacillus Calmette-Guérin (BCG)	Artificial culture	±	Local lesion	Very rare	S	
M. kansasii	Environmental	+	Tuberculosis-like	No	S	37
M. scrofulaceum	Environmental	+	Lymphadenitis	No	S	37
M. avium-intracellulare	Environmental birds	+	Tuberculosis-like	No	S	37
M. fortuitum	Environmental	±		No	F	37
M. marinum	Water, fish	±	Skin granuloma	No	S	30
M. ulcerans	Probably, environmental; tropical	+	Severe skin ulceration	No	S	30
M. leprae	Human	+++	Leprosy	Yes	None	Not applicable

[a] This table omits many essentially saprophytic mycobacteria.
S, slow; F, fast.
INAH and rifampin make the most effective combination for treatment of tuberculosis.

THE MYCOBACTERIA

Tubercle bacilli belong to a distinctive genus of bacteria, *Mycobacterium*. This genus includes several species that are closely related (Table 22.1). Species other than *M. tuberculosis* were first called "atypical mycobacteria" because they only partially resembled the tubercle bacillus; they are now known to cause a variety of diseases. These diseases are related to tuberculosis and are sometimes referred to as *nontuberculous mycobacterioses* (NTM). Also included in this genus is the agent of leprosy, *Mycobacterium leprae*. Several mycobacteria are harmless organisms, some of which live on the human body without causing disease (e.g., the smegma bacillus), or in the environment, especially the soil. The genus is distinguishable because of two characteristics: acid fastness and slow growth.

Acid Fastness—A Mycobacterial Hallmark

Mycobacteria belong to a small group of bacteria that have the unusual ability to retain dyes when treated with acid solutions. The reason for this acid fastness is that mycobacteria are surrounded by unique chemical components, namely waxes. Mycobacterial waxes are long-chain hydrocarbons (incidentally, one of the leading researchers in this field is an ex–petroleum chemist). The main wax is called *mycolic acid*, and is a β-hydroxy fatty acid linked covalently to murein. The waxes of mycobacteria are also important in pathogenesis, as will be discussed later.

As can be expected, the waxy barrier makes a big difference in the permeability properties of these organisms. Common stains do not penetrate the wax layer; for instance, mycobacteria do not take up the dyes used in the Gram stain and therefore cannot be labeled Gram positive or Gram negative. It is possible, however, to stain them using special techniques. One is to melt the wax temporarily by heating a smear of the bacteria while it is covered with a saturated solution of a basic dye, such as fuchsin. Alternatively, one can add a detergent to the stain. The stained smear is then treated with 3% hydrochloric acid in ethanol, which decolorizes nearly all organisms but the mycobacteria. The smear is then counterstained with a blue dye to provide a contrasting background.

Resistance of mycobacteria to chemical and physical agents helps them survive both in the body and in the exterior environment. Thus, they are unusually resistant to killing by phagocytes. Since they are also highly *resistant to germicides*, preparations used to disinfect surfaces must be tested by the manufacturer for their power to kill mycobacteria (mycobactericidal disinfectants usually contain iodine or strong detergents). Mycobacteria are also highly *resistant to drying*, which contributes to their potential for transmission. The wax coating does not, however, help them withstand heat. For instance, they are killed during pasteurization of milk (e.g., heating to 60°C for 30 minutes).

Slow Growth

Mycobacteria grow very slowly. Their generation time is measured in hours, not minutes; it is not uncommon for pathogenic members of the genus to require 24 hours to double in laboratory media. It is possible that slow growth results from inability to transport nutrients rapidly across the wax layer. Slow growth causes delays in diagnosis by culture; laboratory cultures of clinical material are incubated for up to 8 weeks! (To avoid drying up of the culture medium, the laboratory uses tightly capped test tubes rather then petri dishes.) On agar, colonies of mycobacteria look like irregular waxy lumps and are usually quite raised over the agar surface. Touching colonies with an inoculating needle will show that they stick to the medium, are hard to pick up, and cannot be easily dispersed in a drop of water to make a smear.

Not all mycobacteria can be grown in artificial media. The leprosy bacillus has so far resisted cultivation outside the body of humans or a few animals. The inability to grow these bacteria under routine laboratory conditions continues to impede leprosy research.

ENCOUNTER AND ENTRY

It is likely that Ms. C. contracted tuberculosis by breathing aerosols or dust particles containing tubercle bacilli. Most likely, bacteria-laden droplets were produced by her aunt's frequent coughing bouts. In fact, airborne transmission of tuberculosis is an efficient means to spread the disease for at least two reasons:

- If untreated, the disease can lead to the formation of open pulmonary lesions that contain large numbers of bacteria. Coughing spreads the organisms in the environment.
- Since tubercle bacilli are highly resistant to drying, they are capable of surviving for a long time in the air and house dust. This is important, because most often tubercle bacilli enter into the lung in bacteria-containing, so-called droplet nuclei, the products of dried aerosols. Such particles are effective infectious material because they stay suspended in the air for a long time; not becoming trapped in the mucosal blanket, they can gain access to the alveoli.

These two characteristics account for the epidemiology of tuberculosis: It is widespread in crowded areas, primarily among young children who are exposed repeatedly to the organisms.

The inoculum size of tubercle bacilli required to cause infections is usually high. There is a direct relationship between the number of bacilli in a patient's sputum and the likelihood that exposed family members will contract the disease. The location of the organisms in the body depends largely on the site of entry. For example, infection of the lungs (which is most prevalent in countries such as the United States) results from inhalation of the bacteria. Infection of the intestine or the tonsils is usually due to ingestion of the organisms, because tubercle bacilli may be acquired by drinking unpasteurized milk from infected cows. Cattle suffer from a disease similar to human tuberculosis, but caused by bovine strains of mycobacteria, *M. bovis*.

SPREAD, MULTIPLICATION, DAMAGE

Tubercle bacilli do not produce exotoxins or endotoxin. The severe manifestations of tuberculosis are linked to host reactions to the organisms: Damage is caused by uncontrolled, progressive, chronic inflammation and by organisms living within macrophages. It follows that infection has different manifestations in a "virgin" host than in a person who has been infected previously. Tuberculosis manifests itself in two major forms:

- Primary tuberculosis, the disease of persons who are infected for the first time. It is usually mild and often asymptomatic. Occasionally, however, the primary disease progresses directly to cause systemic diseases, such as tuberculous meningitis, miliary tuberculosis, or both (see below). In these cases, the immune reaction fails to develop.

• Secondary tuberculosis is usually due to the *reactivation* of dormant organisms within the body. This is the distinctive presentation of tuberculosis, a chronic disease associated with extensive tissue damage, often progressing to death if untreated.

Primary Tuberculosis

Pathobiological Characteristics

After Ms. C. inhaled tubercle bacilli as a child she might have developed flu-like symptoms of lower respiratory infection (or she may not have had any symptoms at all). She probably developed an acute localized inflammation that was soon followed by a more chronic inflammatory response.

Primary tuberculosis is characterized by a sequence of pathobiological steps (Fig. 22.4). Tubercle bacilli are ingested by resident macrophages of the pulmonary alveoli (Fig. 22.5). Here the organisms multiply, first within these cells and later, within nonresident macrophages that collect in the area. Loaded with mycobacteria, newly arrived cells migrate through the lymphatics to the hilar lymph nodes, where an immune response develops, dominated by T helper cells (Fig. 22.6). Inflammation will now be present in several places: at the original site of infection, along lymphatic channels, and in the regional lymph nodes. This sequence of events takes about 30 days. Despite their slow growth, the mycobacteria will have multiplied substantially by this time and be found in large numbers.

At this stage of the infection, the tuberculin skin test usually becomes positive and a chest x-ray reveals growing patches of density in the lung. The immune defenses now manage to curb the proliferation of the organisms and retard their local spread, while macrophages, activated by T cells, begin to kill the organisms or to slow down their growth. A certain number of tubercle bacilli will already have disseminated throughout the body (Fig. 22.6). In the tissues, especially the hilar lymph nodes, the organisms are contained in *tubercles*, small *granulomas* consisting of epithelioid and giant cells. (Granuloma formation is partly caused by one of the waxes of the organisms known as *cord factor*, because it is responsible for growth of the organisms in rope-like arrangements. Note: Injection of cord factor results in granulomas indistinguishable from those caused by tubercle bacilli.) With time, the centers of the tubercles become necrotic and advance to form acellular masses of cheesy debris, termed *caseous material*. The combination of tubercles in the lung and caseation in lymph nodes is called the *Ghon complex*.

Primary tuberculosis may take two courses (Fig. 22.4): In people who are otherwise healthy, the lesions heal spontaneously and become *fibrotic* or *calcified*. These lesions usually persist for a lifetime and can be seen years later in chest x-rays as radioopaque nodules. In immunocompromised persons, the organisms may invade the bloodstream. The organisms can then localize and cause disease in almost any organ of the body. This can lead to a potentially fatal generalized infection known as *disseminated miliary tuberculosis*. In this case, tubercles are visible in many organs, including the liver, spleen, kidneys, brain, and meninges. The name "miliary" is derived from the resemblance of the tubercles to grains of millet (bird seed).

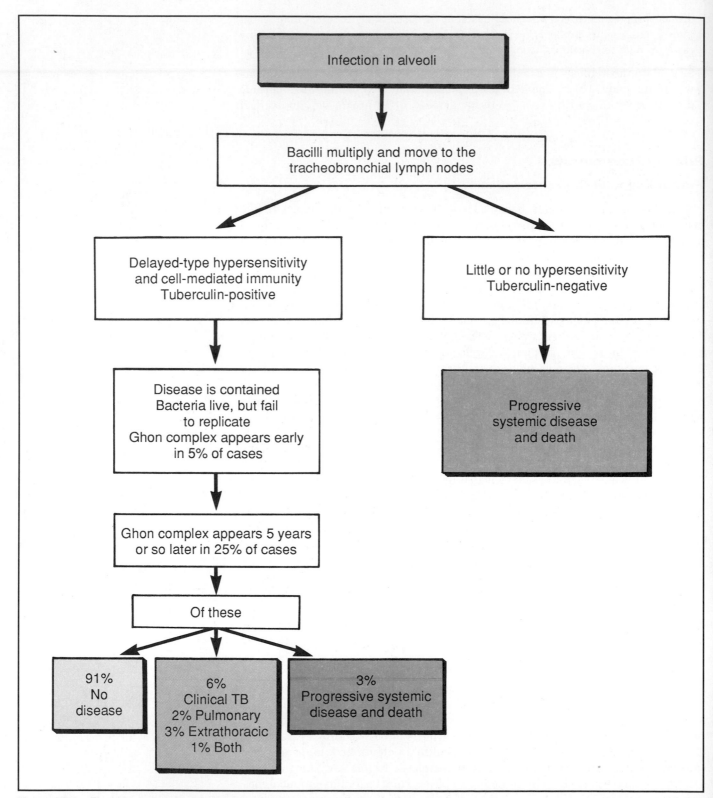

Figure 22.4.   The history of untreated tuberculosis. (Adapted from Myers JA: The natural history of tuberculosis in the human body. *JAMA* 194: 1086, 1965.) We have to depend on older studies to understand the natural course of tuberculosis in humans. It is not ethically justifiable to observe untreated persons over a long period of time.

Figure 22.5. Tubercle bacilli enter through the respiratory tract.

Tracheobronchial lymph node

Bacilli inhaled as droplet nuclei

Resident macrophages in alveoli

Neutrophil

Bacilli in phagocytes

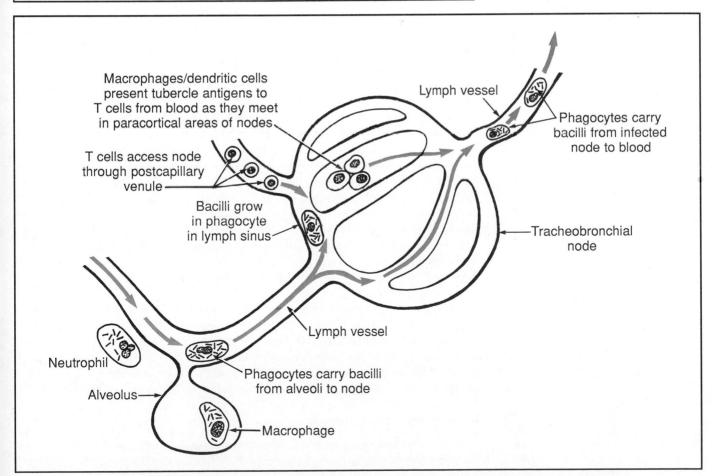

Macrophages/dendritic cells present tubercle antigens to T cells from blood as they meet in paracortical areas of nodes

Lymph vessel

Phagocytes carry bacilli from infected node to blood

T cells access node through postcapillary venule

Bacilli grow in phagocyte in lymph sinus

Tracheobronchial node

Lymph vessel

Neutrophil

Alveolus

Phagocytes carry bacilli from alveoli to node

Macrophage

Figure 22.6. Tubercle bacilli multiply in phagocytes and spread to lymph nodes and the circulation.

How does primary tuberculosis come to a halt? Clearly, the original cellular response fails to curb the multiplication of the organisms. However, with time, *cellular immunity* to the organisms develops. Macrophages which become activated by lymphokines produced by T lymphocytes can now inhibit the intracellular growth of the tubercle bacilli. (A review of the complex topic of cell-mediated immunity might be helpful at this time—see Chapter 5.) As might be expected from the intracellular location of the organisms, humoral immunity does not play a major role in the immune response to tuberculosis. Antibodies appear in the circulation but do not seem to play an effective defensive role, nor are they useful as a diagnostic tool.

Although activated macrophages usually kill intracellular bacteria, they cannot always destroy the exceptionally hardy tubercle bacilli. Intracellular organisms may however be kept in check for long periods of time. An uneasy equilibrium is reached: some macrophages kill the organisms, others are themselves killed and release their bacterial contents, still others are in a state of balance and contain within them dormant bacteria for a long period of time. Immunological processing of those bacteria that are killed leads to continued antigenic stimulation.

The involvement of macrophages has its price. Two substances produced by these cells, *interleukin-1* and *tumor necrosis factor* (Chapter 4), are known to contribute to the symptoms of the disease. Among its various activities, interleukin-1 acts as the mediator of the fever experienced by patients with tuberculosis. Tumor necrosis factor, or *cachectin*, interferes with lipid metabolism and leads to severe weight loss.

Delayed-Type Hypersensitivity and the Tuberculin Reaction

Immunological reactivity to tuberculosis can be demonstrated by the *tuberculin skin test*. The test is carried out by injecting proteins made by tubercle bacilli, known as tuberculin. (The material commonly used is not an isolated protein molecule, but a mixture known as PPD, which stands for "purified protein derivative".) A positive reaction indicates cellular immunity to tubercle bacilli and is indicated by reddening and thickening of the skin 2 to 3 days later. This delayed type hypersensitivity reaction reflects the local events that take place in the infected tissue. Depending on the site of the reaction, delayed type hypersensitivity may account for diverse manifestations, e.g., pleurisy with effusion (the sometimes massive accumulation of exudate in the pleural cavities) or the sudden inflammation of the meninges in *tuberculous meningitis*. Surprisingly few tubercle bacilli are present in the pleural fluid or the cerebrospinal fluid during these infections, but they are able to cause a severe inflammation as the result of a local tuberculin reaction. Likewise, the number of inflammatory cells is also very small. Aspects of the pathogenesis of tuberculosis are depicted in Figure 22.4.

Tubercle bacilli not only elicit cell mediated immunity but also raise the general level of immunological responsiveness. This *adjuvant* effect is used experimentally to increase immunostimulation to other antigens. A mixture of killed tubercle bacilli, mineral oil, and a surfactant is known as *Freund's adjuvant*. Its active component is a fragment of the organisms' murein, a *muramyl dipeptide*, or MDP.

Secondary Tuberculosis

Years after acquiring primary tuberculosis, some people (such as Ms. C.) develop the chronic, progressive symptoms that characterize secondary tuberculosis

(Fig. 22.4). The flare-up can sometimes be blamed on impairment of immune function: Clearly, any compromise of the T cell-macrophage immune system may render a person abnormally vulnerable to mycobacterial infection. Certain infections, such as measles, are known to transiently depress cell-mediated immune responses, including the tuberculin reaction, and are known to predispose patients to reactivation of tuberculosis. It is likely that other common agents have similar effects but are less clinically evident. Patients receiving corticosteroids for inflammatory diseases, undergoing cancer chemotherapy, or suffering from AIDS may become afflicted with tuberculosis. In other cases, the precipitating cause of reactivation of the disease is not known.

Subtle depression of the immune system due to hormonal or other causes may go undetected. Ms. C. did not suffer from malnutrition, which has also been shown to elicit reactivation disease. A contributing factor in her case may be that dark-skinned persons are more susceptible to the disease (Fig. 22.3). The existence of genetic factors is inferred from the high incidence of clinical disease in persons with a specific histocompatibility type, HLA-BW15. The reason that the disease becomes active in older people may possibly be due to a poorly understood loss of immune competence that occurs with aging.

The most common location of secondary tuberculosis is the apex of the lungs. This may be due to the greater level of oxygenation at this site, which gives the highly aerobic tubercle bacilli an edge in growth. Lesions slowly become necrotic, caseate, and eventually merge into larger lesions. With time the caseous lesions liquefy and discharge their contents into bronchi. This event has several serious consequences. It results in a well-aerated cavity, where the organisms can actively proliferate. The discharge of caseous material also distributes the organisms to other sites in the lung, which can lead to rapidly progressing disease known as "galloping consumption". In addition, the bacteria-laden contents of caseous lesions are coughed up and become a source of environmental contamination. Since inflammation of the surface of the bronchi causes increased mucus secretion and stimulation of the cough reflex, patients cough up sputum. Destruction of tissues results in bloody sputa. In advanced tuberculosis, blood vessels may become exposed to the cavities produced by necrosis and patients may die of hemorrhage if these vessels rupture.

What accounted for the various symptoms of Ms. C.? Her fever, weight loss, and night sweats may have been due to the release of interleukin-1 and tumor necrosis factor from the many macrophages involved. Her sputum probably included mucus from inflamed bronchi and material from caseous lesions. Bronchial inflammation may have been caused by a local tuberculin reaction, due to the tuberculoprotein in the caseous material. At this time she became infectious and able to transmit tuberculosis to others.

THE RANGE OF MANIFESTATIONS OF TUBERCULOSIS

Tuberculosis is insidious (Fig. 22.4). Most people are unaware of their initial encounter with the organisms. This group includes those unfortunate patients who do not develop sufficient cellular immunity in time to contain the organisms and who develop miliary tuberculosis. This rampant infection is very different from secondary reactivation tuberculosis (although it is sometimes manifested in patients with this condition as well).

Secondary tuberculosis usually becomes noticeable 1 or 2 years after the primary disease, probably because it takes that long to develop full blown delayed-type hypersensitivity. Although it is most commonly localized in the lung, secondary infection may affect the genitourinary or gastrointestinal tracts, the testicles, the fallopian tubes, the ovaries, or the skin (in other words, almost any organ). Tuberculosis of bone is especially debilitating when it involves the spine, which may collapse as the result of tissue destruction, resulting in lifelong disability. It is clear that the *course of the disease is unpredictable on anatomical grounds alone since the organisms have the ability to colonize practically any site of the body.*

In view of the damage caused in tuberculosis by the immune responses of the host, one may well ask which is worse: the severe cell-mediated immune response to the disease and its resulting damage, or no immune response to tuberculosis at all. Without cellular immunity and delayed hypersensitivity there would be no development of caseation necrosis. However, the tubercle bacilli would not be held in check and would proliferate unimpeded. The result could be, for example, miliary tuberculosis, a disease that can kill much more rapidly than chronic pulmonary tuberculosis. Thus, the immune response serves to contain the disease, even if it eventually causes a great deal of damage. In fact, the body relies on three defensive strategies. One involves the antimicrobial action of activated macrophages. The second consists of walling off and containing the lesion by fibrosis and calcification. The third, which may be called "self-debridement", consists of attempts by the body to expel the caseous material through the bronchotracheal tree or other ducts. The upshot is that defense mechanisms allow a large proportion of patients with tuberculosis to curb progression of the disease for life. Some, because of evident immune compromise or for undefined idiosyncratic features of their immune system, fail to deal with the organisms. They develop clinical disease and many die of tuberculosis.

DIAGNOSIS

The Tuberculin Skin Test

The tuberculin skin test is the most widely used tool to diagnose tuberculosis in the U.S. It only detects delayed hypersensitivity however and does not indicate the presence of active disease. The tuberculin test is usually performed by injecting a small amount of PPD, a mixture of proteins from tubercle bacilli, into the skin of the forearm. A positive test is indicated by reddening and thickening of the skin 48 to 72 hours after injection. The most important criterion for a positive test is the thickening and hardening (induration) of the skin at the site of injection. This is due to infiltration of the area by mononuclear phagocytes and T cells.

The reason this test is so useful in countries such as the United States, where tuberculosis has become rare, is that less than 1% of children and young adults now give a positive test. On the other hand, the test is much less useful in regions where a high proportion of the population is tuberculin positive or has received the BCG vaccine (see "Prevention"). A positive test in the wake of an earlier negative one indicates recent exposure to tubercle bacilli, which constitutes a call for therapeutic intervention (see below). Medical personnel are definitely at risk, especially when exposed to infectious patients. This is why medical students should be tested at intervals for tuberculin reactivity.

There are certain caveats to remember regarding this test. Patients that are immunocompromised may fail to give a positive reaction. Such people are said to be *anergic*, or *unresponsive*. A control test is usually carried out to determine if the person being tested is generally anergic. This is done by injecting small amounts of antigens from the yeast *Candida*, an organism so ubiquitous that most people have developed delayed hypersensitivity to it before reaching adulthood. Positive tuberculin tests may also be caused by cross reactive immunity to mycobacteria other than the tubercle bacillus. Thus, a person infected with *atypical mycobacteria* may give a positive tuberculin test. This is important to recognize, since mycobacteria of this group are often resistant to antitubercular drugs.

Microscopic and Cultural Diagnostic Tests

A rapid diagnostic approach includes a careful history, direct microscopic examination of sputum or exudates, a tuberculin test, and a chest x-ray (Fig. 22.1). Although direct examination is a simple, easily learned procedure, it requires guidance because tubercle bacilli are sometimes so slender that they may escape casual examination. Fortunately, they stand out because they are the only red objects in a smear stained by the most common procedure, the Ziehl-Neelsen method. Direct examination of sputum is especially important because the infectiousness of a patient is dependent on the presence of "red bugs", tubercle bacilli, in the sputum. *Because of its usefulness, every medical student should know how to carry out an acid-fast stain.* In the future, more sensitive methods of rapid diagnosis may become generally available. Such methods are particularly useful in the diagnosis of tubercular meningitis, and include the detection of a tubercle bacillus-specific antigen and a lipid, tuberculostearic acid in the cerebrospinal fluid.

The only rigorous diagnostic method is the cultivation of the organisms. The problem is that it takes 4 to 8 weeks before a positive culture can be read with assurance. Despite this, culturing may be crucial when microscopic examination is negative. Sputa from patients with active tuberculosis may have too few organisms to be detected microscopically but may still give rise to a positive culture. Lastly, if there is growth of tubercle bacilli, it is important to test them for antibiotic sensitivity.

What other conditions resemble tuberculosis? Table 22.1 shows that they are numerous. The main ones are those caused by the so-called atypical mycobacteria, the most common of which are *M. intracellulare* and *M. kansasii*. Diseases caused by these organisms tend to be less severe and more indolent, but they can also lead to disability and even death. Both are important complications in AIDS patients. Other diseases that must be included in the differential diagnosis are those caused by actinomycetes, *Nocardia*, and systemic fungi (see Chapter 38).

TREATMENT

We now have excellent therapeutic resources against tuberculosis, which include several highly effective drugs that can be administered by mouth to ambulatory patients. Among these are *rifampin* and *isonicotinic acid hydrazide* (INAH) (Table 22.1). These drugs are relatively inexpensive (by the standards of affluent countries) and work well if taken for the recommended length of time. Treatment quickly renders the patient noncontagious, so that quarantine is no longer required. Since instituting therapy is an urgent matter, it is advisable to start it before the results of cultures are obtained, as long as the clinical findings (history, examination, x-ray), a positive smear, and a positive tuberculin test suggest the disease.

Thirty years of clinical investigation have uncovered the importance of *multiple drug therapy*. The reason is that tubercle bacilli readily become resistant to antimycobacterial drugs. Chromosomal mutations yield levels of resistance up to 1000-fold greater than the wild type, and arise in one of every 10^6 to 10^7 bacteria. Not surprisingly, drug-resistant mutants appear more frequently in patients with advanced disease. Unfortunately, drug-resistant organisms arise frequently in certain underdeveloped countries, where up to 60% of the isolates of *M. tuberculosis* are resistant to one of the major antitubercular drugs. The solution is clear: Give two drugs. The chance that one organism will become resistant to two drugs simultaneously is infinitesimally small (Chapter 3). However, this simple measure can be too costly in economically poor countries. The economic impasse can be illustrated by the following: In some countries it takes the total economic output of one worker to support the drug therapy of just one patient with tuberculosis.

Another reason for multiple drug therapy of tuberculosis is that some of the agents used may act synergistically. For example, INAH acts on intracellular mycobacteria, while rifampin works both on intracellular and extracellular organisms, including slow-growing strains. Administered together, these drugs are much more effective than given alone. Another drug, pyrazinamide, is also used for chemoprophylaxis. A newly introduced derivative of rifampin, rifabutin, appears to be effective against rifampin-resistant tubercle bacilli. This drug also shows promise for the treatment of infections by the *M. avium-intracellulare* complex.

PREVENTION

The history of tuberculosis strongly suggests that it can be effectively controlled by sanitary measures and improved standards of living. For now, in disadvantaged parts of the world, we must rely on other measures. One problem is that we have no effective vaccine made from killed organisms. The immunology of tuberculosis tells us why: By and large, killed vaccines produce circulating antibodies, which are of limited importance in this disease. In order to elicit a cell-mediated immune response, antigens must be present for long periods. This is best accomplished with vaccines that contain live organisms, which can persist in the body for long times.

There is such a live mycobacterial vaccine, known as *BCG* or bacille Calmette-Guérin, after its French discoverers. It consists of a bovine strain of tubercle bacilli that lost its virulence after prolonged cultivation in vitro. It appears to be a reliably avirulent mutant and has given no signs of reverting to a virulent form. It is still considered useful in parts of the world where tuberculosis is endemic and where other measures are not generally available. BCG vaccine causes the recipient to "convert" to tuberculin positive (in fact, this is a criterion for successful immunization). BCG vaccination thus eliminates a valuable clinical indicator, since conversion to tuberculin positivity is an early warning of infection. To preserve tuberculin conversion as a clinical indicator of new cases, BCG is not used in the United States or other countries with low incidence of tuberculosis. It has become standard practice to administer INAH to personnel at risk or to selected persons who have converted to a positive tuberculin reaction. Such treatment is called *chemoprophylaxis*.

Because tuberculosis is communicable, and not everyone with the disease is aware that they can infect others, it is a dangerous public health hazard. Consequently, Ms. C. and her contacts should be followed. Because her husband had a positive tuberculin test and a negative chest x-ray, he was placed on a prophylactic treatment with INAH. The students who came in contact with Ms. C. were tuberculin tested. Two pupils in her class were tuberculin positive and were also started on INAH prophylactically. The rest of the class remained tuberculin negative, and were retested several months later. For details of chemotherapy and chemoprophylaxis, you may wish to consult a clinical text.

LEPROSY

Leprosy shares some of its pathobiological features with tuberculosis but differs in its clinical manifestations. The contrast in the social response to the two diseases could not be greater or more paradoxical. Because lesions found in leprosy are far more visible, the victims of this disease were long shunned with great vehemence, even though they are much less infectious than patients with tuberculosis! Tuberculosis, the more "sociably acceptable" of the two diseases, is actually far more contagious. Leprosy is rare in the United States today, but is still of worldwide importance. There are an estimated two million patients, mainly in tropical Third World countries, where the disease causes economic loss and human misery.

Leprosy is caused by *Mycobacterium leprae*, which has been studied less extensively than the tubercle bacillus because it cannot be cultivated in vitro. The genes of this organism have been cloned into *Escherichia coli*, and the gene products are being intensively studied. The organism does grow in mice that are inoculated through their tails or footpads. Recently, armadillos have been found to be susceptible to *M. leprae*, and are now also used in leprosy research. The ability to grow *M. leprae* in animals has accelerated important studies on drug sensitivity—prior to this, studies depended largely on observing the responses of human patients. Animal experimentation has established the importance of several drugs, e.g., dapsone and rifampin, in the treatment of leprosy (here again, it is important to use two drugs at the same time to avoid selection of drug-resistant organisms).

Leprosy bacilli grow best at low temperatures. Accordingly, they appear to multiply most rapidly in the skin and appendages of human hosts. There are two types of leprosy, *lepromatous* and *tuberculoid*. Intermediate forms occur as well. Lepromatous leprosy causes loss of eyebrows, and thickened and enlarged nares, ears, and cheeks, resulting in a lion-like appearance ("leonine facies"). Both skin and nerves may be involved. With time, the loss of local sensation leads to inadvertent lesions in the face and extremities. These may become secondarily infected, eventually resulting in bone resorption, disfigurement, and mutilating lesions. Lepromatous leprosy is associated with diminished delayed hypersensitivity to *lepromin*, which is a preparation of antigens of the leprosy bacilli extracted from human lepromatous tissue. Tuberculoid leprosy often appears with red blotchy lesions with anesthetic areas on the face, trunk, and extremities. It causes palpable thickening in peripheral nerves because the bacilli grow in the nerve sheaths. Patients with these symptoms are usually sensitive to lepromin.

Thus, lepromatous leprosy is the malignant form of the disease; it is analogous to systemic progressive (miliary) tuberculosis, where the organisms grow profusely. In both these instances, the cell-mediated immune response is weak. It is not clear why cell-mediated immunity is decreased in leprosy patients; the suspicion lingers that the infecting organisms themselves play a role in this immunosuppression. There is recent evidence that persons belonging to the histocompatibility haplotype HLA-DR3 are more likely to develop to tuberculoid leprosy, and those with the HLA-MT1 class, to lepromatous leprosy. The degree to which cell-mediated immunity is impaired determines the extent of the lepromatous manifestations. Whereas full-blown cases of lepromatous leprosy show no reactivity to lepromin, borderline cases show some.

Tuberculoid leprosy is analogous to secondary tuberculosis in that this form of leprosy provokes vigorous cell-mediated immunity and exaggerated allergic responses. To further the analogy, lesions in lepromatous leprosy are filled with leprosy bacilli, whereas the organisms are hard to find in the tissues in tuberculoid leprosy. The prognosis with tuberculoid leprosy tends to be better than with lepromatous leprosy. In some cases, tuberculoid leprosy is a self-limiting disease; it may, however, progress to the lepromatous form.

The epidemiology of leprosy is not well understood. Clearly, it is a communicable disease. It appears that infected persons must live in close contact with potential victims for long periods in order to transmit the disease. Victims of lepromatous leprosy tend to shed bacilli from their nasal septa. This is undoubtedly one source of contagion; it is not known if there are others.

The prognosis of leprosy patients has dramatically improved with the introduction of effective drugs, such as dapsone, rifampin, rifabutin, and ethionamide. Paradoxically, some of these drugs cause such effective destruction of the organisms that the antigens released cause a distressing inflammation called erythema nodosum leprosum. With appropriate treatment, however, patients can be cured with few residual effects. Unfortunately, drug resistance is a serious problem for some patients with leprosy. Because of this, efforts are being made to develop a vaccine using antigens produced from cloned *M. leprae* genes. Efforts to produce cross-immunity in children of lepromatous patients using BCG have given disappointing or inconclusive results. New drugs are also being tested for the treatment of the disease.

CONCLUSION

Tuberculosis is one of the best studied examples of a human disease caused by facultative intracellular pathogens. An essential point to remember about tuberculosis is that the major lesions of the established disease are due to the hypersensitivity developed from previous exposure to the organism. They are different on the first and on subsequent encounters.

The tubercle bacillus, because of its unusual waxy envelope, grows slowly and is a highly successful parasite, usually sparing the life of its victim for many years. By eventually damaging the lungs, it ensures its spread from the body into the environment and increases its chances of infecting other people. The availability of modern antitubercular drugs places control of the disease within reach. Achieving this goal requires sanitation measures coupled with screening, detection, and prophylactic chemotherapy. Where economical and political reasons make it difficult to mount such an effort, vaccination with BCG can help reduce the burden of this disease.

Many of these considerations apply to cases of leprosy as well. However, the two diseases differ significantly in their clinical manifestations. The two forms of the disease, tuberculoid and lepromatous leprosy, are caused by the presence or absence of cell-mediated immunity to the organisms.

SUGGESTED READINGS

Anonymous: Mycobacterioses and the acquired immunodeficiency syndrome. Joint position paper of the American Thoracic Society and the Centers for Disease Control. *Am Rev Respir Dis* 136:492–496, 1987.

Dannenberg AM: Pathogenesis of tuberculosis. In Fishman AP (ed): *Pulmonary Diseases and Disorders.* New York, McGraw-Hill, 1980, pp 1264–1281.

Kaplan G, Cohen ZA: The immunobiology of leprosy. *Intern Rev Exp Pathol* 28:45–79, 1986.

Mitchison DA: Drug resistance in mycobacteria. *Br Med Bull* 40:84–90, 1984.

Rook GA: Progress in the immunology of mycobacterioses. *Clin Exp Immunol* 69:1–9, 1987.

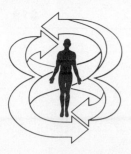

Syphilis: A Disease with a History

E.N. Robinson, Jr.
Z. McGee

Syphilis is one of the classical sexually transmitted diseases. It occupies central stage in the history of medicine, although it has waned in importance in recent years. It remains, however, a puzzling and mystifying infection, characterized by several stages with dramatically different clinical presentations. The first two stages (primary and secondary) manifest themselves as acute and subacute disease, while tertiary syphilis is a chronic disease of many years' duration. The disease may be transmitted from an infected mother to her fetus and cause congenital syphilis.

The agent of syphilis is a spirochete, *Treponema pallidum*, which so far has not been readily cultivated in artificial media. It does not produce toxins and little is known about its pathogenic attributes or the reason why it survives for a long time in the body. Fortunately, it is very sensitive to penicillin, which is why the disease is less prominent today.

CASE

Mr. B., a 24-year-old homosexual, came to the clinic with fever, swollen lymph nodes, and spotty discolorations of the skin of the palms of his hands and the soles of his feet. He had recently noted a penny-sized gray, translucent lesion on the inner aspect of his lower lip. The physician recognized the "macular rash" on the palms and the soles and the lesion on his lip as characteristic of secondary syphilis. Mr. B. reported that he engages in anal-receptive intercourse.

A scraping of Mr. B.'s lip lesion was examined under a dark-field micro-scope; it revealed the presence of large numbers of corkscrew-shaped spiro-chetes. The laboratory reported "positive serology", which indicated the presence of the characteristic antibodies in syphilis. These findings confirmed the diagnosis of secondary syphilis. Mr. B. was treated with a course of penicillin, and his lesions and symptoms abated. He was considered cured even though his "serology" remained positive for several years.

HISTORY OF SYPHILIS, OR, "FOR ONE SMALL PLEASURE I SUFFER A THOUSAND MISFORTUNES"

Christopher Columbus brought back to Spain more than dreams of riches and stories of newly discovered trade routes. His ships' crew probably also returned with *Treponema pallidum*, the causative agent of syphilis. Prior to the first voyage of Columbus, Europe had no record of a disease resembling syphilis. Bones containing gross evidence of syphilis are few and their authenticity is debated. Some authorities consider that "pre-Columbian bones" that show signs of syphilis have been frequently found in the Americas. Thus, it is argued that syphilis was transmitted from native Americans to the sailors on Columbus' ships and there-after to the people of Spain and the rest of Europe. (In exchange, native Americans received smallpox, measles, etc.)

The spread of syphilis through Europe was rapid and, for the first few decades, it was accompanied by a very high mortality rate. In 1494, King Charles VIII of France invaded Italy with an army of mercenaries from many countries, including Spain. Since little actual fighting took place, at first much of the campaign was spent in the consortium of female camp followers. The attacking forces were devastated and the mercenaries dispersed to their home countries, carrying syph-ilis to all of Europe. What the defending army was unable to accomplish, syphilis did. Understandably, nobody wanted to claim syphilis as their own:

The Italians called it the Spanish or the French disease; the French called it the Italian or Neapolitan disease; the English called it the French disease; the Russians called it the Polish disease. And . . . the first Spaniards who recog-nized the disease called it the disease of Hispaniola, which meant at that time the disease of Haiti.

Fracastorius' poem, *Syphilis Sive Morbus Gallicus*, published in 1530, assigned to the "venereal pox" a nonpolitical name, that of the shepherd Syphilos. Ambroise Paré, in 1575, referred to it as "Lues Venerea", the lover's plague. During the 16th and 17th centuries, many clinical manifestations of syphilis were observed and catalogued. One of the most puzzling aspects of the disease is that within a few years of its emergence it ceased to be a rapid killer and acquired the complex clinical manifestations by which we know it now (Fig. 23.3).

As a general rule, sexually transmitted diseases do not "travel alone". Thus, it was difficult to separate the manifestations of one disease (gonorrhea) from an-other (syphilis) since one person might be infected with both at the same time. However, most of the physicians who studied these diseases thought they were separate entities. Unfortunately, John Hunter confused the issue for six decades. In 1767, Hunter, in a courageous but ill-conceived experiment, placed onto his skin pus taken from the urethra of a man with gonorrhea. A chancre ensued. Undoubtedly Hunter had taken pus from a man that was coinfected with both *Neisseria gonorrhoeae* and *Treponema pallidum*. Sixty years later Philippe Ricord

Figure 23.1. In previous years, syphilis stirred the imagination to extremes of gloom and hysteria. This French illustration ascribes to syphilis a degree of mortality that has not been seen since the advent of serologic testing and penicillin therapy.

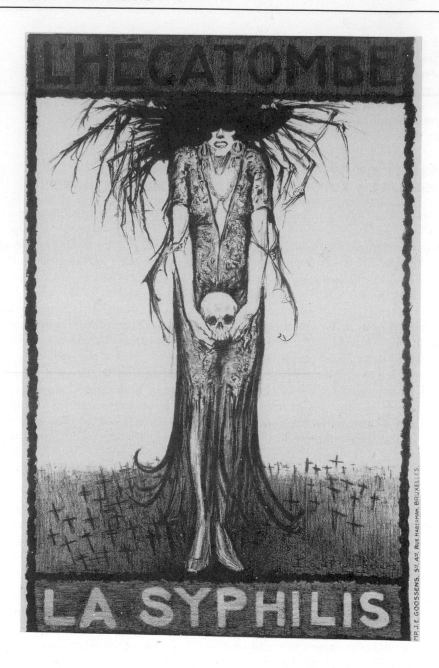

correctly distinguished the two diseases from one another. Ricord also classified the manifestations of syphilis into three stages (primary, secondary, and tertiary).

How Has Syphilis Changed in Recent Decades?

Syphilis has not shared many epidemiological features with other sexually transmitted diseases. Since 1947 there has been a dramatic decline in the cases of syphilis reported in the United States. However, the incidence of primary and secondary syphilis has increased from about 4 cases per 100,000 in 1965 to about 15 per 100,000 in 1982. Demographic data indicate that the disease is being increasingly reported in homosexual males. Homosexual males are now thought to be a significant reservoir of syphilis in the United States. With changing behavior dictated by the fear of AIDS, e.g., reduced number of sexual partners and increased use of condoms, this may be expected to change as well. Rectal intercourse results in the localization of the syphilitic chancre, the primary lesion, in the rectal mucosa. Since this is hidden from sight and chancres are usually painless, the chancre is often overlooked by both patient and physician. The case of Mr. B. illustrates the need to periodically screen sexually active male homosexuals for latent syphilis. Fortunately, if recognized, the disease can be readily treated with penicillin.

THE TREPONEMES

The agent of syphilis belongs to the *spirochetes*, a group of bacteria with a highly characteristic appearance. They are helical, slender, relatively long cells (Fig. 23.2). Spirochetes are widespread in nature; only a few cause disease in humans and animals. The principal human spirochetoses are syphilis, *Lyme disease* (Chapter 60) and *relapsing fever* (caused by members of the genus *Borrelia*), and *leptospirosis* (due to *Leptospira*). The treponeme of syphilis has some close relatives that cause other diseases (yaws, pinta, bejel), mostly in tropical countries.

T. pallidum are so thin (0.1 to 0.2 μm) that they cannot be seen by standard microscopic techniques. They can be visualized by special stains (silver impregnation or immunofluorescence) or special lighting (dark-field microscopy). When observed in a wet mount under the dark-field microscope, they exhibit a characteristic corkscrew-like movement and flexion. They resemble Gram negative bacteria in having an outer membrane, but they do not contain lipopolysaccharide. Their motility is due to flagella that are contained within the periplasm, rather than protruding freely into the medium, as in other motile bacteria.

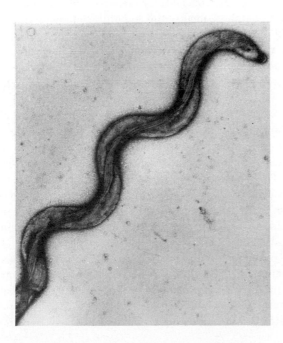

Figure 23.2. Electron photomicrograph of *Treponema pallidum*, negatively stained. Note at the end of the organism, the insertion points of the periplasmic flagella (rope-like contractile structures), which enable the organisms to engage in their typical corkscrew-like motility. (Courtesy of Dr. E.M. Walker, Department of Microbiology and Immunology, UCLA School of Medicine, Los Angeles, CA.)

The amount of information regarding the mechanisms by which *T. pallidum* cause disease is limited primarily by the inability of researchers to readily cultivate the organisms in artificial media, despite many attempts. They can be kept alive to undergo a few divisions. Recent information, especially about their antigenic components, has been obtained by producing *T. pallidum*-specific proteins from genes cloned into *Escherichia coli* vectors.

ENCOUNTER, ENTRY, SPREAD, AND MULTIPLICATION

T. pallidum are very sensitive to drying, disinfectants, and heat (as low as 42°C). Therefore, they are unlikely to be acquired by means other than by personal contact. Neither the toilet seat nor the hot tub can be blamed. The two major routes of transmission are sexual and transplacental. It is estimated that the chances of catching the disease from an infected partner is about 10% per coitus.

The organisms enter a susceptible host through the mucous membranes or the minute abrasions in the skin surface that occur during sex. Once in the subepithelial tissues, the organisms replicate locally in an extracellular location (Fig. 23.3). In culture, they adhere to cells by their tapered ends and probably stick to cells in tissue by the same means. Not all of them stick, and many are soon carried through lymphatic channels to the systemic circulation. Thus, even if the initial manifestation of the disease consists of an isolated skin lesion, syphilis is a systemic disease from the outset.

Treponemes can cross the placental barrier from the bloodstream of an infected mother and cause disease in the fetus. It is not known how the organisms cross this barrier, but Chapter 53 has a general discussion of the issue.

DAMAGE

Initially, neutrophils migrate to the area of inoculation; later, they are replaced by lymphocytes and macrophages. The result of the battle between the locally replicating treponemes and the cellular defenses of the host is the lesion of *primary syphilis*, a painless ulcer—the syphilitic chancre (Fig. 23.3). The time between the initial introduction of the organisms and the appearance of the ulcer depends on the size of the inoculum. The more treponemes that enter, the earlier the chancre appears. This lesion heals spontaneously in 2 to 6 weeks, but by this time the spirochetes have spread and may be causing damage to other parts of the body.

Three to six weeks after the ulcer heals, the secondary form of the disease occurs in about 50% of the cases. *Secondary syphilis* is the manifestation of the systemic spread and involves replication of the treponemes in the lymph nodes, liver, joints, muscles, skin, and mucous membranes distant from the site of the primary chancre. The signs and symptoms of secondary syphilis may be so varied and involve such different tissues and organs, that the disease has been called "the great imitator". The rash and other manifestations of syphilis resolve in the course of weeks to months, but recur within 1 year or so in about one fourth of affected individuals (Fig. 23.3).

This biphasic course of the disease is puzzling for various reasons. Why does the primary chancre heal? Why do the defense mechanisms that are so successful in resolving the primary chancre not function as well systemically? How does the organism survive in the body for long periods of time despite its apparent extracellular location? We do not have answers to these questions or to others

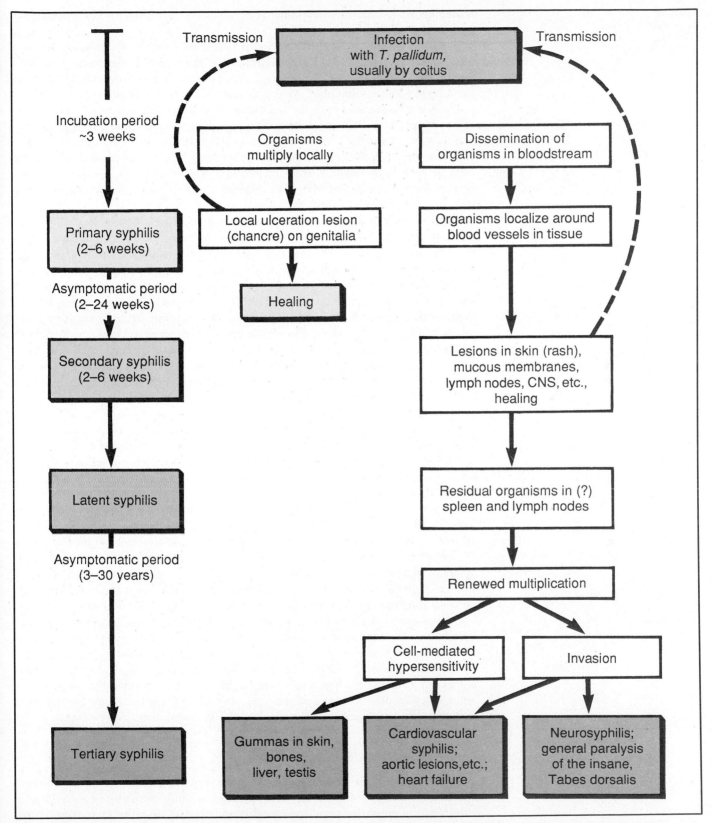

Figure 23.3. The pathogenesis of syphilis. (From Taussig MJ: *Processes in Pathology and Microbiology*, 2nd ed. Oxford, UK, Blackwell Science Publications, 1984.

regarding other aspects of syphilis. It remains one of the more fascinating and puzzling of infectious diseases.

The mechanisms whereby treponemes evade host defenses for years are not well understood. One hypothesis suggests that the ability of treponemes to shed their outer membrane may throw host defenses off target (an analogy might be the release of aluminum chaff by war planes to confuse enemy radar).

The mystery deepens with the resolution of the secondary phase. In about one third of individuals the organisms disappear and the person is cured. In the remaining two thirds the treponemes remain latent for years without causing signs or symptoms (Fig. 23.3). In about half this group, the manifestations of *tertiary syphilis* eventually develop, sometimes after years or decades. Tertiary syphilis is responsible for the majority of the morbidity and mortality associated with the disease. Fortunately, tertiary syphilis is very uncommon in the United States, where routine serologic screening discovers most cases before this stage can develop. The hallmark of tertiary syphilis is the destruction of tissue from a host response to the presence of treponemal antigens. The clinical manifestations are *vasculitis* and *chronic inflammation*. Soft masses composed of few treponemes and inflammatory cells, the gummas, are lesions that commonly destroy bone and soft tissue ("late benign syphilis"), but may involve vital organs as well. In cardiovascular syphilis, vasculitis involves the nutrient arteries supplying the thoracic aorta. Destruction of the elastic tissue in the media of the aorta leads to dilatation of the wall and eventually to aortic valve insufficiency, or the formation of aortic aneurysms and rupture. The central nervous system may also be involved, either by direct invasion of the parenchyma by treponemes or by brain infarction due to vasculitis.

The clinical findings of syphilis can be subtle. Severity of the manifestations depends on the location of the secondary or tertiary lesions in the brain or the spinal cord. Involvement of the dorsal columns of the spinal cord results in loss of position sensation, a classic condition known as *tabes dorsalis*. It is often manifested as ataxic gait; in turn, this usually results in a traumatic destruction of the knee joint, the so-called Charcot's joint. There may also be cutaneous sensory loss over the lower chest, inner aspects of the arms, and lower legs. A generalized involvement of the brain leads to impaired motor function (*paresis*) as well as to gradual loss of higher integrative functions and personality. This clinical picture is known as the *general paralysis of the insane*. A physical sign of neurosyphilis is the Argyll-Robertson pupil—the pupil fails to react to light but accommodates when an object is moved from far to near the eye. When left untreated, neurosyphilis may ultimately lead to death of the patient.

The lesions of tertiary syphilis usually contain few or no treponemes. What then causes lesions to tissues? The damage almost certainly reflects some aspect of the immune response to the organisms. Is it an exaggerated hypersensitivity? Or, could it be a cross-reaction between treponemal and tissue antigens, in other words, an autoimmune response? Once again, it is not known. However, cross-reactive antibodies to host antigens are elicited and are the basis for the most widely utilized tool to detect the disease, the serologic test.

Congenital Syphilis

Despite the decline in the prevalence of syphilis, despite the availability of inexpensive and safe antibiotics, despite the (gratefully) persistent antibiotic sensitivity of the causative organisms, and despite the availability of serologic tests that can detect latent forms of the disease, about 500 babies are born with congenital syphilis in the United States annually. Sexually transmitted diseases, including syphilis, chlamydial infections, gonorrhea, and genital warts, may be silently harbored by women, who then transmit them to their infants, causing morbidity and mortality.

The manifestations of congenitally acquired syphilis are varied; they range from life-threatening organ damage to silent infections. They can also include congenital malformations that are immediately apparent as well as developmental abnormalities that become manifest as the child gets older. The congenital anomalies include premature birth, intrauterine growth retardation, and multiple organ failure (e.g., central nervous system infection, pneumonia, enlargement of the liver and spleen). The most common manifestations of syphilis become evident at about 2 years of age and include facial and tooth deformities (the so-called Hutchinson's incisors and "mulberry" molars). Other less common findings include deafness, arthritis, and "saber shins". These conditions are rare; unfortunately, they have not been entirely relegated to historical textbook descriptions but continue to occur sporadically today. Congenital syphilis is especially tragic because it is completely preventable by penicillin therapy of pregnant women found to have positive serology.

DIAGNOSIS

Prior to this century physicians relied on the clinical manifestations of the disease to make a diagnosis of syphilis. Therefore, only those with obvious skin or mucosal lesions were considered to have syphilis and thus received therapy. Patients with asymptomatic or latent syphilis were undiagnosed and therefore untreated. In 1906, Wassermann, Neisser, and Bruck reported that visible flocculation occurred when extracts of livers of infants who had died of congenital syphilis were mixed with sera of syphilitic adults. It later developed that the same reaction took place with extracts from normal livers or other tissues. In other words, the sera of patients with syphilis have antibodies that react with normal tissue. The tissue component turned out to be a lipid present in the membranes of mitochondria, called *cardiolipin*. Why patients with syphilis form these curious antibodies is not known. As a matter of fact, these antibodies are produced not only in patients with syphilis; biological false-positive tests for syphilis occur in patients with other diseases or conditions (e.g., systemic lupus erythematosus, leprosy, narcotics abuse, even pregnancy). Cross-reactive antibodies are produced in these diseases.

The original test of Wasserman and colleagues led to the development of more rapid and reproducible tests. There are several variations known by their eponyms [e.g., the venereal diseases reference laboratory test (VDRL) or the rapid plasma reagin (RPR)]. They are cheap and easy to perform, which makes them suitable for the initial screening of large numbers of serum samples, as in premarital "blood tests". However, their relative lack of specificity makes it necessary to test all positive samples by more specific tests directed against treponemal antigens. Two such treponeme specific tests are called the FTA and the TPI tests. The fluorescent treponemal antibody test (FTA) uses indirect immunofluorescence. Patient serum is mixed with a film of *T. pallidum* and allowed to react. Antitreponemal antibodies are detected by adding fluorescent rabbit or goat antibodies against human gamma globulin. These react with bound human antibodies and make the treponemes visible under a fluorescence microscope. Another specific test is called the *T. pallidum* immobilization test (TPI) and relies on the inhibition of treponemal motility by specific antibodies in a patient's serum. These tests require specialized reagents and equipment, and are best performed in reference laboratories.

TREATMENT, OR "ONE NIGHT WITH VENUS, A LIFETIME WITH MERCURY"

Two major advances in the diagnosis and management of syphilis have occurred during the 20th century: the development of serologic tests for diagnosing syphilis and the use of penicillin for treating the disease. Fortunately for Mr. B. and the rest of the world, the organisms are exquisitely sensitive to the drug and have shown no sign of becoming resistant.

Before penicillin, treatment depended on an arsenic-containing compound synthesized by Ehrlich early in this century (it was the first effective synthetic chemotherapeutic agent). It was called "606", in recognition of 605 previous failures in that laboratory. Before the introduction of penicillin, therapy consisted of the tedious, expensive, and dangerous administration of arsenic and mercury or bismuth for a minimum of 2 months and as long as 2 or 3 years. An alternative therapy was the induction of fever, based on the heat sensitivity of *T. pallidum*. Fever was induced by the intravenous injection of killed typhoid bacilli (and their endotoxin), or, in an extreme burst of therapeutic zeal, by deliberately giving a patient malaria! Currently, the treatment of latent syphilis relies on the continued sensitivity of *T. pallidum* to penicillin and on the body's ability to maintain barely detectible blood levels of the drug for long periods of time (intramuscular benzathine penicillin, "bicillin").

CONCLUSIONS

The story of syphilis constitutes an important chapter in medicine and in human history. Fortunately, the severity of the disease has waned, and we can remain optimistic as long as *T. pallidum* remains obligingly sensitive to penicillin. Few diseases have a more elusive pathobiology and a greater spectrum of clinical manifestations, most of which cannot yet be explained satisfactorily. Syphilis is, to appropriate a quote from Churchill, "a riddle wrapped in a mystery inside an enigma."

SELF-ASSESSMENT QUESTIONS

1. What is the likely role of antitreponemal antibodies in each of the three stages of syphilis?

2. How would you explain the resolution of primary syphilis and the emergence of the secondary stage?

3. In what ways does tertiary syphilis appear to be an autoimmune disease?

4. During which stage of syphilis is a patient most contagious?

5. What would it take to make syphilis disappear from the face of the earth?

6. If you were involved in syphilis research, what problems would you tackle?

SUGGESTED READINGS

Dennie CC: *A History of Syphilis.* Springfield, IL, Charles C Thomas, 1962.

Fichtner RR, Aral SO, et al: Syphilis in the United States: 1967–1979. *Sexually Transmitted Dis* 10:77–80, 1983.

Perine PL, Handsfield HH, Holmes KK, Blount JH,: Epidemiology of the sexually transmitted diseases. *Ann Rev Public Health* 6:85–106, 1985.

Pussey WA: *The History and Epidemiology of Syphilis.* Springfield, IL, Charles C Thomas, 1933.

Rathburn KC: Congenital syphilis. *Sexually Transmitted Dis* 10:93–99, 1983.

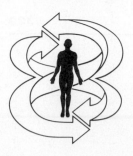

Chlamydiae and a Common Sexually Transmitted Disease

E.N. Robinson, Jr.
Z. McGee

Chlamydiae cause the most frequent sexually transmitted disease, a so-called nongonococcal urethritis that has important consequences in women, namely pelvic inflammatory disease and its attending infertility, ectopic pregnancy, or chronic pelvic pain. Chlamydiae can also cause infections of the eye and other organs. These organisms are strict intracellular bacteria and cannot be grown on cell-free media. They have a complex life cycle, having one form for intracellular multiplication and another for transit between hosts and their cells.

CASE

A 23-year-old male, Mr. C., complained to a physician of a purulent discharge from his penis. The diagnosis of gonorrhea was made (see Chapter 14) and he was given amoxicillin (an oral penicillin) along with probenecid (a drug that blocks the excretion of amoxicillin and increases its blood level). He improved initially, but over the last 3 days noticed a milder but persistent urethral discharge and pain on urination. Worried that he might not have been cured, he went to the Sexually Transmitted Diseases Clinic for evaluation. He reported having had no sexual intercourse since his last visit. His latest sexual partner, Ms. G., accompanied him to the clinic, although she had no complaints of pain, vaginal irritation, or discharge.

On physical examination, Mr. C. had a small amount of clear urethral discharge. Ms. G. was found to have a greenish discharge emanating from her cervical os. Her cervix was inflamed and bled easily when a swab was used to remove adherent secretion. Gram stains of the secretions of both persons revealed numerous neutrophils and no evidence of Gram negative cocci.

Mr. C. was told that he had "postgonococcal urethritis", a condition that may be caused by Chlamydia trachomatis. The incubation time of infections with chlamydiae is generally longer than with gonococci. He may therefore have experienced the overlapping manifestations of two infectious agents acquired simultaneously. Ms. G. was told that she had "mucopurulent cervicitis", the female counterpart of chlamydial urethritis.

The resident physician explained that the original treatment received by Mr. C. did not follow the current recommendations of the U.S. Public Health Service, which take into account that about 45% of the cases of gonorrhea have coexisting chlamydial infections. The recommended treatment of uncomplicated gonorrhea is the administration of both a penicillin for the gonococcus and a tetracycline for the chlamydiae. Both patients were treated with tetracycline and were strongly advised to return after finishing therapy to ensure that they had been cured of both the gonococcal and the chlamydial disease.

Questions that arise include: what are chlamydiae and what diseases do they cause? How frequent are these infections? How do chlamydiae cause lesions? How are these infections diagnosed? How are they differentiated from gonorrhea? What is the best treatment and prophylaxis?

DISEASES CAUSED BY CHLAMYDIAE

Chlamydiae are small bacteria that can only grow inside host cells. These strict intracellular parasites cause many different diseases (Table 24.1). There are at least two species of chlamydia, trachomatis and psittaci. C. trachomatis, the agent involved in these cases, is the more diversified of the two species in humans; it causes diseases (some acute, some chronic) of the mucous membranes of the eye, the lungs, the genital tract, and others. It would be misleading, however, to think that all these diseases are caused by the same organism. C. trachomatis can be divided into different serotypes (Table 24.1) that are associated with different spectra of diseases. One of the most serious is trachoma, an infection of the eye that can readily lead to blindness if untreated. It used to be very common in the Middle East and other parts of the world, and it is still the leading cause of blindness in some developing countries. Psittacosis, a form of pneumonia, is the major disease caused by the other species of chlamydia, C. psittaci.

Table 24.1

Human syndromes due to *Chlamydia trachomatis*

Serotype	Syndrome
A, B, C,	Trachoma
D through K	Nongonococcal urethritis, epididymitis, Reiter's syndrome, proctitis, mucopurulent cervicitis, endometritis, salpingitis, perihepatitis, neonatal inclusion conjunctivitis, infant pneumonia
L1, 2, 3	Lymphogranuloma venereum

Although chlamydial infections are not reported to the health departments, it has been recognized that *C. trachomatis* infections are the most common of the sexually transmitted diseases in the United States, even surpassing gonorrhea and herpes. Genital chlamydial infection is usually manifested as a mild urethritis, often with little pain and minimal recurrent exudate. It is usually self-healing. The mildness of the disease may explain why it often goes unrecognized. It is estimated that three to five million new cases arise each year in the United States alone. It is likely that the number of people who carry the organism in this country is much higher, the vast majority without realizing it.

What is this sexually transmitted disease called? Whereas other chlamydial infections have names, such as lymphogranuloma venereum or inclusion conjunctivitis, the more common disease, like that illustrated in our cases, has no distinctive name. Together with urethritis caused by some other agents (e.g., mycoplasma, trichomonas), it is referred to by the generic term nongonococcal urethritis, or NGU.

The most important aspect of this infection is that it can lead to serious complications, such as ectopic pregnancy (lodging of the embryo in a site such as a fallopian tube, other than the uterine cavity), infertility, or recurrent pelvic inflammatory disease. These complications arise only in a small percentage of the total number of infected individuals, but, given the wide distribution of the organisms, they affect many people.

THE ORGANISMS

Chlamydiae are very small and it took researchers a long time to recognize that they have a typical bacterial structure (Fig. 24.1). They have two membranes, in the fashion of Gram negative bacteria. A murein or peptidoglycan layer has not been demonstrated, despite intense efforts. Nonetheless, the suspicion that

Figure 24.1. **A**, Metabolically active and dividing reticulate bodies of *Chlamydia trachomatis* contained in a phagosomal vesicle. **B**, Late, mature *C. trachomatis* inclusion containing both reticulate bodies (RB) and elementary bodies (EB). (Courtesy of Drs. L. Hodinka and P.R. Wyrick.)

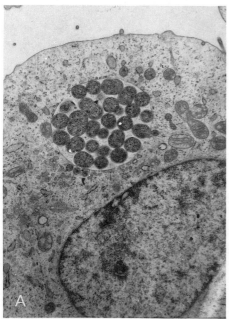

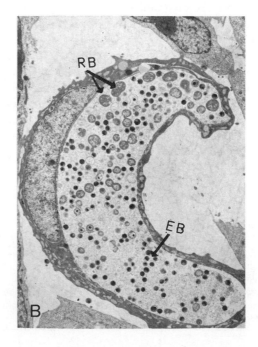

chlamydiae have murein remains, in good part because the organisms are some-what sensitive to penicillin in vitro and have penicillin-binding proteins in their membrane (see Chapter 2). On the other hand, in a clinical setting chlamydia are not sensitive to penicillin (as seen by the failure of this drug to cure Mr. C. and Ms. G). This lack of efficacy is thought to be due to the inability of penicillin to penetrate human cells.

The genome of chlamydiae is about 25% the size of that of *Escherichia coli*. Chlamydiae are strict intracellular parasites; that is, they cannot multiply outside host cells. Why? One suggestive fact is that they cannot generate their own ATP. They do not have oxidative enzymes such as flavoproteins or cytochromes, and apparently rely on their host cells for energy-rich compounds. They are thus energy parasites par excellence. Other factors, as yet unknown, must contribute to their intracellular parasitism, because they do not multiply extracellularly when provided with ATP. Intracellularly, they can synthesize their own macromolecules and do so without losing their cellular integrity. Thus, for all their obligate intra-cellular parasitism, they are true cellular forms of life and are entirely different from their viruses. Their procaryotic nature is emphasized by the important fact that they are sensitive to typical antibacterial antibiotics such as sulfonamides and tetracycline.

ENTRY, MULTIPLICATION, AND SPREAD

Chlamydiae enter host cells by phagocytosis; that is, they are taken up within membrane-bound vacuoles like most intracellular parasites (Figs. 24.1–24.3). In the course of human infection, chlamydiae enter epithelial cells very quickly. Since these cells are nonprofessional phagocytes, the chlamydiae may provide the impe-tus for their own uptake. Apparently this comes from a ligand on the surface of chlamydiae that has high affinity for some receptor on the host cell.

Once inside phagosomal vesicles, chlamydiae grow into microscopic colonies (known as *intracytoplasmic inclusions*) that eventually can occupy more than half the cell's volume. Chlamydiae avoid being killed by the enzymes of the lysosomes by inhibiting their fusion with the phagocytic vesicles. If the ingested chlamydiae are coated with specific antibodies, phagolysosomal fusion is not inhibited; in-

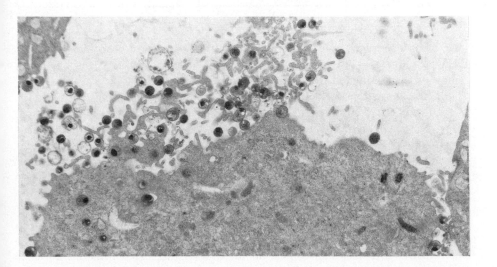

Figure 24.2. The infectious process is initiated by absorption of the chlamydiae to microvilli of columnar epithelial cells. The elementary bodies appear to travel down the microvilli to their base, where they enter via specialized coated pits. (Courtesy of Drs. R.L. Hodinka and P.R. Wyrick.)

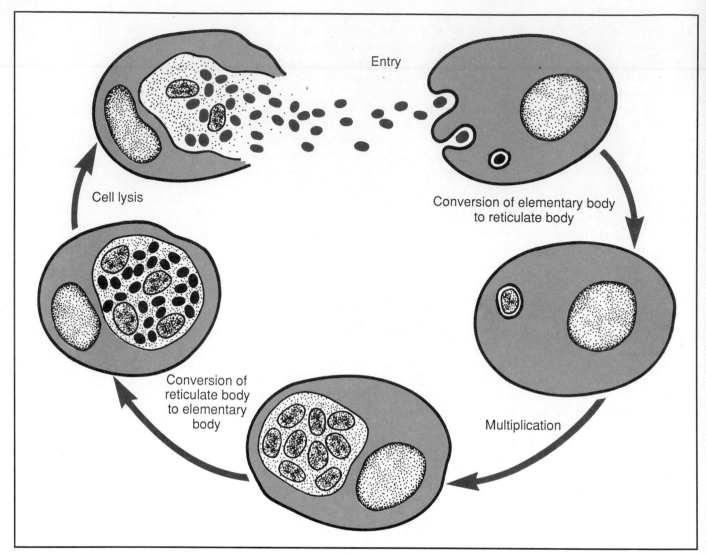

Entry

Conversion of elementary body
to reticulate body

Multiplication

Conversion of
reticulate body
to elementary
body

Cell lysis

Figure 24.3.   The life cycle of
chlamydiae.

stead, lysosomes pour their contents into the phagosome, and the organisms are
killed. This suggests that some surface component of the chlamydiae (which can
be masked or inactivated by antibodies) prevents the fusion.

For a small procaryote, the life cycle of a chlamydia is unusually rich in events.
The free forms of the organisms, those which go from cell to cell and from host
to host, are small tight spheres called *elementary bodies* (Fig. 24.1). Once these
enter the host cells they become larger and metabolically active and begin multiplying by binary fission. These forms of chlamydiae are called *reticulate bodies*,
from their mesh-like appearance in stained preparations. Reticulate bodies are
very fragile and must differentiate into elementary bodies before they are able to
invade new host cells.

This unusual life cycle may be easier to understand if the following is kept in
mind: Reticulate bodies do not survive well outside cells, and they quickly lose
their infectivity. Elementary bodies, on the other hand, can withstand all sorts
of damaging conditions. These bodies are functionally akin to bacterial spores—

structures designed for survival but not for growth. The analogy is not so far-fetched since, like spores, elementary bodies are covered with layers of tough proteins highly cross-linked by disulfide bridges. The reversibility of these linkages is crucial to the transformation from elementary bodies to reticulate bodies when the chlamydiae enter host cells. If the phagosomes in which they are lodged had strong reducing conditions, the disulfide bridges of the envelope proteins could be broken, unraveling the outer shell of the elementary bodies and converting them to reticulate bodies. Unfettered, they could then begin to multiply. This series of events has not been convincingly demonstrated. The reverse process, the conversion of reticulate bodies into elementary bodies, may well be due to oxidizing conditions that can arise late in infection, but this is just a guess at present. The point to keep in mind is that these organisms are dimorphic in their life cycle. That is, they have one morphological form for reproduction and another one for extracellular survival.

DAMAGE

How do chlamydiae damage their host cells? They contain endotoxin (LPS), but it is not really known how this contributes to the lesions. Host cells can tolerate a large load of chlamydiae before damage becomes apparent. Even so, the organisms multiply rapidly and reach large numbers rather quickly. In culture, infected host cells lyse within 20 to 40 hours and release a large number of elementary bodies. These invade adjacent cells or, if carried to other parts of the body by blood or other fluids, attack distant cells.

The genital lesions of chlamydial disease are those typically found in acute inflammation. The symptoms described by both Mr. C. and Ms. G. at the beginning of this chapter can be ascribed to this process. Neutrophils are probably called up by chemotactic substances produced by the ruptured host cells and by the alternate activation of complement (most likely set in motion by the endotoxin).

When the disease is located in the urethra it is usually self-limiting. It can also recur after asymptomatic periods, suggesting that humoral and cellular immunity are insufficient to combat these organisms in their intracellular location. The location of the organisms during periods of remission is not known. If the lesions are located in deeper tissue, fibrotic scarring can occur after the lesions heal, sometimes causing serious consequences. Thus, the infection of fallopian tubes can cause infertility, which results from the loss of ciliated cells that propel the egg toward the uterus. Infection at this site can also facilitate the entry of other organisms into the peritoneal cavity, where they cause recurrent *pelvic inflammatory disease*.

As for trachoma, blindness in patients with this disease is the result of inflammation of the conjunctiva followed by vascularization and scarring of the cornea. Eventually the cornea is so infiltrated by blood vessels and scar tissue that it becomes opaque. The inflammation of tissues in the region interferes with the flow of tears, which is an important defense mechanism. A common result is secondary infection by other bacteria. Together they may lead to blindness.

DIAGNOSIS

Venereal chlamydial infections must be differentiated from gonorrhea and other purulent infections because the drugs of choice are different for each disease (penicillin for those caused by penicillin-sensitive gonococci, tetracycline for those due to chlamydiae). Since chlamydiae cannot develop outside of cells, their detection in clinical specimens requires expensive and time-consuming cell cultures. Instead, a diagnostic tool that is becoming available is the direct microscopic demonstration of the organisms in exudates, using fluorescence antibody techniques. While this is a somewhat specialized procedure, it is quick, and an increasing number of clinical laboratories are becoming equipped to perform it. Eventually, detection of chlamydiae may become even more rapid and convenient using specific DNA probes.

TREATMENT

Two aspects of the life cycle of chlamydiae have a direct impact on how chlamydial infections are treated. First, since the organisms are metabolically active only intracellularly, antibiotics must penetrate the host cells if they are to find their targets. Penicillin, for example, has some antichlamydial activity, but its inability to penetrate mucosal cells severely limits its effectiveness. As illustrated in the case of Mr. C., single-dose penicillin treatments for gonorrhea do not affect the commonly coinfecting chlamydiae. Only extended therapy with alternative agents can result in the eradication of these organisms. Among the effective drugs are tetracycline, erythromycin, sulfonamides, or quinolones.

The second aspect of the chlamydial life style relevant to therapy is that infection by these organisms is a destructive process, whether it occurs in the male urethra, the female cervix, the fallopian tube, or the conjunctiva of neonates. Therefore, individuals shown to be infected with chlamydiae or their known sexual contacts can be sources of infection and should be treated even if asymptomatic. The recommended list of those who should receive antibiotics against chlamydiae is presented in Table 24.2.

CONCLUSIONS

Despite the minimal symptoms which they usually provoke, chlamydiae are important agents of disease since their infection can lead to significant complications.

Chlamydiae have an intriguing life cycle that is likely to yield further surprises. We still do not know much about the details of their metabolic dependence on host cells, the way in which they impede the fusion of lysosomes with phagosomes, or how they transform into the elementary bodies, the "transit" form. Also open for investigation are the precise mechanisms that lead to cell damage and to the symptoms of disease.

SELF-ASSESSMENT QUESTIONS

1. How do replicating chlamydiae differ from chlamydiae "in transit" between hosts? What is the biochemical basis for the changes?

2. What is known about the strict requirement for intracellular multiplication of these organisms? And how do they survive in macrophages?

3. Why are genital infections by chlamydiae a public health problem? What threat do they represent to the individual patient?

Table 24.2
Who should receive antichlamydial therapy?

- Patients with gonorrhea

- Patients with any of the diseases listed in Table 24.1

- All their sexual partners

- Neonates born to women with untreated chlamydial infections

4. Awareness of sexually transmitted chlamydial infections alters the therapeutic strategy for all sexually transmitted diseases. Why? How does it alter it?

5. What aspect of "chlamydology" would you select for further study?

SUGGESTED READINGS

Moulder JW: Comparative biology of intracellular parasitism. *Microbiol Rev* 49:298–337, 1985.

Perine PL, Handsfield HH, Holmes KK, Blount JH: Epidemiology of the sexually transmitted diseases. *Ann Rev Public Health* 6:85–106, 1985.

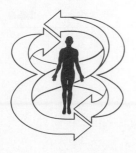

Rocky Mountain Spotted Fever and Other Rickettsioses

M. Schaechter

Rickettsiae are specialized, strictly intracellular bacteria that cause epidemic typhus and related diseases. Rickettsiae are transmitted by lice, fleas, mites, etc. Although it has played a major role in human history, epidemic typhus can be controlled by delousing the population. The principal rickettsiosis in the United States is Rocky Mountain spotted fever. Rickettsiae have a particular tropism for vascular endothelial cells and the symptoms of the diseases are due in part to local damage to small blood vessels, local inflammation, and extravasation of blood.

CASE

Nancy, an 8-year-old, was admitted to a hospital in Cape Cod, Massachusetts in July with a skin rash, most pronounced on the arms and legs, involving the palms and soles. She had a fever of 42°C and appeared listless and confused. The history obtained from the mother indicated that the family had been camping on Cape Cod for the previous 2 weeks. The whole family, including Nancy and her younger sister, found ticks on their bodies almost every day. Three days before admission Nancy complained of a severe headache, muscle pains, and a fever. The rash appeared the day she was brought to the hospital. Her sister and father also had muscle pains, headache, and fever, but no skin rash. At this point the differential diagnosis included either an infection or a noninfectious inflammatory allergic or toxic reaction.

Blood was drawn for culture and serologic tests for rickettsiae. A skin biopsy from the area of the rash was obtained for histological examination and direct immunofluorescence. The laboratory reported negative blood cultures. Pathological examination of the biopsy revealed accumulation of neutrophils *and macrophages and extensive extravasation of blood from damaged small vessels—in other words, a vasculitis accompanied by acute inflammation. Smears from the lesions were positive when treated with a fluorescein-tagged antirickettsial antibody. These findings together with the history of infestation by ticks suggest the diagnosis of Rocky Mountain spotted fever.*

Ponder the following questions:

- How can one catch a disease called Rocky Mountain spotted fever in the eastern United States? How are ticks involved?

- How does the disease affect parts of the body distant from the entry site of the microorganism?

- What causes the vasculitis, and is that causative factor also responsible for the symptoms of the disease?

THE RICKETTSIOSES

This group of related diseases includes various forms of typhus and the so-called spotted fevers. They vary in severity from the extremely severe *epidemic typhus*, one of the scourges of mankind, to diseases which are fairly mild and not often seen in the United States. Epidemic typhus caused many fatalities as recently as World War II. The most common rickettsiosis in the United States is Rocky Mountain spotted fever. It affects some 1000 people annually. It is more

Figure 25.1. Cases of Rocky Mountain spotted fever reported in 1985 by counties in the United States. (Data from the Centers for Disease Control: Rocky Mountain spotted fever—United States, 1985. *MMWR* 35:247–249, 1986.)

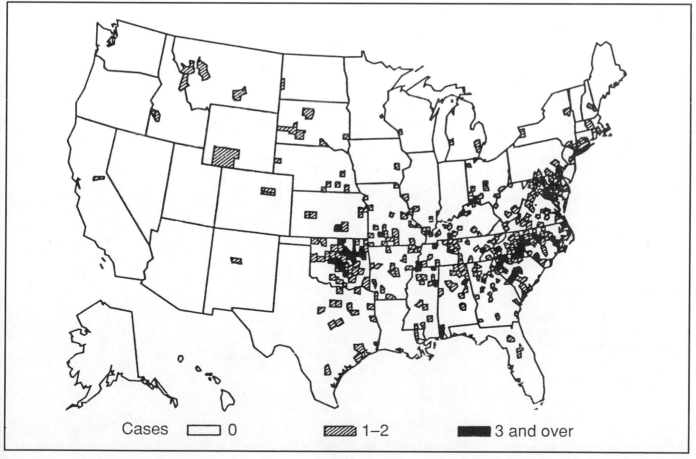

Cases ☐ 0   ▨ 1–2   ■ 3 and over

Table 25.1
The principal rickettsioses of the U.S.

Disease	Rickettsia or Coxiella	Approximate No. Reported Cases/yr in U.S. (in recent years)	Vector	Reservoir
Rocky Mountain spotted fever	R. rickettsii	1000	Ticks	Various rodents
Endemic typhus	R. typhi	60	Fleas	Rats
Rickettsial pox	R. akari	Few	Mites	Mice
Epidemic typhus	R. prowazekii	Very few	Lice	?Humans ?Squirrels
Q fever	C. burnetii	50	Ticks or none	Many mammals

common in the eastern and southern states than in the Rocky Mountains, where it was first described. The likely reason is that humans and ticks come in contact with one another more frequently in densely populated areas (Fig. 25.1). This can be an extremely serious disease, with a mortality rate of about 10% if untreated. Because it responds well to either tetracycline or chloramphenicol, especially in the early stages, a speedy diagnosis is essential.

Most rickettsioses are transmitted by the bite of arthropods such as lice, fleas, mites, or ticks (in microbiological language, they are "arthropodborne"; see Table 25.1 and Chapter 55 on the zoonoses). The reason arthropod vectors are required for transmission seems to be that free rickettsiae do not fare well in the environment.

THE RICKETTSIAE

Because of their small size and their intracellular life-style, rickettsiae were thought at one time to be something between a bacterium and a virus, which is no longer a tenable concept. It is now clear that they are actually small bacteria that do not grow freely. They are strict intracellular parasites—with one excep-

Figure 25.2. Electron micrograph of a thin section of a human endothelial cell infected with *Rickettsia rickettsii*, the agent of Rocky Mountain spotted fever. The rickettsiae are the dark rod-shaped bacteria in the nucleus, about the same size as the mitochondria. Note that these rickettsiae have a predilection for the host cell nucleus. This is an unusual localization for intracellular bacteria; other species of rickettsiae, tubercle bacilli, Salmonella, etc., are usually found in the cytoplasm. (Courtesy of Dr. D.J. Silverman, School of Medicine, University of Maryland, Baltimore, MD.)

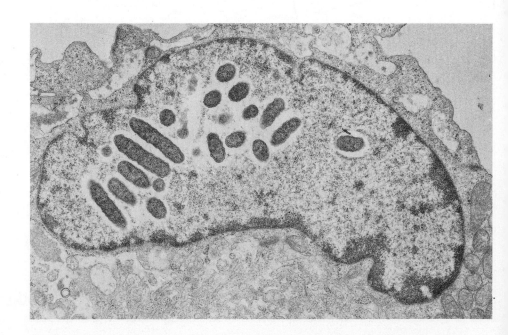

tion: an organism related to this group, which causes a disease called "trench fever", has been cultured in a cell-free medium (blood agar). Like other bacteria, rickettsiae divide by binary fission, make their own proteins and nucleic acids, and are sensitive to protein synthesis-inhibiting antibiotics. In thin sections rickettsiae look like small but fairly typical bacteria (Fig. 25.2). Befitting their rigid rod shape, they contain murein. Like Gram negative rods, they possess two membrane systems.

Rickettsiae can generate their own energy, but they also depend on their host cells for some ATP. These organisms have unusual ATP permeability. Suspensions of rickettsiae lose viability after storage, apparently due to the loss of their intracellular pool of ATP and several coenzymes. Unlike typical bacteria, they can actually exchange their internal ADP for ATP from the host cell. It is possible that this property explains why they are strict intracellular parasites. In regard to this "energy parasitism", rickettsiae resemble the chlamydiae, which are even more strict in requiring energy from their host cells.

ENCOUNTER AND ENTRY

Rocky Mountain spotted fever is acquired by the bite of certain species of ticks. Ticks are not harmed by their rickettsiae and can pass them to their young by a transovarial route. This increases the chances of spreading the organisms. In addition, many different animals can serve as reservoirs of these rickettsiae in the wild. Thus, this disease cannot be eradicated by public health measures. Risk of transmission can be eluded by the use of protective clothing (though lovers of the outdoors may find this annoying).

SPREAD, MULTIPLICATION, AND DAMAGE

The classical rickettsioses are disseminated diseases whose local symptoms can usually be attributed to damage to small vessels (Fig. 25.3). Rocky Mountain spotted fever is therefore a *vasculitis* and its symptoms reflect damage to the

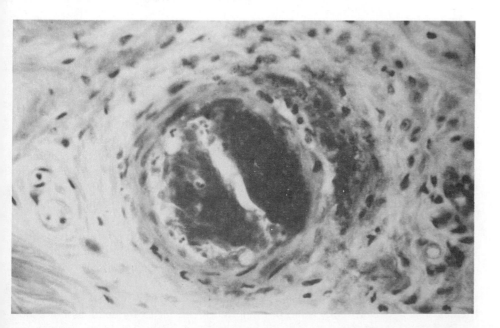

Figure 25.3. Arteritis with a thrombus and red blood cell extravasation in a patient with Rocky Mountain spotted fever. (Courtesy of Dr. Gustav Dammin, Harvard Medical School.)

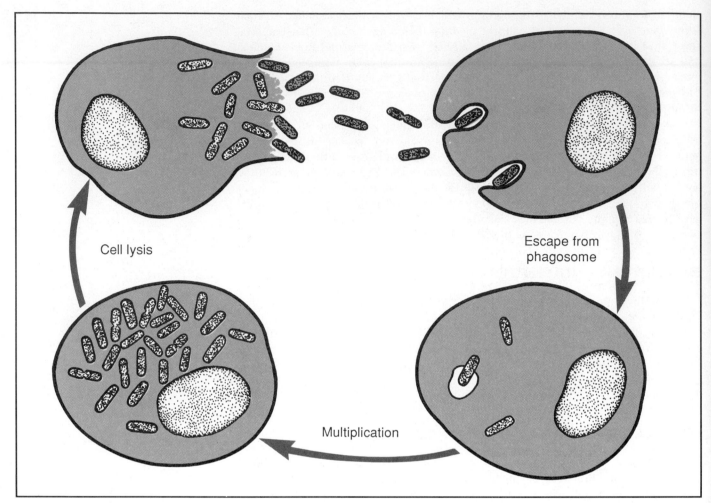

Figure 25.4. The life cycle of
rickettsiae.

integrity of the vessels of important organs. Rickettsiae do not make powerful
exotoxins; most likely they cause damage by directly killing the cells that harbor
them. Lysis of endothelial cells leads to rupture of capillaries and small vessels.
Nancy's rash can be attributed to extravasation of blood into the subcutaneous
tissue. Her mental confusion results from damage to the vessels of the brain.
Other organs are similarly affected.

Rickettsiae can readily penetrate many types of mammalian cells, yet they are
seen mainly in the vascular endothelium. The reason for this striking tropism is
unknown. Could their localization result simply from hematogenous spread,
which places them in frequent contact with the walls of small vessels? In any
event, rickettsiae must be counted among the microorganisms with the greatest
ability to enter nonprofessional phagocytic cells, such as those of vascular endothelia (Fig. 25.4).

These organisms grow slowly, with doubling times of about 8 hours. In stained
preparations or in ultrathin sections, cells are often filled wall to wall with rickettsiae. Interestingly, in culture, cells containing enormous numbers of rickettsiae do not lyse for several days, although eventually they break open and release
their cargo of organisms. Some species of rickettsiae show variations on these
themes. The agent of Rocky Mountain spotted fever, for example, does not accu-

mulate in such large numbers inside cells but is shed gradually. For reasons unknown, rickettsiae of this group have a predilection for the nuclei of their host cells. It is rather startling to see dozens or more such rickettsiae lying within otherwise intact-appearing nuclei.

Rickettsiae enter cells by phagocytosis. The process requires active participation of the host cell's cytoskeleton, as in other examples of phagocytosis. Rickettsiae must contribute actively to this process because nonmetabolizing rickettsiae are not ingested. Once inside the host cell, rickettsiae penetrate the membrane of the phagosome and are seen in the cytoplasm a short time after being taken up. This demonstrates their great capacity for passing through membranes. Possibly a rickettsial phospholipase is involved in weakening or perforating the host cell membranes.

Does escape from the phagosomal vesicles permit rickettsiae to escape destruction by lysosomal enzymes? The ability of rickettsiae to enter the host cell cytoplasm is impaired when they are coated with antirickettsial antibodies. Under these conditions they are taken up by phagocytes, but cannot escape into the cytoplasm. Remaining in the phagosomal vacuole, they become prey to lysosomal enzymes. Circulating antibodies and cellular immunity probably play an important role in the course of the disease. In most patients, the outcome is determined within a few weeks, by which time active immunity is built up. In view of the importance of specific immunity in this disease, it is not surprising that rickettsial vaccines can be effective. The importance of circulating antibodies in determining the outcome of the disease suggests that rickettsiae spread freely through the blood.

Q FEVER

A different type of disease is placed here because the causative agent is related to the rickettsiae. The disease is called *Q fever* (after Queensland, Australia) and is more commonly acquired by inhalation rather than by the bite of arthropods. The organisms that cause Q fever are also small, strict intracellular bacteria, but are sufficiently different from rickettsiae in other regards to have been placed in a different genus, *Coxiella*. In keeping with their mode of transmission, coxiellae readily survive the environment. In fact, they are released from their host cells as a structure that resembles a bacterial spore. Unlike the typical rickettsioses, Q fever results mainly in pneumonia, although endocarditis and hepatitis are also seen. It is often acquired from sheep, and sheep farmers and laboratory workers who use sheep as experimental animals are at risk.

RICKETTSIAE AND HISTORY

Until about 100 years ago, Western societies lived under the threat of epidemic diseases. The most deadly example is the Black Plague, which in the late Middle Ages killed perhaps one third of the population of Europe. The assumption that most of us normally make, that we are likely to conclude a particular day, month, or year in reasonable health, was not tenable at the height of such epidemics. Rather, each day must have offered prospects of a kind of Russian roulette, with the odds on the side of the Grim Reaper.

Among the modern day vestiges of those diseases is *epidemic typhus*. Prevalent in Europe during both World Wars, it is a disease of the trenches, prisons, and concentration camps—truly a disease associated with human misery. In WWII uncounted numbers of civilians and soldiers contracted this disease. It came under control about the time of the invasion of Italy by Allied troops, when they and the civilians of the region were liberally doused with DDT, a pesticide that kills the vector of the disease, the *human body louse*.

Knowledge of the microbiological basis of epidemic typhus has lagged behind that of other important infectious diseases. The most salient reason is that the causative rickettsiae cannot be cultivated outside living cells. Like all strict intra-cellular parasites, rickettsiae are harder to work with than organisms that can grow readily on agar. Among other things, this makes it difficult to provide a simple diagnostic test. Serological tests depend on a source of antigen to detect specific antibodies in patients' sera. Suitable antigens are now prepared by purifying rickettsiae from infected, fertilized chicken eggs. These antigens are used for complement fixation tests to detect antirickettsial antibodies in patients' sera (Chapter 59). They can also be used to produce specific antibodies in animals for the direct detection of rickettsiae in tissues or blood smears using micro-scopic immunofluorescence.

Until recently, laboratory diagnosis of some rickettsioses depended on an indirect and nonspecific test that has been the subject of a remarkable historico-microbiological vignette. Patients with epidemic typhus produce antibodies not only against the elusive rickettsia but, coincidentally, also against the readily cultivable enteric bacillus, *Proteus vulgaris*. The basis for this serological cross-reactivity is not well known, but such "sharing" of antigens occurs in other pairs of microbial species as well. Sera from epidemic typhus patients agglutinate suspensions of *Proteus*; this can be used as a simple diagnostic test.

Knowledge of this serological cross-reactivity was put to a humanitarian use by two Polish physicians in WWII who were aware that the occupying Germans did not send to labor camps people suspected of having epidemic typhus. Inge-niously, these doctors inoculated the people of several villages with an innocuous vaccine made up of killed *P. vulgaris*. The high titer of the serum of these people was taken by the German medical staff to indicate that these villages were hotbeds of epidemic typhus. The inhabitants were spared, thanks to the microbiological acumen of the two physicians.

MORE ON TYPHUS: A CASE OF BRILL'S DISEASE

A 78-year-old man of Eastern European origin had a fever of 43°C, severe headache, mental confusion, rash of the upper torso, and pain in the joints. He had no history of traveling to regions with epidemic typhus since he emigrated to the United States some 50 years ago. He was free of body lice and appeared to be scrupulous in his personal hygiene. His serum fixed complement in the presence of rickettsial antigens at a dilution of 1:32, suggesting a fairly high titer of antirickettsial antibodies. This laboratory finding and the rather typical array of symptoms allowed the diagnosis of Brill's disease, a rare form of recrudescent epidemic typhus seen in persons who had lived years ago in areas where the disease was prevalent at the time. When Dr. Brill, a physician practicing in New York City, examined a case similar to this one, he is reported to have muttered something like: "If this were the Old Country, I'd say the patient has epidemic typhus!"

The following questions arise:

• Where did the patient acquire the rickettsiae?

• Did the rickettsiae lie dormant for 50 years in his body?

Like all rickettsiae, those of epidemic typhus must reside in a living reservoir during interepidemic periods. The disease is apparently confined to humans, and the common way of contracting it is via the bite of human lice. Yet, unlike the ticks involved in Rocky Mountain spotted fever, the lice become sick and succumb to the rickettsiae in about 7 days. Thus they are not the likely repository of the organisms. It has often been remarked that since natural selection favors peaceful coexistence, a disease that is lethal for both host and vector is probably of recent historical origin.

For epidemic typhus the interepidemic reservoir can only be surmised. Possibilities include both humans and animals with which we come in contact. The case for *animal reservoirs* is based on the isolation of epidemic typhus rickettsiae from flying squirrels. The case for *human reservoirs* is suggested by Brill's disease. The epidemiological history of this disease strongly points to the ability of the organisms to survive for long periods in the human body in a state of latency. Indeed, rickettsiae have been found in the lymph nodes of elderly New Yorkers who had no symptoms of the disease but who had spent their early years in Eastern Europe. Only when the rickettsiae succeed in breaking through a state of equilibrium and grow out do they cause symptoms. Even without the manifestations of Brill's disease, rickettsial carriers may conceivably be bitten by lice at times when an occasional rickettsia finds itself in the bloodstream. Fortuitously, these lice could then spread the disease to other persons.

CONCLUSIONS

Rickettsial infections are not very common but some of them can be life threatening. They must be diagnosed promptly and antibiotic therapy must be instituted with due speed. The main disease caused by these organisms, epidemic typhus, has receded in importance due to louse control.

Rickettsiae are delicate organisms but are well adapted to intracellular life and to passage from reservoir to host via arthropods. Their localization in blood vessels causes local inflammation and hemorrhages, sometimes with severe consequences.

SELF-ASSESSMENT QUESTIONS

1. What epidemiological features are shared by all rickettsioses but not necessarily by Q fever?

2. Describe three characteristics of rickettsiae that set them apart from other groups of bacteria.

3. What are the characteristics of the pathogenesis of Rocky Mountain spotted fever?

4. How could one study pathogenic properties of rickettsiae even though they cannot be grown in cell-free media?

SUGGESTED READINGS

Burgdorfer W, Anacker RC: *Rickettsiae and Rickettsial Diseases*. New York, Academic Press, 1981.
Moulder JW: Comparative biology of intracellular parasitism. *Microbiol Rev* 49:298–337, 1985.
Zinsser H: *Rats, Lice and History*. Boston, Little, Brown, 1935. Reprinted 1965, Bantam edition.

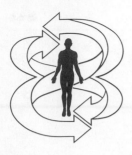

Legionella: An Environmental Pathogen

V.L. Yu

Legionnaires' disease, a recently recognized pneumonia, is caused by aerobic Gram negative rods called *Legionella*. These organisms live in natural bodies of water, including lakes and rivers. They have been isolated from water distribution systems and air conditioning cooling towers linked to outbreaks of pneumonia. The organisms have special nutritional requirements and require media that are not normally used in a hospital microbiological laboratory. The organisms are intracellular parasites that can evade host defenses by entering mononuclear phagocytes and resisting killing.

CASE

Mr. L., a 53-year-old, was admitted to the hospital with high fever, cough, and chest pain. He had attended the 1976 American Legion Convention in Philadelphia 1 week prior to admission. Approximately 3 days after leaving Philadelphia, he complained of malaise, headache, cough, and fever. Over the next 2 days he became febrile (40°C), disoriented, and lethargic. Before this episode, he had been in good health, except for a history of occasional upper respiratory tract infections. He had smoked cigarettes for more than 30 years. On admission he was in a stupor.

A chest x-ray showed a patchy alveolar infiltrate on the right side, indicative of a pneumonia. A Gram stain of sputum was notable for the absence of visible bacteria despite the presence of many neutrophils. Multiple cultures of blood, sputum, and urine were negative. His white cell count was 12,000/μl with 70% neutrophils, which is slightly elevated. His serum sodium level was 129 mEq/liter, which is low. (It was later learned that low sodium levels occur more frequently in Legionnaires' disease than in other pneumonias.)

Lacking a bacteriological diagnosis a broad-spectrum antibiotic, cephalothin, was administered. Despite this therapy Mr. L. continued to deteriorate, with evidence of decreased function of the liver and kidneys. The pulmonary infiltrate progressed to involve both lungs. Two weeks after admission, Mr. L. suffered cardiac arrest and, despite resuscitative measures, died.

Pathological examination showed diffuse inflammation of the lung consistent with a necrotizing pneumonia. Cultures and Gram stain of the lung were again negative. Many months later, tissue sections that had been stored were treated with fluorescent antibodies against Legionella pneumophila. They were positive against serogroup 1 of this species. Stored sera obtained from the patient before death showed a significant antibody titer against the same organism at a 1:512 dilution. This confirmed the clinical diagnosis of Legionnaires' disease.

HISTORICAL PERSPECTIVE

In 1976 the American Legion held its annual convention in a Philadelphia hotel. After the delegates returned home many showed symptoms of fever and severe respiratory distress. Over 200 delegates were afflicted and 34 died.

This epidemic became the object of much public concern and was covered intensively in the media. Considerable fear was sparked by the realization that this seemed to be a new life-threatening disease and that the extent of its spread could not be foreseen. The etiology of this disease became the focus of an intense investigation followed closely by the lay media. The etiology remained elusive, with a toxin or a microbial agent the prime suspects.

Six months after the outbreak, investigators from the Centers for Disease Control isolated bacteria from lung tissue obtained from patients who had died from Legionnaires' disease. They used a variety of techniques developed for the isolation of viruses, fungi, spirochetes, and rickettsiae. The method that worked, borrowed from rickettsial technology, consisted in inoculating the lung tissue into the peritoneal cavity of guinea pigs, waiting for the animal to become ill, removing the spleen, and injecting that tissue into fertilized chicken eggs. Only then could the researchers detect the organisms.

The delay in the identification of the causative bacteria derived from the fact that they do not grow in standard bacteriological media used in hospital laboratories and are difficult to stain. The organisms were found to be distinct from any known bacteria, which led to the creation of a new taxonomic family, the Legionellaceae; a new genus, *Legionella*; and a new species, pneumophila ("lung loving"). Interestingly, a retrospective serologic study conducted after the American Legion outbreak showed that an undiagnosed outbreak of this disease had occurred 2 years earlier among delegates to an Odd Fellows convention held in the same hotel.

The experience with the Philadelphia epidemic and with Mr. L. suggests a number of questions:

• Why had Legionnaires' disease not been recognized before?

• The environmental source of the organism in the hotel was never found since the organism was not discovered until months after the outbreak. Speculate where the organism may have been lurking in the hotel and how it gained access to Mr. L.

• Why did Mr. L. deteriorate so rapidly? How does the causative agent produce the symptoms of the disease?

• How is the disease best diagnosed and treated?

THE LEGIONELLACEAE

Legionella pneumophila is a nutritionally demanding aerobic Gram negative rod. DNA hybridization studies have shown that they are not closely related to any other group of bacteria. These organisms do not grow in the media commonly used to isolate respiratory bacterial pathogens, e.g., blood agar. The reason is that they have an unusual set of nutritional preferences. They require a high concentration of cysteine and are inhibited by sodium ions and aromatic compounds. The media that have been developed for their cultivation contain charcoal to remove the aromatic inhibitors, a non-sodium ion buffer, plus certain antibiotics to suppress competing bacteria and dyes to make the colonies more visible.

Structurally, the legionellae are typical Gram negative bacteria, with an outer membrane, flagella and pili. It is not clear why they do not take up stains readily, especially in tissue. Special techniques (the so-called Gimenez or Dieterle silver stain) are required to visualize them, although they are faintly Gram negative in culture. The difficulty in staining them and their unusual nutritional requirements conspired to make them so hard to detect in the original American Legion outbreak.

Following the discovery of *L. pneumophila*, a number of other legionellae have been found to be human pathogens. They can be definitively identified by DNA hybridization techniques, gas liquid chromatography of the cell wall lipids, or direct immunofluorescent antibody methods.

ENCOUNTER

Legionellae are aquatic organisms, widely distributed in the environment and found in lakes and rivers. They can be isolated in large numbers from thermally polluted streams near power stations. The organisms are relatively resistant to chlorine and can persist in drinking water. When they enter a building via the water mains, they find the hot water tanks particularly to their liking. Their optimum temperature is in the 30 to 40°C range. Thus, they can proliferate in large hot water tanks, as found in large buildings such as hospitals; these sites are also common locales for outbreaks of Legionnaires' disease.

The organisms are readily distributed through the hot water system. Although the water itself may contain only small numbers of legionella, the organisms lodge and multiply in the sediment, with predilection for sites of low flow or obstruction (Fig. 26.1). Over a period of years, large numbers of organisms may accumulate in sediment deposits. The use of water from these sites, including faucets and ice machines, could lead to expulsion of large numbers of legionellae that could thus get to susceptible persons. This may well have been the way Mr. L. acquired the organisms. The fact that legionellae do not spread from person to person explains why the original Philadelphia outbreak did not spread to the legionnaires' families back home.

The combination of sediment and commensal water bacteria interacts synergistically to stimulate the growth of *L. pneumophila*. The sediment provides a shelter for legionella as well as nutrition for other environmental bacteria, which in turn may provide necessary growth factors (e.g., cysteine). The disease caused by

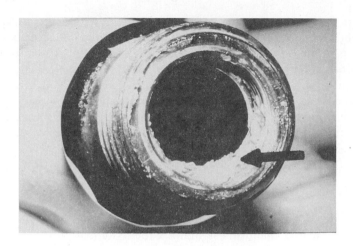

Figure 26.1. Sediment (*arrow*) harbors legionellae in the water fixture. The sediment is composed of mineral deposits (scale) and organic particulate matter (detritus).

L. pneumophila may have emerged with the advent of hot water distribution systems.

ENTRY, SPREAD, AND MULTIPLICATION

Water containing legionellae is delivered to humans via water distribution systems or cooling devices (cooling towers, evaporative condensers, air conditioners). Since the target site in people is almost always the lung, it follows that the primary mode of entry is via the respiratory tract, either by aspiration or by aerosolization. Other ways of acquiring the organisms include inhalation of aerosols from respiratory devices, such as humidifiers and nebulizers, and instillation of contaminated water during respiratory tract manipulations. Wound infections have also occurred following exposure of wounds to water contaminated with legionellae.

As seen in the case of Mr. L., the incubation period from exposure to the organisms to the signs of pneumonia ranges from 2 to 10 days. The initial host response is an acute inflammatory response, first in the pulmonary alveoli and then in the bronchioles. Neutrophils predominate in the early phase of the infection and are followed by macrophages. So far, the infection closely follows the sequence seen in pneumonias caused by other bacteria such as the pneumococcus.

However, there are some important differences. The most obvious difference from many other acute bacterial pneumonias is that in this disease the organisms are located intracellularly in macrophages (Fig. 26.2). Thus, organisms are shielded

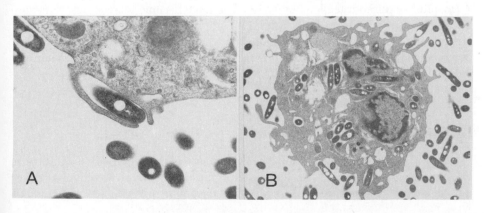

Figure 26.2. Phagocytosis *gionella pneumophila* by macı (From Elliot JA, Winn WC Jr: of alveolar macrophages chalasin D inhibits uptake a quent growth of *Legionella pn Infect Immun* 51:33, 1986.)

from neutrophils and circulating antibodies. Patients with Legionnaires' disease develop both humoral and cell-mediated immune responses. Humoral immune responses may play only a minor role in host defense; in experimental studies antibody does not promote killing of *L. pneumophila* by complement, promotes only modest killing by phagocytes (neutrophils, monocytes, or alveolar macrophages), and does not inhibit intracellular multiplication in monocytes. Cell-mediated immune responses appear to play a primary role: In experimental studies, activated circulating and alveolar macrophages can inhibit the intracellular multiplication of the organisms.

DAMAGE

L. pneumophila elaborates several exotoxins, including proteases, hemolysins and other cytotoxins. One of these inhibits the oxidative killing by neutrophils and impairs their bactericidal activity. These toxins not only permit the bacteria to withstand killing by neutrophils but may also damage tissue directly.

In most cases the manifestations of the disease are those of a typical acute pneumonia. Once the organisms have become established in lung tissue, they may spread rapidly, as in the case of Mr. L. Serial chest x-rays typically show first a localized patchy infiltrate and then progression to other lobes. In immunosuppressed patients, microabscesses may progress to cavities. Pleural effusion is common, and the organisms may be isolated from pleural fluid obtained by needle aspiration.

The protean clinical manifestations of Legionnaires' disease, including the neurological symptoms and diffuse metabolic abnormalities seen in Mr. L., probably result from bloodstream invasion. Other target sites include the heart (endocarditis and pericarditis), kidney (nephritis), lymph nodes, spleen, liver, and brain.

The symptoms of the disease directly reflect the pathologic processes. Cough, chest pains, and abnormal sounds on breathing ("rales"), are all due to the inflammatory disease in the lungs. In some patients the most striking symptom is pain in the chest accentuated by breathing. Fever is seen in the majority of patients. Neurologic symptoms, including confusion and delirium, are poor prognostic signs. Some patients have prominent gastrointestinal symptoms, especially diarrhea.

Since legionellae are ubiquitous in water, why are there not more cases of Legionnaires' disease? From experience we can infer that healthy persons rarely become ill after exposure to the organisms. Most of the patients in the Philadelphia outbreak were in their late middle age or older. Many, including Mr. L., had been heavy smokers and had a history of respiratory disease.

Hospital-acquired infections by legionellae have become increasingly common. These patients are generally compromised by underlying respiratory disease or are immunosuppressed. A newly appreciated risk is transplant surgery. Infection in patients receiving organ transplants may come about by the defects in immunity induced by antirejection drugs or by respiratory tract therapy that employs contaminated water.

DIAGNOSIS

When a Gram stain of sputum from a patient with Legionnaires' disease is viewed microscopically (a classical test for the diagnosis of pneumonia), large numbers of neutrophils are seen, as is typical for pneumonias of bacterial etiology.

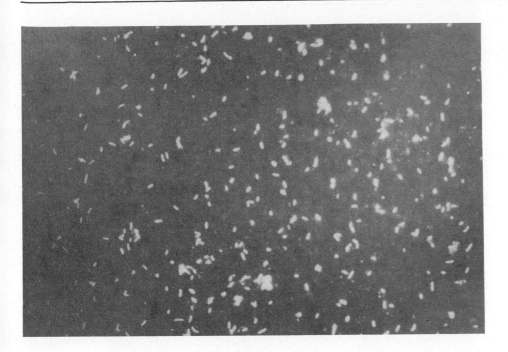

Figure 26.3. Sputum from a patient with Legionnaires' disease was stained with fluorescent-tagged antibodies against *Legionella pneumophila* and examined under a fluorescent microscope.

However, it is notable that few if any organisms are seen, because of the difficulty in staining legionella.

The sputum specimen may also be treated with fluorescent antibodies; the bacteria, if present, will become visible under a fluorescent microscope (Fig. 26.3). A nucleic acid hybridization test using a radioactive-labeled probe for the detection of legionella DNA may also be applied to sputum and other specimens. Unfortunately, neither the fluorescent antibody test nor DNA hybridization are particularly sensitive; both tests require the presence of a large number of organisms, which may occur late in the disease. The most reliable and definitive diagnosis is the isolation of the organisms from respiratory secretions.

The serologic detection of antibodies in patients' sera is useful chiefly for epidemiological studies. A significant titer does not appear until late in the disease, often 4 to 8 weeks after the onset of symptoms. This method allowed the definitive identification of the causative agent in the original Philadelphia outbreak. After the organisms were cultivated, they were used to detect antibodies in the sera of the patients. Legionella antigen can also be detected in the urine of patients with Legionnaires' disease, and this is the most rapid diagnostic test available.

THERAPY AND PREVENTION

A number of antibiotics is available, but erythromycin is the drug of choice. A key factor is its ability to penetrate white cells and affect the organisms in their intracellular location. Antibiotics that are active against the organisms in vitro but which fail to penetrate leukocytes have been less effective in this disease. Had this been realized early on and had Mr. L. received erythromycin soon after the onset of symptoms, he might well have survived the disease.

The organisms can be eliminated from hospital water supplies by heating water to 60°C and flushing outlets with hot water, chemical disinfectants, or ultraviolet light.

PONTIAC FEVER

Legionella also causes an illness called *Pontiac fever*. This syndrome, which resembles an allergic disease more than an infection, is characterized by an abrupt onset of fever, headache, dizziness, and muscle pains. Pneumonia does not occur. It resolves spontaneously within 2 to 5 days. The attack rate after exposure is high, approaching 90%.

This syndrome was first described in an outbreak in, of all places, a county health department building in Pontiac, Michigan. Ninety five percent of the employees became ill and eventually showed elevated serum titers against *L. pneumophila*. The organisms were later isolated from the lungs of guinea pigs exposed to the air of the building. The likely source was water from a defective air conditioner. At the time of the outbreak (1968) no organisms were isolated. The patients' sera and guinea pig lungs had been kept frozen in anticipation that a new bacterial agent might be discovered. This proved to be the case.

CONCLUSIONS

Several characteristic distinguish *L. pneumophila* from other bacterial agents of pneumonia. The organisms are acquired by inhalation from the environment rather than from other humans, as with pneumococci or *H. influenzae*. These organisms can survive intracellularly within macrophages, which is likely to help in their dissemination throughout the body. Thus, legionellosis is not limited to the lungs but may involve a variety of other tissue and cause a wide variety of manifestations. *L. pneumophila* produces a variety of toxins (proteases, hemolysis, cytotoxins) that contribute to destruction of neutrophils and tissue cells.

The diagnosis of legionellosis may be hampered by the variety of its clinical manifestations and by the need to use special bacteriological media to grow the organisms from clinical specimens. Thus, this disease may present a significant diagnostic challenge.

SELF-ASSESSMENT QUESTIONS

1. Discuss the ecological characteristics of *L. pneumophila* and their relation to the epidemiology of legionellosis.

2. Why does legionellosis tend to manifest itself in outbreaks?

3. Contrast pneumonia due to legionella with that due to pneumococci (Chapter 13).

4. Why don't all of us come down with legionellosis, given the widespread occurrence of the organisms?

5. What other pathogenic bacteria are acquired from the water supply by routes other than ingestion?

SUGGESTED READINGS

Cunha B (ed): Legionnaires' disease symposium. *Semin Resp Infect* 2:189–279, 1987.

Fraser D, McDade J: Legionellosis. *Scien Am* 241:21–99, 1979.

Muder RR, Yu VL, Woo A: Mode of transmission of *Legionella pneumophila*: a critical review. *Arch Intern Med* 146:1607–1612, 1986.

Thornsberry C, et al (eds): *Legionella—Proceedings of the Second International Symposium*. Washington DC, American Society of Microbiology, 1984.

Winn WC: Legionnaires' disease: historical perspective. *Clin Microbiol Rev* 1:60–81, 1988.

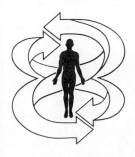

Mycoplasma: A Curiosity and a Pathogen

27

G.A. Storch

The mycoplasmas belong to a highly distinct group of bacteria which lack a cell wall and require sterols for growth. Most of the species associated with the human body are innocuous, but one causes a distinct form of pneumonia, while others are suspected of causing infections in the genitourinary tract and elsewhere. The organisms are sensitive to certain broad-spectrum antibiotics that inhibit functions other than cell wall synthesis.

CASE

Michelle, a 7-year-old who previously had been in good health, developed fever, headache, and a dry cough. Her 12-year-old brother had had similar symptoms 2 weeks earlier. Over the next 2 days, her temperature increased and the cough worsened, becoming productive of small amounts of clear sputum. Her physician noted that she appeared slightly pale, had a temperature of 41.3°C and a respiratory rate of 40 per minute. Scattered rales (abnormal respiratory sounds) were heard through the stethoscope over the right posterior lung.

Her white blood cell count was in the normal range, 8600 per μl, with a normal differential (the ratio between the various cell types). She was slightly anemic (hematocrit of 29%) and had an increased number of reticulocytes. A Gram stain of her sputum revealed only rare neutrophils and no bacteria. Her chest x-ray showed a right lower lobe infiltrate (Fig. 27.1). A special test to detect so-called cold hemagglutinins was positive. This finding and the clinical picture allowed the tentative diagnosis of primary atypical pneumonia caused

Figure 27.1. Chest x-ray reveals an infiltrate in the left mid-lung field. (Courtesy of Dr. Gary Shackleford.)

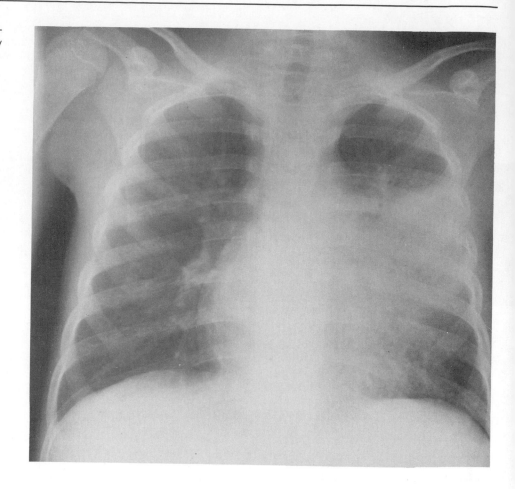

by Mycoplasma pneumoniae. *Michelle was treated with erythromycin and made an uneventful recovery.*

Questions that arise from this case include the following:

1. How did Michelle acquire the organism?

2. What are the distinguishing features of the mycoplasma?

3. What is known about the pathogenic properties of these organisms?

4. How could a definitive diagnosis be made?

5. What can Michelle's family do to avoid spreading the organisms to other family members?

Mycoplasma pneumoniae is a common cause of pneumonia in children and young adults, although it is rarely also seen in other age groups. As in Michelle's case, the illness usually has a less abrupt onset and is milder than pneumococcal pneumonia. Occasional cases may be quite severe, especially in individuals with sickle cell disease. Headache and cough are prominent clinical features. Before the etiology of this disease became known, it was referred to as "primary atypical pneumonia", to distinguish it from "typical" cases of lobar pneumonia (usually caused by pneumococci). Clinicians knew that patients with typical pneumonia responded to penicillin, while those with atypical pneumonia did not.

Table 27.1
Common mycoplasmas and diseases they cause

Organism	Disease	Site
M. pneumoniae	Primary atypical pneumonia	Respiratory tract
M. hominis	Pelvic inflammatory disease, other	Genitourinary tract
U. urealyticum	Urethritis	Genitourinary tract
M. salivarium⎫	None	Mouth, oropharynx
M. orale ⎭		
Others (less common)	None	Genitourinary tract, oropharynx

THE ORGANISM

The mycoplasmas have a number of unusual features:

• They are the smallest organisms capable of growth on cell-free media. They are classified with the bacteria because, in general, they have the structure and composition of procaryotes.

• They are unique among the bacteria in that they lack a rigid cell wall (no murein) and can assume a variety of shapes. This characteristic has important implications for antibiotic therapy, because many commonly used antibiotics (especially the β-lactams) act by inhibiting cell wall murein synthesis, and thus are ineffective against mycoplasmas.

• Their cell membrane contains sterols, which with some exceptions, must be supplied in the medium in order to support their growth.

• Mycoplasmas are common in nature and capable of living in unusual environments, such as high-temperature springs and the acid outflows of mining wastes.

Only three species are known to cause human disease (Table 27.1): *Mycoplasma pneumoniae*, a common cause of respiratory disease, and two organisms that probably account for some cases of nongonococcal urethritis, *M. hominis* and *Ureaplasma urealyticum*. Other species are commonly found as part of the normal human flora but have not been linked to disease. On the other hand, different species cause a number of severe diseases in domestic animals.

Mycoplasmas can be readily cultivated in the laboratory using special media that contain sterols. *M. pneumoniae* grows slowly, and several weeks may be required for colonies to become evident. The colonies are much smaller than those of the common bacteria and have a dense center which gives them a fried egg appearance (Fig. 27.2).

ENCOUNTER AND ENTRY

Infected humans constitute the only known reservoir of *M. pneumoniae*. Patients become ill following exposure to the respiratory secretions of persons harboring the organism. In contrast to the pneumococcus, prolonged asymptomatic colonization with *M. pneumoniae* is uncommon. In most cases the source of the infection is not recognized because most mycoplasma infections are mild. *M. pneumoniae* infections are moderately contagious and spreading within household or residential institutions is sometimes observed. In these situations, an interval between cases of 2 to 3 weeks is sometimes discerned.

Figure 27.2. Colonies of *mycoplasmas*. **A**, *Mycoplasma pneumoniae*; **B**, *Mycoplasma salivarium*. Note their small size and "fried egg" appearance, especially in **B**. (Courtesy of W.A. Clyde, Jr.)

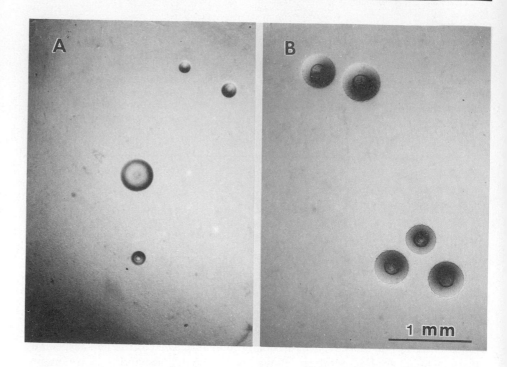

Mycoplasma infection begins with the binding of mycoplasma organisms to the respiratory epithelium. Microscopic studies of *M. pneumoniae* have revealed a specialized terminal attachment structure. A special protein is found in this structure and is thought to mediate attachment of the organisms to a receptor on the respiratory epithelium. Monoclonal antibodies to this protein inhibit the attachment of *M. pneumoniae*.

SPREAD, MULTIPLICATION, AND DAMAGE

The pathogenesis of *M. pneumoniae* infection differs markedly from that of the other forms of pneumonia, such as that caused by the pneumococcus or *Legionella pneumophila*, because it is largely limited to the respiratory mucosa that lines the airways. There is no evidence of involvement of the lung alveoli. An infiltrate of mononuclear cells is present, surrounding infected bronchi and bronchioles. The pattern of involvement is that of a bronchopneumonia rather than a lobar process.

In experimentally infected tracheal organ cultures the organisms are seen lined up along the mucosa, oriented with the terminal attachment structure in contact with the epithelium (Fig. 27.3). Mycoplasma infection is not highly destructive of tissue, but ciliary function is impaired in cells with mycoplasma bound to their exterior. This is thought to result from local elaboration of tissue-toxic substances, probably including hydrogen peroxide. The main cells in the inflammatory response elicited by *M. pneumoniae* are lymphocytes, with very few neutrophils. Some immunocompromised patients with mycoplasma infection do not have visible pulmonary infiltrates, which suggests that the immune response may play a role in causing the manifestations of disease.

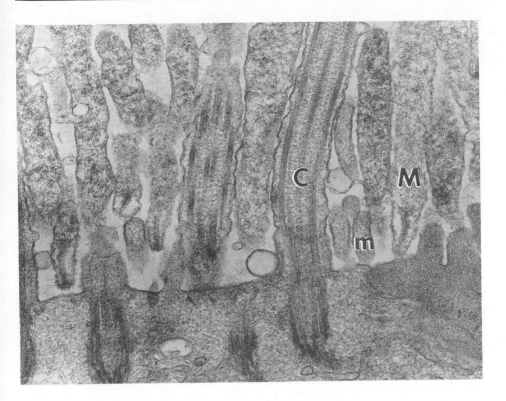

Figure 27.3. Transmission electron photomicrograph of a hamster tracheal ring infected with *Mycoplasma pneumoniae*. Attachment of *Mycoplasma pneumoniae* to hamster tracheal explant. Note the orientation of the mycoplasmas via their specialized tip-like organelle which permits close association with the respiratory epithelium (×50,000). M, *Mycoplasma*; m, microvillus; c, cilia. (From Hu PC et al: Surface parasitism by *Mycoplasma pneumoniae* of respiratory epithelium. *J Exp Med* 145:1328, 1977.)

DIAGNOSIS

Culturing mycoplasma takes a week or more and requires special media and experienced personnel. Consequently, the diagnosis of mycoplasma pneumonia is usually suspected from clinical features and confirmed by serologic tests. This has the undesirable feature that the diagnosis cannot be made until convalescent phase serum becomes available, long after therapeutic decisions about the patient must be made. Thus, *M. pneumoniae* is an attractive target for the development of rapid diagnostic tests that do not involve culture, such as immunoassays to detect mycoplasma antigens or nucleic acid hybridization to detect specific mycoplasmal nucleic acids.

In contrast to pneumococcal pneumonia, sputum production is scanty and the sputum nonpurulent. The peripheral blood usually does not show the leukocytosis and marked increase in young forms characteristic of pneumococcal infection. The chest x-ray in mycoplasma pneumonia is highly variable but most commonly reveals a patchy infiltrate suggestive of bronchopneumonia.

The clinical manifestations of mycoplasma infections are generally limited to the respiratory tract but other organs are occasionally involved. Michelle, the patient described above, had a mild hemolytic anemia, which was caused by an antibody stimulated by mycoplasma. This is an IgM antibody that binds to red blood cells and at reduced temperatures causes them to agglutinate (stick together). These antibodies are called *cold hemagglutinins* and are detectable in about 50% of severe mycoplasma infections. Only a small minority of these patients actually experience clinically significant hemolysis. The reason why *M.*

pneumoniae infection stimulates the production of cold agglutinins is not currently known. Cold hemagglutinins can be rapidly demonstrated at the bedside: Blood drawn from the patient into a tube containing an anticoagulant will look clumpy when placed in an ice bucket. The clumps disappear when the tube is warmed up again.

PREVENTION AND TREATMENT

No vaccine is currently available to prevent mycoplasma infections. Treatment with erythromycin and tetracycline is usually effective.

CONCLUSIONS

Only one human disease, mycoplasma pneumonia, is known with certainty to be caused by this bizarre group of bacteria. Mycoplasmas call attention to themselves because they lack a cell wall, many species require steroids, show marked tropism for different mucous membranes, and produce characteristic clinical manifestations.

SELF-ASSESSMENT QUESTIONS

1. What distinguishes the mycoplasma from other bacteria?

2. Discuss the pathophysiology of mycoplasma pneumonia.

3. Compare the epidemiology of pneumonia due to mycoplasma with that due to pneumococci or *Legionella*.

4. Why do you think it has been difficult to establish definitely the role of other mycoplasmas in disease?

SUGGESTED READINGS

Foy HM, Kenny GE, Conney MK, Allan ID: Long-term epidemiology of infections with *Mycoplasma pneumoniae*. *J Infect Dis* 139:681–687, 1979.
Levin S: The atypical pneumonia syndrome. *JAMA* 251:945–948, 1984.
Cassell CH, Cole BC: Mycoplasmas as agents of human disease. *N Engl J Med* 304:80–89, 1981.
Murray HW, Masur H, Senterfit LB, Roberts RB: The protean manifestations of *Mycoplasma pneumoniae* infection in adults. *Am J Med* 58:229–242, 1975.
Barile MF, Razin S, (eds): *The Mycoplasmas*. New York, Academic Press, 1979.

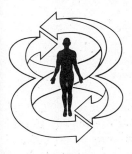

Strategies to Combat Bacterial Infections

28

F.P. Tally

O ver the last one or two centuries health and longevity of people living in developed countries have taken a quantum jump forward. The younger ones among us may not be fully aware of the fundamental changes this has made in the quality of our lives. We take it for granted that we, our relatives, and our acquaintances have survived infancy and will reach a ripe old age. Disease is the exception and premature death relatively uncommon. Two interrelated factors have contributed to this: improvement in nutrition and control of infectious diseases. The greatest initial strides in reducing the incidence of infectious disease were due to preventive measures, largely purification of the water supply and control of human wastes and disease vectors. Later on, in the last 100 years, these measures were joined by medical intervention: vaccination and antimicrobial therapy. Preventive measures, not therapy, have played the greatest role in the control of infectious diseases.

This chapter deals with the strategies that have been developed for prevention and therapy of infectious diseases. The emphasis here is on bacteria, but the same principles apply to all other infectious agents.

PREVENTION

Sanitation

Most public health measures are designed to avert encounters with infectious agents by excluding them or minimizing their spread in the human environment. Sanitary strategies have been used sporadically since antiquity, but only with the

Table 28.1
General types of public health measures

General
  Water purification
  Sewage disposal
  Waste disposal
  Pest control
  Animal control
Protection of food supply
  Refrigeration and freezing
  Pasteurization
  Food inspection
  Adequate cooking of meats

unfolding of the germ theory of disease have they been used in a rational and planned manner. Sanitary measures include personal hygiene and community sanitation (Table 28.1).

Much of personal hygiene is intended to prevent the accumulation of microorganisms or debris on the skin and mucous membranes. These measures never totally eliminate bacterial contamination (despite advertisements to that effect), but they tend to reduce the local microbial load. Among the most successful of the personal measures is dental hygiene, which assists in the prevention of dental caries and periodontal disease. Indeed, together with fluoridation of the water supply, preventive dental care has resulted in an amazing decrease in the incidence of caries. Until recently, the consequence of extensive caries—dentures—was seen as an inevitable accompaniment of old age.

Community sanitary measures include avoiding contamination of the drinking water supply, disposal of sewage, protection of the food supply, and control of insect vectors. Breakdown of any of these steps may lead to outbreaks of epidemic diseases. If we consider, for example, the water supply, relevant sanitary steps include:

• Obtaining water from a source as removed as possible from human and animal wastes.

• Processing drinking water to remove pathogenic microorganisms (usually chlorination).

• Distributing it through a closed system that prevents contamination.

Immunization: Antibodies and Vaccines

Immunity adequate for the prevention of infectious diseases may be accomplished in two ways: by administering specific antibodies (passive immunization) or by vaccination (active immunization).

Passive Immunization

Passive immunization is carried out by the injection of suitable immunoglobulins. It is used mainly when there is exposure to an infectious agent and not enough time for those exposed to develop their own antibodies by active immunization. It is also used if a vaccine is not available. Protection is immediate but usually short lived, depending on the clearance of the injected immunoglobulins from the circulation (Table 28.2).

To minimize immune reactions, immunoglobulins are usually derived from human plasma. This has some disadvantages, among them the fact that suitable donors with appropriate antibody titers to a given agent may be hard to find. Still, this is an improvement over the previous practice of using sera from immunized horses, which resulted in the allergic reaction to foreign proteins known as serum sickness.

Human gamma globulin is used to prevent hepatitis and other viral infections in exposed persons, including both medical personnel and persons at risk because of immune deficiencies. One of the most common injuries to medical personnel is accidental puncture with a syringe needle that has been used on a patient and is therefore contaminated with the patient's blood. It has been reported that needle punctures occur approximately at a rate of one needle stick per 10 hospital employees per year. The viruses that can be transmitted by

Table 28.2
Types of available immunizations

Passive	Active	
	Disease	Vaccine
Viral		
Hepatitis A, B,	Measles	Live
	Mumps	Live
CMV	Yellow fever	Live
Rabies	Smallpox	Live
	Rubella	Live
	Polio	Live (Sabin), killed (Salk)
	Influenza	Killed
	Rabies	Killed
	Hepatitis B	Recombinant, killed
Bacterial		
Gas gangrene	Tetanus	Toxoid
Tetanus	Diphtheria	Toxoid
	Pertussis	Killed
	Meningococcal	Killed, 2 serotypes
	H. influenzae	Killed
	Pneumococcus	Killed, 23 polysaccharides
	Typhoid	Killed (live in trial)
	Typhus	Killed
	Cholera	Killed
	Tuberculosis	Live (BCG)

puncture wounds from contaminated needles include HIV, hepatitis B, and hepatitis non-A, non-B. The incidence of hepatitis in medical personnel who have had an accidental puncture wound with a contaminated needle is sufficiently high that preventive measures are called for. Passive immunization of personnel immediately following the needle stick has a demonstrated benefit in preventing the development of subsequent disease. In a randomized prospective study of medical personnel, the incidence of hepatitis B was 8% in a placebo group and 2% in a group treated with hepatitis B hyperimmune immunoglobulin. Passive immunizations have also been used to protect travelers from acquiring hepatitis A in countries where the disease is endemic.

Vaccines

There are several classes of antimicrobial vaccines, including those that contain purified immunogens, whole killed organisms, or live attenuated organisms (Table 28.2). Their use depends in part on the pathobiology of the infection. For example, in diseases due to the action of exotoxins, such as tetanus or diphtheria, the aim is to induce the production of antitoxins. Tetanus or diphtheria vaccines contain purified *toxoids*, chemically modified forms of the toxins that are still immunogenic but are no longer toxic. If invading organisms have an antiphagocytic capsule, as with pneumococci or meningococci, the vaccine may consist of purified capsular polysaccharides. It is clearly a good idea to include in the vaccine as few extraneous microbial components as possible since some may be toxic. Thus, the use of whole killed Gram negative bacteria means that the vaccine will probably contain endotoxin. Indeed, the traditional typhoid vaccine, which consists of killed *Salmonella typhi*, produces fever and local inflammation in many of the recipients. On the other hand, in many viral and/or chronic diseases, circulating antibodies play a minor role and the aim of vaccination should be to strengthen cell-mediated immunity. Here effective vaccines usually contain live, attenuated microorganisms. The advantages and disadvantages of live versus killed vaccines are discussed below.

Antigenic Specificity

Antigenic specificity may be an important concern when the infecting organisms make several varieties of the same antigenic component. For example, different strains of pneumococci make distinct types of capsular polysaccharides that differ antigenically and do not cross-react immunologically. Thus, a vaccine made against one type would not protect against another type. In this case an effective vaccine must be *polyvalent*, that is, contain several different antigens. The initially marketed pneumococcal vaccine contained 14 capsular serotypes, four of which accounted for more than 75% of the clinical disease. The vaccine in present use in the United States contains the 23 serotypes that are currently causing the majority of cases. This illustrates the need for constantly updating polyvalent vaccines.

Determining which serotypes are involved in current epidemics is particularly important for influenza vaccines. Outbreaks of influenza correlate with changes in the surface hemagglutinin and neuraminidase antigens of the virus (Chapter 30). The development of new vaccines for the prevention of the disease in the elderly and debilitated patients has demanded a substantial effort. Surveillance centers around the globe are constantly searching for the emergence of new strains of the virus, so that a suitable vaccine may be rapidly produced and distributed. With advances in virological and production methods, a new vaccine may be available in as little as 4 months.

Live versus Killed Vaccines

The advantages of a live vaccine are well illustrated with the Sabin polio vaccine. The protection it affords includes local immunity in the intestine, where the virus first multiplies. Immunity is also longer lasting than that elicited by the killed virus vaccine, probably because of the persistence of the virus in the host. Most important, the virus of the vaccine spreads to other people in the community to give herd immunity. (These positive aspects and some possible drawbacks of live vaccines are discussed in detail in Chapter 35). Note that a live vaccine will not "take" if the recipient has a sufficient titer of neutralizing antibodies. This is the case in newborn infants, who may have acquired such antibodies from the mother. For this reason, live polio vaccine is not given until 3 to 6 months of age, after which maternal antibodies are no longer present. In addition, live vaccines should not be given to immunocompromised patients because they may cause the disease they are designed to prevent (as in the example of vaccine induced polio).

If prevention of a disease depends on cell-mediated immunity, the injection of soluble antigens or even killed whole organisms is generally unlikely to be successful. Cell-mediated immunity is often elicited by intracellular agents, and a suitable vaccine should contain *attenuated live organisms* that can reside inside host cells for sufficient time to elicit this slower type of immunity. An example is the tuberculosis vaccine BCG, which consists of an attenuated strain of *Myco-*

bacterium bovis (Chapter 22). This vaccine has had a checkered career but has been shown to be effective in certain regions where the disease is prevalent. However, a recent study has shown that BCG is ineffective in parts of India. The reason for this failure is not known with certainty, but there is an interesting possibility: In India many people become infected with other mycobacteria that cross-react immunologically with BCG. In such a population, BCG may not "take".

The development of both killed and live vaccines has already benefited from the newer tools of molecular genetics. Relevant genes have been cloned into suitable organisms for the purpose of making large amounts of antigens. This has been used to advantage for the production of a vaccine against hepatitis B, the first recombinant DNA vaccine approved for human use by the U.S. Food and Drug Administration. The virus cannot be readily cultivated, and the use of a genetic surrogate, in this case yeast, has permitted the production of vaccine antigen in industrial quantities. Cloning also permits inserting an antigen into a live vaccine. For instance, genes for antigens of influenza, herpes simplex, and other agents have been cloned into vaccinia, the virus of the smallpox vaccine. Conveniently, this virus has a very large genome that permits the insertion of several foreign genes. This allows researchers to hope for the fulfillment of a dream: a cheap, reasonably stable vaccine that spreads spontaneously throughout a population and is effective against a dozen or more of the important diseases of humanity. It is still on the drawing board, but appears to be within the bounds of reality. Note, however, that many people would currently not "catch" this vaccine because they have already received the regular smallpox vaccine.

Why Are Vaccines Not Always Useful and Why Do They Not Always Work?

Vaccines have played a key role in the control of a number of very important infectious diseases, but are of little use in others. There are many factors at play here: There is some potential risk when a large number of people are vaccinated, as seen with the DPT vaccine. The pertussis component of the vaccine causes infrequent but potentially serious complications (Chapter 20). Consequently, vaccines are used with caution and are not recommended for infrequent or easily treatable diseases. There would be little point, for example, to vaccinate the whole population of a country such as the United States against the plague or Legionnaires' disease, although it may make sense to use a vaccine in specific groups at risk. The desirability of vaccination also depends on just how much suitable therapy is available to the general population. In some parts of the world, it is expedient to vaccinate the population against treatable diseases, because the disease is frequent and drug treatment is more expensive than the vaccine and often unavailable. An example is the use of the BCG vaccine in India but not in the United States. Thus, vaccination practices vary considerably with the state of sanitation and economic development of a given region or country.

In addition to these considerations, vaccines are of little or no use unless the recipient is immunocompetent vis-a-vis the relevant antigens. Thus, vaccinating patients with AIDS against commensal invaders would be pointless. In fact, living attenuated organisms may multiply freely and cause disease in these patients. Another example is the failure of vaccination against *Haemophilus influenzae* in children under 2 years of age (Chapter 15). The polysaccharide antigen of these organisms is processed by a T cell–independent route, which develops at a later age. Other examples of vaccine failure are mentioned above, namely BCG in possibly immunologically tolerant populations, and live polio vaccine in children who still have a high titer of maternal antibodies. One of the most tragic of these considerations is that vaccine failures are often seen in children who are immunodeficient due to malnutrition. Such children often live in regions where the need for vaccination is greatest.

The Prophylactic Use of Antimicrobial Drugs

Soon after the introduction of effective antibacterial agents in the 1930s, it became clear that they could be used not only to treat infections but to prevent them as well. However, this is a complex and controversial subject because the use of antibiotics to prevent infections carries risks as well as benefits. Antimicrobial drugs may be used prophylactically for two purposes:

• To prevent the acquisition of exogenous pathogens. An example is the administration of antibiotics to persons who are exposed to patients with menigococcal infections. The meningococcus spreads rapidly among susceptible individuals but antibiotics such as rifampin can usually forestall its clinical manifestations. Likewise, the antituberculous drug, isoniazid, is given to persons who are at high risk of acquiring tuberculosis, such as the children living in the same quarters as a patient with pulmonary tuberculosis (Chapter 22).

• To prevent commensal organisms from spreading from their usual residence to normally sterile sites of the body. The use of antibiotics to prevent postoperative infections in certain high-risk surgical procedures also falls in this category. An example is the administration of antibiotics to patients with damaged heart valves who are therefore at risk of acquiring endocarditis. The drugs are used here to prevent bacteremia and infection of damaged heart valves when such patients undergo dental or major or minor surgical procedures (see Chapter 12).

The risks involved in antibiotic prophylaxis must be clearly understood. They include allergy or other toxic reactions to the drugs, selection of resistant mutants, and masking or delaying the diagnosis of the infection. Antibiotics should be used prophylactically in situations that fulfill the following criteria:

• A surgical or medical intervention carries a significant risk of microbial contamination. This usually occurs when the surgeon crosses a tissue plane that contains a luxuriant microbial flora, such as the colon or the oral cavity. Here the incidence of infection is unacceptably high and the administration of prophylacic antibiotics is necessary. Antibiotic prophylaxis should also be used when the risk of infection is low but its outcome potentially disastrous, for instance in surgery for the implantation of heart valve or hip prostheses. It is not indicated when the risk is low and the outcome is trivial, such as a hernia operation.

• Antibiotics used prophylactically should be directed against the most likely pathogens. Previous studies should suggest which infectious agents are likely to be involved and to what drugs they are probably susceptible. In operations involving the colon, antibiotics should cover the prime pathogens in fecal material. When surgery crosses the oral mucosa, prophylactic antibiotics with a narrow spectrum are indicated because most of the bacteria in the oral cavity are susceptible to penicillin.

• A suitable concentration of the drug must be achievable at the right time in the relevant tissues. Studies in experimental animals (which have also been confirmed in randomized human studies) have shown that prophylactic antibiotics are of no value if given after surgery is completed. However, their effectiveness could be readily demonstrated if they were given just prior to surgery and adequate tissue levels were achieved. It makes sense that a drug should be present in the body when the wound is likely to get contaminated; once the wound is closed, it rapidly becomes impermeable to exogenous bacteria.

• Antimicrobial drugs should be used for a short time to minimize the emergence of drug resistance. Indications for the prophylactic use of antibiotics are expanding with the occurrence of new diseases, new drugs, and new therapeutic methods. The above guidelines should be applicable in the development of new indications.

THERAPY

Despite the great advances in preventive medicine in the last century, until recently little could be done to treat patients with infectious diseases. The medical literature up to about 1930 is full of vivid descriptions of gruesome infections by streptococci, staphylococci, and clostridia. The dawning of the age of antimicrobial therapy, with the introduction of the sulfonamides in the 1930s, allowed physicians to finally cure many of these fatal infections. Here is a description of the first time penicillin was used clinically:

The time had now come to find a suitable patient for the first test of the therapeutic power of penicillin in man. . . . In the septic ward at the Radcliffe Infirmary (Oxford, England) there was an unfortunate policeman aged 43 who had a sore on his lip four months previously, from which he developed a combined staphylococcal and streptococcal septicaemia. He had multiple abscesses on his face and orbits: he also had osteomyelitis of his right humerus with discharging sinuses, and abscesses in his lungs. He was in great pain and was desperately ill. There was all to gain for him in a trial of penicillin and nothing to lose. Penicillin treatment was started on 12 February 1941, with 200 mg (10,000 units) intravenously initially and then 300 mg every three hours. . . . Four days later there was striking improvement, and after five days the patient was vastly better, afebrile and eating well, and there was obvious resolution of the abscesses on his face and scalp and in his right orbit.

Unfortunately, this first clinical trial of a β-lactam antibiotic terminated abruptly because the total supply of the drug was exhausted by the 5-day course of treatment, despite efforts to recover the drug from the patient's urine. The patient died 4 weeks later.

Although the experiment ended tragically, it served to demonstrate the efficacy and superiority of the new therapy over any that was available until that time. Since then, it has become increasingly more difficult to prove the superiority of new antibiotics over those already in use. Since placebo controls cannot be justified, new drugs have to be compared with the old and, as the old get better, it becomes harder to show differences. In assessing new drugs, pharmaceutical companies must carry out complex and expensive trials that include laboratory work, experimental animals, and lengthy clinical studies. The practicing physician may often find it difficult to evaluate such intricate studies.

The selection of an appropriate drug from those presently available is also not a simple matter. For example, the β-lactam imipenem may be thought to be a true "wonder drug", because it has the widest antibacterial spectrum of any antibiotic presently available and is resistant to inactivating β-lactamases. However, there are specific infections for which penicillin (which has neither of these desirable properties) is far preferable. For example, because of its broad spectrum, imipenem may wipe out other members of the normal bacterial flora, and lead to colonization by resistant species. In addition, imipenem is far more expensive. Thus, pharmacokinetic properties of the drugs, their cost, and many other properties also enter as considerations. The selection of an appropriate drug involves the following criteria:

• What pathogens are causing the infection? If we cannot determine their identity in time, what are the likely possibilities?

• What antibiotics are they susceptible to?

• Will the drug penetrate to the site of infection and will it work under the conditions at that site?

• What is the toxicity of the drug to the patient?

• What is the effect of the drug on the microbial ecology? Will its use lead to the emergence of broadly based antibiotic resistance, and thus pose a threat to the patient being treated and to other infected patients in the community?

• Are other host factors relevant to the proposed therapy?

Note that in many cases the proper conclusion may be that the patient should not be treated with antimicrobial drugs at all because the benefit of such treatment is not likely to outweigh its drawbacks.

The Infecting Organisms

The proper choice of an antimicrobial drug depends on the identification of the infecting organisms. Consider, for example, patients with recurrent urinary tract infection. Often the infection is caused by *E. coli*, but it may be due to group D streptococci, to *Pseudomonas aeruginosa*, or to one of the other enterobacteriaceae, such as *Klebsiella*, *Enterobacter*, or *Serratia*. These organisms have differing susceptibilities, and the determination of their antimicrobial susceptibility is mandatory.

Note that in many cases the physician treating recurrent urinary tract infections can usually wait for the result of laboratory cultures and drug susceptibility testing. This may take two or more days. Such a waiting time is not advisable when the symptoms of the disease are severe. Here, treatment may have to be instituted with only a presumption as to the nature of the causative agents. In such cases, antimicrobial therapy should be broad enough to cover all likely pathogens. To do this, physicians must take into account factors pertinent to the individual patient and the local environment, especially recent experience with similar cases and the antibiotic susceptibility pattern in their hospital or community. Other situations that require empirical therapy are those in which an adequate sample of infected material for direct analysis or culture cannot be obtained.

The following are drawbacks of "shotgun" antibiotic therapy:

• Failure to "cover" the pathogen;

• The synergistic toxicity of multiple drugs;

• Possible antagonism between drugs;

• Increased likelihood of superinfection by resistant bacteria or fungi;

• Increased cost of therapy.

With specific identification of the organism, safer antibiotics may be substituted for broad antimicrobial therapy.

Methods currently available for microbiological diagnosis are described in Chapter 59. In general, the more rapid the diagnosis, the sooner proper therapy can be instituted. Much effort is being expended on the development of rapid diagnostic methods, but most still require one or several days. Some situations are ready-made for a rapid diagnosis. For instance, a Gram stain of spinal fluid showing Gram negative diplococci is highly suggestive of meningococcal meningitis and allows the physician to start specific therapy within minutes. When culturing is requested, it is important that the physician specify if unusual media or handling are appropriate. Unless asked, the laboratory technologist will process samples by methods that will culture many ordinary bacteria, but will certainly not be suitable for viruses, fungi, or even some fastidious or unusual bacteria. Examples of bacteria that will be missed unless cultivated on special media are the tubercle bacilli or *Legionella pneumophila. It is the physician's responsibility to alert the laboratory to such possibilities.*

Antibiotic Susceptibility

Within broad limits, bacteria fall into large groups with regard to antibiotic susceptibility. Gram positive bacteria, possibly because they lack an outer membrane (Chapter 2), are generally more susceptible than Gram negatives, usually because they are more permeable to many of the classical antibiotics. For example, streptococci and pneumococci are generally about 1000-fold more susceptible to penicillin G than *E. coli.* However, the exceptions are too numerous to make these generalizations very useful. Much depends on the presence of antibiotic-resistant strains in a particular environment. Nationwide and local monitoring of resistant strains is helpful in providing general guidelines, but basically, each individual isolate should be tested for susceptibility.

The simplest and most widely used assay for microbial susceptibility is to place a disk containing the antibiotic on an agar plate inoculated with the organisms. As the antibiotic diffuses into the agar, it inhibits bacterial growth up to the limit of the effective concentration (Fig. 28.1). This is not, however, a truly quantitative technique, because many factors influence the diffusion of the drug. Quantitative techniques require the use of dilutions of the drug in liquid media. They provide an estimate of the *minimum inhibitory concentration* (MIC) a parameter that is useful to ascertain whether an effective concentration is attainable in body fluids.

The importance of microbial drug resistance is illustrated by the catastrophic outbreaks of chloramphenicol resistance that occurred in Mexico in the late 1960s and the early 1970s with *Shigella* dysentery and subsequently with *Salmonella* infection. In the initial epidemics it was not recognized that the reason patients

Figure 28.1. The disc diffusion method for determining antibiotic susceptibility. Bacteria were uniformly seeded on the surface of a nutrient agar plate, and filter paper discs containing different antibiotics were placed at intervals over the surface. After incubation, susceptibility to some of the antibiotics is indicated by clear areas around the discs. The diameter of the clear area depends on the extent of diffusion of the drug through the agar. Resistance to other antibiotics is indicated by growth (turbidity) up to the edge of the discs. (Courtesy of Dr. D.J. Krogstad.)

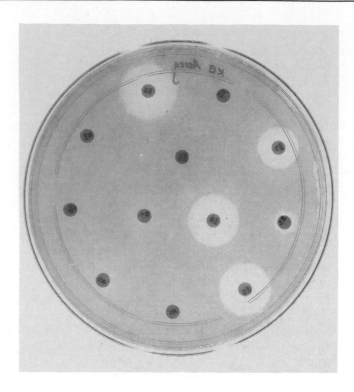

failed to respond to chloramphenicol was that the bacteria had become resistant. Rather, it was thought that the disease was caused by a protozoan parasite. Subsequent analysis revealed that the *Shigella* was chloramphenicol resistant. A similar scenario occurred 2 years later in outbreaks of typhoid fever, with *Salmonella typhi* that was also chloramphenicol resistant. Before the resistance was recognized, a number of people had died from the disease because they were treated with chloramphenicol alone. It is estimated that upwards of 30,000 people died in each of these outbreaks in Mexico and Central America. For this reason it is extremely important that drug resistance be monitored on a nationwide and local basis and that the information be made readily available to medical personnel.

Static versus Cidal Drugs

The minimum inhibitory concentration (MIC) tells us the *bacteriostatic* concentration of a drug but not the *bactericidal* one. The two are not usually the same: Most agents that are bactericidal are bacteriostatic at lower concentrations. The minimum bactericidal concentration (MBC) is determined by subculturing the tubes or microtiter plates that have no visible growth into antibiotic-free media (which, obviously, allows replication of bacteria whose growth was inhibited but which are still alive.) This is a time-consuming technique with some technical problems. It may, however, yield important information. Why? Whereas it is true that bactericidal and bacteriostatic drugs are often equally effective, this is not always the case. For example, in patients with endocarditis and meningitis, the outcome with bactericidal drugs is frequently more satisfactory. Moreover, bactericidal drugs tend to be superior in immunocompromised patients, especially those who are neutropenic. In such cases, it is appropriate to determine the MBC for the causative bacteria.

Multiple-Drug Therapy

The use of combinations of antibiotics (usually two drugs) has evoked comments of "reckless poly-pharmacy", but is clearly needed in a number of clinical situations. As discussed in Chapter 3, when drugs are combined, there are three main possible results:

- *Synergism*, where the two in combination work better than one. An example is the use of trimethoprim and sulfamethoxazole for *E. coli* and *Shigella* enteric infections. The two drugs work on folate metabolism but inhibit different steps (Chapter 3). Synergistic action may also be indirect, for example, by one drug preventing the inactivation of another, as in the case of inhibition of β-lactamases by clavulanic acid.

- *Antagonism*, an undesirable effect that may lead to treatment failure. An example is the combination of penicillin and any of a number of protein-synthesis inhibitors (chloramphenicol, tetracycline) for the treatment of pneumococcal meningitis. The fatality rate among patients treated with the drug combination has been shown to be significantly higher than with penicillin alone. For reasons unknown, antagonism that can be readily demonstrated between two drugs in vitro, often fails to be manifested with the same pair of drugs in clinical situations.

- *Indifference*, in which case each drug acts independently of the other.

There are various indications for combined therapy, e.g.,

- To prevent the emergence of resistant organisms, e.g., in tuberculosis, where this has proven particularly effective;

- To treat polymicrobial infections such as intra-abdominal abscesses, where each organism may be susceptible to different drugs;

- As initial empiric therapy to "cover" multiple potential pathogens.

In other instances, the reason for multiple therapy may be more subtle. For instance, the use of several drugs may allow a lower dosage of each one, which may avoid problems of toxicity. It may also be necessary in order to achieve drug synergy for the treatment of severe, particularly recalcitrant, infections such as endocarditis or bacteremia in a granulocytopenic patient.

Local Factors and Pharmacokinetics

In the early steps of many infections there is tissue inflammation, which changes the environment in which an antibiotic is to work. If the infection is not controlled, cell death and tissue necrosis change conditions even further. In an abscess caused by staphylococci or a mixed anaerobic-aerobic flora, the environment will become anaerobic and the pH may drop as low as 5.5. Antibiotics must be selected for their ability to function under these conditions. As shown in Table 28.3, the function of aminoglycosides is diminished at low pH or in the presence of a high concentration of divalent cation.

The pharmacokinetic factors that should be considered in the choice of drugs include (a) absorption, (b) distribution in tissues, and (c) excretion. The *absorption* profile of a drug dictates its route of administration. The most convenient route is usually by mouth, and is used with highly absorbable antibiotics such as the quinolones or chloramphenicol. Many antibiotics, such as vancomycin, the aminoglycosides and the newer β-lactams, are not absorbed via the gastrointestinal tract

Table 28.3
Physicochemical conditions that affect the activity of antimicrobial agents

	Decrease	Increase
Low pH	Aminoglycosides	Tetracycline
	Some β-lactams (porin changes)	Chloramphenicol
	Erythromycin	
Low redox potential	Aminoglycosides	Metronidazole
High divalent cation concentration	Aminoglycosides	
	Tetracycline (Ca^{++})	

and must be given by parenteral injection. A major exception to this rule is the use of nonabsorbable antibiotics to treat infections limited to the gastrointestinal tract. A good example is the use of oral vancomycin to treat *Clostridium difficile*-induced diarrhea or colitis. Also, drugs cannot be given orally if the patient is vomiting or in shock because absorption becomes unreliable.

Distribution of drugs takes place via the circulation and is followed by entry into tissues by passive diffusion. The diffusion and polarity properties of antibiotics are relevant here, as they are with all drugs. Some antibiotics bind to plasma proteins, which has a good and a bad side. On the one hand, this limits the amount of unbound drug that is available for diffusion, on the other hand the drug remains available for a much longer time.

A vital consideration is the barrier that must be crossed by the drug. Drugs that cross the blood-brain barrier most readily are nonpolar at neutral pH. This is critically important because of the seriousness of infections of the CNS. Note, however, that the permeability properties of the blood-brain barrier may become modified during infection. Two other organs with important barriers are the eye and the prostate, and infections at each of these sites require careful selection of drugs. Infections of the interior of the eye may require direct injection of drugs into the tissue. Similar considerations regarding the placental barrier are discussed in Chapter 53.

Lastly, consideration must be given to the speed of excretion of the drug. Most drugs are excreted by the kidney. Certain drugs (e.g., chloramphenicol, erythromycin, lincomycin) are excreted by the liver via the biliary tree. Some of the newer cephalosporins are excreted via both liver and kidneys. This pattern of excretion can be used to advantage in infections of the urinary tract or the biliary tree. However, the level of renal or hepatic function must be taken into account because an effective level may only be reached if the excretion mechanisms are working properly. You should consult a pharmacology text for a detailed discussion of the pharmacokinetics of antimicrobial drugs.

Antibiotic Toxicity

Antibiotics, like all drugs, have toxic side effects as well as beneficial properties. Toxicity is sometimes so severe as to limit the general usefulness of some of them. For example, chloramphenicol is associated with cases of fatal aplastic anemia and is used only in life-threatening infections, such as meningitis with ampicillin resistant *H. influenzae*. It must be kept in mind that, as with all drugs, antibiotic toxicity is generally dose dependent. As mentioned already, the toxic level of a drug may be avoided on some occasions if it is given in combination with other drugs. The main types of toxic manifestations discussed below represent an overview of the subject. Practicing physicians need more detailed information and must constantly update it.

Allergy

Antimicrobial agents may be recognized as foreign substances by the immune system, resulting in sensitization of some individuals. The most common antibacterial drugs associated with severe allergic reactions are the penicillins, cephalosporins, and sulfonamides. A likely reason why penicillins lead this list is that they readily bind to proteins and function as haptens to elicit IgE antibody responses. The most severe reactions result in immediate hypersensitive responses: hives, angioneurotic edema, and anaphylactic shock. These complications may be fatal. Mild to fairly severe allergic reactions range from rash, urticaria (hives), lymphadenopathy, asthma, and fever. In some cases, fever may confuse the clinical picture because it may be attributed to the infection and not to the drug. Previous history of drug sensitivity often dictates the choice of other agents. If a history of allergy is questionable, the patient may be skin tested with the drug in question.

Other Systemic Reactions

All major organs of the body may be affected by toxicity from antimicrobial drugs. The most frequent reactions involve the *gastrointestinal tract*, ranging from mild distaste to perforation of the colon. Gastrointestinal distress and diarrhea are the most common reactions and often require that the drug be discontinued. These manifestations are often due to a direct stimulatory effect of the drugs on the sympathetic nervous system. More troublesome is diarrhea associated with changes in the intestinal flora. This usually occurs late in the course of treatment and may be manifested only after treatment is stopped. About a third of the cases of antibiotic associated diarrhea have been associated with the toxin produced by *Clostridium difficile* (Chapter 21). The spectrum of diseases caused by this organism ranges from the trivial and self-limiting diarrhea to a severe and life-threatening pseudomembranous colitis.

The *liver* is the major site of drug metabolism and is frequently affected. Many drugs induce mild alterations of function of the hepatic parenchyma, usually manifested by an increase in the serum level of certain transaminases. Some drugs affect biliary excretion. Most of these manifestations are mild and reversible, although cases of liver failure have been reported in pregnant women treated with tetracycline.

The *kidney* is also a frequent site of adverse reactions, resulting in decreased renal function. These are caused by three general mechanisms: (*a*) immunological damage to the glomeruli, blocking filtration; (*b*) damage to the tubules; and (*c*) obstruction of the collecting system by crystals of the drug. This is an important problem because many drugs are excreted via the urinary tract. Unrecognized decrease in renal function may result not only in ineffective levels in the urine but also in toxic serum levels of the drug. The aminoglycosides are the most important class of drugs and cause these side effects. They also cause eighth cranial nerve toxicity (deafness and imbalance). The frequency of these toxic reactions is so high that it requires frequent monitoring of renal function and of the blood levels of the drug.

Other organs that are sometimes affected by antimicrobial agents include the *skin*, which may be affected by allergic reactions or, more seriously, by exfoliative dermatitis and a disease known as the Stevens-Johnson syndrome that leads to the formation of bullae, large vesicles on the skin and inflammation of the eyes and mucous membranes. The *hemopoietic system* may be adversely affected, leading to decreased production of red and white blood cells in the bone marrow. Furthermore, peripheral red and white blood cells may become immunologically sensitized, resulting in their hemolysis or sequestration by fixed macrophages. Also affected at times are the circulatory system, the CNS, the musculoskeletal system, and the respiratory tract. Most of these manifestations are specific to individual drugs. The information about them is made available to physicians in reference manuals published periodically, which should be consulted prior to prescribing medication.

Interactions with Nonantimicrobial Drugs

Antimicrobial drugs sometimes interact with other medications a patient may be taking. The drugs may interact directly or by affecting an enzyme that influences their pharmacology. The drugs most commonly affected are anticoagulants and anticonvulsants. An example follows:

A 67-year-old woman with recurrent thrombophlebitis and pulmonary embolism had been asymptomatic on an oral anticoagulant (warfarin) that maintained her clotting or prothrombin time at 24 seconds (twice the normal value). She had been recently found to have pulmonary tuberculosis and was placed on isoniazid and rifampin. Several days later she required hospitalization for recur-

Table 28.4
Some examples of interaction of antimicrobial agents with other drugs

Antimicrobial Agent	Interacts with	Effect
Aminoglycosides	Anesthetics	Neuromuscular blockage (additive)
	Ethacrynic acid	Ototoxicity
Amphotericin B	Digitalis	Decreases potassium concentration, enhances digitalis toxicity
Ampicillin	Oral contraceptives } Antacids }	Decreases gastrointestinal absorption
Erythromycin	Carbamazepine	Increases activity (nausea, vomiting, diplopia, drowsiness)
	Digitalis	Increases concentration and toxicity
	Theophylline	Increases activity
Griseofulvin	Anticoagulants	Decreases activity
Ketoconazole	Cyclosporine	Increases activity (immunosuppression)
	Antacids and histamine blockers	Decreases activity
Rifampin	Anticoagulants Digitoxin β-blockers Oral contraceptives Ketoconazole Corticosteroids }	Decreases activity
INH	Ketoconazole	Decreases absorption
Sulfonamides	Anticoagulants	Increase activity
	Methotrexate	Increases activity
Tetracyclines	Digitalis	Increases concentration and toxicity
	Methoxyfuran	Increases nephrotoxicity
	Oral contraceptives	Decrease gastrointestinal absorption

rence of her thrombophlebitis. Laboratory evaluation revealed that her prothrombin time was only 2 seconds above normal, despite taking the same amount of warfarin. Her physician then learned that rifampin induces the liver to make a warfarin-inactivating enzyme. Rifampin was stopped and the patient was treated with intravenous heparin to raise her clotting time.

This is an example of the numerous interactions that occur between drugs. The potential consequences may be catastrophic for the patient, particularly if the therapy affected is life-saving, as in the example above. Imagine the problem if the patient had required anticoagulation therapy to prevent clotting on an artificial heart valve. The converse effect, prolongation of clotting time, may also occur with sulfonamides and metronidazole and lead to massive gastrointestinal bleeding. A list of prominent adverse drug interactions that involve antimicrobial agents is listed in Table 28.4. The severity of such complications cannot be overestimated and the message must never be lost on the practitioner.

SUGGESTED READINGS

Drug Evaluation, 6th ed. Chicago, American Medical Association, 1986.

Ginsberg MB, Tager IB: *Practical Guide to Antimicrobial Agents*. Baltimore, MD, Williams & Wilkins, 1980.

Handbook of Antimicrobial Therapy. New Rochelle, The Medical Letter, (Published yearly.)

Moellering RC: Principles of anti-infective therapy. In Mandel GL, Douglas, RG, Bennett JE, (eds): *Principles and Practice of Infectious Diseases*, 2nd ed. New York, John Wiley & Sons, 1985.

Sande MA, Mandel GL: Antimicrobial agents: General considerations. In Gilman AG, Goodman LS, Rall TW, Murray F (eds): *Pharmacological Basis of Therapeutics*, 7th ed. New York, MacMillan, 1985.

Review of Main Pathogenic Bacteria

These charts are intended to review the general features of the main human pathogenic bacteria. Included are the organisms of greatest medical relevance.

Many of the bacteria that cause relatively uncommon diseases were not included. Complete this chart as a method of reviewing this subject matter.

Organism	Gram Reaction and Morphological Type	Common Habitat and Mode of Encounter	Virulence Factors (Toxins, Adhesins, Mechanisms of Resistance to Host Defenses)	Disease(s) and Systems Involved	Relevant Chapters
Staphylococcus aureus					11, 49, 50, 57
Staphylococcus epidermidis					11, 57
Group A streptococci					12, 49, 51
Other β-hemolytic streptococci					12, 53
α-Hemolytic streptococci					12, 51
Pneumococcus (S. pneumoniae)					13, 45
Meningococcus (Neisseria meningitidis)					14, 47
Gonococcus (N. gonorrhoeae)					14
Haemophilus influenzae					15, 45, 52
Bacteroides sp.					16, 49
Escherichia coli					17, 46, 48, 53
Shigella sp.					17, 46
Klebsiella pneumoniae					17, 45

Organism	Gram Reaction and Morphological Type	Common Habitat and Mode of Encounter	Virulence Factors (Toxins, Adhesins, Mechanisms of Resistance to Host Defenses)	Disease(s) and Systems Involved	Relevant Chapters
Proteus sp.					17, 48
Vibrio cholerae					17, 46
Salmonella sp.					18, 46
Pseudomonas aeruginosa					19, 51, 54
Bordetella pertussis					20
Clostridium botulinum					21, 58
C. tetani					21
C. perfringens					21, 58
Listeria monocytogenes					58
Mycobacterium tuberculosis					22, 45
Atypical mycobacteria					22
Treponema pallidum					23
Chlamydia trachomatis					24
Rickettsia sp.					25
Legionella pneumophila					26
Mycoplasma sp.					27, 45

The following charts refer to pathogenic characteristics of bacteria. Complete these charts as a method of reviewing this subject matter.

Capsulated Bacteria of Medical Importance

	Genus and Species	Disease(s)	Organ Systems Involved
1.			
2.			
3.			
4.			
5.			
6. (more if known, but not essential)			

Medically Important Strict Anaerobes

	Genus and Species	Disease(s)	Organ Systems Involved
1.			
2.			
3.			
4.			
5.			
6.			

Typically Pyogenic (pus-producing) Bacteria

	Genus and Species	Disease(s)	Organ Systems Involved
1.			
2.			
3.			
4.			

Major Bacterial Toxins

Bacterium	Site of Action in the Host	Known or Suspected Mode of Action
1.		
2.		
3.		
4.		
5.		
6.		
7.		
8.		

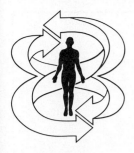

Introduction to the Viruses

29

C. Meissner
M. Schaechter

The fundamental difference between viruses and all other infectious agents is in their mechanism of reproduction. Unlike cellular forms of life, viruses do not simply divide in half. The ditty "when they divide, they multiply" applies to cells, not to viruses. Viruses replicate by synthesizing multiple copies of their genome and their proteins, which assemble spontaneously within the host cell to form progeny virus particles. Viruses have no means to produce energy and contain at most a few enzymes. Thus, viruses are totally dependent on a host cell: They are *obligate intracellular parasites*. Because they are relatively simple and rely on the host for their multiplication, viruses play a key role as models in molecular biology.

The answer to the question: "are viruses alive?" depends on the criteria used to define life. A virus particle by itself cannot be considered to be alive. However, inside a suitable host cell, viruses replicate, mutate, and recombine, which are all properties of living things. In their simplest forms, viruses may be considered as vehicles for transporting genetic material between cells. Viruses are small, although the largest ones (e.g., the smallpox virus) are just visible with the light microscope and fall within the lower range of size of bacteria (e.g., the mycoplasmas or chlamydiae). They vary in volume over a 1000-fold range in structure, from relatively simple to very complex (Fig. 29.1).

Viruses are important pathogens of virtually all forms of life, including humans and other animals, plants, fungi, and bacteria. At a cellular level the outcome of a viral infection shows surprising diversity. When a cell is infected by a virus

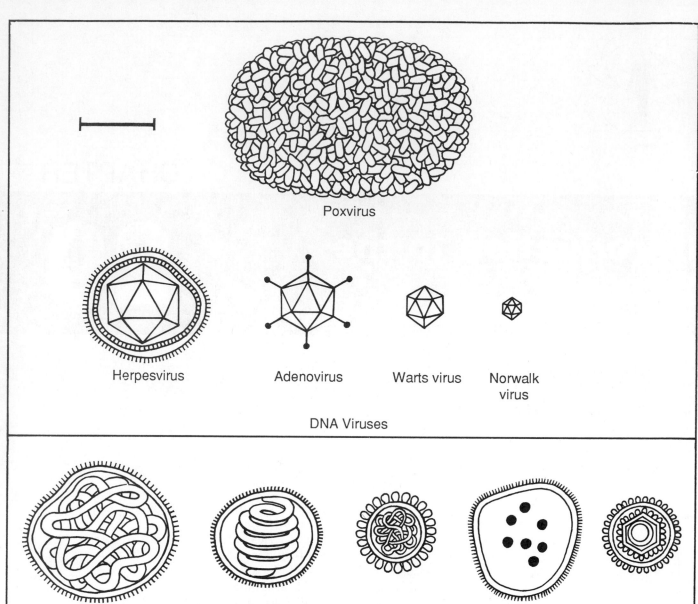

Poxvirus

Herpesvirus   Adenovirus   Warts virus   Norwalk virus

DNA Viruses

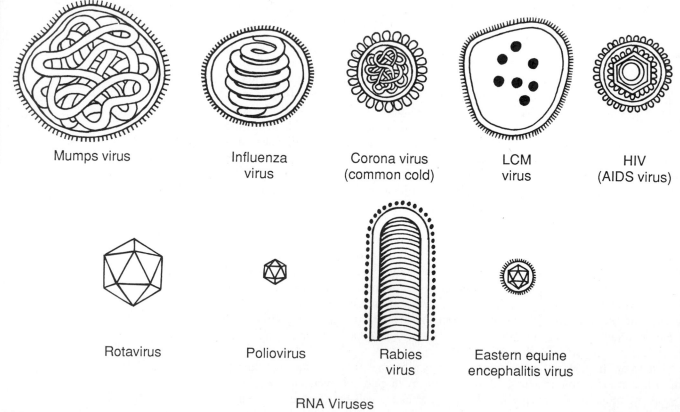

Mumps virus   Influenza virus   Corona virus (common cold)   LCM virus   HIV (AIDS virus)

Rotavirus   Poliovirus   Rabies virus   Eastern equine encephalitis virus

RNA Viruses

Figure 29.1. Examples of viral morphology. (From White DO, Fenner F: *Medical Virology*, ed 3. New York, Academic Press, 1986.)

there are three possible consequences. In a *lytic infection* the virus undergoes multiple rounds of replication. This results in the death of the host cell, which has acted as a factory for virus production. The number of viral particles produced in a single cell in a lytic infection vary from a few with some viruses to thousands for others. This outcome is typical of infections with polio or influenza viruses.

At the opposite end of the spectrum is a *latent infection*, which does not result in the immediate production of progeny virus. The genetic material of the infecting virus may become incorporated into the genome of the host cell or may exist as an extrachromosomal element. During cell growth the genetic material of the virus is replicated along with the chromosomes of the host cell. Herpes viruses, for example, produce latent infections that result in well-known human diseases such

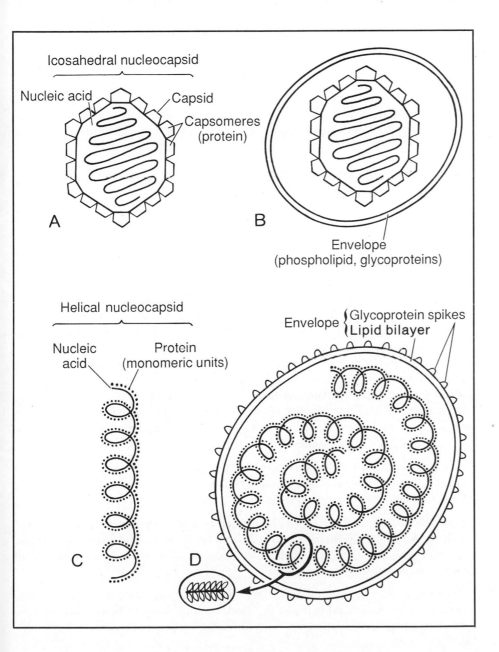

Figure 29.2. Basic viral forms. *A*, Icosahedral, nonenveloped. *B*, Icosahedral, enveloped. *C*, Helical, nonenveloped. *D*, Helical, enveloped. (From Taussig MJ: *Processes in Pathology and Microbiology*, ed 2. Oxford, UK, Blackwell Scientific Publications, 1984.)

as fever blisters and zoster. In the cases of a retrovirus, this may result in *trans-formation* of the cell, a cancer-like state.

A *persistent infection* differs from a lytic and a latent infection in that virus particles continue to be shed after the period of acute illness has passed. It is marked by a slow release of virus particles without death of the host cell. The amount of virus produced is usually lower than in lytic infections. Often, persistent infections do not result in overt diseases, while in other instances clinical disease may be present. Hepatitis B virus is well recognized to cause a persistent infection in the liver that may lead to chronic hepatitis and even liver cancer.

A few definitions should be learned: The term used to denote a single virus particle is a *virion*. The *capsid* is the protein coat that surrounds the viral nucleic acid and is made up of subunits called *capsomeres*. The nucleic acid and the capsid combine to form the *nucleocapsid*. The nucleocapsid of many animal viruses is surrounded by an *envelope* usually made up of lipids and glycoproteins. Viruses display considerable variation on this structural theme (Fig. 29.2). Many fall within this general outline, others will be quite unexpected. The reader may want to keep in mind that the structure and mode of replication of a particular virus give important clues to its pathogenic mechanism. This chapter is intended as a brief introduction to the general characteristics of animal viruses. Specific aspects related to individual viruses will be discussed in subsequent chapters.

AN EXAMPLE OF THE VIRAL REPLICATION CYCLE: ADENOVIRUS

We will use an *adenovirus* as a typical DNA-containing virus to illustrate the steps in viral replication. Adenoviruses derive their name from the fact that they were first isolated from human adenoids. They are important causes of respiratory tract infections, primarily in young children and military recruits. Adenoviruses fall about midway in the range of sizes of animal viruses. Their genome contains about 50,000 base pairs of DNA, enough to code for about 20 to 50 average-size proteins. Under the electron microscope virions of adenovirus are seen as complex particles (Fig. 29.1). They have 20 triangular faces (each an equilateral triangle) and 12 vertices in a symmetrical arrangement that gives them a hexagonal profile. This *icosahedral structure* is characteristic of a number of viruses. Unique to adenoviruses are protein fibers that stick out from each vertex, giving the appearance of a space satellite. Adenoviruses have no envelope.

Adenoviruses multiply in cells of human origin such as HeLa cells, the commonly used line derived from human cervical carcinoma tissue. The replication cycle has several distinct stages that in general terms are common to all viruses:

- First virions *adsorb* to the surface of host cells at specific receptors. These are chemically defined sites on the plasma membrane of the host cell. Adenoviruses bind to these receptors by their fibers.

- The viruses are then internalized by the cell and *enter* the cytoplasm, where *uncoating* occurs: The protein capsid is selectively degraded by cellular proteases, releasing the nucleic acid, which in the case of adenoviruses is a molecule of double-stranded DNA.

- Once uncoated, the virus particles *lose their infectivity*. No longer are they distinct particles recognizable under the electron microscope. The interval between uncoating and the emergence of new infective virions is known as the *eclipse*

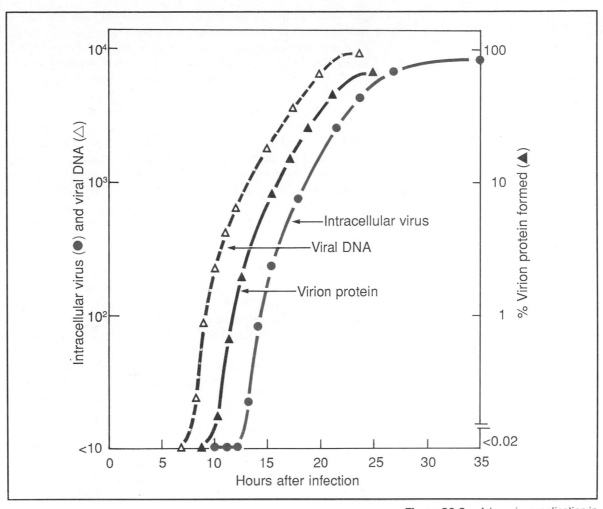

Figure 29.3. Adenovirus replication in cell culture. (Modified from Wold S *et al.* in Nayak DP (ed): *Molecular Biology of Animal Viruses*, vol 2. Marcel Dekker, 1978.)

phase. It can be followed experimentally by assaying the number of infective particles in the cell. For several hours after infection, little if any infectious virus can be detected. During this phase, viral DNA within the cell is sensitive to digestion by nucleases because it is not protected by the capsid.

- After uncoating, the replication phase begins (Fig. 29.3). Uncoated viral DNA is transported to the nucleus, where DNA synthesizing enzymes of the cell are located. As with many viruses, the biochemical details of adenovirus DNA replication differ from conventional DNA replication. This point should be appreciated because, at least in theory, it suggests therapeutic strategies.

Adenovirus replication has two unusual aspects: First, the genome has a protein covalently attached at the 5′ ends of the linear DNA molecule. A precursor of this protein serves in lieu of an RNA primer for the elongation of daughter molecules. Second, DNA replicates one strand at a time, making single-stranded copies that are themselves used for making double-stranded molecules. The final outcome is the same as with DNA replication in cells, namely parental molecules are replicated in semiconservative fashion. Overall,

$$\text{DNA} \longrightarrow \text{DNA}$$

Another major difference between viral and cellular DNA replication is its timing: Host chromosomes replicate by a well-regulated process that occurs once in a division cycle; viral replication, on the other hand, is uncoordinated and takes place continuously over a period of time. Replication of viral DNA is independent of host DNA synthesis, although host enzymes are utilized. About 6 hours after infection, adenovirus DNA synthesis begins and host DNA replication is gradually inhibited by poorly understood mechanisms (Fig. 29.3).

One of the first events to take place after adenovirus DNA reaches the nucleus, but before viral DNA synthesis begins, is the synthesis of viral messenger RNAs that code for *regulatory proteins*. These proteins help *redirect* the protein-synthesizing machinery of the cell toward synthesis of viral proteins. Host mRNA on polyribosomes is gradually displaced by viral mRNA. At this time, only these virus specific proteins are synthesized. The capsid proteins are not needed and their genes are not yet transcribed. It is customary to speak of this class of messenger RNA molecules as "early messengers" and of the proteins as "early proteins".

Several hours after viral DNA replication has started, synthesis of "late" or structural proteins begins (Fig. 29.3). The complete adenovirus capsid is constructed from three major proteins, the *hexons*, each of which touch six other proteins in the icosahedral shell, and the *pentons*, which are surrounded by five hexons each and make up the apices of the capsids. A *fiber* protein projects from each penton.

Synthesis of viral proteins can only take place in the cytoplasm, where the ribosomes and the rest of the protein synthesizing machinery are located. Once made, viral proteins are transported into the nucleus. On the way to the nucleus they begin to copolymerize into capsomeres and arrive there already partly assembled. They now finish their *self-assembly* process to make empty capsid shells. Viral DNA that has accumulated in the nucleus now fills the capsid, together with so-called core proteins. Further protein cleavage takes place, and mature virions are finally *assembled*. This marks the end of the eclipse period. If the cells were opened at this time, a mixture of infectious and noninfectious particles would be found. The synthesis of viral protein and nucleic acid does not take place in an efficient manner, and many capsid particles are defective—that is, they are not filled with a complete viral genome. The number of particles made per cell can be as high as 7000, with less than 10% being infectious (Fig. 29.3). This suggests that efficiency is not of paramount importance for the survival of these and many other viruses.

After mature virions are assembled in the cell, they are *released* into the extracellular environment. The time from the beginning of infection to the emergence of progeny viruses in the medium is known as the *latent period*. With many other viruses, the end of the latent period is heralded explosively by lysis of the host cells and the release of the virions contained within the cell. This is not the case with adenoviruses, which do not lyse the cells, but cause them to become rounded and to clump together. Eventually the cells die, but only after a long period of time during which they may even continue some metabolic activities.

Replication of adenoviruses can be summarized as follows:

• Viruses *enter* the cell.

• The nucleocapsid is *uncoated* in order to present a "readable" nucleic acid template.

- The cell's machinery is *redirected* preferentially toward the synthesis of viral components.

- Viral components are *assembled* into mature particles.

- Progeny virions *exit* the cell. These steps are illustrated in Figure 29.3, which shows a so-called viral growth curve.

VARIATIONS ON THE THEME OF REPLICATION

Replication of Single-Stranded DNA Viruses

The smallest of all viruses are the parvoviruses, some of which have barely enough genetic material to replicate. Some of them in fact do not have enough, and require the presence of coinfecting *helper viruses* to supply some of the functions needed for replication. An example of such a *defective virus* is the so-called *adeno-associated virus*, which requires the presence of adenovirus helper in order to replicate.

A self-replicating parvovirus has been recently identified as the cause of "fifth disease", or erythema infectiosum, a common skin rash of childhood. The genome of this virus is so small that it codes for only three or four proteins. Replication of this virus requires rapidly dividing cells, ostensibly because only in this stage can the host cells supply all the needed constituents.

DNA Synthesis in the Cytoplasm

Unlike other DNA-containing viruses, smallpox and other poxviruses *multiply in the cytoplasm*. This suggests that pox viruses do not require host cell enzymes for their nucleic acid synthesis (since these are located in the nucleus). Smallpox virions also carry their own RNA polymerase as well as the enzymes needed for processing of RNA transcripts into functional mRNA (i.e., those involved in capping the messengers at the 5′ end and polyadenylating the 3′ end). Thus, without help from the host, pox viruses can synthesize mRNA for the production of their own proteins, including DNA polymerase and other enzymes involved in DNA synthesis. At first glance the concept of a *virion-associated enzyme* may seem novel. Actually, many types of viruses use this strategy and finding enzymes associated with virions is not unusual. These enzymes are usually coded by the viruses themselves and not by the host cells.

Given this genetic and biochemical load, it follows that poxviruses are structurally highly complex and are among the largest of all the viruses. Are they really different from bacteria? The seminal difference is that they lack the capability for protein synthesis and contain no RNA. Thus, their genes can only be expressed when the viruses become uncoated, synthesize RNA, and present their messenger RNAs to the protein-synthesizing machinery of the host. Their dependence on the synthesizing capability of the host is barely greater than that of small intracellular bacteria such as the chlamydiae, but they are typical viruses because *they do not maintain their structural integrity during replication.*

RNA Virus Replication

In normal cells RNA is not made from an RNA template. Thus, RNA-containing viruses must use a different biosynthetic strategy than do DNA viruses or host cells. Their replication depends on an RNA-dependent RNA polymerase, or *RNA replicase*. This enzyme carries out the reaction

$$RNA \longrightarrow RNA$$

Because RNA replicase is not present in uninfected cells, it must be supplied by the virus in one of two ways: It is either synthesized from viral genes, or it is carried into the cell by the infecting virus, having been synthesized in the previous round of infection. Many RNA viruses are single stranded. Their genome may be either of the same polarity or "sense" as messenger RNA, or of complementary polarity. If the genome is of the same sense as messenger RNA, it can be used directly as messenger RNA. These viruses are called *positive stranded*. An example is poliovirus, which replicates as follows: After entry and uncoating, viral RNA is translated, using host ribosomes and other components of the protein synthesizing machinery. One of the products of translation is the poliovirus RNA replicase, which uses the genomic RNA molecules as templates. The first RNA molecules made by this replicase are complementary to the genome and of negative sense. These transcripts in turn serve as template for repeated replication of positive-sense RNA molecules, which function as messengers to synthesize a large amount of capsid protein molecules. In time, the newly made viral RNA and the capsid proteins will self-assemble into mature virions that are eventually released from the host cell.

Other RNA viruses are *negative stranded*, that is, the RNA contained in their virions is complementary to messenger RNA. These viruses have a problem: How can they replicate their RNA? They cannot immediately make RNA replicase since their RNA cannot serve as messenger. The solution is that they carry preformed RNA replicase in the virions and introduce it into the host cells upon infection. Examples of negative-stranded viruses are influenza, rabies, mumps, and measles, all of which contain an RNA replicase associated with the virions.

A third class of RNA viruses has *double-stranded* RNA. How do they replicate? One might think that they would follow the plan of the positive-stranded RNA viruses, since one of their two strands is already the same sense as messenger RNA. However, the protein-synthesizing machinery cannot use double-stranded RNA as a template; in order to become translatable these viruses must first make single-stranded RNA. For this purpose they also carry RNA replicase molecules in the virion, and start their cycle with RNA replication rather than protein synthesis. An example of a segmented double-stranded RNA virus is the rotavirus, a frequent cause of diarrhea in children.

Lastly, some RNA viruses replicate via a DNA intermediate. They have not evolved a gene for RNA replicase and cannot make RNA from an RNA template. These are the *retroviruses*, which include the agent of AIDS and several others that cause tumors in animals. How can a DNA intermediate be made from RNA? None of the enzymes of normal cells nor of the viruses mentioned above do this. Retroviruses carry in their virions the special enzyme RNA-dependent DNA polymerase, or *reverse transcriptase*, an enzyme that performs the unique task of making DNA using RNA as a template. The result is that the viral genome is copied into a DNA version, and this is integrated into the host chromosome. It becomes part of the genetic component of the host and is replicated along with the host genes by host DNA polymerase. At a later time it is copied by host DNA-dependent RNA polymerase into viral RNA to make mRNA or progeny virions. The viral genome then undergoes a circle:

$$RNA \longrightarrow DNA \longrightarrow RNA$$

The complex subject of these viruses is treated further in Chapter 33.

THE ENVELOPED VIRUSES: A STRUCTURAL COMPLEXITY

For the enveloped viruses the final stage of assembly takes place when the nucleocapsids "bud" out from a host cell membrane. Some envelope proteins are encoded by the virus, others derived from the host. The lipids, on the other hand, are distinctly of host origin and have the same composition as the host's membrane from which they were coopted by the virus. Envelope formation may take place at the level of the nuclear membrane, as, for instance, with the herpesviruses, or at the cytoplasmic membrane, as with the viruses of measles or mumps (Fig. 29.4). As a result, herpes virions have the lipids characteristic of the nuclear membrane, while measles viruses have those of the cytoplasmic membrane. In nearly every case, viral-encoded and host cell-derived proteins are glycosylated, a general characteristic of membrane proteins. Viruses that become enveloped at the cytoplasmic membrane do not become infective until they are released from the

Figure 29.4. Viral budding through the cytoplasmic membrane. (From Taussig MJ: *Processes in Pathology and Microbiology*, ed 2. Oxford, UK, Blackwell Scientific Publications, 1984.)

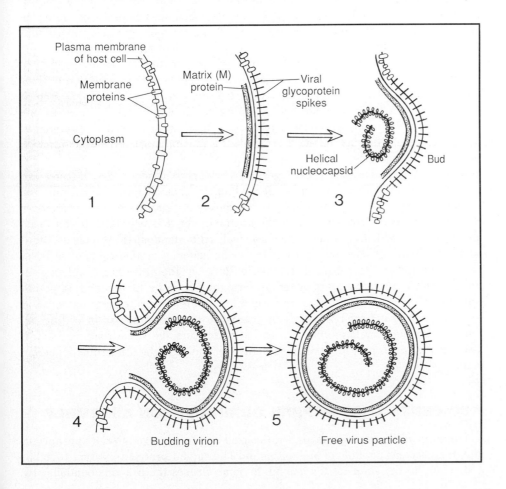

cell; infective particles are not found in the cytoplasm because these viruses require their envelope in order to attach and infect new host cells.

The envelope endows viruses with special properties. For example, enveloped viruses can escape from the cell without damaging it. Virus release is therefore not necessarily accompanied by cell destruction. In fact, viral production may be a gradual process that extends over a long period of time. With regard to viral entry, the envelope allows penetration of some viruses into the cell without phagocytosis, by fusion of the envelope with the plasma membrane. At first glance it may be thought that the envelope plays a protective role in the extracellular environment, but it turns out that it is usually a liability instead. Broadly speaking, enveloped viruses are less able to survive in the environment than the nonenveloped ones. For example, many enveloped viruses are inactivated by gastric acidity or in the small intestine by pancreatic enzymes and are unable to use the gastrointestinal tract as a portal of entry. They are also more sensitive to drying. It follows that nonenveloped viruses can be transmitted more frequently via the environment, while the enveloped ones often require person-to-person contact, insect vectors, or some other means of direct inoculation into a susceptible host.

ECONOMY AMONG THE VIRUSES

Some viruses have a small genome and must make efficient use of the amount of genetic information they carry. The smallest genomes tend to be found in viruses with single-stranded nucleic acids. Thus, the parvoviruses have about 1.5×10^6 daltons of DNA, enough to code for a few proteins only. As we have seen, they may require specific cellular conditions for replication.

Polyoma viruses display a special degree of efficiency in the utilization of their genetic material. They code for more than one protein from the same stretch of nucleic acid. These viruses have *overlapping genes*, which can be used in one of two ways: The same sequence can be read in different frames, or proteins of different size may be made in the same reading frame but start and end in different places in the sequence.

Viruses may *splice* their messenger RNA. Noncoding sequences, *introns*, are removed from precursor RNA molecules, which are then cleaved, leaving only the mRNA sequence that is expressed in protein synthesis, the *exons*. Messenger RNA splicing was discovered with the adenoviruses and was later found to be characteristic of eucaryotic cell systems as well. At first glance this seems wasteful because it requires carrying extra DNA in the genome for the segment of RNA that is cut out and is not used to make mRNA. On the other hand, splicing allows the virus to derive more genetic information from its limited coding potential. By a shift in reading frame, splicing allows different proteins to be encoded by the same stretch of DNA. Splicing can also remove stretches of coding sequences, so that smaller proteins can be made from the same reading frames. These mechanisms may result in considerable economy in the utilization of genetic coding potential.

ACCIDENTS THAT HAPPEN DURING VIRION ASSEMBLY

Once the viral constituents are synthesized and transported to the appropriate site, they become capable of self-assembly. The capsid proteins interact to make a structure in the shape of the capsid. In some viruses the proteins condense by themselves, while in others this only takes place when the nucleic acid is present. In bacterial viruses, the bacteriophages, this morphogenetic process has been studied in detail. It sometimes happens that the bacteriophage capsid incorporates not viral nucleic acid, but pieces of the host chromosomes that have been generated by breakage from nucleases. If bacteria become infected with a virus that contains chromosomal genes, they may become *transduced*; that is, they may acquire genes from the virus' previous host. This kind of erroneous packaging is also seen during assembly of some animal viruses, where the particles are known as *pseudovirions*.

Adenoviruses and other animal viruses frequently package less than a complete copy of the viral genome. The result is the formation of incomplete particles known as defective viruses. Although defective particles are incapable of replication on their own, they may adsorb to host cells at specific receptors and thus interfere with the replication of full virus particles. A virus known as hepatitis delta is another example of a defective but pathogenic agent. This RNA containing virus requires the helper function of hepatitis B virus in order to replicate and cause disease. In order to develop hepatitis D, the disease caused by the delta virus, an individual must be coinfected with both hepatitis B and D viruses.

OTHER SURPRISES: PRIONS AND VIROIDS

Recent years have seen the development of an astonishing new field of microbiology, based on the discovery of new classes of infectious agents, *prions* and *viroids*. These are the smallest known agents of disease. Viroids cause disease in plants and consist of naked, covalently closed circles of single-stranded RNA, less than 300 to 400 nucleotides in length. In spite of this extraordinarily small size, they replicate without the help of viruses. Some evidence suggests that they do not code for proteins at all. How they replicate and cause disease remains a mystery.

Prions are thought to differ from both viruses and viroids in that they consist of proteins and not nucleic acids. Presumably, the prion proteins are encoded by cellular genes. There is evidence to suggest that the degenerative diseases, Creutzfeldt-Jakob disease and kuru, may be caused by prions. These diseases, as well as the so-called slow virus diseases (Chapter 36), remind us to be ready for further surprises.

WHERE ARE VIRUSES FOUND IN NATURE AND HOW DO THEY INFECT PEOPLE? THE PATHOBIOLOGY OF VIRAL INFECTIONS

Many viruses, especially the nonenveloped ones, are tough and can survive in many environments. They are found in drinking water and food, often because of fecal contamination from carriers or patients. One important group of viruses acquired by the *oral-fecal route* is the rotaviruses. These viruses cause a serious infantile diarrhea in millions of infants growing up, not only in some of the developing countries but also in countries with more privileged socioeconomic status.

Enveloped viruses have two main modes of transmission: *direct from person to person*, via contaminated secretions, fomites, or droplet nuclei, or through the *bite of insects*. There are many examples of the first: Measles or mumps viruses are spread in respiratory droplets from one person to another. Herpes simplex viruses tend to be spread by direct contact between mucous membranes. In contrast, transmission via insects is the rule among certain viruses capable of causing encephalitis, an infection of brain tissue. These viruses are grouped together under the name of arthropodborne viruses, or arboviruses, where the first two letters come from "arthropod", the second two from "borne". The list of vectors is a long one, the main ones being mosquitoes and ticks. This mode of transmission suggests that the diseases may be controlled by containing or limiting the arthropod population. A grander example of a bite that may lead to encephalitis is seen in rabies, which usually results from contact with infected saliva of dogs, bats, or raccoons.

How Do Viruses Cause Damage to Cells and Tissues?

Nearly all tissues and organs of the body are susceptible to damage by viruses. In general, viruses have marked tissue tropism and have specific target organs. As with other infectious diseases, the extent of damage depends on the inoculum size and on the target cells and tissues. Infection of relatively few cells can result in the devastating complications of AIDS or paralytic polio. In contrast, many cells may be affected by influenza virus, yet this disease is relatively milder. Damage caused by viral replication may be due to one of several mechanisms.

Host Cell Damage

Viruses do not produce soluble toxins. Many cause damage directly by redirecting the host cells' synthetic activities into viral replication and preventing normal cell function. In many instances, such as infection with poliovirus or herpesvirus, the result is lysis of the host cell due to damage to the cytoplasmic membrane. Viral growth may also result in damage to lysosomes, with the spillage of damaging lysosomal enzymes into the cytoplasm.

In some instances, pathologists are able to recognize viral multiplication by the presence of *inclusion bodies*, which are dense concentrations of virions at their site of assembly. They appear as highly stained particles in characteristic locations. Thus, herpesviruses make intranuclear inclusion bodies, whereas those formed by poxviruses are typically cytoplasmic. These morphological features are often helpful in diagnosis. For example, detection of the inclusion bodies seen in the neurons of people or dogs infected with rabies (known as *Negri bodies*) allows a more rapid diagnosis than attempts at cultivation of the virus.

Immunopathology, Tumorigenesis, and Cell Fusion

Viral infections may cause damage by immunopathological mechanisms, such as immune complex formation or immunological destruction of infected cells. These will be discussed in more detail in the chapters on individual agents, especially hepatitis B (Chapter 32).

Certain forms of damage are virtually unique to viruses. One is virus-induced hyperplasia, which ranges from relatively benign warts to frank tumors. Viruses appear to cause tumors in association with environmental and host factors. The process results in *cell transformation*, which is discussed in the chapters on warts and retroviruses. Also characteristic of certain viral infections is the fusion of certain host cells to form *syncytia* or *multinucleated giant cells*. Involved are proteins on the surface of virions known as *fusion proteins*. These are typical of enveloped viruses, and function to "melt" together the viral capsule and the cytoplasmic membrane during viral penetration. Cells infected with such viruses express fusion proteins on their surface. Thus, these cells act as "megaviruses" and fuse with adjacent cells (see Chapter 36 on measles). In this manner, the virus may spread to new cells without an extracellular phase. Note that this virus-induced fusion is the same one exploited to produce hybridomas for the production of monoclonal antibodies (see Chapter 5).

Host Defenses Against Viruses

The Interferons

In addition to the humoral and cellular defense mechanisms, viral infections elicit an inducible defense mechanism, the interferons. These proteins are encoded by the host cells and their formation is induced by viruses and other agents. They inhibit viral replication in infected cells by inducing a state which will not support viral replication. Interferons do not interact with viruses directly; rather, they induce the synthesis of cellular proteins that minimize viral replication. Their discovery and practical applications are discussed in the chapter on antiviral strategies (Chapter 37).

There are three main kinds of interferons (Table 29.1), named α, β, and γ. Viruses are important inducers of the first two. Interferons are also readily induced by double-stranded RNAs and synthetic double-stranded ribonucleotide polymers. It is thought that double-stranded RNA produced during some viral infections may be the normal inducers. As to γ-interferon, it is usually induced by the activation of T cells by specific antigens, but can also be induced by other compounds, including bacterial endotoxin.

The mode of action of the various interferons is only imperfectly understood, in part because thay have several different activities in cells. They inhibit viral replication by promoting degradation of messenger RNA and interfering with viral and host cell protein synthesis. One enzyme induced by interferon is known as *2',5' oligoadenylate synthetase*, which makes a short polymer made up of 2',5' adenylate residues. This compound activates a specific ribonuclease known as *RNase L*, which can degrade viral and host mRNA. In addition, interferons induce a *protein kinase* that phosphorylates protein factors needed for protein synthesis, thus inactivating them.

The role of interferons in attenuating viral infections has proven difficult to determine. Most likely, infected cells secrete interferon molecules that are taken up by adjacent cells, which are then protected from the infecting virus. Since interferons are not specific, the cells will also be protected from infection by other viruses. However, interferons are short lived in the circulation. For this reason

Table 29.1
Human interferons

Current Name	Produced by	Typical Inducers
IFN α	Leucocytes	Viruses
IFN β	Fibroblasts	Viruses
IFN γ	T cells	Antigens
		Mitogens

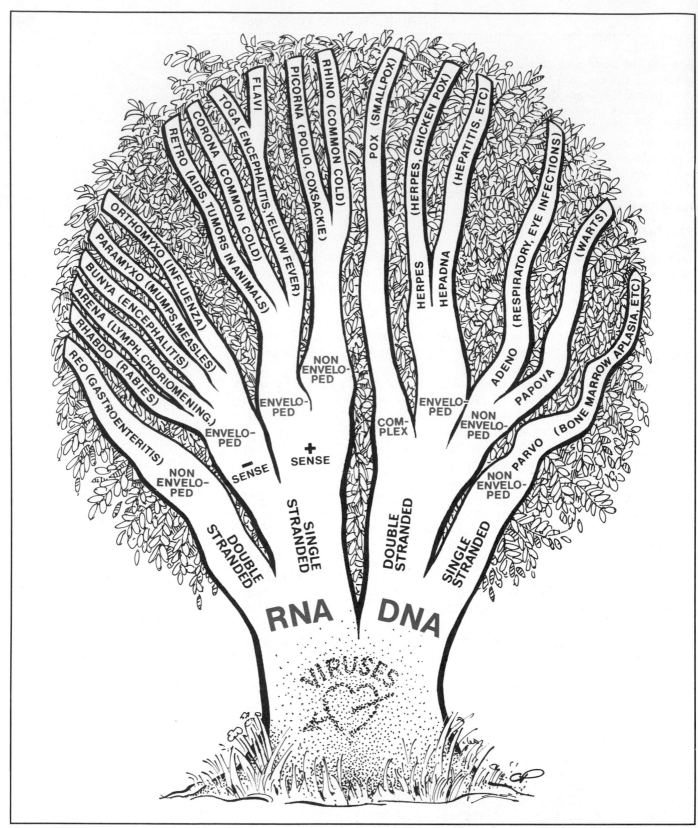

Figure 29.5. The main groups of human viruses. (This is a practical representation and does not represent phylogenetic relationships.)

and because they may have toxic side effects, interferons have not yet lived up to initial expectations in therapeutic applications (Chapter 37).

How Do Antibodies Inhibit Virus Infections?

Individuals with congenital hypogammaglobulinemias are more susceptible to certain viral diseases, such as paralytic polio, despite the fact that they are able to mount normal cellular immunity and synthesis of interferons. The role of circulating antibodies in preventing disease is also demonstrated by the success of vaccines that induce their formation, such as in polio.

Antibodies bound to viral antigens expressed on the surface of infected cells may lead to complement-mediated cytolysis. Virus-infected cells may also be killed by *antibody-dependent cell-mediated cytotoxicity* (ADCC), the mechanism whereby K lymphocytes bind to the Fc fragment of antibody molecules that are attached to antigens on the surface of infected cells. In most viral infections, the role played by circulating antibodies is considerably less important. They may contribute to the inflammatory response seen in some viral diseases (e.g. smallpox) by activating complement by the classical pathway and by eliciting the formation of chemotaxins and the recruitment of phagocytic cells.

Cell-Mediated Immunity in Viral Infections

Viruses are often shielded from antibodies by virtue of their intracellular habitat. However, infected cells are susceptible to the action of cytotoxic T cells, which recognize viral antigens on their surface. This mechanism is particularly important with enveloped viruses, although it also operates in infections by certain nonenveloped viruses, such as the adenoviruses, which induce the expression of viral antigens on the cell's surface.

T cells are more effective in killing virus-infected cells than is antibody-mediated lysis (whether by formation of the membrane attack complex of complement or by ADCC). Deficiencies in T cell function, either congenital or acquired as in AIDS, lead to serious and often persistent viral infections.

TAXONOMY OF VIRUSES

The main viruses that affect humans belong to about a dozen separate genera and hundreds of individual species. As in the case of bacteria, it may be helpful to place the main groups in larger categories (Fig. 29.5). In virology, the division is along structural and molecular lines. One convenient and popular method of classification is by nucleic acid content: DNA viruses and RNA viruses. Each category can then be subdivided into viruses with single-stranded and double-stranded genomes. RNA viruses may be further subdivided into those with positive- and negative-stranded genomes. Alternatively, viruses may be classified by morphological characteristics, such as the presence or absence of an envelope. The major groups of viruses are described individually in the chapters that follow.

Why is there such a rich variety of viruses? We can answer in the most general terms only: Make the assumption that each virus represents an evolutionary solution to particular problems of selection and survival. Since these problems have many forms, the number of particular solutions must also be large. In some instances aspects of the disease they cause help to explain the strategy used by the virus. This will be discussed in the chapters on individual agents.

SELECTED READINGS

Belshe RB (ed): *Textbook of Human Virology*. Littleton, MA, PSG Publ., 1984.

Fields B (ed): *Virology*. New York, Raven Press, 1985.

Mims CA, White DO: *Viral Pathogenesis and Immunology*. Boston, Blackwell Science Publications, 1984.

Primrose SB, Simmock NJ: *Introduction to Modern Virology*. New York, John Wiley & Sons, 1980.

Rothschield H, Cohen JC: *Virology in Medicine*. Oxford, UK, Oxford University Press, 1986.

White DO, Fenner F: *Medical Virology*, ed 3. New York, Academic Press, 1986.

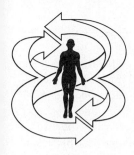

Influenza and Its Viruses

S.E. Straus

I nfluenza (the "flu") ranks among the major epidemic diseases in developed countries. It may even spread throughout the world, causing pandemics. In healthy adults, it is a relatively mild disease, but it contributes significantly to the mortality of the elderly and of persons with respiratory illness. The main reason why influenza has not been eradicated is that the viruses have the ability to change their main antigens, hemagglutinin and neuraminidase. Thus, previous exposure or vaccination does not ensure immunity against newly emerging strains of the virus. Up-to-date vaccines, containing different combinations of antigens, are administered during epidemics to persons at risk. Several drugs are effective in the treatment of this disease.

Influenza viruses are enveloped and belong to the *Orthomyxovirus* group. Their RNA genome is divided into eight segments of negative polarity. It is not known how these segments are assembled in the progeny virions to ensure that each viral particle contains a complete copy of the genome.

CASE

When Ms. I., a healthy 40-year-old, was told by her doctor that she probably had influenza she realized that she has never forgotten the early winter of 1957. It seemed as if everyone in her entire family had developed the flu. With all of the coughing, chills and aches, it was hard to get any sleep. Everyone had to take turns getting out of bed to get aspirin or fluids for the ones who were the weakest. Schools were closed for several days during the outbreak because so many teachers and students had become ill. But the most upsetting recollection was the death of her grandfather. He was a smoker and had a little heart trouble, but basically he was quite sound. And then the flu came on. His illness began like it did in the rest of the family although he coughed and spit a bit more. One night his fever increased and he started to get very short of breath. He was rushed to the hospital but died in 2 days despite antibiotics and oxygen.

Now the news reports indicate that a new strain of flu has gotten a foothold in the United States, this one apparently from the Far East. Ms. I. is apprehensive about the possible effects of this new Asian flu and concerned that she, and particularly her aging parents, may be vulnerable. Her own symptoms are those of the classic upper respiratory infection. She has a runny nose, mild sore throat, cough, fever, muscle aches and fatigue. Her doctor did not carry out laboratory tests but based a tentative diagnosis on the clinical picture and on an alert he received from the State Board of Health about the presence of a new strain of influenza virus. If the course of her disease is typical, Ms. I. will feel sick for 4 to 7 days, but the fatigue and dry cough may last for days or even weeks thereafter.

This chapter will explain why the 1957 influenza epidemic was so severe. Influenza is usually regarded as a bothersome but minor illness. Is this true in the light of Ms. I.'s childhood experience? Ms. I. is probably also asking several other questions, including:

1. How do new influenza strains arise?

2. Why are people susceptible to repeated influenza infections?

3. What makes some strains of influenza more dangerous than others?

4. What can be done to prevent influenza?

5. Why are vaccines recommended every year instead of once or a few times in a lifetime as with other virus vaccines?

6. How can influenza infection be treated?

Beyond the classic presentation of influenza, such as that in Ms. I.'s case, lies an entire spectrum of pulmonary complications that are more likely to develop in certain settings: during pregnancy, in the elderly, and in any individual with congenital or acquired cardiopulmonary diseases. A few such individuals are at risk for the development of either primary influenza pneumonia, a devastating virus infection of the lung parenchyma, or more typically, secondary bacterial pneumonia.

Influenza has many imitators. Similar but less severe illnesses caused by other viruses are all commonly called the "flu". Gastrointestinal symptoms such as cramping, nausea, vomiting and diarrhea are not common features of influenza (except in children), and the term "intestinal flu" is a total misnomer.

HISTORY OF INFLUENZA

Epidemics of brief illness with fever, cough, and severe weakness were described by Hippocrates in the 5th century BC and reported repeatedly throughout the Middle Ages. Since 1173 more than 300 outbreaks of influenza-like illness have been recorded at an average interval of 2.4 years. The development of intercontinental travel and commerce made possible the first known pandemic (global epidemic) of influenza, which occurred in 1580 and originated in Asia, spreading to Europe and later to the Americas. Twenty-two pandemics of influenza illness have been recorded since the early 18th century; the most dramatic of these was the Great Spanish Influenza Pandemic of 1918–1919, in which more than 20 million died worldwide.

Influenza is an Italian word used in the belief that the illness resulted from the "influence" of atmospheric factors. An infectious etiology for influenza was not seriously espoused until the end of the last century when a bacillus, now known as *Haemophilus influenzae*, was recovered from the sputum of patients with this syndrome. The viral etiology of influenza was finally proven in 1933. The virus was first grown in the laboratory in 1940 (in fertilized chicken eggs), and by 1950 the three serologic types of influenza known to infect people were recognized.

THE INFLUENZA VIRUSES

Influenza viruses belong to the family *Orthomyxoviridae* and include three types, A, B, and C. The minor structural differences and the major epidemiologic and clinical differences among the three types are summarized in Table 30.1. Influenza viruses are enveloped RNA viruses (Figs. 30.1 and 30.2). The viral envelope is covered with spikes, or *peplomers*, which in the cases of influenza A and B strains are made up of two different proteins, the *hemagglutinin* and the *neuraminidase*. Influenza C viruses have a single protein with both hemagglutinin and neuraminidase activity. Matrix proteins line the inner aspects of the viral envelope while other internal proteins, polymerases and nucleoproteins, are associated with the viral RNA.

Influenza A viruses are among the best studied human RNA viruses. The entire amino acid sequence and the three-dimensional structure of some of their proteins are known, as are the sequences of all their RNA segments. The influenza A virus genome consists, surprisingly, of *eight discrete segments* of single-stranded RNA of *negative polarity*. The size, coding assignment, and function of each of these segments, and most of their gene products, are known (Table 30.2).

Table 30.1
Comparison of influenza A, B and C viruses[a]

	A	B	C
Severity of illness	+ + + +	+ +	+
Animal reservoir	Yes	No	No
Spread in humans	Pandemic, epidemic	Epidemic	Sporadic
Antigenic changes	Shift, drift	Drift	Drift
No. of RNA segments	8	8	7
No. of surface glycoproteins	2	2	1

[a] Adapted from B. Murphy, unpublished data.

Figure 30.1. The structure of influenza virus detailing its surface proteins and segmented genome.

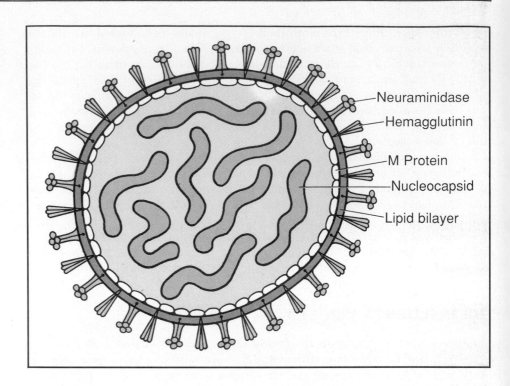

Neuraminidase

Hemagglutinin

M Protein

Nucleocapsid

Lipid bilayer

Table 30.2
Influenza virus RNA segments and their protein products

RNA Segment	Protein	Function and Location in Virion
1	Polymerase-B1	RNA synthesis; core protein
2	Polymerase-B2	RNA synthesis; core protein
3	Polymerase-B4	RNA synthesis; core protein
4	Hemagglutinin	Attachment to cell receptor; envelope
5	Nucleoprotein	RNA synthesis; core protein
6	Neuraminidase	Release of virus from cell; envelope
7	Matrix-1	Virus maturation? envelope
8	Nonstructural-1	RNA synthesis? nonstructural
	Nonstructural-2	? Nonstructural

How Do These Viruses Replicate?

Many biochemical and molecular aspects of the replication cycle of influenza virus have been elucidated. They illustrate important aspects of virus-host cell interaction and will be presented in some detail. Influenza infection starts with binding of the viral hemagglutinins to specific cell surface glycoprotein and/or glycolipid receptors. After binding to these receptors the viruses are engulfed in phagosomes, where they become uncoated. The acidic milieu of the lysosomes (which fuse with the phagosomes) alters the conformation of the viral hemagglutinins, uncovering peptide sequences that stimulate fusion of membranes. The result is that the viral membrane fuses with the phagolysosomal membrane, releasing the nucleocapsid cores into the cytoplasm. The next events, further uncoating of the virus and transport of the viral RNAs to the nucleus for replication, are not well understood.

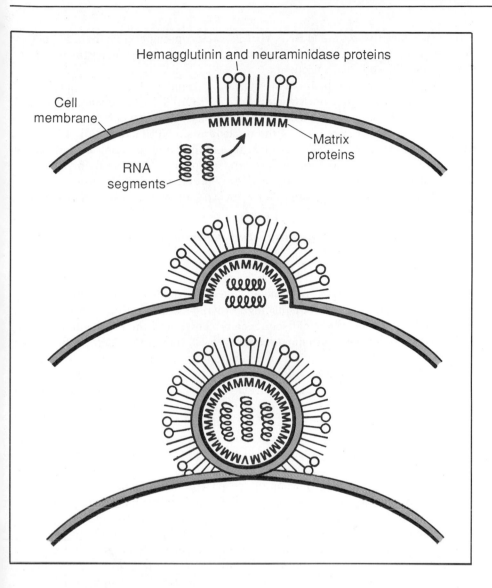

Hemagglutinin and neuraminidase proteins

Cell membrane

MMMMMMM

RNA segments

Matrix proteins

Figure 30.2. Assembly of influenza virus at the cell surface and subsequent release.

Replication of influenza viruses is set in motion within an hour after infection and begins with RNA transcription that uses the infecting RNA genome as the direct template. This cannot be carried out by any known host cell enzymes and requires an RNA-dependent RNA polymerase activity provided by components of the infecting viral core (polymerase proteins PB1 and PB2). The transcripts made are of positive polarity and serve as messengers for protein synthesis. Each is longer than the parental negative strands because after transcription its 5′ end is "capped" by the addition of methylated nucleotides and its 3′ end is polyadenylated.

Some of the details of the posttranscriptional modification of influenza mRNAs have been elucidated, and are revealing of how host cell and viruses interact. Influenza virus replication takes place in the nucleus. Apparently influenza mRNAs "steal" the methylated caps plus 10 to 13 of the first nucleotides from the 5′ ends of cellular mRNAs that had been synthesized and modified in the nucleus. The influenza viral enzymes involved in transcription, unlike those of many other negative-stranded RNA viruses, lack capping and methylating activities. Thus, as behooves an efficient parasite, this virus has evolved the ability to use some of the cell's own products.

Ultimately 10 transcripts are synthesized and translated in the cytoplasm into seven structural and three nonstructural proteins (Table 30.2). How are the special RNA molecules destined for packaging in progeny virions made? Apparently two viral proteins (polymerase PA and the nucleoprotein NP) facilitate the transcription of a special type of RNA, identical in length to the infecting strand. These full-length positive strands are neither capped nor polyadenylated and therefore cannot direct protein synthesis. Instead, they are copied directly, to yield RNAs of negative polarity that are suitable for incorporation into new virus particles.

Influenza Virus Hemagglutinin and Neuraminidase

The hemagglutinin and neuraminidase of these viruses are two of the best studied of all viral proteins, and are the most important determinants of influenza virulence. They migrate to the cell membrane to assemble in patches on the outer surface of the cell membrane, displacing normal cellular membrane proteins (Fig. 30.2). Their complete amino acid sequence is known and their three-dimensional conformation has been determined by x-ray crystallography. Each of the 400 or so hemagglutinin spikes of a virion are composed of three identical polypeptides. Each spike has a hydrophobic end, which is embedded in the lipid envelope, and a hydrophilic end, which projects outward. The hemagglutinin attaches to the cell receptor and antibodies directed against it neutralize virus infectivity. Some of the hemagglutinin sequence is highly conserved between influenza strains, but specific regions vary greatly, allowing serologic discrimination between virus types. These antigenic differences among hemagglutinins determine the extent of cross-reactive immunity, and therefore the severity of disease.

The other peplomer, the neuraminidase protein, looks like a square-topped, mushroom-like projection from the cell surface. Each peplomer comprises four identical peptides with hydrophobic feet embedded in the viral envelope, and a stalk with a hydrophilic head that projects outward. As with the hemagglutinin, variable domains of the neuraminidase are important for serotyping and immune recognition. The function of the neuraminidase is unknown but it seems to be important for releasing the virus from the infected cell, perhaps by removing receptors for the hemagglutinins on the cell surface. Antibodies to neuraminidase decrease the efficiency of virus spread both in culture and in tissues. Operationally, neuraminidase is recognized and defined by its ability to enzymatically cleave glycosialic bonds. This is assayed by addition of red blood cells to an influenza virus suspension. The red cells agglutinate but then disaggregate spontaneously at 37°C. Disaggregation is due to the neuraminidase, which cleaves the glycosialic bonds that formed between N-acetylneuraminic acid on the red cell surface and the viral hemagglutinin.

A third envelope-associated protein, the matrix protein, attaches to the inner aspect of the membrane, perhaps recognizing the presence of the viral polypeptides beyond. It might be considered a "scaffolding" protein on which viral nucleocapsids are constructed. As new copies of the viral genome are synthesized, they assemble together with the polymerase proteins and nucleoproteins at the inner cell membrane sites coated with the matrix protein. The virus gradually takes shape by the evagination of the altered cell membrane around the developing viral core. Ultimately, a new particle buds off from the cell surface.

How Do Influenza Viruses Get Assembled?

The assembly of infectious viruses that have multiple genome segments is a remarkable process. At least one copy of each of the different RNA segments must be packaged for the virion to be infectious. How a complete set of RNAs is selected is not known, but several possibilities can be imagined. If it were an entirely random process in which the assembling nucleocapsid were to entrap the first eight RNA segments that come along, the proportion of infectious virions would be very small. It has been estimated that this proportion is reasonably high for animal viruses, about 10% of the total particles, so this model cannot be correct. How, then, is it done? If all the segments were linked to each other by proteins they could be replicated together and then drawn into an assembling nucleocapsid like links of sausage. No evidence for such a nucleoprotein complex has been found. The hypothesis that is currently favored suggests that the influenza virus is so flexible in construction that it can package more than eight RNA segments. Some of the larger virions contain 15 segments or more. The probability of including a complete complement of gene segments into an assembling particle thus becomes much greater.

Antigenic Variation Among the Influenza Viruses

To understand intelligently the features of influenza epidemiology, you must understand one molecular feature of this virus that has been alluded to previously, namely, its seemingly unlimited capacity for antigenic change. While strains of many other viruses remain nearly identical year after year, influenza virus strains vary—sometimes slightly and sometimes enormously—from one year to the next. Variety is the way of life among these viruses.

Changes actually occur in several of the viral proteins, but the most easily assayed ones take place in the two outer envelope proteins, hemagglutinin and neuraminidase. The strains of virus involved in infection in any given outbreak are identified by the serologic properties of the two proteins. Slight variations in either protein are said to represent *antigenic drift*. A major change in the neuraminidase or hemagglutinin is termed *antigenic shift*.

Antigenic drift takes place in nature by changes in small, highly variable domains of the proteins, presumably through random point mutations in the nucleic acid and selection of strains that escape neutralization by the antibodies of the host. Major antigenic shifts are believed to result from an entirely different process, involving the mixture of genes from different virus strains. To understand this process, it is useful to recall that influenza virus contains a multisegmented genome. If a cell is infected simultaneously with two or more different influenza viruses, the RNA segments from each parental strain become shuffled and are dealt out to the progeny in random order. Each developing virus particle encapsulates some segments from both parental strains (Fig. 30.3). This process of *genetic reassortment* occurs with very high frequency. Successful reassortants in nature are ones that escape serological neutralization.

These mechanisms would be of no epidemiologic relevance unless people are likely to become infected with different influenza strains. What evidence is there that these processes occur in nature? What is the origin of the different coinfecting strains? First, we know that human influenza A strains are similar to animal influenza strains. In the laboratory, human and animal strains reassort readily

Figure 30.3. Genetic reassortment of influenza viral RNA segments. In this study, human (H) and avian (A) strains of influenza virus were used together to infect cells in culture. A recombinant (R) strain of progeny virus was derived. Each individual segment makes a separate band in gel electrophoresis (RNA 1, 2, 3). The recombinant strain contains some human and some avian RNA segments. Protein bands specific for each strain are also seen: HA (hemagglutinin), NA (neuraminidase), NP (part of nucleoprotein complex), M (major virion protein), NS (nonstructural protein).

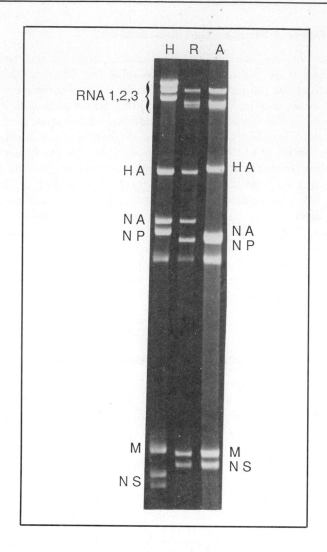

to generate hybrid progeny. Second, human influenza A strains have been re-covered from animals in the field. The influenza virus strain associated with the Great Spanish Influenza Pandemic of 1918–1919 apparently became adapted to infect swine, because pigs were later found to be infected with viruses related to the 1918 human strains. Third, strains recovered from wild ducks and horses are antigenically similar to strains later recovered during human epidemics. Thus, it is believed that animals provide a reservoir for influenza strains from which new genetic variants of human influenza virus can be drawn.

To understand this better, imagine a cell that is coinfected with a human and an avian influenza A virus. The hybrid that arises may contain the avian hem-agglutinin and neuraminidase genes but the remainder of the genes may be of the human virus type. Such a hybrid virus has no problem replicating efficiently in human cells. If humans had never been exposed to the avian hemagglutinin and neuraminidase antigens, such a hybrid virus would not be recognized by the immune system and could spread rapidly in the population. The possible result: an epidemic.

ENCOUNTER

With these molecular features as a background, it is possible to comprehend the complex pattern of influenza infection over the ages. More than a century ago, it was recognized that some epidemics of the disease are associated with higher than usual mortality from cardiopulmonary disease. This allows the tracking and recognizing of types of influenza epidemic from year to year. The Centers for Disease Control tabulates the total cardiopulmonary mortality for each week in each region of the United States. Almost every winter the expected mortality increases. When deaths in a region of the country exceed the expected level by a certain amount, an influenza epidemic is suspected in that region (Fig. 30.4). More precise characterization and proof of the onset of an epidemic are based on the recovery and antigenic typing of virus strains at sentinel clinics in each region of the country.

Through these surveillance mechanisms we have learned that influenza infection occurs in the United States on an annual basis, beginning typically in the fall and generally terminating in the late winter. In most years the influenza outbreaks are mild and sporadic, but every few years more severe epidemics develop. Pandemics (causing frequent disease worldwide) appear less frequently; in this century they arose in 1918, 1957, and 1968.

Thus, influenza may be *endemic* (present but causing relatively few cases), *epidemic* (affecting many people in one area), or *pandemic*. Why does this illness

Figure 30.4. The rate of death from respiratory disease in the United States from 1973 to 1976. A higher than expected rate of respiratory deaths indicates the occurrence of influenza epidemics.

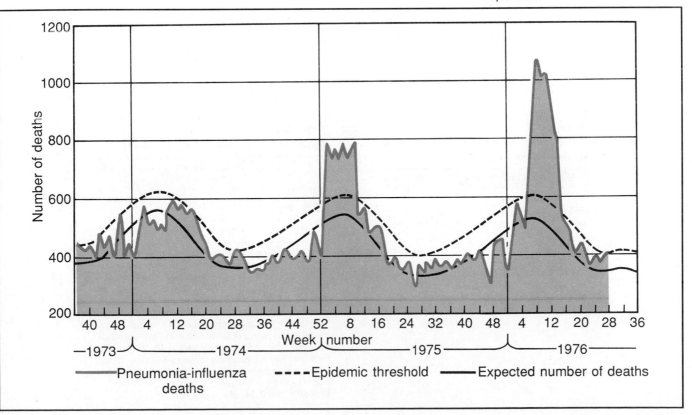

have three different patterns? The answer lies in the distribution of immunity in the population. Individuals who have been infected in the past with a specific strain of influenza virus become immune to that strain. If the same strain were to be reintroduced the next year, it would cause disease mainly among those who missed the earlier outbreak. For that year, influenza would be endemic. When antigenic drift occurs in the circulating influenza strains, the antigenic differences are sufficient to permit epidemics, because illness occurs even among those who developed some immunity from earlier infections. Major antigenic shifts, however, lead to pandemics. Since nearly the whole population is susceptible, many are likely to be infected.

The strains that cause illness each year are identified by the serologic properties of their neuraminidase and hemagglutinin. A uniform classification scheme has been adopted internationally for these antigens. New influenza strains are named by their type, city or country of first isolation, year of recovery, and hemagglutinin and neuraminidase subtypes. An example is the Hong Kong 1968 H3N2 strain. Thirteen different hemagglutinins (H1–H13) and nine different neuraminidase subtypes (N1–N9) have been recognized in viruses recovered from humans, swine, horses, and birds. Table 30.3 lists the influenza A virus strains associated with the most serious pandemics in this century. The influenza pandemic of 1957 that led to Ms. I.'s grandfather's death was associated with H2N2 virus. It was particularly severe and widespread because this virus was antigenically quite different from the earlier H1N1 virus.

Table 30.4 shows how minor and major antigenic changes can be measured and how these findings are reflected in the virulence of a circulating influenza A strain. In this example, stored sera collected from a large group of individuals in 1968 and 1972 were tested for their levels of antibodies directed against influenza A hemagglutinins. Lack of prior immunity to the new H3 strains in 1968 led to a pandemic. The partial immunity that existed in 1972 to new H3 strains that appeared by antigenic drift limited the spread and impact of the virus but

Table 30.3

Major antigenic shifts in influenza A strains in recent years

Year	Strain Designation	Common Name
1947	H1N1[a]	
1957	H2N2	Asian
1968	H3N2	Hong Kong
1976	$H_{sw}N1$	Swine
1977	H1N1	USSR

[a] H, hemagglutinin; N, neuraminidase.

Table 30.4

Antigenic change in influenza A strains [a,b]

Sera Tested in Year	Mean Hemagglutination Inhibition Titer to the Indicated Virus Strain		
	H2	$H3_{68}$	$H3_{72}$
1968	1:100	<1:10	<1:10
1972	1:100	1:80	1:30

[a] Each serum was tested against three influenza A virus strains; a strain containing an H2 type of hemagglutinin similar to that associated with the prior 1957 pandemic, the H3-containing strain associated with the 1968 pandemic and the similar but slightly different H3-containing strain associated with the 1972 epidemic. Sera obtained in 1968 prior to that year's pandemic contained, on the average, high levels of antibodies to the 1957 H2 strain but none to the newly appearing H3 strain. By 1972 the sera contained high antibody levels for the 1968 H3 proteins but reacted less effectively with the newly emerging H3 variant of that year.

[b] Adapted from B. Murphy, unpublished data.

an epidemic still occured among those with partial immunity and those (particularly children) who missed the 1968 pandemic.

ENTRY

Influenza can be transmitted to the nasopharynx of susceptible individuals by inhalation of large-particle aerosols, but the major vehicle for transmission is small-particle aerosols liberated during sneezes or coughs. Experimental observations suggest that small droplets are capable of reaching the terminal bronchioles and alveoli. If they contain a single infectious dose of virus, this may be sufficient to induce disease. It is possible that the virus can also be transmitted from hand to nose after touching virus-bearing objects. In general, young children are the most efficient transmitters of the infection, spreading it among their friends and to their families. Thus, in 1957 our patient Ms. I. may have been the index case for influenza in her family, having brought it home from school.

SPREAD, MULTIPLICATION, AND DAMAGE

Influenza viruses infect primarily upper and lower respiratory tract epithelial cells. Viral multiplication leads to lysis of these cells and to the release of viral antigens and destructive cellular enzymes. The host responds with an influx of macrophages and lymphocytes, followed by an outpouring of humoral mediators of inflammation, including interferon. This response helps to clear superinfecting bacteria and fungi, to inhibit virus replication and to destroy virally infected epithelial cells. Release of interleukin-1 from macrophages results in fever, while interferon probably causes the diffuse muscular aches and fatigue that is characteristic of influenza (which is one of the reasons for its limited therapeutic use). The inflammatory mediators provoke vasodilation and edema. In the nose this results in stuffiness and rhinorrhea. In the tracheobronchial tree the irritation caused by the debris and the host responses stimulates mucus production. The remaining undamaged ciliated epithelium and the cough reflexes help propel the mucus and debris upward. In areas where extensive destruction of epithelium has occurred superinfecting bacteria—especially virulent encapsulated ones—can gain a foothold, leading to secondary bacterial bronchitis or pneumonia.

The role of cellular immune responses in influenza is not known. Patients with cellular immune impairment are not at substantially increased risk for influenza infections. The humoral responses to the viral outer envelope proteins seem more important. The example in Table 30.4 shows that the presence of neutralizing antibody to hemagglutinin will protect against or limit infection. Antibody to the neuraminidase seems to modify the spread of virus through the respiratory tract and can prevent illness. Thus, in an individual with partial immunity to neuraminidase the disease may be restricted to the upper respiratory tract.

The bacterial superinfection that accompanies primary influenza pneumonia tends to be diffuse. Even if treated it carries a mortality rate in excess of 10%. More commonly, the bacterial pneumonia that complicates influenza infection is confined to a single pulmonary lobe and typically involves pneumococci, staphylococci, or *Haemophilus influenzae*; hence, the incorrect attribution of the cause of this disease a century ago to H. flu. These bacterial complications account for the increase in mortality associated with influenza each year. The demise in 1957 of Ms. I.'s grandfather was probably due to bacterial superinfection. Figure 30.5

Figure 30.5. The course of the 1918–1920 pandemic in Oregon is suggested by the relative thickness of the books tabulating deaths. In the three pandemic years, when the population of Oregon was under 800,000, there were 28,651 influenza cases, with 3,788 deaths.

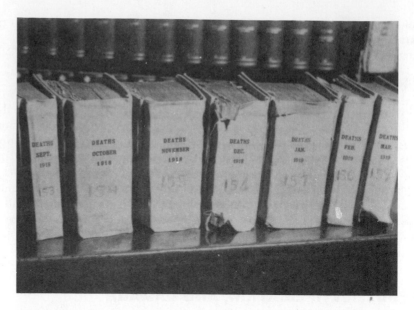

shows in a graphic way the dramatic increase in mortality in Oregon during the 1918–1919 pandemic.

DIAGNOSIS

The clinical manifestations of influenza virus infection strongly suggest the diagnosis. When flu is widespread throughout a community in the winter months, the diagnosis is likely to be correct. Definitive laboratory diagnoses are usually made for purposes of research or for epidemiologic surveillance. The virus can readily be recovered from nasopharyngeal swabs or washes by inoculation into cell cultures. Virus replication is detected by a simple assay for the expression of the viral hemagglutinin. Guinea pig red blood cells are added to the cultures and adhere to the surface of cultured cells in which influenza virus is replicating.

A variety of serologic techniques are available for diagnosing past influenza A infection. Hemagglutination inhibition (as used in Table 30.4) and neutralization are most often utilized. Their major value is in defining the serologic character of new virus strains and for seroepidemiologic surveillance.

PREVENTION AND TREATMENT

The major treatments for influenza infections are the time-proven ones involving hydration, rest, and antipyretics, especially acetaminophen rather than aspirin (to decrease the likelihood of the aspirin-associated postinfluenzal Reyes' syndrome). For most people these conservative measures are adequate. On the other hand, influenza A is the first virus for which successful systemic antiviral chemotherapy was developed. In the early 1960s, it was recognized that *amantadine* (Fig. 37.2), a compound now more widely utilized for the treatment of parkinsonism, effectively diminishes the duration and severity of influenza A infection. It is most effective when given prophylactically, before an individual is exposed to the virus, leading to a 70% to 80% reduction in the development of symptoms. As a therapeutic agent, it decreases the duration and severity of symptoms by about 50% if given promptly at the first signs of illness.

The precise mechanism by which amantadine exerts its antiviral effect is not known. The drug has been shown to interfere with early replicative events, including uncoating of the virions. A related compound, *rimantadine*, appears equally effective and has improved pharmacokinetics, so that there is a lower incidence of the mild confusion and dysphoria that attend amantadine use, particularly in the elderly individual. Unfortunately, both agents are active only against the influenza A strains of virus.

A different class of agent, represented by the nucleoside analog *ribavirin* (Fig. 37.2), is active against both influenza A and B viruses. In early trials of ribavirin in which the agent was inhaled as a fine-particle aerosol, there was evidence of rapid clearance of virus and resolution of symptoms.

Because of the worldwide impact of the disease, control of influenza is a major international effort. Under the auspices of the World Health Organization, sentinel clinics monitor and track the emergence and spread of influenza in both animals and humans. When this becomes evident in a country, local public health authorities announce cautionary warnings that the elderly or chronically impaired patients should avoid contact with individuals with upper respiratory infections. Prophylaxis with amantadine can be initiated in high-risk susceptible people.

The most powerful thrust of the influenza control program focuses on vaccination. The current vaccines contain viral hemagglutinin and neuraminidase proteins from killed virus. These vaccines reduce the incidence and morbidity of influenza by about 75%. The major problem with these vaccines is that they do not provide permanent immunity to the disease. The fault is not with the vaccines themselves, which provide relatively durable immunity, but with the antigenic variations of the virus. Authorities in the United States convene each year to review data on worldwide influenza patterns and attempt to predict the strains that are likely to emerge in the coming season. There is then a frantic effort to prepare adequate vaccine for those strains in time for the onset of the next influenza season. The vaccine formula is altered yearly, and vaccination must be performed annually to afford maximal protection.

Most Americans are not vaccinated and do not require the vaccine. Many of those who would benefit from vaccination are either apathetic or fear federally sponsored vaccine programs. Some of the recent fear stems from the apparent increase in cases of Guillain-Barré syndrome, a rare neurological complication of vaccination, in the year following nationwide use of the swine influenza vaccine in the mid-1970s. The fear that the vaccine was responsible for this serious neurological problem still discourages some individuals from obtaining the appropriate vaccination.

Newer classes of vaccines are being studied. More effective than the killed virus vaccines are live, attenuated vaccines, which can be rapidly prepared for each season. The vaccine viruses grow and divide in the recipient and induce potent cell-mediated, as well as humoral immune, responses. Thus, they are likely to induce greater and more durable immunity than the current influenza vaccines. Further field trials are necessary before these new vaccines are approved.

CONCLUSION

We can now answer all of Ms. I.'s concerns about influenza. It is unlikely that she and her family will experience severe influenza at this time since substantially altered strains enter the community only infrequently. These new strains develop by mutation and genetic reassortment. It is the antigenic differences in these strains that permit them to infect individuals who have had prior influenza infection. Because Ms. I.'s parents are elderly, they should seek medical consultation for annual vaccination, and, if the influenza season has already begun, possibly receive amantadine prophylaxis along with vaccination. If any of the family members become infected, amantadine treatment should be considered on a case-by-case basis.

SELF-ASSESSMENT QUESTIONS

1. Describe the structure of influenza viruses and their replication cycle. What is peculiar about them?

2. Why do influenza epidemics recur? What causes influenza pandemics?

3. What role do hemagglutinin and neuraminidase play in the pathogenesis of influenza?

4. Compare antigenic drifts and shifts in influenza with antigenic variation in the fimbriae of the gonococcus (Chapter 2) and with the generation of immunological diversity (Chapter 5).

5. Discuss the immune response in influenza.

6. How would you counsel elderly patients about the need for influenza vaccination?

SUGGESTED READINGS

Crosby AW, Jr: *Epidemic and Peace, 1918.* Westport, CT, Greenwood Press, 1976.

Dolin R, Reichman RC, Madore HP, et al: A controlled trial of amantadine and rimantadine in the prophylaxis of influenza A infection. *N Engl J Med* 307:580–584, 1982.

Kilbourne ED (ed): *The Influenza Viruses and Influenza.* New York, Academic Press, 1975.

Louria DB, Blumenfeld HL, Ellis JT, Kilbourne ED, Rogers DE: Studies on influenza in the pandemic of 1957–1958. II. Pulmonary complications of influenza. *J Clin Invest* 38:213–265, 1959.

Palese P, Young JF: Variation of influenza A, B, and C viruses. *Science* 215:1468–1474, 1982.

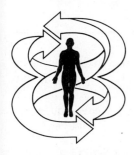

CHAPTER 31

Herpes Simplex Virus and Its Relatives

S.E. Straus

The term "herpesvirus" refers to several human and animal viruses, the most widely known of which is the causative agent of herpes simplex. This disease has two main manifestations, fever blisters and a genital infection. Other herpesviruses cause important diseases, including infectious mononucleosis, cytomegalovirus infection, and chickenpox. These viruses persist for life in cells of the host, producing a latent infection that can be reactivated at intervals.

CASE

Mr. H., a 26-year-old graduate student, returned home from his first real vacation in years. A lot of rest, fresh air and a new love. But now, several days after his last sexual contact he notices painful, itchy sores are developing on the shaft of his penis. He had engaged in oral sex as well and among his other symptoms is a sore throat. During a difficult telephone call his new girlfriend admits to past episodes of genital herpes. "Could this be herpes?" he wonders. He has heard a lot about herpes infections and knows there are several types and that some recur.

What do you need to know to help Mr. H. with his many questions?

1. Many microorganisms can cause genital lesions.

2. Two types of herpes simplex viruses can cause genital lesions.

3. These viruses are both fundamentally similar to and yet different from other herpes viruses.

407

4. Herpes infections are unique in their ability to recur many times.

5. Treatment is still limited, and we do not know how to prevent the infections.

These and other aspects of herpesvirus infections will be covered in this chapter.

Despite recent public awareness, herpesviruses are not new causes of human disease. Oral infections similar to what we recognize as being associated with herpes simplex were well described in ancient Greek medical texts. Herpes is probably what Shakespeare had in mind in Romeo and Juliet (Act I, scene iv):

> O'er ladies' lips, who straight on kisses dream
> Which oft the angry Mab with blisters plagues

Today we know that most humans become infected with herpesviruses during their lifetime. The herpesviruses that cause common oral and genital infections are called herpes simplex viruses. They are the best understood of all herpesviruses and are the major focus of this chapter; but there are other herpesviruses. In fact, there are dozens of different ones capable of infecting just about every animal from oysters to humans, causing a varied repertoire of diseases. Two *herpes simplex* virus types cause common infections of the skin and mucous membranes. The *varicella-zoster* virus causes chickenpox and shingles. *Cytomegalovirus* causes hepatitis, pneumonia, and serious congenital infections. The *Epstein-Barr* virus is best known as a cause of infectious mononucleosis, but is also thought to be involved in certain human cancers. A sixth herpesvirus called the *human herpesvirus type 6* has been recently described but little is known of the spectrum of disease it may provoke.

Herpesviruses are among the most frequent and constant viral companions of human beings. It is not surprising that they are also among the most interesting.

Table 31.1
Human herpesviruses

Herpes simplex virus 1 (HSV 1)
Herpes simplex virus 2 (HSV 2)
Varicella-zoster virus (VZV)
Cytomegalovirus (CMV)
Epstein-Barr virus (EBV)
Herpesvirus type 6 (HHV6)

THE HERPESVIRUSES

Herpesviruses are relatively large, complex viruses with a double-stranded DNA molecule that is able to code for 50 to 80 proteins (Fig. 31.1, Table 31.1). They replicate and assemble in the nuclei of cells; they then bud through and become enveloped in portions of the nuclear and cytoplasmic membranes. One cannot distinguish between different herpesviruses by electron microscopy—they all look alike (Fig. 31.2). They can be distinguished, however, by serological and DNA hybridization tests. Most herpesviruses are relatively unrelated, either by their antigens or their DNA homology. The exceptions are the two herpes simplex viruses, types 1 and 2, which are quite similar to each other. Antibodies raised to proteins of type 1 react with many of the proteins of type 2 virus. Proteins that are totally unique to each type have been identified recently. The DNA of one herpes simplex type hybridizes to DNA of the other type with about half the avidity that it hybridizes to itself. The issue of the relatedness of herpes simplex viruses 1 and 2 is not merely academic. The two viruses cause nearly identical diseases, but the reason for their different but overlapping clinical manifestations is still a mystery, despite our knowledge of much of their genetic makeup.

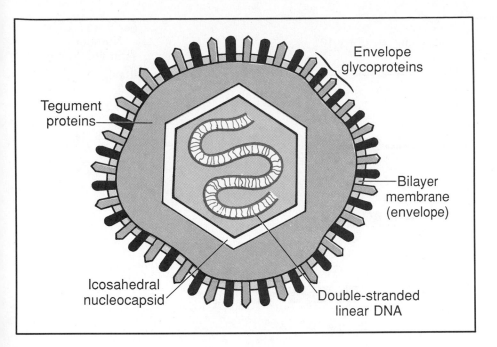

Figure 31.1. Schematic drawing of a herpesvirus.

The genomes of the five well-defined human herpesviruses have a unique organization: They are long, double-stranded linear molecules with several repeated and inverted sequences (Fig. 31.3). The DNA can be conveniently considered as having two stretches of unique sequence, one long (*unique long sequence*, U_L) and one that is much shorter (*unique short sequence*, U_S). Each of these is bracketed by short, identical DNA repeats. For example, at the left-hand end of the herpes simplex U_L is a short terminal repeat. An exact copy of this sequence is repeated backwards at the right-hand end of the U_L segment. (A perusal of Figure 31.3 is recommended.) To complicate things further, in some

Figure 31.2. Electron micrograph of a herpesvirus.

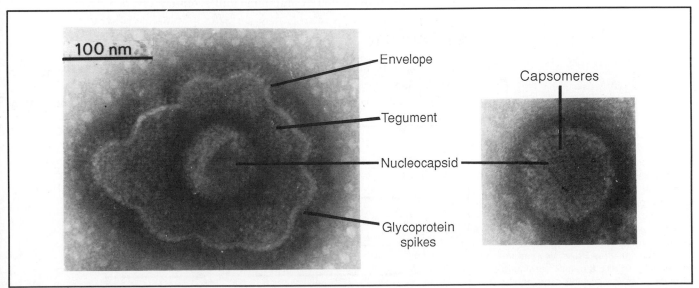

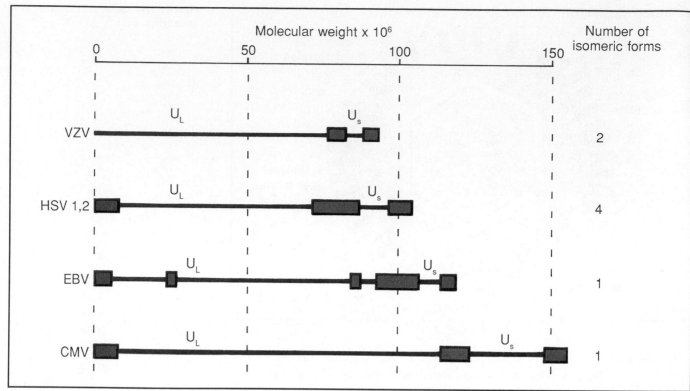

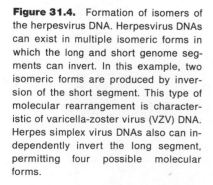

Figure 31.3. The size and organization of herpesvirus genomes. The five human herpesviruses are compared by size, in megadaltons; organization of the unique long (U_L), unique short (U_S), and repeat sequences; and the number of isomeric forms of the genome.

herpesviruses, each major segment (U_L or U_S) and its terminal repeats can be rearranged in the DNA either in the forward or the backward direction (Fig. 31.4). In herpes simplex, the various arrangements of the major segments result in four isomeric forms of the genome. All of the sequences are present, whatever the isomeric form of each herpesvirus. We have no idea why this has evolved, but the rearrangements of the DNA during viral replication may provide greater opportunity for the introduction of mutations and evolution of the genome.

ENCOUNTER

Infection with one or more herpesviruses probably occurs sooner or later in every human. Herpes simplex virus type 1 is often spread by kissing or exchange of saliva very early in life. Most children acquire the virus, but if they

Figure 31.4. Formation of isomers of the herpesvirus DNA. Herpesvirus DNAs can exist in multiple isomeric forms in which the long and short genome segments can invert. In this example, two isomeric forms are produced by inversion of the short segment. This type of molecular rearrangement is characteristic of varicella-zoster virus (VZV) DNA. Herpes simplex virus DNAs also can independently invert the long segment, permitting four possible molecular forms.

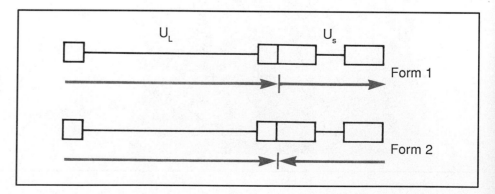

have avoided doing so they have another opportunity to do so when they become sexually active, either through oral-oral or oral-genital contact. Two-thirds to three-fourths of adults possess antibodies to herpes simplex 1, indicating prior infection. Herpes type 2 is also spread by oral-oral and oral-genital contact, but is primarily spread by genital-genital contact. It is uncommon before adolescence, but the prevalence of infection rises rapidly with sexual activity. About one-fourth to one-half of all adults have experienced infection with this virus.

Most infections with herpes simplex viruses are asymptomatic. Perhaps only a fourth of the individuals who harbor the virus recognize symptoms from it. Clinically evident infection with herpes type 2 is increasing, however. Rough estimates suggest about a 10-fold increase from about 1965 to 1985.

ENTRY

Herpesviruses are very fragile and susceptible to drying and inactivation by heat, mild detergent, and solvents. This susceptibility is imposed by their membrane envelope. Because the viruses do not survive well on environmental surfaces, infection with the herpesviruses requires *direct inoculation* of virus into areas where they can replicate. Herpesviruses can infect humans by a variety of different routes (Table 31.2). Mucous membranes of the mouth, eye, genitals, respiratory tract, and anus are the sites most readily infected by herpes simplex viruses. The first line of defense we mount against herpes simplex is our skin. Normal skin is not readily penetrated or infected by herpes simplex viruses. It is likely that the thick, horny keratin layer of the superficial epidermis prevents access of these viruses to their receptors. The mucous membranes do not represent such a formidable barrier, and hence are more readily infected. Thus, our patient, Mr. H., probably acquired genital herpes during sexual contact with the infected tissues of his girlfriend.

Cytomegalovirus and EBV can be transmitted by infected leukocytes during transfusion with blood products, or through saliva and probably semen as well. It is believed that saliva is the most common vehicle for transmitting Epstein-Barr virus, which is why the major disease associated with this virus, *infectious mononucleosis*, is occasionally called the "kissing disease". Inhalation of viruses borne in aerosols seems to be the way most individuals contract chickenpox (varicella). However, direct inoculation is possible here too. Thus the mucous membranes of the respiratory tract provide the primary line of defense. Direct

Table 31.2
Transmission of human herpesviruses

Virus	Means of Transportation	Portal of Entry	Initial Target Cells
HSV 1	Direct contact	Mucous membranes, skin	Epithelial
HSV 2	Direct contact	Mucous membranes, skin	Epithelial
VZV	Inhalation, direct contact	Respiratory tract, ? mucous membranes	Epithelial
CMV	Saliva, blood, ? urine, ? semen	Bloodstream, mucous membranes	Neutrophil, monocyte, others
EBV	Saliva, blood	Mucous membranes, blood stream	B lymphocyte, salivary glands

inoculation or ingestion of virus-bearing materials would first challenge either mucosal or circulating defenses, as the case may be.

MULTIPLICATION AND SPREAD

The replication of herpesviruses is complex and not completely understood, but it resembles that of other large DNA viruses (Fig. 31.5). A *lytic* or *productive cycle* of infection begins with the attachment of virus particles to susceptible cells. The virions interact with specific receptors via glycoproteins that project from the viral envelope. As with most viruses, we do not know much about these receptors nor why they have evolved at all. In the case of the Epstein-Barr virus they are present on B lymphocytes, where they also serve as receptors for complement proteins.

Following binding of the virus to the cell surface, the viral core is transported to the cell nucleus where virus-specific synthetic processes are orchestrated. As with all other viruses, the herpes simplex virus genes are transcribed and translated into proteins in an orderly program, leading ultimately to the production of new progeny virions. Unlike many other viruses, newly formed herpesvirus particles are not efficiently released into the extracellular space. Rather, *virions spread from cell to cell* at points of contiguous cell contact. This phenomenon has several important implications for the pathogenesis of disease associated with each herpesvirus and the host responses to infection by them. Diseases induced

Figure 31.5. Productive infection of a cell by a herpesvirus.

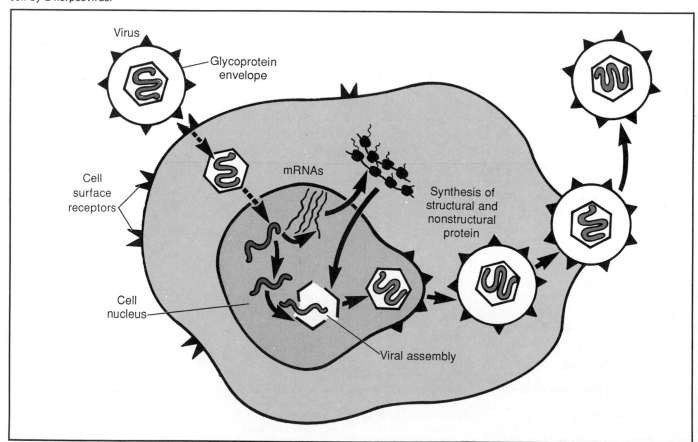

by herpes simplex virus, for example, involve local spread and progression of lesions. These are not systemic illnesses. Infection at multiple distant sites is rare with herpes simplex and probably requires the circulation of infected cells rather than of free virus. Chickenpox, cytomegalovirus, and Epstein-Barr viruses induce multisystem diseases—a feature that may be due in part to their ability to infect and be transported in circulating leukocytes.

Viruses that are released from cells into the extracellular space can be neutralized by circulating antibody. Because herpesviruses are hardly ever found outside of cells, antibody is of little value in limiting the duration or severity of infections by these viruses.

How Do Host Defenses Limit the Severity of Infection?

The immune response to herpes infections is multifaceted and incompletely understood. Host defenses are adequate to limit the duration and severity of infection and, in some people, are capable of preventing symptomatic recurrences. Within several days of the onset of a herpesvirus infection, antibodies to some of the viral proteins appear in the circulation. However, these antibodies develop too late to modify the infection and have no role in its recurrence. In fact, persons who fail to make antibodies, the agammaglobulinemics, have no special problems with herpesviruses. The likely reason is that these viruses spread from cell to cell and provide little opportunity for antibodies to come in contact with them. The only phase in the cycle of herpesvirus infection when the virus is extracellular virus is during the initial encounter. At that time antibodies can prevent infection. For this reason, antisera to herpesviruses are administered prophylactically to persons who are at risk of severe infection (see "Prevention"). Overall, cellular immune mechanisms are the more important determinants of the severity of the infection and of the likelihood of recurrence.

Certain lymphocytes can lyse cells in which herpesviruses are replicating. They do so by detecting the "foreign" viral antigens that are displayed on the surfaces of the infected cells. Between infections the herpesviruses remain hidden from immune recognition and establish a latent infection. The virus of herpes simplex, for example, persists in cells of neural ganglia. Somehow, neurons seem to avoid immune recognition and killing by lymphocytes, possibly because part of each neuron is protected by the blood-brain barrier and most of each axon is sheathed in myelin layers. Whatever the reason, the viruses here dwell in a stable privileged reservoir.

The ability to mount an adequate cellular immune response to herpesviruses changes with age. The relevant immune effector cells gradually mature during the first month of an infant's life. Until this maturation is complete, herpes infections can be devastating. Neonatal herpes simplex infection is often fatal. By 1 month of age, however, the infant tolerates the virus well. On the other hand, reactivation of varicella virus to give the so-called zoster infection occurs with increasing frequency as the patient ages, perhaps providing another indicator of the changes in the immune response with age. The likelihood of having zoster is about 10 times greater at age 80 than at age 8.

Do interferons play a role in these diseases? These proteins are found in the blood of some patients who are infected systemically with herpesviruses, and they can be detected in the fluid of herpes simplex-induced blisters. Interferons are released both from virally infected epithelial cells and from defending lymphocytes, but their role in the spontaneous limitation of herpesvirus infections in humans is not known. However, large doses of interferon preparations can ameliorate serious varicella, zoster, and cytomegalovirus infection, indicating that these proteins have defensive value.

DAMAGE

Herpes simplex viruses can be destructive. Epithelial cells in which the virions replicate are ultimately lysed. Under the microscope, changes can be observed in such productively infected cells: Their nuclei become enlarged and distorted by viral cores and aggregates of nucleoproteins. Gradually the nuclear membrane dissolves and the cell swells and ruptures, but not before virus spreads to infect contiguous cells. Thus, a major component of the symptoms and signs of herpes simplex virus infection is the destruction of superficial epithelial cells in skin and mucous membranes. The spreading viruses quickly affect regional nerve cells as well, and some of the symptoms of herpes infections may result from damage to these nerves or from the inflammation that surrounds them. The symptoms include itching, tingling, burning, and pain. The host defenses mounted to limit the infection may also contribute to the severity of symptoms and lesions. Degranulation of leukocytes and release of mediators in response to local viral infection augment the tissue swelling and inflammation.

Herpes Simplex Virus Infections

Now to return to your patient, Mr. H. Because immune responses take time to evolve, it can be predicted that healing of all his lesions will require 2 to 3 weeks in a primary infection. Although the outward manifestations of infection disappear completely, Mr. H. will still carry the virus in the sacral ganglia and he may have recurrent sores in the genital area an average of three to four times per year for many years (Table 31.3). Because antibody- and cellular-mediated immune responses are elicited during the primary infection, these later recurrences are typically briefer and milder, lasting an average of 7 to 10 days in all. The immune responses, however, are not adequate to prevent recurrent infection in all individuals.

Table 31.3

Stages in herpes simplex infection

1. Acute mucocutaneous infection
2. Spread to local sensory nerve endings
3. Establishment and maintenance of neuronal latency
4. Reactivation of virus and distal spread
5. Recurrent cutaneous infection

Table 31.4

Infections associated with herpes simplex viruses

Infection	Predominant Virus Type	Frequency	Age Group	Usual Outcome	Recurrence
Ocular herpes	1	Common	All	Resolution, visual impairment	Yes
Oral herpes	1 > 2	Very common	All	Resolution	Yes
Genital herpes	2 > 1	Common	Adolescents, adults	Resolution	Yes
Neonatal herpes	2 > 1	Very rare	0–4 weeks	Developmental impairment	No
Meningo-encephalitis	2	Uncommon	Adolescents, adults	Resolution	No
Encephalitis	1	Very rare	All	Severe neurologic impairment, death	No
Disseminated herpes	1 > 2	Rare	All	Resolution or death	No

This describes a typical genital herpes infection in an adult. Herpes simplex virus may induce somewhat different conditions depending upon the body site, age, and general host immune capacity (Table 31.4). Herpes simplex viruses may infect nearly any area of the skin. A common site of infection, particularly in health care workers, is the finger tip, acquired by touching active herpetic lesions in patients. These infections, known as *herpetic whitlows*, can be exceedingly painful because there is little room in the finger tip for swelling of inflamed tissues.

Herpes can infect the conjunctiva and cornea of the eye, a condition known as *herpetic keratoconjunctivitis*. This infection causes inflammation and swelling in the superficial tissues of the anterior eye, with potential scarring and loss of vision.

Under special circumstances, herpes can cause severe and life-threatening infections. Like the newborn, patients with lymphomas, leukemias, or AIDS have inadequate cellular immune defenses. In these individuals, the infection can spread widely across the skin and to vital viscera, especially the lungs, esophagus, liver, and brain.

A rare form of herpes simplex virus disease involves reactivation of virus, presumably from the trigeminal ganglion, and its ascent into the brain, rather than the usual descent to the mouth. *Encephalitis* ensues, characterized by an unusually progressive and destructive inflammation of a unilateral and focal nature. This condition is usually deadly if untreated.

WHY DO HERPES INFECTIONS RECUR?

Perhaps the most remarkable aspect of herpesvirus infection is the ability of the virus to persist in humans for life. The reason for this persistence is that the virus can initiate a *latent* type of infectious cycle in selected cells, one which is distinct from the productive type just reviewed. In the case of herpes simplex the virus spreads to infect nerve endings early in the course of the initial mucocutaneous infection (Table 31.3). As hosts for herpes simplex virus, nerve cells are very different from epithelial cells. Rather than permitting a full replicative cycle culminating in the release of progeny virions, most infected neurons develop an abortive or latent infection. The process is not well defined, but it appears that only one or a few viral genes are expressed. Viral DNA is not synthesized in this process, nor are progeny virions produced. The viral DNA remains stably associated with the neuronal nucleus. It is not known whether it is physically integrated into the chromosomes or remains a separate plasmid-like element, replicating rarely if at all in these nondividing cells.

Similar types of latent infections occur with each of the other human herpesviruses. Varicella-zoster viruses also reside in sensory neurons, while cytomegaloviruses reside in neutrophils and monocytes. The Epstein-Barr viruses are harbored in B lymphocytes and salivary gland cells. This latent infection *persists for life*. Autopsy studies reveal that nearly all individuals who have been infected with herpes simplex virus harbor the viral DNA in selected nerve ganglia. The trigeminal (V) ganglia are the most commonly affected sites (Fig. 31.6), followed by certain sacral root ganglia. These are the nerves that serve the ocular and oral (trigeminal) and genital (sacral root) regions, the sites of most common herpes simplex infection. Under certain circumstances, such as when there are breaks in the skin or open wounds, herpes simplex can penetrate and infect any body site.

Figure 31.6. The sites of active and latent facial herpes simplex infections.

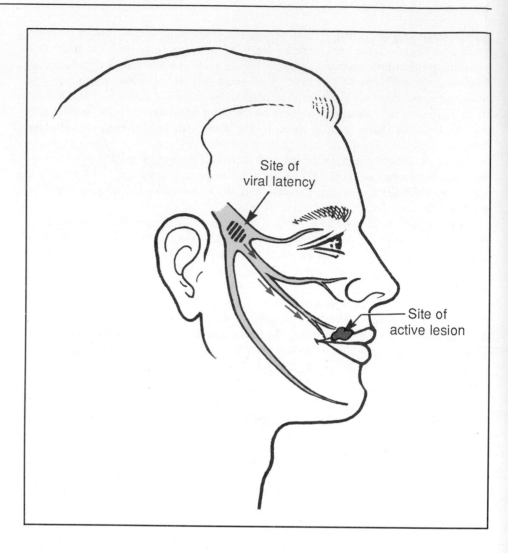

The virus will establish a latent infection in the sensory nerves serving any such area.

Occasionally, latency is interrupted. Certain factors trigger the *reactivation* of latent herpes simplex virus and produce symptoms. These stimuli include sunburn, systemic infections, immune impairment, emotional stress, and menstruation. We do not know how these seemingly unrelated factors induce viral reactivation. Reactivated herpes simplex viruses travel down the axonal processes and bud off from the nerve endings to spread to and infect contiguous mucocutaneous epithelial cells. If the amount of newly replicated virus is small, symptoms are less likely to develop. As you may know personally, symptomatic recurrences of fever blisters are common.

The ability of herpes simplex to establish a lifelong latent infection and to undergo episodic reactivation is one of the most fundamental facts that must be imparted to your patient, Mr. H. He must know that he is likely to experience repeated episodes of genital herpes, each of which renders him potentially contagious.

INFECTIONS CAUSED BY OTHER HERPESVIRUSES

Each of the other herpesviruses causes important and unique clinical syndromes that will be reviewed briefly (Table 31.5). Varicella-zoster virus, as the name implies, is associated with only two diseases, *chickenpox* (varicella) and *shingles* (zoster). Chickenpox is a familiar, annoying disease of childhood which results in the appearance of vesicles in the skin. It can be serious in immunodeficient patients. Eighty to 90% of all Americans experience chickenpox by adult age. The infection is rarely asymptomatic. Shingles is caused by the reactivation of latent varicella virus in less than 10% of infected people. It generally involves a rash similar to that of varicella, but it is painful and restricted to the skin area served by a single sensory nerve root in which the virus had lain dormant. The risk of this disease rises sharply with age. In the compromised host, zoster infection can disseminate to cause severe infections.

Most *cytomegalovirus* infections result in few if any symptoms. However, there is a series of well-defined syndromes associated with this in individuals of different age and risk category. About 1% of infections occur in utero, due to transplacental transmission of virus from a mother experiencing primary or reactivation cytomegalovirus infection. The newborn may suffer from hemolytic anemias, thrombocytopenia, hepatitis, splenomegaly, rash and developmental disorders. Infection is common in early childhood, particularly in day-care settings. In the population as a whole about 60% have been infected by age 40.

Severe visceral infections with cytomegalovirus also occur in transplant recipients, leukemia and lymphoma patients, and AIDS patients. Adolescents and young adults with cytomegalovirus infection develop hepatitis or a mononucleosis-like illness with fever, sore throat, enlarged lymph nodes, and an increase

Table 31.5
Infections associated with other herpesviruses

Virus	Syndrome	Frequency	Age Group	Tissues Involved	Usual Outcome
Cytomegalovirus	Congenital infection	Uncommon	Newborn	Brain, eye, liver, spleen, others	Developmental problems, death
	Mononucleosis	Common	Adolescent, adult	Lymph nodes, liver	Resolution
	Hepatitis	Uncommon	Adolescent, adult	Liver	Resolution
	Pneumonia	Very common	All	Lung	Death
	Retinitis	Very common	All	Eye	Blindness
Epstein-Barr virus	Mononucleosis	Common	All	Lymph nodes, liver, spleen	Resolution
	Lymphomas	Very rare	All	Lymph nodes, liver, spleen, brain	Death
Varicella-zoster virus	Chickenpox	Very common	All	Skin, others uncommon	Resolution, rarely death
	Shingles (zoster)	Common	Older adults	Skin, nerves, others very uncommon	Resolution, chronic pain, Rarely death

in the number of circulating lymphocytes, some of which have an atypical appearance. These disorders are particularly prevalent in young homosexual men, nearly all of whom eventually acquire the virus.

Epstein-Barr virus is also very common. Nearly all children in developing nations are infected before age 5. In industrialized countries the infection is delayed, occurring in only one-half of people by college age, but in more than 90% by age 40. Epstein-Barr virus infection in early childhood tends to be mild or asymptomatic. However, if the first exposure to Epstein-Barr virus is delayed until adolescence or early adult age, the expression of the infection is dramatically different. *Infectious mononucleosis* often ensues. This syndrome is similar to that caused by cytomegalovirus, with sore throat, fever, and swollen glands. Atypical lymphocytes (reactive T cells) circulate in high number, as do "heterophile" antibodies, which, as the name implies, have broad reactivities and are not specific for Epstein-Barr virus antigens. The appearance of heterophile antibodies reflects the general (polyclonal) stimulation of B lymphocytes to start synthesizing immunoglobulin of diverse specificity, including antibodies to the red blood cells of several different animals. These serve as the basis for simple and rapid diagnostic tests involving hemagglutination.

A new B-lymphotropic virus, herpesvirus type 6, has been recently discovered. Little is known about it, but it appears to be associated with lymphoproliferative disorders. Thus, the herpesviruses as a group have many features in common. They are ubiquitous, generally cause mild diseases that can recur, and are especially problematic for patients with cellular immune deficiencies.

HERPESVIRUSES AND CANCER

Earlier, we reviewed two major types of infection with herpesviruses, namely, productive and latent infections. In vitro most herpesviruses can also initiate an additional and important type of infectious cycle known as a *transforming infection*. Herpesviruses (especially the Epstein-Barr virus) transform cells in culture, causing them to take on features of malignant tissues. The cells are morphologically altered, become "immortalized," and have different nutritional requirements. It is not really known if this type of infectious cycle actually takes place in humans and leads to malignant disease. Herpesviruses, or at least their proteins or genes, have been found in human cancer cells, but we are not certain whether they induce cancer themselves, participate in cancer induction, or are merely not-so-innocent bystanders. Cytomegalovirus is found in many cases of Kaposi's sarcoma. Herpes simplex type 2 infection has been linked to cervical carcinoma, but it is likely that other factors such as papillomaviruses are more important in the pathogenesis of this cancer. The Epstein-Barr virus has been found in the cancerous cells in Burkitt's lymphoma and nasopharyngeal carcinoma. Burkitt's lymphoma is a common tumor of children in central Africa. In fact, the nearly universal association of African Burkitt's lymphoma with the Epstein-Barr virus is the strongest reason for believing that a human cancer may be caused by a herpesvirus.

DIAGNOSIS

The astute clinician who understands the biology and pathophysiology of herpes simplex virus infection will have little difficulty in diagnosing herpes. In the case of Mr. H. the history and physical examination were all that was required

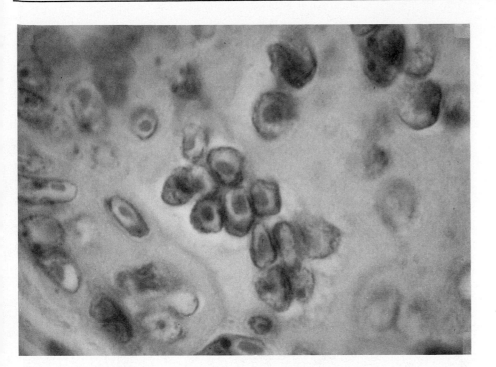

Figure 31.7. Photomicrograph of a biopsy of a skin lesion from a patient with herpes simplex infection. Numerous multinucleated cells containing eosinophilic intranuclear inclusions are apparent.

to suggest herpes. To establish the diagnosis one must demonstrate the presence of virus or its components in active lesions. Scrapings of lesions like Mr. H.'s can be examined microscopically for multinucleated giant cells whose nuclei contain *eosinophilic inclusions* (Fig. 31.7), the hallmark of herpes replication in tissues. Scrapings can also be stained with specific fluorescein-labeled antisera, which will bind to viral proteins and fluoresce when examined with a microscope with an ultraviolet light source.

The definitive diagnostic tool is virus isolation in cell culture (Fig. 31.8). Herpes simplex virus grows well in a wide variety of fibroblastic and epithelial cell lines from animals or humans. Replicating viruses induce the type of deformity and cell destruction described earlier. The appearance of these cytopathic changes characteristic of herpes simplex allows definitive diagnosis.

PREVENTION

Herpesviruses are ubiquitous, and it is not practical to avoid contact with all individuals with herpes infections. It is appropriate, however, to avoid sexual contact during active genital herpes infections. Unfortunately, safe and effective vaccines have not been developed for herpes simplex viruses. Even if an effective vaccine were available, it would probably not help those with existing infection. It is unlikely that a vaccine could induce a better immune response than a natural infection, which does not suffice to prevent recurrence.

Other herpesvirus infections can be prevented in selected situations. Severe chickenpox in immunodeficient children can be partially prevented by administration of specific human immune globulin promptly after exposure. A live, attenuated varicella vaccine has proven effective in normal and immunologically impaired (leukemic) children. For it to be safe and sufficiently effective in

Figure 31.8. Rabbit kidney cells (**A** and **B**) and human diploid fibroblasts (**C** and **D**) before (**A** and **C**) and after (**B** and **D**) inoculation with herpes simplex virus type 2. (From Hsiung GD, Mayo DR, Lucia HL, Landry ML: Genital herpes: pathogenesis and chemotherapy in a guinea pig model. *Rev Infect Dis* 6:33–50, 1984.)

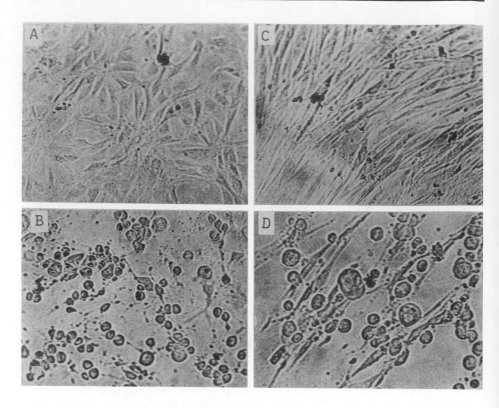

leukemics, the vaccine must be administered at times when there are reasonable numbers of circulating lymphocytes, such as after a course of chemotherapy has been completed. Live, attenuated vaccines for cytomegalovirus are being studied and may be useful for certain high risk individuals.

TREATMENT

Antiviral therapy is still a primitive science. The first glimmers of hope, however, have been in the treatment of herpes simplex virus infections. Nucleoside analogs (see Chapter 37) have been developed that are preferentially utilized by viral synthetic pathways. The most useful drug to be studied extensively in man is *acyclovir*.

Mr. H. should be given acyclovir because treatment significantly decreases the duration and severity of first episodes of genital herpes. Acyclovir, however, is not a cure. It does not prevent entry of virus into nerve ganglia nor does it remove virus once there. Therefore, patients treated with acyclovir remain susceptible to later recurrences. Long-term treatment with acyclovir pills will suppress most recurrences, and this regimen would be useful for Mr. H. if his recurrences were very frequent.

Severe varicella-zoster infections in the immunocompromised host can be ameliorated by intravenous acyclovir or vidarabine, another nucleoside analog with antiherpes activity. Treatment of Epstein-Barr virus infections has not been widely explored, but the available agents are not likely to be potent enough to affect these diseases significantly. There is a desperate need for effective treatments for cytomegalovirus infections, as they contribute significantly to the morbidity and mortality of transplant recipients and patients with AIDS. At present we have one drug for cytomegalovirus infection. It is an analog of acyclovir that is effective in preventing retinal infections by this virus in AIDS patients. Unfortunately, it is too toxic for use in milder infections by cytomegalovirus.

CONCLUSIONS

Mr. H. has genital herpes, one of the common sexually transmitted diseases, most often caused by herpesvirus type 2. His symptoms may become ameliorated with acyclovir but recurrence of the disease at a later time is likely. His sexual partners should avoid contact with sites of active infection.

Herpesviruses display a wide range of biological and medical manifestations. They illustrate an important correlation between the life cycle of the viruses and the clinical manifestations of the diseases they cause. This is a fertile area for the study of viral pathogenesis and oncological transformation.

SELF-ASSESSMENT QUESTIONS

1. What are the main types of herpesviruses?

2. Describe the reproductive cycle of a typical herpesvirus, including the latency stage.

3. What is the role of the host defenses in herpesvirus infections? Are there generalizations that apply to most of these infections?

4. What are the main problems in therapy of herpes simplex?

5. If you became involved in work on prevention of herpes simplex infections, how would you go about it?

6. How would you counsel a young person suffering from genital herpes?

SELECTED READINGS

Hirsch MS, Schooley RT: Treatment of herpesvirus infections. *N Engl J Med* 309:963–970, 1034–1039, 1983.

Klein RJ: The pathogenesis of acute, latent and recurrent herpes simplex infections. *Arch Virol* 72:143–168, 1982.

Mandell GL, Douglas Jr RG, Bennett JE: *Principles and Practice of Infectious Disease*, ed. 2. New York, John Wiley & Sons, 1985, p 1282–1341.

Nahmias AJ, Dowdle WR, Schinazi RF: *The Human Herpesvirus: An Interdisciplinary Perspective.* New York, Elsevier Press, 1981.

Weller TH: Varicella and herpes zoster. Changing concepts of the natural history, control, and importance of a not-so-benign virus. *N Engl J Med* 309:1362–1434, 1983.

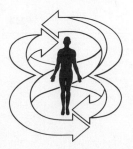

Viral Hepatitis

S.E. Straus

Viral infections of the liver are serious diseases caused by several unrelated viruses. They usually have an acute phase that is sometimes followed by a chronic debilitating condition. At least one of these viruses is associated with an increase in liver cancer. These diseases resemble each other clinically and can only be differentiated with the aid of laboratory tests. They differ in their mode of spread: Some are acquired by ingestion of contaminated food and water, while others are acquired by injection with contaminated needles or via blood transfusions. All the viruses that cause hepatitis are difficult to study in the laboratory, and our knowledge of many of them is superficial. Some of the most important ones replicate by unique molecular mechanisms.

CASE

Mr. P., a 23-year-old grocery clerk, came to the emergency service of the city hospital because he was worried about his jaundice. For several days he had felt increasingly weak, nauseated, and feverish. He felt pain in the right side of his abdomen and his joints. He had no appetite. Mr. P. thought that he had picked up a bad case of the "stomach flu" until, while shaving, he noted that his eyes were yellow. He reported that he had experimented with a variety of oral and injectable drugs, but denied being addicted. He had a stable job, and a girlfriend with whom he was sexually active.

The emergency room physician suspected that Mr. P. had hepatitis B virus infection, and that he may have acquired it from contaminated needles. The *laboratory reported elevation of several indicators of liver injury, namely serum aminotransferases, bilirubin, and alkaline phosphatase. Antibodies to hepatitis A virus were absent, but an antigen associated with hepatitis B, called HBsAg, was detected in his serum. These findings confirmed the diagnosis of* acute hepatitis B virus infection.

The following questions suggest themselves:

1. What were the key elements in the diagnosis of Mr. P.'s disease?

2. Why did the physician suspect that the disease was acquired from contaminated needles?

3. What caused Mr. P.'s symptoms?

4. What is his prognosis? What treatment could be instituted?

5. Can Mr. P. transmit the disease to others? What counsel can he be given to avoid further transmission?

THE VIRAL HEPATITIDES

The disease known as epidemic jaundice has been recognized since ancient times and large outbreaks have been observed, particularly during wars and other conditions of deprivation. Not until the middle of this century was it appreciated that the viral hepatitides have multiple causes and that they are distinct from two other forms of "infectious jaundice", namely yellow fever and leptospirosis. The disease that follows the injection of blood and blood products has a long incubation period, while that associated with ingestion of contaminated food or water has a shorter incubation period. The first became known as *serum hepatitis*, the second as *infectious hepatitis*. Today, these are called *type B* and *type A hepatitis*, respectively.

The distinction between types A and B hepatitis depended on several findings. In a series of elegant studies involving institutionalized retarded individuals, it was shown that there must be more than one etiologic agent: The same person could be sequentially infected with different viruses, since they do not induce cross protection. In the 1960s to early 1970s tests for both hepatitis A and B viruses became available, permitting an accurate distinction between the two diseases.

It soon became apparent that many hepatitis cases had still another etiology. This disease became known as *non-A, non-B hepatitis* because there was no serologic evidence of recent infection with hepatitis A or B in these patients. This disease is also associated with blood transfusions and the use of parenteral needles.

In the late 1970s, Italian scientists described a previously unrecognized antigen in the liver of some individuals with type B hepatitis. Further work found that the antigen belongs to a separate agent, the *delta virus*. Delta is a distinct virus that only infects patients who are also actively infected with hepatitis B virus.

Many other viruses are capable of producing liver inflammation and jaundice (including yellow fever virus, lassa virus, herpes simplex virus, varicella-zoster virus, adenoviruses, Epstein-Barr virus, and cytomegalovirus). However, many of these cause other diseases as well, whereas the liver is the primary target organ for hepatitis viruses.

Table 32.1
Properties of human hepatitis viruses

Agent	Size (nm)	Nucleic Acid Composition	Virus Family
Hepatitis A	27	Single-stranded linear RNA	Picornaviridae (enterovirus 72)
Hepatitis B	42	Nicked, circular, mostly double-stranded DNA	Hepadnaviridae
Non-A, non-B	?	?	?
Delta agent (hepatitis B virus coat)	37	Single-stranded RNA	?

Table 32.2
Epidemiology and transmission of hepatitis viruses

	A	B	Non-A, non-B	Delta
Epidemiologic patterns				
Epidemic	Yes	No	Yes	Yes
Sporadic	Yes	Yes	Yes	Yes
Transmission				
Fecal/oral	Yes	No	Probable	No
Sexual	Yes	Yes	Probable	Probable
Vertical[a]	No	Yes	Probable	Yes
Parenteral	Rare	Yes	Yes	Yes

[a] Includes transmission in utero and perinatally.

Table 32.3
Clinical comparison of diseases associated with hepatitis viruses

	A	B	Non-A, non-B	Delta
Incubation period (days)	15–40	60–180	28–112	?
Asymptomatic infection	Usual	Common	Common	?
Chronicity	No	Yes (10%)	Yes (30–60%)	Yes
Long-term sequelae	No	Cirrhosis, hepatocellular carcinoma	Cirrhosis	Exacerbation of chronic HBV infection

HEPATITIS B VIRUS

The four viruses that infect the liver as their primary target (Table 32.1) differ in structure and replicative strategy. Each exhibits a particular epidemiologic profile and mode of transmission (Tables 32.2, 32.3). We will first describe the hepatitis B virus and then compare it with the other hepatitis viruses.

Hepatitis B virus belongs to a family of *enveloped DNA viruses*, the Hepadnavirus (Fig. 32.1). Related viruses in this group cause chronic hepatitis, cirrhosis, and liver cancer in ground squirrels, woodchucks, and ducks. Hepatitis B virus contains several proteins useful in diagnosis:

• An envelope protein called *hepatitis B surface antigen* (HBsAg) or "Australia" antigen

• The *core antigen* (HBcAg)

• The *e antigen* (HBeAg)

• A viral *DNA polymerase*

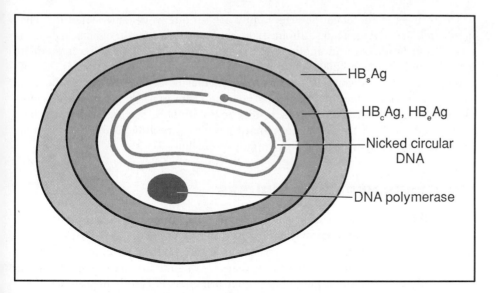

Figure 32.1. The structure of the hepatitis B virus.

- HB$_s$Ag
- HB$_c$Ag, HB$_e$Ag
- Nicked circular DNA
- DNA polymerase

HBsAg circulates freely in the blood in long linear or small circular aggregates of 22 nm in diameter, or as part of the virions, the so-called Dane particles (Fig. 32.2). The blood of infected patients contains enormous numbers of the HBsAg aggregates, as many as 10^{13} particles per milliliter. The aggregates vastly outnumber the complete virions in the circulation. Complete virions only attain titers of 10^5–10^7/ml of serum, but are what make blood infectious.

HBsAg is made up of three antigens in various combinations, comprising a number of subtypes that do not appear to differ in virulence or chronicity. They are, however, useful for epidemiologic studies of the spread of a strain of virus in a community. Serologic analysis of other cases of hepatitis B among our patients' contacts could link them to Mr. P.'s.

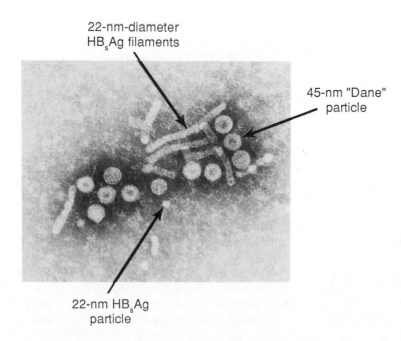

22-nm-diameter HB$_s$Ag filaments

45-nm "Dane" particle

22-nm HB$_s$Ag particle

Figure 32.2. Electron micrograph of 22-nm-diameter spherical aggregates of hepatitis B surface antigen (HB$_s$Ag) particles, 22-nm-diameter filamentous aggregates of the antigen, and several 42- to 45-nm hepatitis B virus ("Dane") particles. (Courtesy of Dr. John Jerin.)

The viruses of the hepadnavirus family are unique in genome structure. They have circular DNA genomes, about 3200 base pairs in length, consisting of one strand that is nicked and another that is incomplete (Fig. 32.1). The incomplete strand is only 1700 and 2800 bases long. From in vitro studies it appears that the endogenous DNA polymerase synthesizes the missing stretch during replication. The evolutionary value of this unique genome structure is unknown, but it has obviously not impaired this virus' ability to establish a secure ecological niche for itself. Aspects of the biology of hepatitis B virus are difficult to study because the virus cannot be grown reliably in cultured cells.

THE OTHER HEPATITIS VIRUSES

The other hepatitis viruses differ considerably from the hepatitis B virus. *Hepatitis A virus* is an enterovirus, one of a family of small RNA viruses (Picornaviridae) related to the coxsackieviruses and polioviruses. Progress in studying this virus was also hampered for many years by its limited host range. This virus infects only humans and a few other higher primates. Recently, hepatitis A virus was shown to replicate in cultured marmoset liver cells and rhesus kidney cells, a discovery that is being exploited for vaccine development.

Hepatitis A virus is a positive-stranded virus since its genome RNA serves directly to encode proteins as messenger RNA. The replication of hepatitis A virus is not well understood, but it appears to involve a strategy similar to that employed by other picornaviruses, Replication of hepatitis A takes place in the cytoplasm and involves a double-stranded RNA intermediate.

The *non-A, non-B hepatitis viruses* have not been definitively identified or characterized. Several studies were performed with chimpanzees inoculated with blood from patients with non-A, non-B hepatitis infections. The infectivity of some non-A, non-B hepatitis-inducing material appears to resist organic solvents, implying that these viruses are not enveloped. Other preparations have proven solvent sensitive, suggesting that some of these viruses may be enveloped. Clearly, this is a heterogeneous group of agents.

The *delta virus* has a remarkable replicative strategy, at least for human viruses. It is a small defective RNA virus that *can replicate only in the presence of hepatitis B virus*. The RNA genome has long stretches of self-complementary sequences that allow base pairing within the strand. The resulting partially double-stranded structure is unique among known human viruses, and resembles the genome of plant pathogens known as *viroids*. Viroids are "naked viruses" that lack the protein coat; the delta virus, on the other hand, is not naked RNA, but "borrows" the surface antigen of hepatitis B virus for its own coat. Thus, delta virus may be considered to be a "parasite's parasite."

The remarkable dependence of delta virus on another virus has a precedent among human viruses: The so-called adeno-associated parvovirus is also defective and replicates only in cells coinfected with adenoviruses.

ENTRY

There are four routes by which hepatitis viruses can be transmitted from human to human (Table 32.2). Transmission of hepatitis B virus takes place largely by exchange of virus-containing blood and blood products. It is most likely that Mr. P. acquired hepatitis from a contaminated needle that had been previously used by another actively infected drug user. Nonparenteral transmission also occurs: Semen, saliva, and vaginal secretions have been shown to contain hepatitis B virus, so that sexual transmission is common. Thus it is also possible that Mr. P. contracted hepatitis from his girlfriend, or that he might transmit the infection to her. The inoculation of hepatitis B virus-containing fluids into open wounds or direct injection into the bloodstream is the most efficient means of spreading the infection. In areas where hepatitis B is endemic, such as parts of Africa and Asia, it is also possible that some cases are transmitted by arthropods.

In developed nations antibodies to hepatitis B virus are found in about 5% of all adults. The highest prevalence is among intravenous drug abusers and promiscuous homosexual men, more than 80% of whom are seropositive. Antibodies to this virus are commonly found in developing nations. Among African and East Asian nations about 50% or more of all people are antibody positive, and 5% to 15% are chronically infected. Thus, there is an enormous reservoir for this virus. *At least one quarter of a billion humans are potentially infectious at any time.*

A major problem with hepatitis B virus infection is transmission to the neonate. In Taiwan, for example, one-third of infants born to HBsAg-positive mothers become infected. Transmission apparently does not occur in utero, but during delivery or through contact with the mother's blood or milk, or minor skin wounds.

MULTIPLICATION AND SPREAD

The target of hepatitis B virus is the hepatocyte. Although recent findings suggest that hepatitis B virus can replicate in pancreatic and bone marrow cells, nearly all that is known about this virus and its infectious processes comes from studies of hepatocytes. As with some other viruses, hepatitis B virus can initiate a number of different types of infection. *Acute productive infection* leads to synthesis of viral DNA. HBcAg can be detected in the nucleus, and HBsAg in the cytoplasm, and infected virions are subsequently released into the circulation. Studies of hepatitis B replication are limited to infected liver tissues because the virus has not yet been grown in cultured cells. The restricted tropism of the virus seems to be due to the existence of specific receptor sites for HBsAg in the liver and few, if any, in other tissues.

Hepatitis B virus replicates in a unique way among DNA viruses (Fig. 32.3): it is the only known human DNA virus that replicates via an RNA intermediate. This is its sequence:

$$\text{partly dsDNA} \longrightarrow \text{dsDNA} \longrightarrow \text{ssRNA} \longrightarrow \text{ssDNA} \longrightarrow \text{partly dsDNA}$$

$$\text{step 1} \qquad \text{step 2} \qquad \text{step 3} \qquad \text{step 4}$$

The virion contains a single-stranded DNA molecule and only part of its complementary strand. The first step in replication consists in filling in the incomplete strand of the infecting DNA molecule. (step 1). This is carried out by the polymerase contained in the virion. The completed molecule then serves as a template for the synthesis of a full length RNA intermediate of positive polarity (step 2). The viral polymerase, which possesses reverse transcriptase activity, then synthesizes a complementary negative DNA copy on the RNA strand (step 3). The RNA strand is now degraded and the DNA is used to make its complementary strand (step 4).

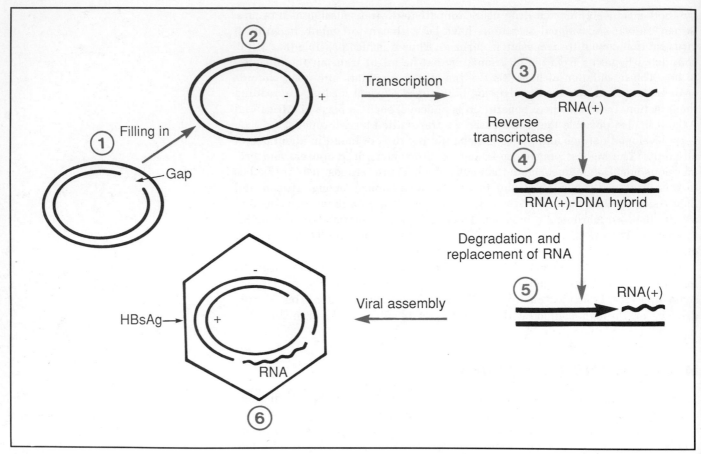

Figure 32.3. Proposed mechanism of hepatitis B virus DNA replication.

The reason for this convoluted replicative strategy is not known, but it may be related to the fact that at some point during acute hepatitis B virus infection of hepatocytes, the viral genome integrates into the host cell chromosome. Liver specimens from patients or experimental animals with chronic hepatitis B virus infection, especially those that have undergone cancerous transformation, contain one or more copies of the viral DNA integrated in seemingly random fashion into the host cell DNA.

DAMAGE

Replication of hepatitis B virus in the liver results in hepatocyte injury and the release of progeny virions into the bloodstream. Cell injury is not due to cytopathic properties of the virus itself but is apparently caused by the activation of cytotoxic immune mechanisms. Hepatitis B virus replicates prolifically but inefficiently. Trillions of particles can be detected in the serum, but only a very small fraction of the particles are complete virions rather than HBsAg envelope aggregates (Fig. 32.2).

In addition to the productive replication process that characterizes the acute infection, hepatitis B virus may also cause a lifelong, chronic infection of the liver. In about 10% of cases the virus or HbsAg alone circulates in the bloodstream for more than 6 months after the acute infection. Chronic hepatitis B virus infection most often leads to a *persistent hepatitis*, with mild periportal inflammation.

Alternatively, it may result in a *chronic active hepatitis* with more widespread inflammation and necrosis. Chronic active hepatitis leads to cirrhosis and hepato-cellular carcinoma. In Taiwan the risk of developing primary hepatocellular carcinoma is over 200 times greater in HBsAg carriers than in noncarriers. It is not known if hepatitis B virus causes the cancer, if the inflammatory process of the chronic infection promotes the cancerous change, or if there are local predisposing causes.

THE OTHER HEPATITIDES

Hepatitis A

Hepatitis A infections are acquired mainly through ingestion of fecally con-taminated food and water. It is presumed that, as with other enteroviruses, they are absorbed through the intestine and gain access to the liver directly through the portal circulation. This is its only known site of hepatitis A replication and the place where virus particles are released into the bloodstream and possibly also into the bile. This would explain why feces are so infectious. A brief viremic phase occurs during the incubation period and may account for the few docu-mented bloodborne cases of hepatitis A.

The likelihood of experiencing hepatitis A infection, and the age of occurrence, are highly dependent on socioeconomic factors. In countries with primitive sanitary facilities, nearly all the people become infected before age 10. In the developed nations, early acquisition of infection is only common in poorer segments of the population. An increased risk of hepatitis A is associated with homosexuality because of oral-anal sex, and with institutionalization because of fecal contamina-tion of the environment.

In terms of the damage inflicted by these other viruses the hepatitis A virus is more cytopathic than is hepatitis B virus. However, the extent of acute hepatic injury in hepatitis A infection is usually more limited than that seen in hepatitis B. Presumably, this difference results from the greater amount of immune damage in type B hepatitis.

Non-A, Non-B Hepatitis

Until the serodiagnosis of non-A, non-B infections can be reliably carried out, the incidence and prevalence of infection by these viruses can only be surmised. In developed nations, most cases of non-A, non-B hepatitis are acquired from transfused blood; some are waterborne. About 5% of all individuals who receive blood transfusions develop non-A, non-B hepatitis.

The pathogenesis of non-A, non-B hepatitis has not been well studied, largely because it is impossible to carry out in vitro work with these agents. Non-A, non-B infections result in chronic infection more frequently than hepatitis B, but patients with this disease generally have a better prognosis. There is no proof that non-A, non-B infection leads to an increased risk of liver cancer, as does hepatitis B.

Delta Hepatitis

The epidemiology of hepatitis delta infection is changing rapidly. First recog-nized in southern Europe in the early 1970s, it has been associated with epidemics of unusually severe hepatitis B infections throughout the world and is becoming increasingly prevalent in northern Europe and in North America. At present 20%

to 30% of all HBsAg-positive intravenous drug abusers in the United States are infected with delta. For this reason Mr. P. is at risk of acquiring both hepatitis B virus and delta virus by sharing needles with other infected drug abusers.

As mentioned above, the delta agent only replicates in liver cells in which hepatitis B virus is also actively replicating. Coinfection of the liver with delta agent and hepatitis B virus may lead to more serious acute or chronic infection than with hepatitis B virus alone. There are no data to indicate whether coinfection with delta agent affects the risk of hepatocellular carcinoma.

MANIFESTATIONS AND DIAGNOSIS OF HEPATITIS

Most infections with hepatitis viruses throughout the world are asymptomatic, particularly in children (see Table 32.3). These infections differ mainly in their epidemiology. Thus, Mr. P. was suspected of having hepatitis B because he was an intravenous drug user. Otherwise, the clinical features of all acute viral hepatitides are so similar that an accurate diagnosis cannot be made on clinical grounds alone (Fig. 32.4). Apparent infection is often milder and briefer with hepatitis A than with hepatitis B (Fig. 32.5). Fulminant or fatal hepatitis A infection is rare.

Mr. P.'s symptoms and jaundice can be expected to resolve in 2 to 3 weeks, but fatigue may persist for weeks or months. Mild to moderate elevation of the serum level of certain enzymes released from damaged liver cells can continue from months to years for patients who do not clear the virus. These enzymes include serum alanine and aspartate aminotransferases and alkaline phosphatase.

The diagnosis of hepatitis B infection depends on finding components of virus or specific antibodies in the blood (Table 32.4). Assays that detect the presence

Figure 32.4. Typical course of acute hepatitis A virus (HAV) infection.

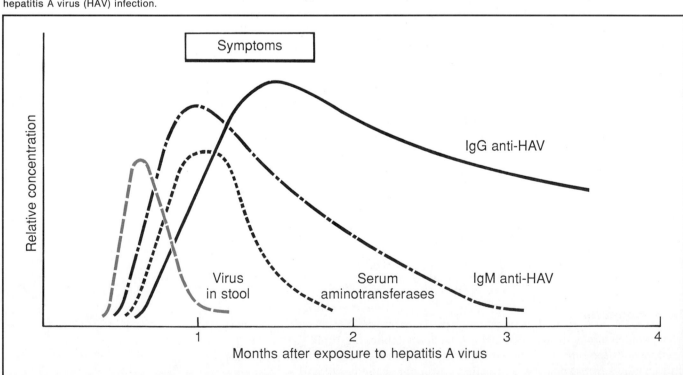

Table 32.4
Interpretation of serologic assays for hepatitis B virus (HBV)[a]

HBsAg	HBeAg	anti-HBc	anti-HBe	anti-HBs	Interpretation
−	−	−	−	−	No evidence of present or past HBV infection
+	−	−	−	−	Incubation period of HBV
+	+	+	−	−	Early in acute infection with HBV or chronic HBV infection with high infectivity
+	−	+	+	−	Later in acute infection, or chronic HBV infection with lower infectivity
−	−	+	±	−	"Window" period late in acute HBV infection
−	−	+	+	+	Convalescent from HBV
−	−	+	−	+	Later in convalescence (anti-HBe has waned)
−	−	−	−	+	Response to HBV vaccine, or recent administration of hyperimmune anti-HB's immunoglobulin

[a] Adapted from Lutwick L.I., unpublished data.

of either circulating HBsAg, HBeAg, and DNA polymerase, or antibodies against these antigens, are widely available. This extensive diagnostic armamentarium is usually not required, but it permits a detailed determination of the stages of hepatitis B. For example, if HBsAg, but not HBeAg, is detected chronically in Mr. P.'s serum, we expect a mild, inapparent, nonprogressive infection that is relatively noncontagious. Were HBeAg and polymerase to persist in his circulation (reflecting release into the circulation of complete infectious particles), Mr. P. would be relatively more contagious (Fig. 32.6, Table 32.4).

Figure 32.5. Typical course of acute hepatitis B virus infection. Note the window of time in which HB$_s$Ag is no longer found, but IgG anti-HBs has not yet developed in detectable levels.

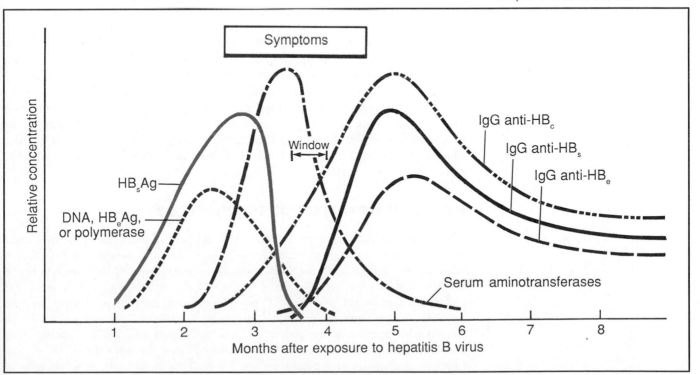

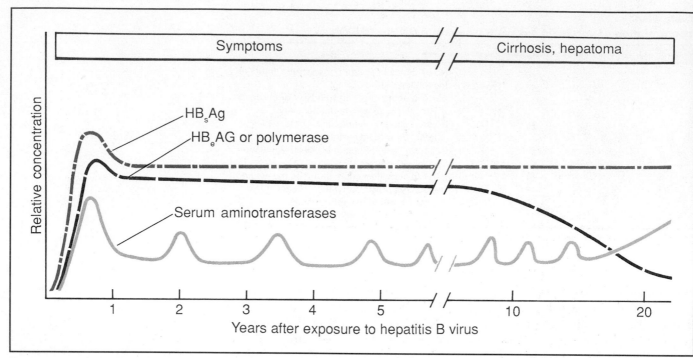

Figure 32.6. Typical course of chronic hepatitis B virus infection. After years of undulating symptoms and aminotransferase levels the circulating Dane particle activity, as reflected in levels of viral DNA, HB$_e$Ag or polymerase may fall or even disappear, but cirrhosis, and ultimately hepatoma, may still evolve.

Hepatitis A virus is shed in the stool late in the incubation period of the infection and persists briefly after the onset of symptoms (Fig. 32.4). There are, however, no convenient assays for hepatitis A virus in the stool or blood. For this reason, the laboratory resorts to the detection of IgM and IgG antibodies to this virus. These antibodies are already present at the onset of symptoms.

Non-A, non-B hepatitis is also indistinguishable clinically from type A or type B hepatitis. Typically, the patient has constitutional symptoms and jaundice for 2 to 3 weeks, but 30% to 60% of all cases suffer from a mild, chronic infection. There are no serologic markers to follow the course of this disease.

Acute delta hepatitis is recognized by the presence of delta antigen in the liver and of hepatitis B antigens in the circulation, and subsequently by the emergence of antibodies to delta antigen (Fig. 32.7). In individuals with mixed chronic infections with delta agent and hepatitis B, high titers of IgM and IgG antibodies to the delta agent persist.

HOW CAN HEPATITIS BE PREVENTED?

There is no clearly effective treatment for acute viral hepatitis, thus preventive measures are of paramount importance. An experimental vaccine for hepatitis A virus has been developed from virus grown in marmoset cell cultures. However, because this virus generally causes low morbidity and mortality it is unclear if such a vaccine would be utilized. Currently, the best preventive strategy against hepatitis A is adequate sanitation and sewage treatment. Those exposed may be treated with immune serum globulin. It has been known for several decades that globulin administration either prevents or reduces the severity of infections. Immune globulin is also recommended for passive immunization of persons at

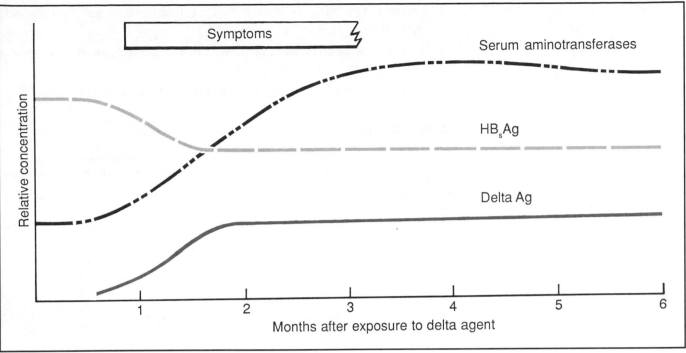

Figure 32.7. The course of chronic hepatitis B infection exacerbated by infection with delta agent. The aminotransferases may rise and the liver histology may shift from that of a chronic persistent to that of a chronic active hepatitis.

risk of hepatitis B, namely intravenous drug users, such as Mr. P., and sexual contacts such as his girlfriend.

A safe, effective and widely available vaccine for hepatitis B contains surface antigen purified from the pooled sera of chronically infected donors. A newer form of hepatitis B vaccine contains hepatitis B surface antigen that has been produced in a recombinant yeast vector containing the cloned viral gene. This was the first recombinant DNA-generated vaccine to be used in people.

No vaccines are available for non-A, non-B, or delta hepatitis (although vaccination for hepatitis B should protect against delta infection), and the efficacy of immune serum globulin for these infections is unproven.

Hepatitis B virus and non-A, non-B viruses are often transmitted by transfusions. Mr. P. must be advised never to donate blood. Cases of transfusion-associated hepatitis have been reduced significantly by the use of volunteer donor blood and by universal screening of blood donors for HBsAg. More than 90% of the remaining cases are now associated with non-A, non-B hepatitis, for which there is no specific screening test available. Posttransfusion hepatitis may be decreased by excluding blood donors with elevated aminotransferases.

SELF-ASSESSMENT QUESTIONS

1. How do the acute viral hepatitides differ epidemiologically?

2. Discuss the replication cycle of hepatitis B virus. In what ways is this unusual? Why is this hard to study? Can you think of ways to facilitate such investigations?

3. How do hepatitis A and hepatitis B differ in the way they cause tissue damage?

4. Discuss the problems associated with the differential diagnosis of the viral hepatitides.

5. What are the distinguishing features of non-A, non-B hepatitis and of delta virus hepatitis?

6. Discuss the prophylactic measures available for the viral hepatitides.

SELECTED READINGS

Dienstag JL: Hepatitis A virus: Identification, characterization and epidemiologic investigation. In Popper H, Schaffner F (eds): *Progress in Liver Disease*. New York, Grune & Stratton 1979, vol 6, pp 343–370.

Lutwick LI: Hepatitis B virus. In Belshe RB (ed): *Human Virology*. Littleton, MA, PSG Publishing Co, 1984, pp 729–756.

Szmuness W (de): *Proceedings of the 1981 International Symposium on Viral Hepatitis*. Philadelphia, Franklin Press Institute, 1982.

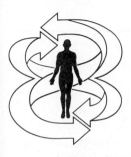

CHAPTER

The Retroviruses and AIDS

33

C. Meissner
J. Coffin

It is difficult to overestimate AIDS. C. Everett Koop, the former Surgeon General of the United States, has written:

AIDS is a life-threatening disease and a major public issue. Its impact on our society is and will continue to be devastating. By the end of 1991, an estimated 270,000 cases of AIDS will have occurred, with 179,000 deaths within the decade since the disease was first recognized. In the year 1991, an estimated 145,000 patients with AIDS will need health and support services at a total cost of between $8 and $16 billion.

Two attributes make AIDS unique among infectious diseases: It is uniformly fatal and most of its devastating symptoms are not caused directly by the causative agent. With suppression of the host's immune response by the AIDS virus (or human immunodeficiency virus, HIV), opportunistic organisms are free to cause disease. Most symptoms seen in an AIDS patient result from secondary infections.

THE HISTORY OF RETROVIRUSES

Understanding the role of retroviruses as the etiologic agents of AIDS requires a historical detour through the puzzling connection between viruses and cancer. It includes a challenge to a traditional tenet of molecular biology, that genetic information flows from DNA through RNA intermediates to protein. In the late 1960s, an unusual class of viruses was recognized that carried genetic information

435

in molecules of RNA. While RNA-containing viruses were not a novelty, these viruses were unique because they contained the formerly unrecognized enzyme, *reverse transcriptase*. This enzyme uses RNA as a template and reverses the conventional flow of genetic information by synthesizing a copy of complementary DNA that ultimately integrates into the genome of the host cell. This DNA, called the *provirus*, serves as an intermediate stage in the replicative cycle.

Some of these viruses (now called *retroviruses* in recognition of their reverse or "retro" mode of replication) are capable of causing tumors. A virus of this type was first isolated in 1911, when Peyton Rous reported that tumors in chickens could be caused by a virus (later known as *RSV*, for Rous sarcoma virus). Since then, hundreds of retroviruses have been isolated from virtually all groups of vertebrates. In the early 1960s, a cancer-inducing cat virus was discovered, now called the *feline leukemia virus*. This virus proved to be important in understanding the biology of retroviruses for two reasons. First, it induces in cats an immunodeficiency similar to the one later observed in AIDS patients. Second, feline leukemia virus is transmitted among cats in a household setting, providing a valuable model for epidemiological analysis of retrovirus infection.

Until the late 1960s, there was considerable skepticism that a virus could mediate the transmission of cancer. Since cancer appeared to be a genetic alteration, it was difficult to conceive how an RNA-containing virus could interact with the DNA of the host cell to produce oncogenic changes. The discovery of reverse transcriptase suggested a route by which this may happen.

THE ISOLATION AND CHARACTERIZATION OF HIV

Since 1980, two groups of retroviruses capable of causing disease in humans have been isolated and characterized (Table 33.1). For several years before 1980 there had been suspicion that retroviruses may be agents of human disease, but the point could not be proved because these viruses did not grow in cultured cells. Several advances in cell culture technology overcame this obstacle. One of the most important was the discovery of *T-cell growth factor* (or interleukin-2, II-2), which stimulates the growth of T-lymphocytes in vitro. These lymphocytes could then be used for the isolation of several *human T-cell lymphotropic viruses* (HTLV). The first, HTLV-I, was isolated from the cells of two patients with adult T-cell lymphoma. Subsequent HTLV-I isolates from other leukemia patients were shown to be closely related, as determined by serology and nucleic acid hybridization. Epidemiologic studies suggested a causal relationship between in-

Table 33.1
The pathogenic human retroviruses

Oncoviruses	
HTLV-I	Causative agent of certain cutaneous T-cell lymphomas; implicated in HTLV-I myelopathy (also called tropical spastic papaparesis)
HTLV-II	Not conclusively linked to a specific disease; found in cases of hairy T-cell leukemia
HTLV-V	Associated with certain cutaneous T-cell lymphomas and leukemias (including mycosis fungoides)
Lentiviruses	
HIV-1	Causative agent of AIDS; formerly called HTLV-III, ARV, LAV
HIV-2	Related to, but distinct from, HIV-1; described as a cause of AIDS, particularly in West Africa

fection by HTLV-I and the development of lymphoma in a few percent of infected individuals as many as 40 years later. A similar virus, *HTLV-II*, was later isolated from a patient with hairy cell leukemia but its role in human disease is less clear at the present time.

The disease caused by HTLV-I is uniformly fatal but is relatively rare (even in infected individuals) and has been limited to certain specific populations. Nevertheless, this virus attracted considerable attention, both because it was the first known human retrovirus and because of the novel features of its biology. Although uncommon in the United States, there is concern about the spread of this virus through the blood supply, and there is consideration for routine screening of donated blood for evidence of infection by this virus. Fortuitously, studies of this virus provided the technology needed for the isolation of the AIDS agent several years later. Thus, AIDS was shown to be caused by a human lymphotropic retrovirus within 3 years after the first description of the disease in 1981. Since it was first isolated, this virus has had several names (lymphadenopathy-associated virus, LAV; AIDS-related virus; ARV; and human T-cell lymphotropic virus, HTLV-III). Recently, it has been agreed that it will be referred to as the *human immunodeficiency virus* (HIV). The remainder of this chapter will focus on this virus.

RETROVIRUS STRUCTURE

Retroviruses have a small spherical virion surrounded by a lipid envelope (Figs. 33.1 and 33.2). The genome contains two identical RNA molecules linked in a dimeric structure (Fig. 33.3). These molecules resemble eucaryotic mRNA because

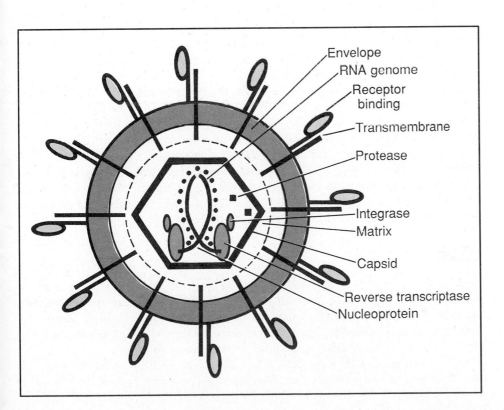

Figure 33.1. Retrovirus structure. Schematic drawing shows the virion proteins and other structures.

Envelope
RNA genome
Receptor binding
Transmembrane
Protease
Integrase
Matrix
Capsid
Reverse transcriptase
Nucleoprotein

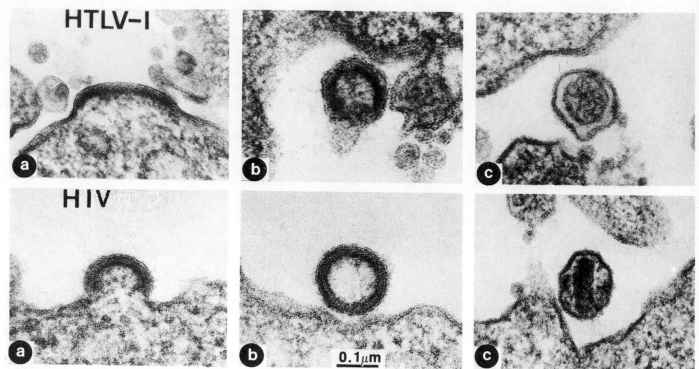

Figure 33.2. Electron micrographs shows successive stages (*a–c*) in the assembly and budding of the human retroviruses HTLV-I and HIV. Note the difference in structure of the core in the negative virion (*c*). (Courtesy of Dr. M. Gonda.)

they contain a *cap structure* at the 5′ end and *poly A sequence* at the 3′ end. Three viral genes are necessary for the replication of retroviruses (see Fig. 33.4). The *gag* gene codes for four or five core proteins. The *pol* gene codes for the *reverse transcriptase* or *polymerase*, the enzyme responsible for replication of the genome, as well as *integrase*, a function necessary for integration of viral DNA into the host of cell genome. The *env* gene codes for the two envelope glycoproteins. Non-coding sequences include terminally redundant regions and unique regions near the ends of the genome. Reverse transcriptase (RNA-dependent DNA polymerases) molecules are associated with the genome and are carried within the virion.

In addition to the genes common to all retroviruses *gag*, *pol*, and *env*, the HIV genome contains at least four other genes (see "The Virus Life Cycle"). These encode functions that seem to be important in regulating the complex replication cycle of this virus, both in maintaining a latent state in the infected cell and in permitting rapid replication at the appropriate time.

CASE

Baby boy G. was born by cesarean section after a 36-week gestation to a 19-year-old prostitute with terminal AIDS. The mother had developed a second episode of Pneumocystis carinii pneumonia 2 weeks prior to delivery. Despite intensive therapy including intubation and mechanical ventilation, the mother died 2 hours following delivery because of respiratory failure.

IgG antibodies to HIV were detected in the infant both by an ELISA test and by Western blot analysis (see "Diagnosis"). The infant received no blood or blood products. By 4 months of age he experienced poor weight gain, exten-

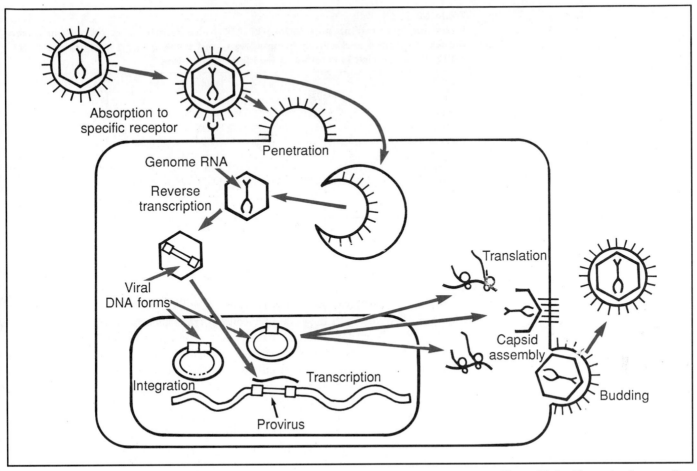

Figure 33.3. The retrovirus replication cycle.

sive thrush (oral candidiasis), diffuse lymphadenopathy (enlargement of lymph nodes), and persistent diarrhea. He developed a rapidly progressive pneumonia and died of **Pneumocystis** pneumonia. Cytomegalovirus was cultured from lung tissue obtained at autopsy.

The diagnosis of AIDS in this infant was based on his birth to a known HIV-infected mother and on the absence of findings that suggest a neonatal immunodeficient state. The infant's positive HIV serology (i.e., antibodies to HIV), however, may have been due to maternal antibodies transmitted transplacentally. Passively acquired maternal antibodies to HIV may persist until 15 months of age, thus positive serology in young children alone does not mean that they are infected with the virus. Since the child was born by cesarean section, had no contact with his mother after delivery, and had received no blood products, it is most likely that his infection was acquired by transplacental passage in utero.

ENCOUNTER

AIDS was recognized in the United States in 1978 and the syndrome was described among homosexual men with multiple sexual partners in 1981. There is evidence that unrecognized cases may have occurred earlier. By late 1981, the

Table 33.2

Incidence (per million population) of AIDS and relative risk (shown in parentheses) by racial and ethnic groups, age, and transmission categories, 1981–1987. Relative risk is relative to incidence in whites.[a]

Category	White	Black	Hispanic	Other
Adult men	380.8(1.0)	1068.1(2.8)[b]	1036.3(2.7)[b]	141.0(0.4)[b]
Adult women	12.2(1.0)	161.1(13.2)[b]	104.6(8.6)[b]	11.1(0.9)[b]
Homosexual men	298.6(1.0)	413.8(1.4)[b]	513.9(1.7)[b]	94.7(0.3)[b]
Bisexual men	46.8(1.0)	177.7(3.8)[b]	126.3(2.7)[b]	24.9(0.9)[b]
Heterosexual IV drug abusers	10.1(1.0)	201.2(19.9)[b]	195.1(19.3)[b]	4.2(0.3)[b]
Hemophilia	2.6(1.0)	1.4(0.6)[b]	2.7(1.0)	1.7(0.7)
Transfusion	5.1(1.0)	7.5(1.5)	6.5(1.3)	5.0(1.0)
Pediatric (all causes)	3.8(1.0)	46.3(12.1)[b]	26.1(6.8)[b]	3.2(0.8)

[a] Adapted from Curran JW, Jaffe HW, Hardy AM et al. Epidemiology of HIV infection and AIDS in the United States. *Science* 239:610, 1988.
[b] Relative risk significantly different from 1.0 ($P < 0.05$)

disease was reported in heterosexual intravenous drug abusers. The first cases among individuals with hemophilia receiving transfusions of human factor VIII were described in 1982. Soon, transmission of the presumed infectious agent to heterosexual partners of infected intravenous drug abusers and bisexual men was documented. At present, homosexual and bisexual men account for approximately 70% of AIDS cases in the United States (including 8% who are also intravenous drug abusers). The most prominent risk factors for acquisition of infection are a high number of sexual partners and participation in sexual practices that increase the risk of transmission due to damage of the anorectal mucosa (mainly receptive anal intercourse). The incidence of AIDS in various risk groups is shown in Table 33.2.

Intravenous drug abusers represent the second largest group with HIV infection, about 15% to 20% of total cases. Importantly, this group acts as a bridge for the spread of HIV infection to nonhomosexual contacts. Transmission among drug abusers occurs because of sharing of contaminated needles and syringes that contain a residue of blood (including infected white blood cells) from previous users. Major urban areas of the United States, including New York City, Newark, New Jersey and surrounding areas, and Miami, Florida, account for a high proportion of members of this group.

Hemophiliacs have long been identified as a group at risk for bloodborne viruses such as hepatitis B and non-A, non-B. This is because they receive preparations of factor VIII and factor IX obtained from plasma pooled from thousands of donors. Currently, 75% to 90% of frequent adult recipients of factor VIII are positive for antibodies to HIV. The most rapid period of seroconversion among hemophiliacs occurred between 1982 and 1984. At the present time, factor VIII concentrates are unlikely to contain HIV because blood donors are screened for HIV antibodies and because plasma products are treated with heat or chemicals to inactivate contaminating viruses. AIDS is the most common cause of death among hemophiliacs at the present time and is likely to continue to be so for some time to come.

Heterosexual transmission of HIV has been implicated in approximately 4% of reported cases. There is concern that this mode of transmission may increase more rapidly than any other. The proportion of cases of AIDS acquired by individuals who have no known risk factor other than heterosexual contact with HIV-infected persons increased from 1.1% in 1982 to 2.3% in 1986. The Centers for Disease Control estimate that unless there is a change in the present trend, the proportion of AIDS cases acquired by heterosexual contact will continue to increase disproportionately, reaching 5% by 1991. Most of these individuals reported sexual contact with either IV drug abusers or bisexual males. Transmission rates to long-term heterosexual partners of AIDS patients vary widely, between less than 10% and 70%. Of the persons who acquire HIV by heterosexual contacts, 17% are male and 83% female. Thus, transmission occurs more readily from infected males to female contacts than vice versa, but it does take place in both directions. Vaginal transmission from females to males may occur less frequently due to unfavorable factors for HIV survival in the vagina, and because such transmission may require penile ulcerations or damage to the male urethral mucosa.

Heterosexual transfer of HIV is more common in certain countries in Central Africa and the Caribbean. For example, the overall ratio of male to female AIDS cases in Zaire is approximately 1:1 as opposed to 13:1 in the United States. One study showed that heterosexual African males with AIDS had a markedly higher number of sexual partners than matched controls without AIDS. Possible other factors include lowered resistance due to coexistent sexually transmitted diseases. Regardless of differences in rates of transmission in the various groups, the prevention of major heterosexual epidemics must focus on all young, sexually active individuals. HIV has been detected in a number of body fluids including peripheral blood, semen, cervical secretions, breast milk, urine, cerebrospinal fluid, saliva, and tears. It is unlikely that the last four represent an important means of transmission. With few exceptions, HIV transmission in the United States occurs at the present time by one of three routes: sexual contact, intravenous drug abuse, and vertical passage from infected mothers to offspring.

Congenital transmission, as in the case of baby G., is the most important route of transmission of pediatric AIDS. As of the fall of 1987, there were nearly 1000 cases of AIDS in children under 13 years of age in the United States. Many of these children were born into a family in which one or both parents are in high-risk groups for AIDS, while a minority acquired the virus from blood or blood products. Approximately 50% of children with AIDS are born to mothers who are intravenous drug abusers. Congenital infection by HIV has been reported to occur in 30% and 75% of infants born to seropositive mothers. Transmission may also occur during the birth process, as well as via breast milk in the postnatal period.

HIV transmission among health care workers is an area of particular concern. As of July, 1987, 5.8% of adults with AIDS were involved in health care or worked in clinical laboratories. Health care workers make up 5.6% of the labor force, indicating no disproportionate risk among such workers. In addition, 95% of HIV-infected health care workers belong to a recognized high-risk group. *These figures indicate that HIV transmission in a medical setting is an exceedingly rare event.* While HIV transmission has been reported in a small number of instances after contact with contaminated body fluids, HIV is considerably less contagious than hepatitis B virus. With the general adoption of "universal precautions", which assume that blood or other fluids from *all* patients is potentially infectious, HIV spread to health care workers should remain an unusual event.

It is important to emphasize that spread of HIV through nonsexual household contact is exceedingly rare. Several studies involving more than 450 family members of AIDS patients failed to detect a single instance of transmission between them in the absence of sexual or vertical transmission or blood transfusion.

Arthropod vectors have been proposed as a route of transmission, but there is no evidence for this whatever. If arthropods, such as mosquitoes or ticks, were important, children in Third World countries would be frequently infected, as they are often victims of bites. In fact, the occurrence of AIDS in children outside recognized risk groups is highly unusual, making this an unlikely mechanism of transmission.

ENTRY, SPREAD, AND MULTIPLICATION

The mechanism by which HIV establishes an infection in the host is poorly understood because of the variable course of the disease and the scarcity of infected cells, especially during the long latent phase of infection. Most likely, HIV enters the host contained within infected cells, e.g., macrophages, lymphocytes, or spermatozoa. Such cells are deposited in tissues and enter the body either through microabrasions on the surface of mucous membranes or through penetration of intact skin with a needle.

While HIV can infect an expanding list of cell types, two major groups of cells in the body serve as preferred targets for infection by HIV: helper T lymphocytes and monocytes. Both these cells contain on their surface the specific CD4 (or T4) protein which plays an important role in immunological function (Chapter 5). Most of our knowledge of HIV replication comes from studies using cells derived from human T-cell tumors, which can be grown in the laboratory.

The Virus Life Cycle

The replication cycle of HIV (Figs. 33.2 and 33.3) includes the following steps:

- *Binding.* Once in close proximity to a helper T lymphocyte, HIV recognizes and binds to the CD4 receptor molecule via its envelope glycoprotein. Antibodies to either the viral envelope protein or the cell receptor block this interaction and prevent infection.

- *Fusion* of the virus envelope with the cell membrane. As the result, the virion loses its integrity and characteristic morphology. Genomic RNA is released into the cytoplasm within the virus core, which includes molecules of reverse transcriptase.

- *Synthesis of DNA.* Reverse transcriptase now synthesizes a complementary DNA molecule corresponding to the viral RNA genome. The enzyme then synthesizes the second DNA strand (complementary to the first), generating a double-stranded DNA molecule.

- *Integration.* The double-stranded DNA molecule is transported to the nucleus and integrated into host cell chromosomes. A virus-coded enzyme, called *integrase*, is responsible for integrating the double-stranded DNA into the chromosome. In the integrated state, viral genetic material is called the *provirus*. The provirus behaves like a cellular gene in that it is passed to daughter cells at division and contains signals that control its transcription into RNA.

- *Synthesis of progeny virus.* In the "productive phase", viral DNA is transcribed into messenger RNA by host cell RNA polymerase. After transcription, some of

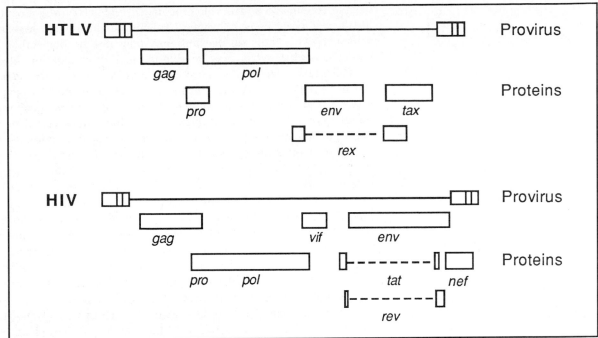

Figure 33.4. The genetic organization of human retroviruses. The *top line* in each case shows the provirus with control sequences shown as *boxes* at the ends. The *lower boxes* indicate the location of the viral genes, with *dotted lines* showing genes which are spaced by introns. Note that both these viruses have several genes in addition to those that code for virion proteins (*gag*, *pol*, and *env*).

these viral RNA molecules are used as messengers for the synthesis of viral proteins. Others become incorporated as genomes into progeny viral particles. Final assembly takes place when these particles acquire their envelope by passage through the cytoplasmic membrane.

• *Latency and transactivation.* The replication cycle described so far is common in outline to all retroviruses. HIV and related viruses are unusual in several ways: (*a*) Infection also involves a *latent* phase in which infected cells contain a provirus but do not express viral RNA or proteins. (*b*) Expression of viral macromolecules is subject to regulation by viral gene products that operate as soluble elements (in "trans"). This phenomenon is known as *transactivation*. At least two HIV genes (called *tat* and *rev*; see Fig. 33.4) function as *transactivating factors* which greatly increase the expression of viral RNAs and proteins. (*c*) Their proviruses contain signals that can turn on expression when HIV-infected cells are stimulated by antigen or infected by some viruses (such as a herpesvirus). These features appear to be related in an important way: after infection of lymphocytes and integration of the provirus, the infection process may be halted, to be re-initiated much later in an explosive way by unknown stimuli. The outcome is a high level of transactivation, resulting in a burst of virus production and rapid death of the cell. The need for secondary stimuli to complete the replication cycle may account for the unpredictable timing of the disease.

Antigenic Variation

A unique characteristic of infection by HIV is that the immune response of the host is unable to curtail viral replication (although it may be important in suppressing it during the latent phase of the disease). This is a paradox, since for most other viral infections the presence of antibody indicates immunity, protection from infection, and a favorable prognosis. How is HIV able to survive despite the host's immune response? Two mechanisms may be at work here: Latently infected cells not expressing surface antigens may not be detectable by the immune response, and the virus may be able to mask or change its antigenic specificity.

Which HIV gene products are important in directing the immune response of the host? HIV genes that code for internal viral proteins (gag and pol) show relative stability from one isolate to the next, but the env gene readily undergoes mutations that lead to variations of its product, the envelope glycoprotein. Antibodies to gag and pol proteins are found in infected individuals, but do not seem to be important. Antibodies to the envelope proteins, on the other hand, neutralize the virus. HIV envelope glycoproteins have two unusual features. First, they are extensively coated with polysaccharide side chains that, because they are added by host enzymes, are antigenically invisible. Second, they contain hypervariable regions that permit the virus to present new antigenic configurations to the host. In contrast, the segments of the surface glycoprotein that are involved in the interaction of cellular receptors must be genetically conserved. Conserved segments may then be hidden and protected from neutralizing antibodies by the hypervariable regions. HIV can constantly vary its surface antigenic composition, which may allow it to avoid inactivation. If this turns out to be an important mechanism, HIV would resemble influenza viruses, and trypanosomes of sleeping sickness in withstanding the immune response by changing major surface antigens. Such a mechanism would hinder the development of an effective vaccine containing the surface glycoprotein.

Recently, a new retrovirus has been isolated from patients with AIDS living in West Africa. This new isolate, called *HIV II*, has an envelope glycoprotein that is more closely related to a monkey virus (simian immunodeficiency virus, SIV) than to HIV. Epidemiological features of this virus, such as its routes of transmission, are not yet known. Major sequence differences exist between the two HIV types. Antibodies against the surface glycoprotein of HIV type I only partially cross-react with HIV type II. Antibodies directed against core proteins of HIV I and HIV II show some cross-reactivity. Thus, AIDS may be caused by one or more distinct but related viruses.

DAMAGE

Our knowledge of the molecular events that modulate lymphocyte damage in HIV-infected patients is still rudimentary. However, on the basis of known abnormalities of humoral and cellular immunity, it is possible to outline a sequence of events that follow HIV infection:

HIV preferentially infects *helper T-cells*, i.e., lymphocytes that express the *CD4* surface antigen. This protein defines this subset of T cells and serves as the receptor for attachment of HIV. Many of these cells are killed by replication of the virus. Even cells that survive can participate in killing, since such cells express viral envelope protein molecules and, in turn can bind to CD4 receptors on other cells. The result is cell-to-cell aggregation and eventual fusion, resulting in the formation of large multinucleated syncytia (Fig. 33.5).

Damage to and depletion of helper T-cells during HIV replication results in a characteristic change in the ratio of helper/suppressor-cytotoxic cells. Depletion of helper T-cells results in a reduction in total circulating lymphocytes (lymphopenia) and a relative increase in the number of suppressor-cytotoxic lymphocytes.

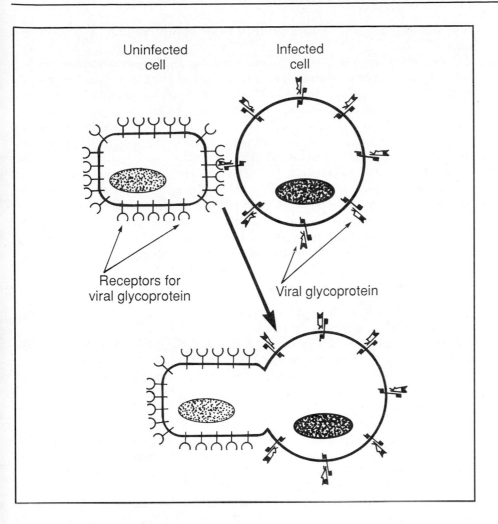

Figure 33.5. Mechanism of HIV-mediated cell fusion.

In addition to quantitative T-cell deficits, HIV induces functional T-cell abnormalities: these cells modulate the function of other cells in the immune system, including B cells, monocytes, and natural killer cells (see Chapter 5).

The impact of the preferential depletion of helper T-cell is multifaceted and explains much of the spectrum of immunologic dysfunction in AIDS. This is only a general scheme and most of the details have yet to be explained. One of the puzzling features is that, at least initially, the proportion of infected helper T-cells is quite small. Presumably, the number of infected helper cells increases as the infection progresses. In the terminal stages of AIDS, most CD4 cells may be gone and it may be more difficult to find HIV.

An important unresolved question is how HIV replication results in dysfunction and death of infected helper T-lymphocytes, a small percentage of which are infected. Various mechanisms that interfere with cell metabolism have been proposed. For example, does the formation of large syncytia of T-lymphocytes sequester a sufficient number to explain their depletion? Is there a toxic protein made by HIV but not by other retroviruses? Does unintegrated HIV DNA build up, with possible disruption of cellular biosynthetic activities? Do the infected lymphocytes undergo premature differentiation and senility? Do helper T-cells become inactivated by loss of CD4 from the cell surface? All these phenomena can be observed in cell cultures but their importance in natural infections is not clear.

Recently, the specific CD4 marker characteristic of helper T-lymphocytes has been found in membranes of other cell types, including circulating monocytes and macrophages, natural killer cells, certain B-lymphocytes and neuronal cells. These cells may also become infected and damaged by viral replication or, in addition, may serve as a reservoir for virus latency. Defects in killing secondary invading microorganisms may be attributes of HIV infection of macrophages and monocytes, as well as by the loss of helper T cells.

Even though many patients with AIDS have elevated immunoglobulin levels in their serum, their ability to produce antibodies against specific antigens may be impaired. For example, children with HIV infections cannot make antibodies against the specific capsular polysaccharide antigens of the pneumococcus and *Haemophilus influenzae* type b. This defect may be due to direct impairment of B lymphocytes as well as to the loss of helper T-lymphocytes.

Some Clinical Consequences

AIDS represents the terminal stage of infection by HIV. Clinical syndromes vary with different stages of infection:

Initial HIV infection (group I) may be associated with a mononucleosis-like syndrome approximately 1 to 2 weeks following exposure. This may include fever, a skin rash, muscle aches, lymphadenopathy, and meningitis. Seroconversion (the development of detectable antibodies to HIV) occurs approximately 2 to 3 months after the initial infection.

Once infected, an individual may become completely asymptomatic (group II) or develop persistent generalized lymphadenopathy (group III). Lymphadenopathy may persist or resolve before progressing over months to years to the *AIDS related complex* (ARC), characterized by diarrhea, oral candidiasis, weight loss, and fever.

Patients with ARC will progress to develop AIDS (group IV) with opportunistic infections, Kaposi's sarcoma, and/or B cell lymphomas (Table 33.3). In the cases

Table 33.3
Secondary infections found in HIV-infected patients with immunodeficiency[a]

Protozoan and helminthic infection
    Intestinal infection with *Cryptosporidium* or *Isospora* causing chronic diarrhea
    Pneumocystis carinii pneumonia
    Strongyloidiasis disseminated beyond the GI tract
    Toxoplasmosis disseminated beyond the liver, spleen, or lymph nodes
Fungal infections
    Candida esophagitis
    Pulmonary candidiasis
    Cryptococcosis of the central nervous system
    Disseminated histoplasmosis
Bacterial infections
    Disseminated infection with *Mycobacterium avium* complex
Viral infections
    Disseminated cytomegalovirus infection
    Herpes simplex virus infection, either disseminated or of the lungs or GI tract
    Progressive multifocal leukoencephalopathy

---

[a] From Lifson AR, Curran JW: Epidemiology of AIDS: current trends and prevention. In Gottlieb MS et al (eds) *Current Topics in AIDS*. New York, John Wiley & Sons, 1987, pp 1–7.

described above, both mother and child eventually died of *Pneumocystis carinii* pneumonia. See Chapter 54 for details on infections of the compromised patient. The majority of AIDS patients develop neurologic symptoms. This may be due to a secondary infection by opportunistic organisms such as the protozoan *Toxoplasma gondii* or the fungus *Cryptococcus neoformans*, or to the development of malignancies of the CNS or, more often, by direct invasion of neurons by HIV. HIV may invade the CNS directly and replicate in. Presumably, the virus is carried to the CNS by circulating monocytes. It is not known if damage to brain cells is due to the release of toxic substances from the monocytes or to direct damage to neurons by replicating virus.

The most important single factor in the development of AIDS in HIV-infected individuals is time. For all risk groups, the percentage of HIV-infected individuals who develop symptoms of AIDS increases with each year. *The precise number of HIV-infected individuals who will ultimately develop AIDS is not known at the present time* because the disease has been studied for only a few years. For the same reason, the mean incubation period (from acquisition of the virus to the manifestation of symptoms) is also not known. A recent study estimates that this period is about 5 years for 40% and 8 years for 99% of AIDS patients. These figures indicate not only the seriousness of HIV infection, but also the magnitude of the health problem in years to come. Even if no one became infected with HIV from now on, the incidence of the disease will continue to increase well into the 1990s. It is not known if the probability of progression to AIDS is increased by "cofactors" (e.g., diseases often seen in some of the risk groups, such as hepatitis, cytomegalovirus, herpes infections) or by genetic determinants.

DIAGNOSIS

Before the viral etiologic agent was identified, diagnosis of AIDS was based solely on clinical findings. The presence of specific opportunistic infections or certain tumors such as Kaposi's sarcoma in high-risk groups was necessary before the disease could be suspected. Patients in the early stages of infection could not be identified. In September, 1987 the Centers for Disease Control issued revised criteria for a *case definition of AIDS* based on the presence or absence of laboratory evidence of HIV infection (Table 33.4). Evidence of infection is generally based on the presence of antibodies to HIV. The presence of virus in blood

Table 33.4
Selected features of the case definition for AIDS[a]

A. **If laboratory evidence regarding HIV infection is not available, several conditions serve as indicators,** including specified manifestations of infections by any of the following: *Candida* (fungus), *Cryptococcus* (fungus), *Cryptosporidium* (protozoan), cytomegalovirus, herpes simplex virus, *Mycobacterium avium* complex (bacteria), *Pneumocystis carinii* (protozoan), *Toxoplasma* (protozoan). Other indicators are specified manifestations of Kaposi's sarcoma, brain lymphoma, leukoencephalopathy, and several others.

B. **If laboratory evidence for HIV infection is present,** any of the above diseases indicates a diagnosis of AIDS. To this list are added here specified manifestations of the following: infections by *Isospora* (protozoan), *Coccidioides* (fungus), *Histoplasma* (fungus), Salmonella (bacterium), plus other lymphomas, encephalopathy, and HIV wasting disease. Some of these conditions serve as indicators even if diagnosed presumptively (i.e., without waiting for definitive tests).

C. **If there is laboratory evidence against HIV infection,** under some conditions, the diagnosis of AIDS cannot be ruled out for surveillance purposes. These conditions are met when the patient is immunodeficient for other causes that cannot be ruled out and has an indicator condition.

[a] 1987 revision by the Centers for Disease Control

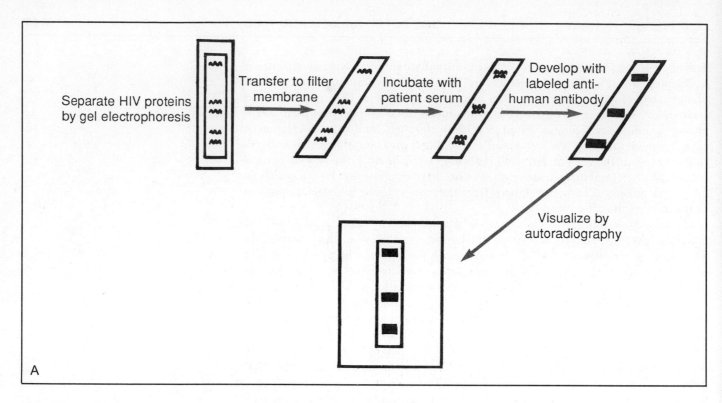

Figure 33.6. Detection of HIV antibodies by Western blot. **A**, Schematic outline of the procedure. **B**, An example of a Western blot exposed to acquired immunodeficiency syndrome (AIDS) patient serum. (Courtesy of Dr. B. Mermer.)

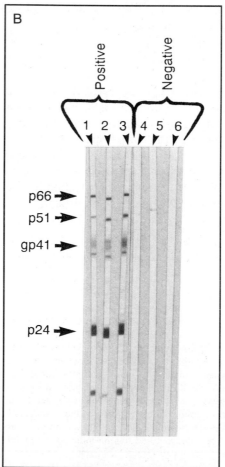

or tissues can be documented by growth of the virus in cell culture or by molecular methods, but these techniques have not been standardized and are not widely available. Remember also that in the early stages viremia is rare and only a small percentage of lymphocytes are infected and that such cells may be hard to find. Therefore, laboratory evidence is generally based on serologic work.

Serologic tests for HIV infection detect and characterize specific anti-HIV antibodies in serum. The ability to grow HIV in culture made such tests possible. It is now clear that close to 100% of HIV-infected individuals have measurable antibodies in their serum. The exceptions are a small group of individuals either in the earliest stages of the disease (before seroconversion) or in the terminal ones (when their B cells are unable to synthesize antibodies). On very rare occasions, certain individuals may "serorevert" (lose detectable antibodies while still carrying the virus). Antibodies may not be detected in an HIV-infected person because of technical problems (false negative). It is important to remember, therefore, that in a very limited number of instances the absence of antibodies does not completely rule out an HIV infection. The persistence of detectable antibodies to HIV is generally accepted as an indication of infection and the ability to transmit the virus.

Initial tests for HIV serology generally are performed by an ELISA test (enzyme-linked immunosorbent assay). This test is carried out by adding a sample of the patient's serum to small plastic cups to which HIV antigen is bound (kits for such assays are commercially available). If antibodies are present, they will complex with HIV antigen. After washing away unreacted components, antihuman immunoglobulin antiserum linked to a readily assayable enzyme, such as a peroxidase, is added. Anti-HIV antibodies in the clinical sample can then be detected by adding a chromogenic enzyme substrate; a positive test is indicated by a suitable color change (see Chapter 59 for details). The test is usually repeated with positive samples and the results confirmed by immunofluorescence or Western blot analysis. The Western blot detects antibodies against individual viral polypeptides that have been separated by electrophoresis and transferred ("blotted") onto a thin membrane filter (Fig. 33.6).

The ELISA test has a false-positive rate of around 0.4%. With confirmatory Western blot tests, the joint false-positive rate approaches a remarkable 0.005%. However, even these low numbers become worrisome when a population with low prevalence of HIV infection is tested. Thus, it has been estimated that among non-high-risk female blood donors in the United States (whose rate of HIV infection is approximately 1 in 10,000) the likelihood that infection is actually present in a woman with a confirmed positive test is only around 70%. In such a low-risk population, the use of the test raises difficult moral and legal issues.

The predictive value of an AIDS test must be carefully weighed in deciding whether low-risk individuals should be tested. The impact of a positive test result on a person's state of mind, social interactions, marriage, insurance eligibility, and employment opportunities is enormous. How many false positives is our society willing to accept in order to identify a relatively small number of infected individuals?

PREVENTION

Control of the spread of AIDS has proved to be difficult because a vaccine is not available. Control of spread of this disease requires a change in the life-style of many individuals. Education appears to be the most important means of reducing the spread of AIDS at the present time. The most important measures include curtailing high-risk practices, such as multiple sexual contacts for both the homosexual and heterosexual population; using condoms; and being aware of the danger of anal intercourse and the danger of using contaminated needles for intravenous drug abusers. Evidence that education has an impact on sexual practices comes from experience in the homosexual community in San Francisco, where transmission of other sexually transmitted diseases, especially gonorrhea, is markedly reduced. While it is not yet known if this has also led to the desired diminution in AIDS cases, it has reduced the spread of HIV in this community.

What problems are encountered in designing an AIDS vaccine? The ability of HIV to change its antigenicity will probably complicate conventional approaches to vaccine development. Antigenic peptides prepared by genetic engineering techniques are currently in the early stages of testing. It should be emphasized that so far there is only a limited understanding of the nature of the immune response to HIV infection. Antibody titers in infected individuals are low compared with other viral infections.

It is not known whether a vaccine-induced immune response would confer protection against primary HIV infection. A problem with an HIV vaccine is that the virus is probably transmitted from person to person mainly within infected cells (lymphocytes or macrophages) and therefore may not be accessible to the immune system. HIV may be transmitted directly from cell to cell, without going through an extracellular phase. The ability of HIV to induce cell fusion may also reduce the importance of extracellular antibodies. Protection may then require a more complex immune response, probably of the cell-mediated type. Lastly, HIV exists in a number of states within a cell: In the latent state infected cells harbor virus without expressing viral antigens.

At the time of writing (June 1988), the development of an effective vaccine remains a distant goal. The availability of an effective vaccine for feline leukemia virus offers some promise. However, testing of an HIV vaccine presents special problems. The chimpanzee is the only animal known to be susceptible to HIV infection (although its disease is different from the human). Once a potential HIV vaccine has been developed, human clinical trials will be extraordinarily difficult to accomplish. Here are some of the problems: Volunteers will have the stigma of becoming HIV antibody positive; what criteria should be established for the volunteers' sexual preference?; how will we determine if a response is protective? To provide a statistically significant answer (in view of the low incidence of infection in the population) a huge number of people will have to be vaccinated. Note that the ability of HIV to establish a latent infection will complicate vaccine trials. If a vaccinated person becomes infected but remains asymptomatic, is that a vaccine failure or a vaccine success? How long should such a person be followed before results can be meaningfully interpreted? None of these questions has easy answers.

THERAPY

There has been some progress in the development of antiretroviral therapy. The life cycle of retroviruses is intimately connected with the replication of mammalian cells, so that only a limited number of metabolic reactions can be singled out for targets of specific chemotherapy. Reverse transcriptase is an attractive target because inhibition of this enzyme should have no effect on the host cell. Many anti-HIV agents now being investigated inhibit this uniquely viral function. *Azidothymidine* (AZT), the only drug licensed for AIDS by 1987, inhibits this enzyme. Initial studies indicate that AZT administration over periods of up to 18 months decreases the frequency of opportunistic infections in selected AIDS patients. In addition, some AZT treated patients show an increase in the number of helper T cells and an improvement in cell-mediated immunity. It has not yet been demonstrated that these effects are due to inhibition of virus replication. Nonetheless, this first-generation compound demonstrates that effective drug therapy can be developed.

CONCLUSIONS

AIDS is a uniquely devastating disease: It kills all those that exhibit symptoms. It is a chronic illness, often becoming manifested years after the virus is acquired and after the individual has had the opportunity to transmit it. Based on estimates of infected individuals, a threefold increase in the number of cases has been projected between 1987 and 1991 (Fig. 33.7). By inactivating a central cellular component of the immune system, the helper T lymphocyte, HIV produces severe impairment of both humoral and cellular immunity. The disease is lethal because defenses against opportunistic pathogens are gone. Diseases that were practically unseen before AIDS (e.g., encephalitis due to *Toxoplasma gondii*), or under reasonable control (e.g., mycobacterial infections), have become common and highly dangerous among AIDS patients (Chapter 54).

AIDS runs counter to the tenet that a successful parasite does not cause lethal injury to its host, suggesting that HIV may be a relative newcomer among human infectious agents. The disease appeared suddenly in the United States and its etiology was established with remarkable speed. We have acquired a great deal of knowledge about HIV and other retroviruses but are still unable to explain many of the features of the disease. We do not understand how helper lymphocytes

Figure 33.7. Incidence of acquired immunodeficiency syndrome (AIDS) in the United States. The number of cases is projected to 1991 based on a statistical extrapolation.

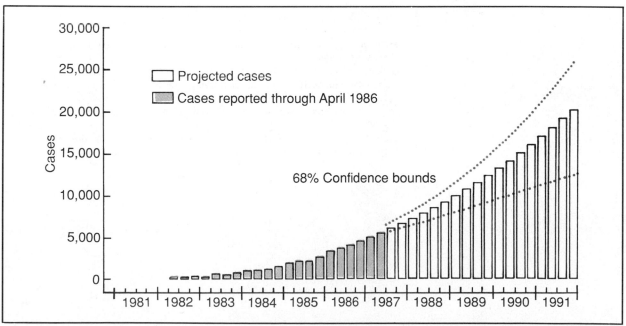

are killed or impaired, or why the infection of a small proportion of them has such devastating effects. Lack of this knowledge hinders the design of drugs and vaccines. The virus is particularly elusive to immunotherapeutic approaches because of variability in surface antigens and other features of its structure and life-style.

Prolonging life among those that have acquired the virus presents a major medical problem. In the absence of an effective vaccine, prevention of HIV transmission among uninfected members of the population depends on public education.

SELF-ASSESSMENT QUESTIONS

1. Discuss the structure and mode of replication of retroviruses.

2. How does HIV differ from the other known retroviruses?

3. Imagine having to address a community group regarding AIDS. What would you say about its history, transmissability in the community, and prospects for prevention and therapy?

4. What important aspects of HIV infection have yet to be elucidated? How could understanding their mechanism help prevent or treat AIDS?

5. What problems are associated with designing an effective AIDS vaccine?

6. If you were asked, what specific areas of research and education on AIDS would you target for the award of research funds?

7. What is your guess about the status of AIDS 10 years from now and 20 years from now?

SUGGESTED READINGS

Coffin J: Genetic variation in AIDS viruses. *Cell* 46:1–4, 1986.

Curran JW et al: The epidemiology of HIV infection and AIDS in the United States. *Science* 239:610–616, 1987.

Friedland GH, Klein RS. Transmission of the human immunodeficiency virus. *N Engl J Med* 317: 1125–1135, 1987.

Gallo RC: The first human retrovirus. *Scient Am* 255: 88-98, Dec 1986.

Ho DD, Pomerantz RJ, Kaplan JC: Pathogenesis of infection with HIV. *N Engl J. Med* 317:278–286, 1987.

Meyer KM, SG Pauker: Screening for HIV: can we afford the false positive rate? *N Engl J Med* 317:238, 1987.

Yarchoan R, Broder S: Development of anti-retroviral therapy for the acquired immune deficiency syndrome and related disorders. *N Engl J Med* 316:557–564, 1987.

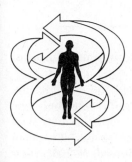

CHAPTER

Warts and Other Transforming Viruses

34

S.E. Straus

Warts result from persistent infections by a group of small DNA viruses. These tumor-like growths of the skin and mucous membranes are sometimes associated with true malignancies. Some of the distant relatives of these viruses, polyoma and simian virus 40 (SV40), produce tumors in animals and are among the best studied models of viral oncogenesis.

CASE

Warren's mother was perplexed. She had taken her 4-year-old to see a throat specialist because of constant hoarseness. After an examination, the physician recommended a biopsy and possible surgery for what he believed were warts of the vocal cords. To her, warts implied little bumps on the hands or other skin surfaces, but nothing as serious as this. Now she had several concerns:

1. How could warts get to Warren's vocal cords?

2. Will they cause further problems?

3. Could there be any relation between Warren's warts and the ones for which she was treated by her gynecologist several years earlier?

In this chapter we will address these issues about wart viruses and review their diversity and oncogenic potential. Since wart viruses cannot be grown in the laboratory, much of our present understanding of these viruses reflects the

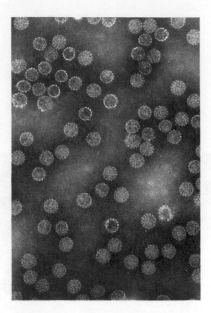

Figure 34.1. Electron micrograph of purified wart viruses. (Courtesy of Dr. K.V. Shah.)

Table 34.2
Human papillomavirus (HPV) types and their associated lesions

HPV-1	Plantar warts
HPV-2	Common warts
HPV-3	Flat juvenile warts
HPV-4	Plantar warts
HPV-5	Macular lesions in EV[a]
HPV-6	Condyloma acuminata
HPV-7	Common warts in meat handlers
HPV-8	Macular lesions in EV
HPV-9	Macular lesions in EV
HPV-10	Flat warts
HPV-11	Laryngeal papillomas
HPV-12	Macular lesions in EV
HPV-13	Focal epithelial hyperplasia
HPV-14	Macular lesions in EV
HPV-15	Macular lesions in EV
HPV-16	Bowenoid papulosis; cervical carcinoma
HPV-17	Macular lesions in EV
HPV-18	Cervical carcinoma
HPV-19–29	Macular lesions in EV
HPV-30	Laryngeal carcinoma
HPV-31	Cervical dysplasia
HPV-32–45	Have not been described

[a] EV, Epidermodysplasia verruciformis, associated with malignant degeneration.

burgeoning application of recombinant DNA technology to problems in medical microbiology and infectious diseases.

Few diseases are fraught with as many folk notions about the cause, transmission, and treatment as warts. They have been endowed with magic and mystery, probably because they may persist for many months or years and then disappear quickly. It was finally shown in our times that warts are not caused by toads' urine but by viruses (Fig. 34.1). In 1894 an investigator demonstrated their contagious nature by inoculating himself with material from his brother's warts. The viral etiology was established by demonstrating that extracts of warts were still infectious after passing them through bacteria-retaining filters.

THE PAPILLOMAVIRUSES

Papillomaviruses are a large group of DNA viruses that include pathogens of humans, mice, monkeys, cattle, birds, fish, and other animals. They belong to a family known as the *papovaviruses*, an acronym for the most famous members of the group, the <u>pa</u>pilloma viruses, the <u>po</u>lyoma viruses and the <u>va</u>cuolating viruses, notably SV40. Papillomaviruses differ sufficiently from the other papovaviruses to be placed in a separate genus within the family (Table 34.1).

Papillomaviruses cannot as yet be cultured in vitro but small quantities of the viruses can be purified from lesions. It is difficult to classify them by the usual serological typing methods, which require large amounts of virus. However, their DNA can be cloned and used in hybridization tests to determine degrees of homology, a process known as *genotyping*. Viruses that have between 50% and 100% homology under stringent conditions are considered to be related subtypes. Greater differences place them in different types. Minor differences within types can be detected by restriction endonuclease analysis. At the time of this writing there are about 45 human papillomavirus types, divided into several subtypes (Table 34.2). It is likely that this number will increase with further studies.

Much of what we know about the structure and replication of wart viruses comes from analogy with the better studied mouse *polyoma* and monkey *SV40 viruses*. All these papovaviruses consist of nonenveloped particles made up of 72 identical capsomeres in an icosahedral array. The amount of DNA of these viruses is not large and it can code for only a few proteins.

Table 34.1
Biological features of various papovaviruses

	Papillomaviruses	Polyomaviruses
Human viruses	Human papillomavirus types 1–45	Human BK virus, human JC virus, human AS virus
Animal viruses	Shope rabbit papillomavirus, bovine papillomavirus, many others	Mouse polyomavirus, simian vacuolating virus 40, and others
Target tissues	Skin, mucous membranes	Brain, kidneys, other organs
Virion size	52–55 nm	43–45 nm
DNA content	$4.55–5.55 \times 10^6$ daltons	$3.0–3.6 \times 10^6$ daltons
Strands transcribed	One	Both
Transforming ability	Yes	Yes
Genome in transformed cells	Usually not integrated	Usually integrated

ENCOUNTER AND ENTRY

Human papillomaviruses are acquired by direct contact with lesions of infected people or with virus-containing material in the environment. They are quite stable and may be transferred via scales of exfoliated skin. The other important mode of transmission is by sexual contact. These viruses are not highly contagious and epidemics are rare, even within a family. The site of entry, as well as virus type involved, determines the location of the lesions. The normal skin is relatively resistant to entry, and infection takes place more readily when the virus comes in contact with mucous membranes or with traumatized skin. Thus, the most frequent sites of lesions are the commonly injured skin surfaces, such as the fingers, hands, soles, knees, elbows, the penis, vulva and cervix, and much more infrequently, the oropharynx and the larynx as in Warren's case. Warts of the soles of the feet, for instance, can result from abrasion on the concrete surfaces of swimming pools. Frequent warts in the hands and fingers of butchers are due to the inoculation of virus into cuts they sustain at these sites. Transmission from mother to child is believed to occur during delivery by direct contact of the newborn with the virus in the cervical or vaginal area. Since Warren's mother had a history of genital warts it is likely that he became infected in this manner at birth.

Recent surveys of patients attending the National Health Service clinics in Great Britain have documented that anogenital warts occur in epidemic proportions. Through the 1970s and 1980s their incidence has risen faster than that of genital herpes. Warts are now the single most common sexually transmitted infection that leads people to seek medical attention in that country. Less complete figures indicate similar trends in the United States, where genital warts vie with chlamydial infections for first place among the sexually transmitted diseases.

Many people become infected with wart viruses during their lifetime without exhibiting symptoms. This is demonstrated by finding antibody against papillomaviruses in serum. The reason why some develop warts or other symptoms is not known, although deficiencies in the immune system can lead to diseases by these viruses—some of them quite serious.

MULTIPLICATION AND SPREAD

The replication of human wart viruses is inferred in part from the better studied polyoma and SV40 viruses. These agents produce two types of infections: a *lytic* one that leads to formation of progeny viruses, and a *persistent* one which may lead to oncogenic transformation of the host cells. The beginning steps are the same in both cases: After binding to cell receptors, the virions traverse the cytoplasm intact and are uncoated in the nucleus. Here they replicate, following a well-timed series of events. Early (or pre-DNA synthesis) messenger RNAs are transcribed from about one half of the genome. These mRNAs exit the nucleus and are translated into early virus proteins in the cytoplasm.

If the infection follows the lytic course, DNA begins to replicate, using one of the early proteins. Replication is not a haphazard process but begins in a defined region of the genome and proceeds bidirectionally for about 180° around the circle, when the two completed progeny molecules separate. This mode of replication resembles that of the chromosomes of bacteria to a greater extent than it does that of most DNA viruses. DNA replication is accompanied by transcription of the late mRNAs that encode the major viral proteins. These proteins are transported back to the nucleus where they assemble with the newly replicated DNA to form progeny virions.

Papovaviruses are extremely efficient in their use of genetic material. They are known to be marvels of economy and squeeze the maximum assistance from their host cells. For example, papovaviruses use cellular histones for their "chromosomes" and cell enzymes for replication and transcription. For these reasons, they are valuable models for studies of mammalian cell function. In addition, they make especially efficient use of the information in their own genome. They use several stratagems to read one stretch of DNA in various ways to produce several different proteins (Fig. 34.2). One strategy is to process a single mRNA molecule in different ways. This is done by the removal of different intervening noncoding sequences ("introns"), leaving more than one type of mRNA coding sequences ("exons"). Another strategy for deriving more information from a DNA sequence is to read the same stretch of DNA in more than one different "frame". DNA is transcribed into mRNA three nucleotides at the time, starting at a fixed point and moving along until termination signals are encountered. If transcription started one or two bases further along the chain, DNA would be read in a different frame, which would normally result in genetic gibberish. In these viruses, however, such shifts in frame are programmed, and result in the synthesis of three different readable mRNAs from the same stretch of DNA. This allows the virus to make more than protein from the same stretch of DNA.

Although the human wart viruses have not been analyzed in the same detail as polyoma and SV40, they use slightly different replication strategies. Wart virus DNAs are larger and contain information for a few more proteins. They also transcribe some of their DNA in all three frames, but from one strand only. This contrasts with the polyoma and SV40 viruses which transcribe "early" genes from one strand and "late" genes from a nonoverlapping part of the other strand. All types of human wart viruses, even those that share little DNA homology, have a similar genetic organization (Fig. 34.2).

Figure 34.2. Open reading frames predicted from analyses of human papillomavirus types 1 and 6. Although these viruses share little DNA homology, they possess similar genomic organization. RNAs are transcribed from each wart virus in only one direction but in all three reading frames. RNAs encoding early (E) and late (L) viral proteins are grouped as shown.

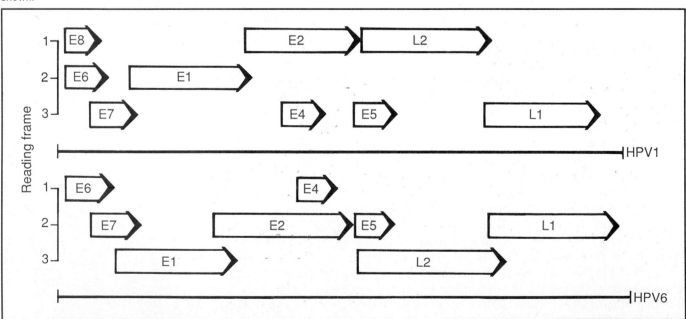

The papillomaviruses establish a lytic or productive infection only in the keratinized cells of the superficial epithelium. In the deeper epithelial layers they establish an abortive form of infection. As these infected cells differentiate and are displaced outward toward the skin surface, the virus can complete its replication cycle. These viruses can persist for many years in the deeper layers of the epidermis. At times these persistent viruses may lead to oncogenic transformation of their host cells.

How do papovaviruses transform cells? Apparently, transformation occurs when these viruses infect cells incapable of supporting the lytic cycle. Often these cells are from a different animal species than one the virus infects naturally. Transformation results from an abortive growth cycle. Neither replication nor translation of late viral proteins is required. The maintenance of the transformed state requires the continued expression of early viral genes.

It is worth digressing for a moment to describe what is known about transformation by SV40 and polyoma viruses. The phenotypes that result from transformation are similar for both, but the mechanisms involved differ in detail. Both these viruses code for a regulatory protein, called *large T antigen*, that is involved in initiation of DNA replication and regulation of transcription during the lytic cycle. It is important to realize that this protein affects not only viral processes, but analogous processes of the host cell as well. In addition, large T antigens are required for the integration of the viral genome into host chromosomes during transformation. The mechanism is not known, but at least in the case of SV40, large T antigen appears to stabilize regulatory proteins of the host cells. Changing the inherent instability of such proteins may well alter the pattern of cellular regulation.

Polyoma virus works differently. Its large T antigen is somehow also required for transformation, but a second protein, called *middle T antigen*, is responsible for altering the cell to the transformed phenotype. Middle T antigen binds to a protein produced by a cellular oncogene, known as $pp60^{c-src}$. Binding results in the activation of $pp60^{c-src}$, which can now phosphorylate cell proteins that are involved in the regulation of cell growth and division. This protein is the cell's homolog of the transforming protein of an RNA retrovirus, Rous sarcoma virus. Thus, polyoma viruses may transform cells in a way that is analogous to that of other transforming viruses, but by activating a host protein instead of coding for such a protein.

Is this scheme of transformation relevant to the human wart viruses? From what we know at present, they use different strategies. A crucial difference is that papillomaviruses induce tumors in their natural hosts. As with polyoma and SV40, continued expression of viral early antigens is required for maintenance of the transformed state. Within benign tumors, papillomaviruses are not integrated in the host cell genome but remain extrachromosomal. Thus, chronic carriage of these viruses is more akin to a latent infection than to classical cell transformation. In fact, entirely normal skin and mucous membranes adjacent to warty growth have been found to contain human papillomavirus DNA within them.

The mechanism of tumor induction by the wart viruses is still murky, but is being studied vigorously. It is thought that some virus-coded proteins interact with host components in a manner similar to the mouse polyoma viruses. However, tumor formation by these viruses may well involve the presence of other factors, such as herpesviruses, chemical and physical carcinogens, and the host immune system.

DAMAGE

Papillomaviruses are thought to infect the cells of the basal layer of the skin and replicate in concert with them. As these cells mature and migrate toward the skin surface, viral replicaton begins. When the cells begin to differentiate and start making keratin, the number of virus genomes in each cell increases. In the outer skin layers the infection becomes manifest and is characterized by proliferation and thickening of the basal cell layer, and vacuolization of the cytoplasm. These changes lead to the appearance of a wart. Thus, the lesion is not caused by cell destruction but by cell proliferation.

Warts look different at different sites. Physicians have no trouble recognizing the common warts of the hands: elevated, firm, fleshy lesions with a sharp border (Fig. 34.3). They range in size between 1 and 10 mm or more in diameter. Proliferation of separate dermal papillae within a lesion results in a coarse cauliflower-like appearance. On the soles of the feet warts tend to be more deeply embedded and more keratotic than those on the hands. Warts of the hand and feet are believed to have long incubation times, between 6 and 18 months.

Elsewhere, on the face, knees, or arms, warts tend to be flat, less distinct and harder to recognize. They are more likely to occur in larger numbers and to be clustered (Fig. 34.4). Anogenital warts (condylomata acuminata) may be either flat or elevated. One or several cauliflower-like lesions may surround the anus, the labia, or the shaft of the penis (Fig. 34.5). Warts of the uterine cervix are usually flat and tend to be missed during casual speculum examinations. Cervical warts have an incubation time of only 2-6 months after sexual contact, perhaps because they do not involve a long maturation process of host cells, as is the case in the skin. They are of special concern, because over 80% of all cervical carcinomas, local or invasive, contain papillomavirus DNA, especially that of types 16 and 18.

Warts of the larynx are most common in preschool age children and can lead to progressive impairment of laryngeal function unless treated. As in the case of

Figure 34.3. Common warts.

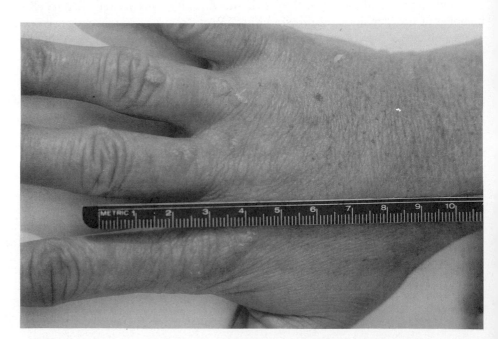

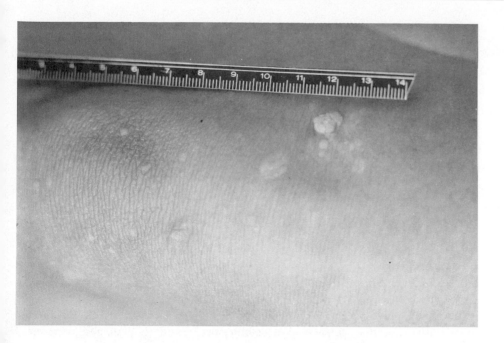

Figure 34.4. Multiple flat warts on knee.

Warren, hoarseness is the usual complaint in children, but respiratory distress and secondary bacterial pneumonias signify the presence of obstructing lesions in the bronchial tree as well. The virus types associated with these lesions as well as those of the oropharynx are the same as those that cause anogenital warts, an observation that, as indicated above, suggests perinatal transmission. Oral-genital transmission is also possible, as seen by the greater incidence of these types of warts in homosexual men.

How does the host respond to infection by these viruses? Both humoral and cellular immunity probably participate, but their respective role has not been fully

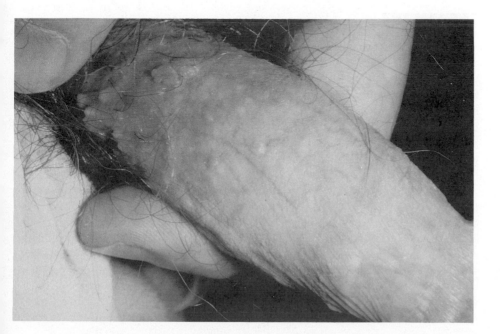

Figure 34.5. Penile warts.

elucidated. Type-specific antibodies to external virion antigens of these viruses can be detected in patients' sera. The infection is primarily controlled by cell-mediated immunity. People who are deficient in their cellular immunity (transplant recipients, patients with AIDS or lymphoma) are more likely to have multiple chronic warts.

A rare but aggressive form of papillomavirus infection occurs in persons with an autosomally inherited defect in cellular immunity. The condition is called EV, or epidermodysplasia verruciformis, a mouthful of words that mean "warty looking changes of the epidermis". It is manifested by hundreds or thousands of flat warts. In 30% of these cases, the disease progresses to squamous cell carcinomas of the skin.

PAPILLOMAVIRUSES AND CANCER

The road from warts to cancer is a short one. Not only are warts themselves a form of tumor, albeit a benign one, but they have been found in a variety of cancers as well. It is currently believed that at least 80% of cases of cancer of the cervix are associated with wart viruses. Certain virus types are more likely to initiate dysplastic than frankly neoplastic changes. Even the virus types associated with malignancy cause benign lesions more frequently than malignant ones. The progression from benign to dysplastic to malignant disease is a slow process that can take decades. It is believed that a consequence of the current epidemic of genital warts among sexually active adolescents and young adults may be a dramatic increase in the incidence of cervical cancer in the first decades of the 21st century. There is mounting evidence that, in addition to genital cancers, a number of other human squamous cell tumors, such as some squamous cell carcinomas of the oropharynx, larynx, bronchi and anus, may be associated with wart viruses. In the absence of specific probes for all possible viruses that may be involved, we cannot know the total spectrum of neoplastic disorders associated with papillomaviruses.

TREATMENT

About 50% of warts regress spontaneously within 1 to 2 years. Treatment is most often considered for cosmetic reasons but more substantial reasons for desiring therapy include the control of pain, bleeding, impairment of laryngeal function (as in Warren's case), or the concern of sexual transmission. Unfortunately there are no specific treatments. Nearly all modes of treatment are ablative, like surgical excision, destruction with laser beams, dry ice or liquid nitrogen, or by the application of strong chemicals. These and other approaches have been used with variable long-term success. In a case like Warren's, the treatment may have to be repeated many times.

In view of the high rate with which warts recur after ablative treatment, attention has turned to biological approaches, but most of these have not been successful. The best hope at present is the administration of interferon into the lesions themselves or systemically. α-Interferon causes significant but transient remission in patients with EV, genital, or laryngeal warts.

An important theoretical factor that limits the potential of some forms of therapy is that the viruses often persist in apparently normal tissue adjacent to the warts. Ablation of the lesion may remove one focus of infection but can leave a residual inoculum nearby, which may later result in local recurrence.

PREVENTION

There is no way to prevent becoming infected with wart viruses other than by avoiding contact with the infected surfaces of other people. This is not a practical suggestion, especially due to the extraordinary measures that would have to be taken to prevent the relatively small number of cases of serious disease caused by these viruses. Condoms may prevent transmission of the virus to or from the penile shaft. In the case of Warren, the laryngeal warts may have been avoided if his mother had been aggressively treated prior to delivery. Some have suggested cesarean sections for pregnant women with genital warts. Unfortunately, genital warts are very common so that this would lead to a large increase in these operations to protect very few children. The risks in most instances certainly outweigh the benefits.

Considering the strong association of genital warts with cervical cancer, one important measure is the regular examination of the cervix. Papanicolaou smears, visual inspection of the cervix (colposcopy), and biopsies of suspicious cervical lesions can detect precancerous changes in time to permit effective treatment.

SELF-ASSESSMENT QUESTIONS

1. Describe the basic properties of wart viruses.

2. Contrast the replication cycle of wart viruses with that of polyoma virus.

3. Why are warts more than a bothersome clinical problem?

4. Discuss the problems in the treatment of warts.

5. Why are warts difficult to prevent, especially in children?

SUGGESTED READINGS

Bunney MH: *Viral Warts: Their Biology and Treatment.* New York, Oxford Univ. Press, 1982, 5–9.

Centers for Disease Control: Condyloma acuminatum—United States 1966–1981. *MMWR* 32:306–308, 1983.

Eron LJ, Tucker S et al: Interferon therapy for condylomata acuminata. *N Engl J Med* 315:1059 1064, 1986.

Genital warts, human papillomaviruses, and cervical cancer (editorial). *Lancet* 11:1045–1046, 1985.

Gissman L, Wolnik L, Ikenberg H et al: Human papillomavirus type 6 and 11 DNA sequences in genital and laryngeal papillomas and some cervical cancers. *Proc Natl Acad Sci USA* 80:560–563, 1983.

Margolis S: Therapy for condyloma acuminatum: A review. *Rev Infect Dis* 4: (Suppl) S829-S836, 1982.

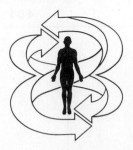

Polio and Other Enteroviruses

35

C. Meissner

Poliomyelitis is no longer a common disease in the United States, although it continues to be important in some developing countries. Paradoxically, its dreaded consequences, paralysis and death, are more common in unvaccinated individuals living in countries with a high standard of sanitation. Polio serves as a good model for understanding the epidemiology and pathogenesis of viral infections because of the tropism exhibited by the virus, the well-understood and comparatively simple replication cycle of poliovirus, and the relative ease with which it can be studied in the laboratory. Furthermore, several related viruses (other enteroviruses) continue to cause important diseases in the United States.

CASE—AN OUTBREAK OF POLIOMYELITIS

In October, 1972, 11 of 130 students attending a private school in Greenwich, Connecticut came down with paralytic poliomyelitis. Three weeks elapsed between the first and the last case. Nine of the 11 cases were boys 12 to 17 years of age, and all were members either of the football or the soccer team. The clinical history of these patients was similar. They reported "flu-like" symptoms: fever up to 39°, sore throat and muscle pains. These lasted 1 to 3 days. Two to 3 days afterwards, they complained of stiff neck, increased muscle pain, and fever up to 41°. This was followed by flaccid paralysis of the legs, which varied in intensity from relatively minor to totally incapacitating. During the first 3 weeks of October 17 other students were seen at the school infirmary with non-specific complaints that suggested an acute viral syndrome.

Poliomyelitis was diagnosed by serologic studies based on a rising titer of antibodies to type 1 poliovirus, but not types 2 and 3. The diagnosis was confirmed by the isolation of type 1 virus from the feces and throat washings of patients with paralytic disease. More than 50% of the students of the school had received no oral polio vaccine because of religious convictions. A small number of day students at the school lived at home, where they interacted with friends from surrounding towns in activities that included swimming classes at the local YMCA. Paralytic disease did not occur among nonmembers of the school. An immunization survey of the public schools revealed that more than 95% of the students had been vaccinated.

Several questions are raised by this outbreak:

• Where did the virus come from and how did it spread among the students?

• What caused the illness among the 17 students who complained of nonspecific signs and symptoms?

• Why did the disease not spread to all the students or to the community outside the school?

• How does poliovirus cause paralysis and the other symptoms of the disease?

• What could have been done to halt further spread of polio in the school?

Poliomyelitis is an ancient disease and has been one of the most dreaded since pre-biblical times. An Egyptian stone slab from about 1350 BC shows a young priest with the typical withered leg of a polio survivor (Fig. 35.1). In the prevaccine era of the early 1950s, there were about 21,000 paralytic cases a year in the United States. The figure is now less than 30 cases a year—a striking testimony to the efficacy of the polio vaccine. The dramatic virtual elimination of this disease from this country and much of Europe is one of the spectacular triumphs of medical research.

The history of poliomyelitis has seen major changes in disease incidence and age distribution. Prior to the 1900s, most infections occurred in infants. Few developed paralytic disease because in infants the virus is not as neurotropic and is more likely to confine its replication to the alimentary tract. Poor standards of sanitation and crowding facilitated transmission of virus, particularly among children in the first year of life. Infection, symptomatic or not, confers lifelong immunity and, if widespread, prevents large outbreaks from taking place in older persons.

Around the turn of the century, the situation changed when improved living conditions limited circulation of the virus. As unexposed children without immunity grew older they entered an increasingly larger pool of susceptible individuals. Introduction of poliovirus into this community resulted in more frequent infections later in life, and resulted in devastating epidemics of paralytic disease. This is because older persons are more likely to develop paralytic disease when infected by poliovirus. In a sense, polio became a disease of affluent societies. This, then, is an example of changes in severity of a disease due to changes in the host rather than in the infectious agent. Underdeveloped countries of the world continue to experience the endemic pattern of poliovirus infection early in life, even today.

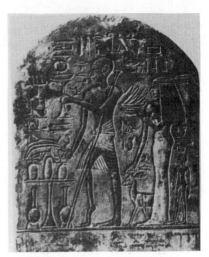

Figure 35.1. An early case of paralytic polio? This Egyptian stele depicting the typical paralysis of a polio victim dates from the 18th dynasty (1580–1350 BC). (From Lyons AS, Petracelli RJ: *Medicine: An Illustrated History*. New York, Harry M. Abrams, 1978.)

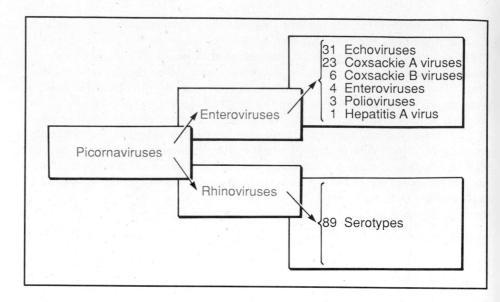

THE ENTEROVIRUSES

Poliovirus belongs to a heterogeneous group of viruses called the *enteroviruses*, which derive their name from their natural habitat, which is the gastrointestinal tract. There are six major groups of enteroviruses. The most notorious member of this group is in fact poliovirus, and more is known about its molecular biology and mechanism of pathogenesis than the other enteroviruses. Polioviruses are divided into three antigenic types. Most epidemics are caused by type 1. Other enteroviruses include coxsackievirus, first isolated during a polio outbreak in New York State, and echovirus (enteric *c*ytopathic *h*uman *o*rphan virus), so called because initially they could not be linked to any human disease, having been isolated from feces of individuals who had no symptoms. This distinction has been dropped for newly discovered enteroviruses and they are now simply assigned a number, e.g., enterovirus 70. For example, *hepatitis A* virus is also known as enterovirus type 72.

Enteroviruses belong to the Picornavirus family (pico = small, rna = RNA containing) (Fig. 35.2). The family contains a second genus, the *Rhinovirus*, which are the most frequent isolates from patients with the common cold. The properties of the two genera of picornaviruses help explain why they cause disease in certain sites of the body. Enteroviruses are resistant to gastric acidity (stable at pH 3.0) and to bile. Rhinoviruses replicate best at 33°C, a temperature found in the nose, while enteroviruses prefer the core body temperature, 37°C. This may help explain why rhinoviruses seldom cause pneumonia and enteroviruses are an infrequent cause of the common cold.

ENCOUNTER AND ENTRY

Enteroviruses are secreted in large amounts in stool. In the outbreak at the school in Connecticut, the likely source of contamination was a single individual who shed high titers of virus from the gastrointestinal tract. A summer or early fall outbreak is typical of countries in temperate climates, while in the tropics the diseases caused by these agents are endemic and occur throughout the year. The major portal of entry is the mouth, and primarily from person to person via the oral-fecal route.

SPREAD AND MULTIPLICATION

Soon after ingestion, enteroviruses replicate in the lymphoid tissue of the pharynx and the intestine. They may then spread throughout the body via the bloodstream. In most cases the infection does not proceed further: Enteroviruses are either contained in the Peyer's patches of the small intestine or are kept in check soon after the onset of the viremia. With poliovirus, the distinction between infection and disease is particularly important.

When viremia persists, distant sites become seeded as the viruses localize in their target organs. Their tropism is due to the presence of specific receptors on the membranes of target cells. All three types of poliovirus share similar receptors since saturation of binding sites with, say, an excess of type 1 virus blocks the binding of types 2 or 3. Binding of coxsackie or other enteroviruses remains unaffected, indicating different binding sites for these related viruses.

Replication of poliovirus is better understood than that of the other enteroviruses, in part because they reproduce rapidly and yield high titers in cell culture. Polioviruses are a prototype of *positive-strand viruses*, meaning that their genomic RNA may act directly as messenger RNA. The first step in their replication cycle is uncoating, which oddly enough begins while the viruses are still extracellular. Once they are taken up, uncoating is completed and their genomic RNA is released into the cytoplasm, where replication and assembly take place. Poliovirus RNA is single stranded and as is typical of eucaryotic mRNAs, has a poly (A) tract at the 3′ end on the genome. A viral protein called VPg is attached to the 5′ end. This protein is not essential for infectivity but may be involved in packaging the genome in the virion and in priming poliovirus RNA synthesis.

Synthesis of poliovirus proteins has been studied extensively and has revealed several unexpected facts. A single long polypeptide, a *polyprotein*, is synthesized in the cytoplasm using the host cells' protein synthesizing apparatus. A series of posttranslational cleavage reactions cut the polyprotein into four structural proteins and about seven nonstructural proteins. After this processing, the structural proteins can assemble to make the capsid. We do not know why poliovirus has evolved to translate its messenger into a polyprotein. By this mechanism each protein is made in equal amounts. At least one of these proteins is an enzyme, while the others are structural constituents of the virions.

Poliovirus RNA is replicated by an unusual enzyme, an *RNA-dependent RNA polymerase*. This enzyme is not found in eucaryotic cells (whose RNA is made from DNA templates) and accordingly is encoded by the viral genome. The enzyme makes complementary negative strands of RNA, which in turn serve as templates for additional positive-strand copies of the genome. As the structural viral proteins accumulate, increasing amounts of viral RNA are encapsidated into mature virions. The viral particles are then released as the host cell is destroyed.

Under optimal conditions of cell culture, roughly 1000 infectious virus particles are released per cell. A complete cycle of replication, from viral attachment to the release of progeny virus, is completed within about 10 hours, which is unusually rapid for animal viruses. Other enteroviruses follow a similar scheme of replication.

DAMAGE

Poliovirus is a typically *lytic* virus and its replication is accompanied by destruction of infected host cells. Enteroviruses typically have 2- to 5-day incubation periods. They may continue to replicate in the intestine and be shed in the stool for weeks or months after all symptoms are gone. In the school outbreak, virus continued to circulate and to infect new students for some time. This explains the onset of symptoms in different students over a 3-week period.

Polioviruses spread from the gastrointestinal tract to the central nervous system, where they replicate in the neurons of the gray matter of both brain and spinal cord. Virus travels via the bloodstream, although spread along neural pathways is also possible. The characteristic flaccid paralysis of limb muscles occurs when anterior horn cells of the spinal cord are destroyed. A most severe form of disease is bulbar poliomyelitis, the paralysis of the respiratory muscles resulting from involvement of the medulla oblongata. It is this type of polio that led to the development of "iron lungs", cumbersome predecessors of modern respirators that made patients inhale and exhale by external changes in pressure. The mortality rate in paralytic cases of poliomyelitis is 2% to 3%.

Why is infection by enteroviruses, and poliovirus in particular, often so mild or asymptomatic? Apparently many factors are at work. They include the size of the viral inoculum, the concentration of viruses in the blood, the virulence of individual virus strains, and the presence of circulating antibodies. The same virus may cause different illnesses in different individuals. In the school outbreak described previously there was a spectrum of disease caused by one strain of poliovirus. Among the host factors involved, physical exertion and trauma correlate with increased risk of paralysis. This may in part explain the observation that 9 of the 11 students affected were actively participating in football and soccer. Another predisposing factor for bulbar poliomyelitis is tonsillectomy, perhaps due to lower titers of antipolio antibodies in the nasal secretions of immunized persons. Circulating antibodies may play an important role, as seen in patients with agammaglobulinemias, who have difficulty in resolving infections by echovirus.

DISEASES CAUSED BY OTHER ENTEROVIRUSES

The most frequent diseases caused by enteroviruses in the United States are attributed to coxsackievirus (Table 35.1). They cause a large number of illnesses, differing somewhat between those caused by group A and group B. Both cause

Table 35.1
Major enterovirus diseases

Disease	Polio	Coxsackievirus Type A	Coxsackievirus Type B	Echovirus	Enterovirus
Asymptomatic infection	+	+	+	+	+
Viral meningitis	+	+	+	+	+
Paralytic disease	+	+	+	+	−
Febrile exanthems (rash)	−	+	+	+	+
Acute respiratory disease	−	+	+	+	+
Myopericarditis	−	+	+	+	−
Orchitis	−	−	+	+	−

so-called *aseptic meningitis*, a term used for nonbacterial meningitis. In addition, group A viruses cause *herpangina*, a fever of sudden onset with vesicles or ulcers on the tonsils and palate. Group B viruses also infect other organs, particularly the heart. In general, echoviruses produce similar diseases (Table 35.1).

Most of these infections are not sufficiently unique to allow a specific diagnosis on clinical grounds alone. For example, the skin rash (exanthem) due to coxsackievirus is indistinguishable from that due to echovirus. One important exception is the so-called *hand, foot, and mouth disease*, a readily identifiable febrile illness that produces blisters in the palate, hands, and feet. It is usually caused by a specific type of coxsackievirus, type A16.

During the viremic phase these enteroviruses infect any of several organs and do not exhibit the same degree of tropism for the CNS as poliovirus. Infected newborns are at particular risk of severe disease, unless they have acquired enough protective antibodies from their mother. Their own immune system may be insufficiently developed to curtail an enterovirus infection. Neonates may acquire coxsackievirus or echovirus by transplacental passage of the virus near term, from contact with maternal fecal material during birth, or from conventional person-to-person passage.

DIAGNOSIS AND THERAPY

Since diseases caused by enteroviruses are seldom sufficiently characteristic to enable a diagnosis on purely clinical grounds, it may be helpful to take into account certain epidemiological features. A person who becomes ill with symptoms of viral meningitis in the early fall during a communitywide outbreak of coxsackievirus is likely to be a victim of that agent.

During endemic months when enteroviruses circulate in a community they can be readily isolated from throat washings or fecal specimens from symptomatic as well as asymptomatic persons. In this setting, recovery of an enterovirus from the throat or feces of an asymptomatic person is consistent with but not diagnostic of acute infection. Definitive proof requires isolation of the virus from the involved site, such as cerebrospinal or pericardial fluids. Isolation of these viruses is expensive and time consuming, as it requires cell culture techniques. Serological tests are not practical here because related enteroviruses do not share common antigens.

At present there is no therapy for infections by enteroviruses, with the possible exception of the administration of gamma globulin to immunocompromised patients suffering from severe echovirus or coxsackievirus infections.

PREVENTION

A disease caused by an agent whose only reservoir is human beings is a candidate not only for control but for elimination. The best example is of course smallpox, which appears to have been erased from the face of the earth. Polio may well be a candidate for this sort of medical success. The issues surrounding polio vaccination merit close examination. Vigorous efforts to develop an effective polio vaccine go hand in hand with seminal developments in virology, mainly the use of cell cultures to study viral multiplication. The killed Salk vaccine was introduced in 1955 and led to a precipitous decline in the incidence of both paralytic and nonparalytic disease (Fig. 35.3). In 1961, the oral live attenuated Sabin vaccine was introduced in this country and it soon replaced the Salk vaccine.

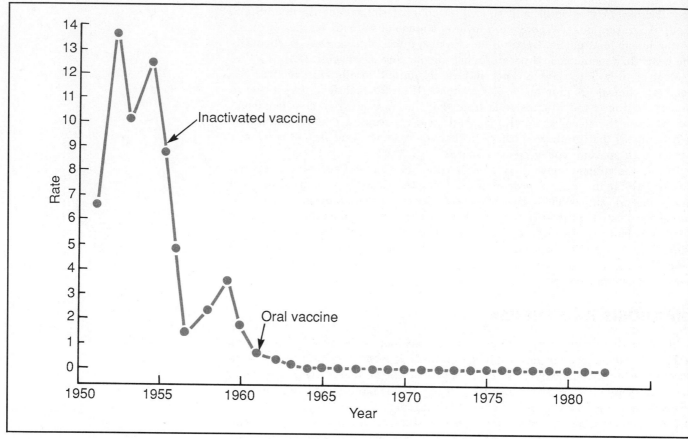

Figure 35.3. The incidence of paralytic poliomyelitis in the United States from 1952 to 1982. Reported cases are per 100,000 population. (Data from the Centers for Disease Control, Atlanta, GA.)

Considerable controversy surrounded the introduction of a live vaccine after the killed vaccine had already demonstrated its effectiveness. A comparison of the two vaccines is shown in Table 35.2.

The original arguments continue to form the basis for the use of the live vaccine (Fig. 35.4). Antibody production by the killed vaccine is not always long lasting and is slow to develop. Repeated booster shots are necessary. Perhaps most important, the immune response elicited by the live, attenuated vaccine closely resembles that brought about by natural poliovirus infection. The reason is that the live, attenuated vaccine is administered orally, resulting in an active infection in the intestine and stimulating the local formation of secretory antibodies. In contrast, the killed vaccine is administered by injection and produces immunity in the circulation but not in the intestine (Fig. 35.4). Thus, a recipient of the killed vaccine, while protected from symptomatic disease, could still propagate and spread the virus.

Because immunization rates in this country never approach 100%, the live vaccine would reduce the number of individuals who may act as reservoirs for poliovirus. Contacts of individuals given the live, attenuated vaccine may be asymptomatically infected, regardless of their immunization status. In most instances, this contact produces a booster response in already immunized individuals. In the infrequent setting where the vaccine strain spreads to nonimmunized persons, the community may benefit from the increased number of immune individuals. However, spread of live virus by this means is not without harm: At

Table 35.2
The poliovirus vaccines

Inactivated vaccine (Salk)	
Advantages	Disadvantages
Cannot undergo genetic mutation to increased virulence.	Fails to elicit gut immunity
	Requires parenteral administration expensive
	Some lots have inadequate antigenic potency
	Confers immunity only after four boosters
	Stringent control of production required to ensure inactivation

Live, attenuated vaccine (Sabin)	
Advantages	Disadvantages
Relatively inexpensive and easily administered	Can mutate to more virulent strain
Induces both systemic and local immunity	Less reliable in tropical climates
Maintains potency without refrigeration	
Prepared in human cells, eliminating risk of latent viruses found in monkey kidney cells	
Induces herd immunity	

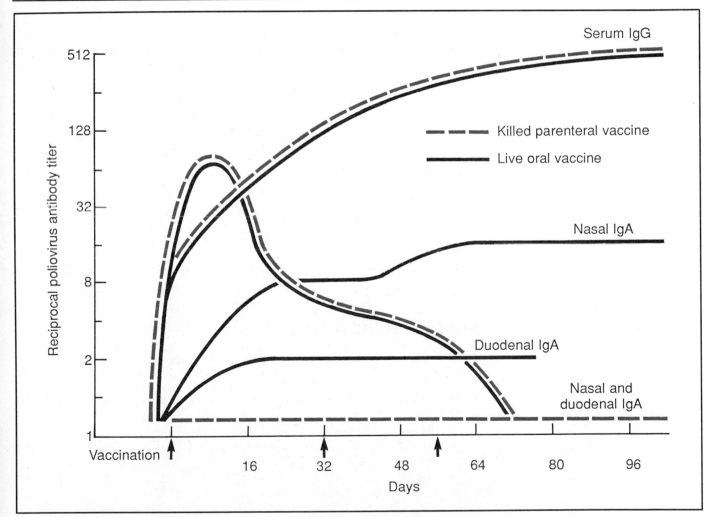

Figure 35.4. The antibody response to the live and killed poliovirus vaccine. The levels of serum IgG and nasal and duodenal IgA are compared as a function of time after vaccination.

least half of the few cases of paralytic poliomyelitis in the United States today are thought to be due to the virus used in the live vaccine. It should be emphasized, however, that the risk of developing polio from the vaccine strain is extraordinarily small, about 1 case of polio per 4 million people vaccinated. Also, at times the live vaccine has been found to contain contaminating viruses from the monkey cells used for cultivation.

The live vaccine should not be used in certain circumstances. Immunocompromised individuals should not receive any live vaccine, including the Sabin vaccine. In some underdeveloped countries, the live, attenuated vaccine has not resulted in an acceptable antibody response. One reason for vaccine failure seems to be interference from other enteroviruses already replicating in the intestine. For this reason, the live vaccine is given to children in five doses, which ought to minimize the likelihood of other enterovirus replicating at the time of vaccination.

CONCLUSIONS

Enteroviruses commonly cause infections in human beings. They are readily communicable but only rarely do they cause severe disease. Illnesses caused by enteroviruses may be highly tissue specific (poliovirus) or they can affect many organs (coxsackievirus and echovirus infections). These diseases are often difficult to distinguish clinically, and a presumptive diagnosis is often based on the epidemiologic picture. The success in eradicating polio with vaccination is providential, since there is no other known way to control this disease.

SELF-ASSESSMENT QUESTIONS

1. Discuss the changes in severity and incidence of polio in the United States in the last 100 years.

2. What diseases do the enteroviruses cause? What are their common clinical features?

3. Discuss the replication cycle of poliovirus.

4. What are the problems associated with vaccination against polio?

5. Discuss how the eradication of smallpox may help us eradicate polio.

SUGGESTED READINGS

Evans AL: *Viral Infections of Humans*, ed 2. New York, Plenum 1982, pp 182–251.
Feigen RD, Cherry JD: *Textbook of Pediatric Infectious Diseases*. WB Saunders, Philadelphia, 1981, pp 1316–1365.
International Symposium on Poliomyelitis Control. *Rev Infect Dis* 6 (Supple 2):1984.

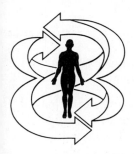

Measles

S.E. Straus

Measles is one of the typical and hazardous childhood illnesses. It can also affect adults. It is on the wane in many parts of the world but is still a major cause of death in children in some developing countries. It is especially associated with high mortality in malnourished persons. The manifestations of measles are not due solely to multiplication of the virus but also to the immune response of the host. An effective live attenuated vaccine helps control the spread of this disease.

CASE

Ms. M., an aspiring journalist, took ill just prior to crucial college midterm examinations. She had looked forward to a relaxed spring break after these exams, but now her ability to take them seems in doubt. She feels miserable, has fever, a runny nose, cough, a blotchy rash, and is told by the health service physician that she might have measles. "That's absurd," she thinks. "Only little kids get measles and I think I had it as a child."

Her rash appeared first on the neck and head, then spread to the trunk and extremities during the next few days. At first the rash was composed of discrete, reddish lesions that blanched on pressure. They then quickly merged together and became increasingly brownish.

If you were the university health service physician, it would be your responsibility to make a definitive diagnosis of Ms. M.'s condition and to take several steps to ensure that if it were measles, she would not contribute to the further spread of this apparent epidemic. What must you know?

1. Given the current rarity of the disease in the United States, is it reasonable to consider measles as a probable diagnosis?

2. What information can be gleaned from the medical history of the patient, her physical findings, and laboratory tests to confirm or rule out the diagnosis of measles?

3. Could Ms. M. have had measles previously and now have it again?

4. What other illnesses are associated with rashes, and could any of them be Ms. M.'s problem?

5. What complications might Ms. M. or others experience from this illness?

6. How can transmission of measles to others be prevented?

HISTORY AND EPIDEMIOLOGY OF MEASLES

The history of measles is one of the most interesting, colorful, and generally underplayed of all infectious diseases. Except for plague, cholera, typhus, and smallpox, measles has perhaps had the greatest impact on people, on the successes or failures of their explorations, their colonization attempts, their military campaigns, and their ability to survive to old age. Curiously, among the general public these facts are little known. The availability of an effective vaccine has so reduced the incidence of measles in developed nations that we have been quick to forget that it is among the most spectacularly contagious of human infections, one which is still a major killer of children in underdeveloped countries.

Measles is an ancient disease. A Moslem physician of the 10th century, Rhazes, is credited with its first recorded accounts. Numerous epidemics swept across Europe through the Middle Ages and Reformation period. Measles accompanied European explorers and immigrants to isolated new lands where the indigenous populations were susceptible to the disease. Among the most dramatic and informative effects of measles in totally susceptible populations was that of the "virgin soil" epidemic in Greenland in 1951. Within 6 weeks, all but five of the 4000 inhabitants of the affected region contracted measles!

The study of measles made a natural progression from the field to the laboratory. In a model of early scientific investigation, Home demonstrated in the mid-18th century that measles could be transmitted by exposure to blood of infected individuals. These findings were confirmed in 1905 and extended several years later through studies of experimental transmission to monkeys. In 1954, Enders and Peebles reported successful growth of measles virus in cultured cells. This paved the way for studies of the molecular biology of measles virus and for the important development of an effective, live, attenuated measles virus vaccine.

THE MEASLES VIRUS

The disease is caused by the measles virus, a *Morbillivirus* of the paramyxovirus family (Table 36.1). The members of this virus family are pleomorphic, meaning that they have a variety of different shapes. The viral genome, composed of RNA, is contained within a helical nucleocapsid that is surrounded by a lipid bilayer envelope (Fig. 36.1). The surface is studded with glycoproteins that project from the envelope surface.

Table 36.1
The classification of paramyxoviruses

Family: Paramyxoviridae
Genus: *Pneumovirus*—respiratory syncytial virus
       Paramyxovirus—mumps virus, parainfluenza virus
       Morbillivirus—measles, canine distemper virus

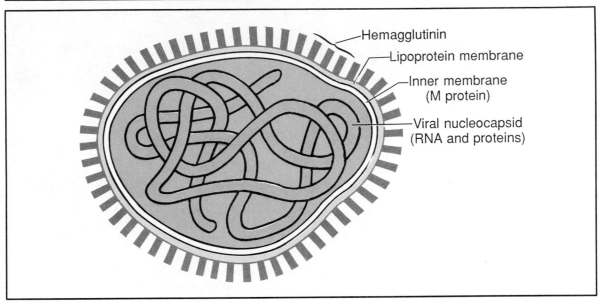

Figure 36.1. Schematic diagram of measles virus. (Modified from Morgan EM, Rapp F: Measles virus and its associated diseases. *Bacteriol Rev* 41:636–666, 1977.)

Measles virus has a single-stranded, nonsegmented RNA genome with negative sense (Fig. 36.2). Individual mRNAs, transcribed from the parental RNA, are translated into measles proteins. This virus replicates in the nucleus—which is unusual for RNA viruses, which more commonly replicate in the cytoplasm. Capsid proteins of *Morbillivirus* include hemagglutinins, whereas those of the related mumps viruses (genus *Paramyxovirus*) have both hemagglutinin and neuraminidase activity (Fig. 36.1). These proteins are named after

Figure 36.2. Transcription and translation of proteins by negative-stranded and positive-stranded RNA viruses.

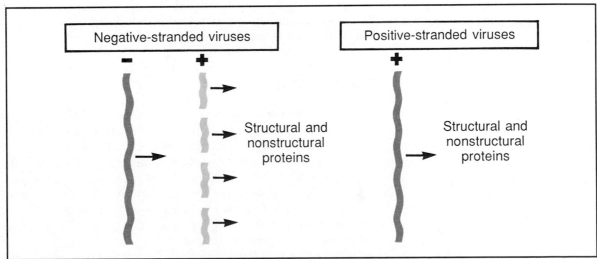

Figure 36.3. Giant cell (syncytium) formation in measles pneumonia. (From Morgan EM, Rapp F: *Bacteriol Rev* 41: 636–666, 1977.

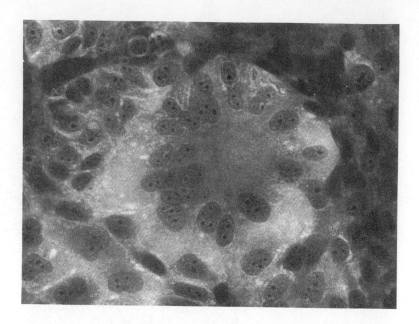

easily identified biological properties and are more fully described in the chapter on influenza virus (Chapter 30).

Measles virus possesses an additional protein known as the *F* (for "fusion") *protein*, which endows the virus with the ability to *cause membranes to fuse together*. Presumably, the F protein participates in fusion of the infecting virus to the cell membrane. Secondarily, its expression on the surface of infected cells during viral replication causes fusion of adjacent cells. This results in one classic hallmark of measles virus infection, namely, the formation of *giant cells*, or syncytia (Fig. 36.3). Measles virus also contains an *M* (for "matrix") *protein* on the inner surface of the viral envelope. This protein is said to participate in the proper envelopment of assembling nucleocapsids. Release of infectious progeny virions is dependent upon the M protein. Other internal proteins, a large protein (L) and the polymerase (P), are believed to participate in transcription and genome replication. Measles replication is manifested not only by formation of syncytia, but also by the appearance of eosinophilic inclusions in the cytoplasm and nucleus. These inclusions are aggregates of proteins that take up the eosin (red) stain commonly used in staining tissue slices.

ENCOUNTER

What do you need to know to consider further if Ms. M. has measles or to discount the possibility? First, did she ever have measles or has she been vaccinated? Before vaccination programs were initiated in this country, measles occurred primarily in 5- to 6-year-old children, and Ms. M. may have been too young to remember her early childhood diseases. A parent or an older sibling might recall; a simple phone call could be of help with her history. Second, we would want to ask whether Ms. M. has recently been in contact with anyone who has this disease. However, patients are not usually aware of measles exposure until a cluster of cases is recognized.

The infection is extremely contagious, maximally so during the 2- to 3-day period prior to the appearance of the rash. Experiments done with virus-containing aerosols have shown that the disease can be acquired through inhalation. Therefore, Ms. M.'s exposure may have involved a seemingly innocuous encounter in an elevator, a bus, or simply anywhere. For instructive purposes, let us assume that other cases of measles have recently been recognized among individuals at Ms. M.'s university.

SPREAD AND MULTIPLICATION

Measles virus is inhaled during exposure to individuals with measles. It is believed that the virus replicates in respiratory epithelial cells and about three days later spreads through the bloodstream to infect distant body sites, including the lung, and lymphoid tissues of the tonsils, lymph nodes, gastrointestinal tract, and spleen. After a few more days, a second, larger wave of virus is released from these sites into the bloodstream, producing maximal symptoms and skin involvement. Infections like measles that involve multiple replicative cycles and spread from the site of inoculation to local and then to distant sites typically have incubation periods of at least 10 to 14 days. Infections that manifest themselves at or near the site of inoculation (e.g., herpes simplex and influenza) and do not disseminate characteristically have short incubation periods (2 to 7 days).

DAMAGE

Most of the pathology associated with measles infection can be attributed directly to viral invasion and *cytopathic destruction of tissues* (Fig. 36.4). It seems likely, however, that some of the features of the disease are attributable to damage inflicted by the host immune responses to the virus. Measles causes the classic

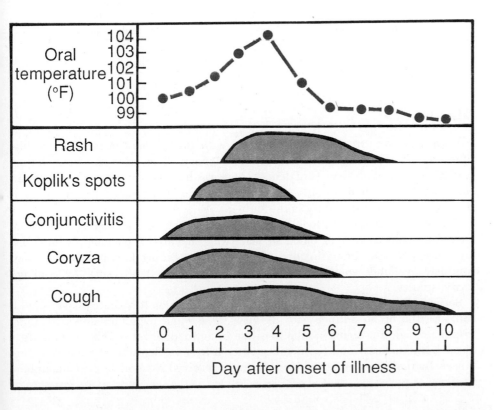

Figure 36.4. Signs and symptoms of measles infection. (From Krugman S. Katz S.: *Infectious Diseases of Children*. St. Louis, CV Mosby, 1981, p 145.

viral *enanthem* (lesions on mucous membranes) in the mouth called *Koplik's spots*, as well as a diffuse *exanthem* (external lesions), the typical measles rash. Biopsies of measles lesions show viral antigens and particles in the tissues but the most prominent finding is an intense inflammatory response with edema and mononuclear infiltration. Immunodeficient children occasionally fail to develop a rash during measles infections, which suggests that the inflammatory response may be a major cause of tissue damage in the mucocutaneous lesions.

Both the humoral and the cellular immune responses modulate the outcome of acute measles infection. Administration of measles-specific globulin to susceptible individuals shortly after exposure to the virus will ameliorate the infection. The cellular immune response, however, is probably the major determinant of protection against severe measles infection and reinfection. Patients with agammaglobulinemia tolerate measles well, while those with congenital or acquired cellular immune deficits, such as those associated with acute leukemia, are prone to severe or fatal infection.

Measles infection itself stresses and further decreases cellular immunity. During measles, patients are at an increased risk of reactivating herpes simplex infections and tuberculosis, and transiently losing their delayed hypersensitivity response to tuberculin and other antigens.

HOW DOES THE HOST RESPOND TO MEASLES?

Acute measles virus infection is nearly always symptomatic and is inevitably accompanied by immune responses in immunocompetent people. IgM antibodies circulate within 2 weeks of development of the rash and persist for several weeks longer. IgG antibodies can be detected in serum shortly after the IgM antibodies, peak within a few weeks and gradually decline, although they persist for life. Secretory IgA antibodies are detectable in nasal secretions. A measles-specific lymphocyte-mediated immune response can be demonstrated in acute infection. So can interferon, whose levels wane rapidly with convalescence. The cellular immunity persists for life; thus Ms. M. probably had neither the vaccine nor the disease in childhood.

DIAGNOSIS

With a known exposure, and certainly with the classic "measly" or *morbilliform* appearance (Fig. 36.5), a tentative diagnosis of measles can be made on clinical grounds with some confidence. There are, however, more precise means of establishing the diagnosis, and it is appropriate to employ such tests whenever the appearance or the history is in doubt.

The definitive diagnostic tool is virus isolation. The virus can be recovered from nasopharyngeal secretions, blood, or urine any time after the onset of symptoms and until the second or third day of rash. The procedure is expensive and not routinely available, so that most physicians appropriately resort to serodiagnostic studies.

Serum collected very early in the course of the infection (the acute phase) would contain little or no antibody to the virus. The rapid evolution of an immune response to viral proteins results in a rise in antibody level so that the quantity of such antibodies would be much greater 2 to 4 weeks after the onset of the illness. By then most measles infections have resolved. Several serologic methods

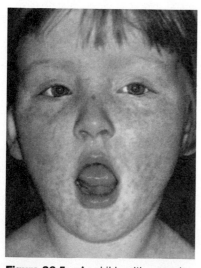

Figure 36.5. A child with measles, showing classic rash, runny nose, and conjunctivitis. (From Emond RTD: *Color Atlas of Infectious Diseases.* London, Wolfe Medical Publications, 1987.

are applicable, but the most widely used tests involve hemagglutination inhibition or an enzyme immunoassay (ELISA test; see Chapter 59).

As the health service physician you can confirm Ms. M.'s diagnosis by collecting and storing serum during her first visit to your office and asking her to return about 2 weeks later to have another serum specimen drawn. At that time you would submit both specimens for testing. A typical confirmatory result might be an eight fold rise in HAI titer, from 1:8 to 1:64, between the samples. These numbers mean the following: In the first sample there was already a sufficient quantity of measles antibody to be detectable in the assay when the serum was diluted eight times, but not more. In the convalescent serum specimen there was so much more measles antibody that it could still be detected in serum that had been diluted 64-fold.

COMPLICATIONS

Immunologically competent individuals experience few complications, although the course of measles infection tends to be more severe in adults than in children. The most common complications involve superinfections of the middle ear and the lung, primarily with pneumococci, staphylococci, or meningococci. Injury to respiratory tract tissues may render a patient more susceptible to bacterial superinfection. Pneumonia is the major reason for hospitalization in measles cases. It can be especially severe if the pneumonia is caused by the virus itself (giant cell pneumonitis) rather than by superinfecting bacteria.

About 1 in 1000 children with measles experience neurological complications. In general, these symptoms appear several days after resolution of the rash and consist of fever, headache, irritability, confusion, and seizures. Most patients survive this meningoencephalitis, but permanent sequelae include deafness, mental retardation, and seizure disorders.

Death from measles, which is rare in developed countries, stems largely from pulmonary and central nervous system complications. In developing nations, measles remains a major killer, felling tens of thousands of infants each year and making measles a major priority of international health programs. There are several reasons for the remarkable prevalence of measles in children of the third world. First, vaccination is expensive and beyond the meager public health resources of many countries. Second, modern diagnostic and therapeutic tools are often not available to limit evolving complications. Third, and most important, the infants of these regions frequently lack the immunological resources to combat the measles virus and other complicating pathogens. Malnutrition impairs cellular immune defenses and poor hygiene favors bacterial superinfection of the skin and respiratory tract (Chapter 61).

PREVENTION

Assuming that our patient, Ms. M., has measles, she may already have exposed others to her virus, at school or elsewhere. Is it possible to break the cycle of the infection in her community? Yes. We noted above that immune serum globulin can modify measles infection. This is appropriate for exposed individuals who are at risk of complicated infection, which includes infants under age 1 and especially children with leukemia or other disorders associated with substantial cellular immune impairment.

Of greater value however, is the measles vaccine. A number of different ones have been developed. The first one, a killed virus vaccine, provided limited protection and only modified the disease associated with subsequent exposure to measles virus. The resulting *atypical measles syndrome* has many clinical features that differ from those of classic measles. Atypical measles occurs in young adults and adolescents and is difficult to diagnose because the exanthem has a highly variable appearance and pleuro-pulmonary complications are frequent.

Antibodies that neutralize virus infectivity are required to limit the spread of measles virus to uninfected cells. Many antibodies can also be induced by viral proteins but fail to inactivate the virus. The killed measles vaccine induces little antibody to the F (fusion) protein but high levels of antibody to the hemagglutinin. Since antibody to the F protein is required to prevent cell-to-cell spread of measles virus, the killed vaccine provided only partial protection against infection.

A live attenuated virus vaccine is well tolerated and confers durable immunity. Currently the recommendation is that it be given at 15 months of age. The reason for this choice is interesting: This age was selected because virtually all maternal antibody to measles vaccine is likely to have disappeared from the child's circulation by that age. Only a small proportion of the children of that age have sufficient residual antibody to prevent the vaccine virus from growing enough to elicit an adequate immune response. The problem with delaying vaccination until 15 months is that it leaves most of the infants at risk for measles from the time their maternally derived protection has waned until they are vaccinated. Were

Figure 36.6. Reported cases of measles (bars) and subacute sclerosing panencephalitis (SSPE) (circles) in the United States, 1962–1979. (From Hinman AR *et al*. Elimination of indigenous measles from the United States. *Rev Infect Dis* 5:538–545, 1983.

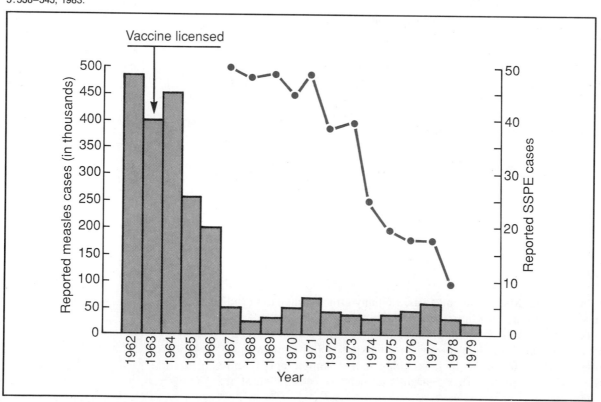

an epidemic to occur, all 12- to 15-month-old children would need immediate vaccination. Measles vaccine is administered together with those against mumps and rubella, all consisting of attenuated live viruses.

Measles vaccination is very successful and is a model for effective prevention of important common viral infections (Fig. 36.6). Current epidemics in the United States and developed countries result from suboptimal vaccination of the population. The Centers for Disease Control has urged universal vaccination, and most states have now mandated that a child must have it before being accepted into primary school. The eradication of measles infection may be within our reach and has been championed by public health authorities in many countries.

SUBACUTE SCLEROSING PANENCEPHALITIS

A process known as a *slow virus infection* consists of the gradual appearance of disease months or years after a virus enters the body. It is to be distinguished from chronic viral infections such as that associated with hepatitis B virus (see Chapter 32) in which the disease progresses steadily after exposure. It is also different from recurrent viral infections like zoster (see Chapter 31), in which the virus can remain dormant for decades before reactivating.

A slow virus infection is unrecognized and undetectable for a long time, until it produces a slowly progressive disorder, one which is characteristically fatal. The best studied slow virus infections of man involve central nervous system degeneration and include *kuru*, *Creutzfeldt-Jakob disease* (CJD) and *subacute sclerosing panencephalitis* (SSPE). Kuru and CJD are caused by "unconventional agents", meaning that their exact nature is undefined.

SSPE is caused by a kind of measles virus and is the best understood of the slow virus infections. Although rare, SSPE has captured the attention of the scientific and medical communities. It is a slowly progressive, unrelenting and untreatable, degenerative neurologic disorder that is characterized by scarring and demyelination of many areas of the brain. Death usually occurs within 2 years of onset. The incidence of SSPE is diminishing in parallel with the decrease in measles cases (Fig. 36.6).

SSPE occurs several years after the initial measles infection and is less likely to occur in individuals who received live measles vaccine. The remarkable aspect of the pathogenesis of SSPE is its association with an *altered measles virus*. How or why the alteration occurs in the virus is unknown, but presumably it results from a spontaneous mutation. Using special techniques, physicians can recover the virus from the brains of some affected patients, but its pattern of replication in brain, cultured cells, or experimental animals is altered. It appears that the measles M protein, normally involved in virus assembly, is not expressed normally; thus the release of infectious progeny virus is impaired.

CONCLUSIONS

On clinical grounds we have been able to determine that Ms. M.'s problem is measles. As her physician you can predict that she will experience a brief illness, one that is likely to be free of complications. The disease will undoubtedly lead to a campus epidemic because about 10% of college students are susceptible to measles. An emergency vaccination program should be initiated without delay. Measles represents a major but now manageable public health menace.

SELF-ASSESSMENT QUESTIONS

1. What peculiar effects does measles virus have on tissue cells?

2. Describe the replication cycle of measles virus.

3. Discuss the role of the immune responses in measles.

4. What problems are associated with vaccination against measles?

5. How could we eradicate measles from the face of the earth?

SUGGESTED READINGS

Hall WR, Hall CB: Atypical measles in adolescents: Evaluation of clinical and pulmonary function. *Ann Intern Med* 90:882–886, 1979.

Katz SL, Krugman S, Quinn TC: International symposium on measles immunization. *J Infect Dis* 5:389–625, 1983.

Modlin JF: Measles virus. In Belshe RB: *Textbook of Human Virology*. Littleton, MA, PSG Publishing Co, 1984, pp 333–360.

Morgan EM, Rapp F: Measles virus and its associated diseases. *Bacteriol Rev* 41:636–666, 1977.

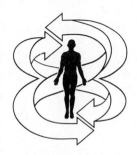

Strategies to Combat Viral Infections

37

S.E. Straus

"There is always some little thing that is too big for us."
(Archy and Mehitabel in Don Marquis' *Archy and Mehitabel*)

The key to successful chemotherapy of viral disease, like all infectious diseases, is drug selectivity. Over the past 50 years the achievements with drugs effective against bacteria, and to a lesser extent against fungi and animal parasites, led to the optimistic assumption that similar chemotherapeutic strategies could be successfully exploited for viruses as well. How much do facts meet these expectations?

Antiviral drugs have been sought since the early days of eucaryotic cell virology. Thousands of compounds have been screened in a random way against viruses in many taxonomic groups. Many substances were found to inhibit virus replication, but mostly because they were toxic to the host cells themselves. It became increasingly clear that virus growth is inextricably tied to host cell processes. The emerging science of animal virology revealed only few points at which one could safely sever the Gordian knots that link viruses and their hosts. Skepticism replaced optimism about the likelihood of obtaining safe and effective antiviral agents.

During the past several years, some cautious advocacy and even occasional enthusiasm have been restored. This has resulted from the sophisticated elucidation of more biochemical targets at which viral replication may be impaired, and more directly, from clear demonstrations that some drugs are safe and effective, at least for a few viruses.

This chapter addresses various strategies by which virus replication can be inhibited, and it summarizes a series of successful applications to human viral disease.

INHIBITION OF VIRUS INFECTIVITY

The most obvious approach to treating viral infections is to block the infectivity of the offending agent. This is easy in the laboratory because many viruses are fragile and easily disrupted. Heating to 50°C, mild detergent, solvents, chelating agents, and numerous other chemical and physical processes all destroy viral infectivity. This results in disinfection, but obviously not therapeutic options. Nevertheless, such measures can be useful to prevent acquisition of infection. Studies have proven that for instance, transmission of the viruses of the common cold by direct contact can be diminished by washing hands or by using iodine-impregnated facial tissues.

Immunologic approaches to blocking viral infectivity are feasible and some are appropriate and effective in humans. Specific antisera can be raised in animals that when mixed with viruses will neutralize viral infectivity. Immune globulins pooled from human sera are commercially available for prophylaxis and therapeutic management of several infections (Tables 37.1, 37.2).

Table 37.1

Use of human immune serum globulins for postexposure prophylaxis of virus infections

Infection	Preparation	Indication
Measles	Pooled human globulin	Susceptible immunodeficient patients
Rubella	Pooled human globulin	Pregnant susceptibles
Poliovirus	Pooled human globulin	Susceptibles
Varicella	Varicella-zoster human immune globulin	Susceptible immunodeficient and pregnant patients
Rabies	Rabies human immune globulin	All cases
Smallpox	Vaccinia human immune globulin	Susceptibles
Hepatitis A virus	Pooled human globulin	All susceptibles
Hepatitis B virus	Pooled human globulin	All susceptibles,
	Hepatitis B human immune globulin	High-risk susceptibles
Cytomegalovirus[a]	CMV human immune globulin	Susceptible transplant patients

[a] Experimental.

Table 37.2

Use of human immune serum globulins for treatment of viral infections

Infection	Preparation	Indication
Vaccinia	Vaccinia human immune globulin	Progressive infection
Echoviruses	Pooled human globulin	Chronic myositis or meningoencephalitis
Arenaviruses	Lassa human immune plasma	Lassa fever
	Junin human immune plasma	Argentinian hemorrhagic fever
	Machupo human immune plasma	Bolivian hemorrhagic fever
Hantaan virus	Hantaan human immune plasma	Korean hemorrhagic fever

There are, however, practical and theoretical limitations to the use of immune globulins for managing human viral diseases. First, many sera are not readily available in large amounts or with adequate antiviral antibody titers. The development of human monoclonal antibody technology provides a way to circumvent this limitation. Second, sera may be contaminated with viruses or other infectious agents. The methods by which the serum immunoglobulins are purified and stabilized kill many known agents, but unknown or nonconventional viruses may resist the process. A classic example of this type of problem occurred during World War II. Several thousand soldiers in the U.S. Army developed hepatitis after receiving a yellow fever vaccine that had been stabilized by the addition of contaminated human serum. Third, the successful prophylactic use of these sera depends on early recognition of exposure. Later in the incubation period of virus infection sera are of no practical value. Chickenpox represents a practical situation in which the timing of immunoglobulin prophylaxis is critical. Human immune globulin pooled from patients recovering from zoster (shingles) infection is effective for preventing severe varicella (chickenpox). A series of clinical studies have proven that the antisera can prevent infection reliably only if they are administered within the first 3 to 4 days after exposure.

Other imaginative immunoglobulin-based approaches to management of viral infections are being developed. Theoretically, monoclonal antibodies directed at the cellular receptor for a virus could sterically hinder virus binding. Unfortunately the nature of the receptor is not known for many viruses, making it impossible to produce the desired monoclonal antibodies since this requires screening a large number of hybridoma cells with a suitable antigen. Without the antigen, this methodology cannot be used. On the other hand, one immediately applicable case is that of AIDS, where the cellular receptor is known to be the CD4 antigen, for which monoclonal antibodies already exist. It has been suggested that treatment with anti-CD4 antibody may prevent the growth and spread of the AIDS retrovirus.

Conventional immunoprophylactic and immunotherapeutic interventions all require an extracellular phase of virus infection. Indeed, most viral infections are initiated by extracellular attachment of free virus. Once the infection is established, however, the therapeutic effects of immunoglobulins are limited to those viruses that freely traverse the extracellular space to infect neighboring or distant cells. The enteroviruses are clear examples (Chapter 35). Immunoglobulins provide effective therapy for some enterovirus infections, such as the serious but rare form of enteroviral encephalitis that develops in patients with agammaglobulinemia. In contrast, infections with herpesviruses, which typically spread directly from cell to cell, cannot be ameliorated by specific immunoglobulins.

INHIBITION OF VIRUS REPLICATION

For most viral infections exposure cannot be determined soon enough to permit effective immunoprophylaxis. Thus a more practical and flexible approach is treatment of infected individuals with substances that inhibit the viruses at a specific point in the viral replicative cycle. A review of the relevant discussion of viral replication in Chapter 29 would be appropriate at this point.

Every step and every biochemical reaction involved in virus replication is conceivably a target for intervention. But for many processes that depend on cellular metabolic pools, energy sources, and enzymes, inhibition of cellular processes is likely to result in unacceptable cell toxicity. It is easy to see why no "penicillin"

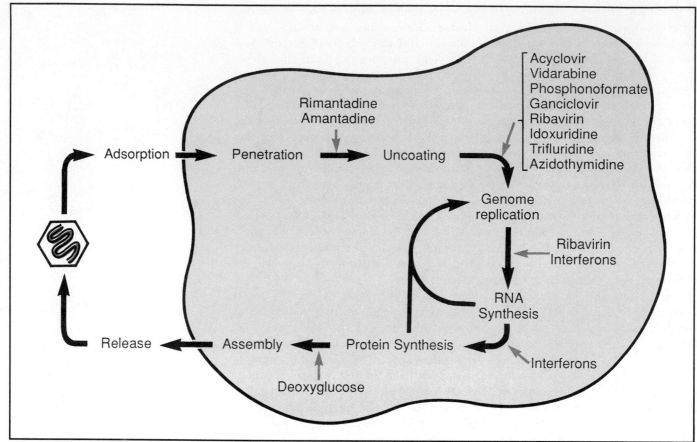

Figure 37.1. Schematic life cycle of viruses showing the steps at which replication can be inhibited by various drugs.

has yet been discovered for viruses. Fortunately, some steps in virus replication differ sufficiently from the cellular ones—they can be inhibited with little or no impact on the host cell. Examples of such specific processes include penetration or uncoating of the virus, synthesis of viral enzymes necessary for viral nucleic acid synthesis, translation, modification, or assembly of viral proteins, and release of the virus from the cell. Figure 37.1 shows the steps in an idealized virus growth cycle where various agents have been found to act.

There are two points to be aware of in considering the current state of antiviral drug development. First, most compounds available have very *narrow spectra of activity*. Very few useful substances inhibit more than one class of viruses. The reason for this may lie in the enormous diversity of viral structures and replicative strategies. In contrast, it is not surprising that antibacterial drugs can have broad activity spectra. Except for differences in the cell envelopes, most bacteria utilize much the same replicative strategies, often different from those of eucaryotic cells. Thus, bacteria have many potential targets in common with one another. Second, few substances that impair virus uncoating or penetration are available. Even worse, we have no substances that safely inhibit virus assembly. These early and late phases of the viral replicative processes are most dependent on the proper association of viral structural elements with cellular ones rather than on de novo synthetic events. To date nearly all of the potentially useful antiviral substances inhibit nucleic acid synthesis. The following is a survey of some of the major compounds being investigated or in clinical use for viral infections.

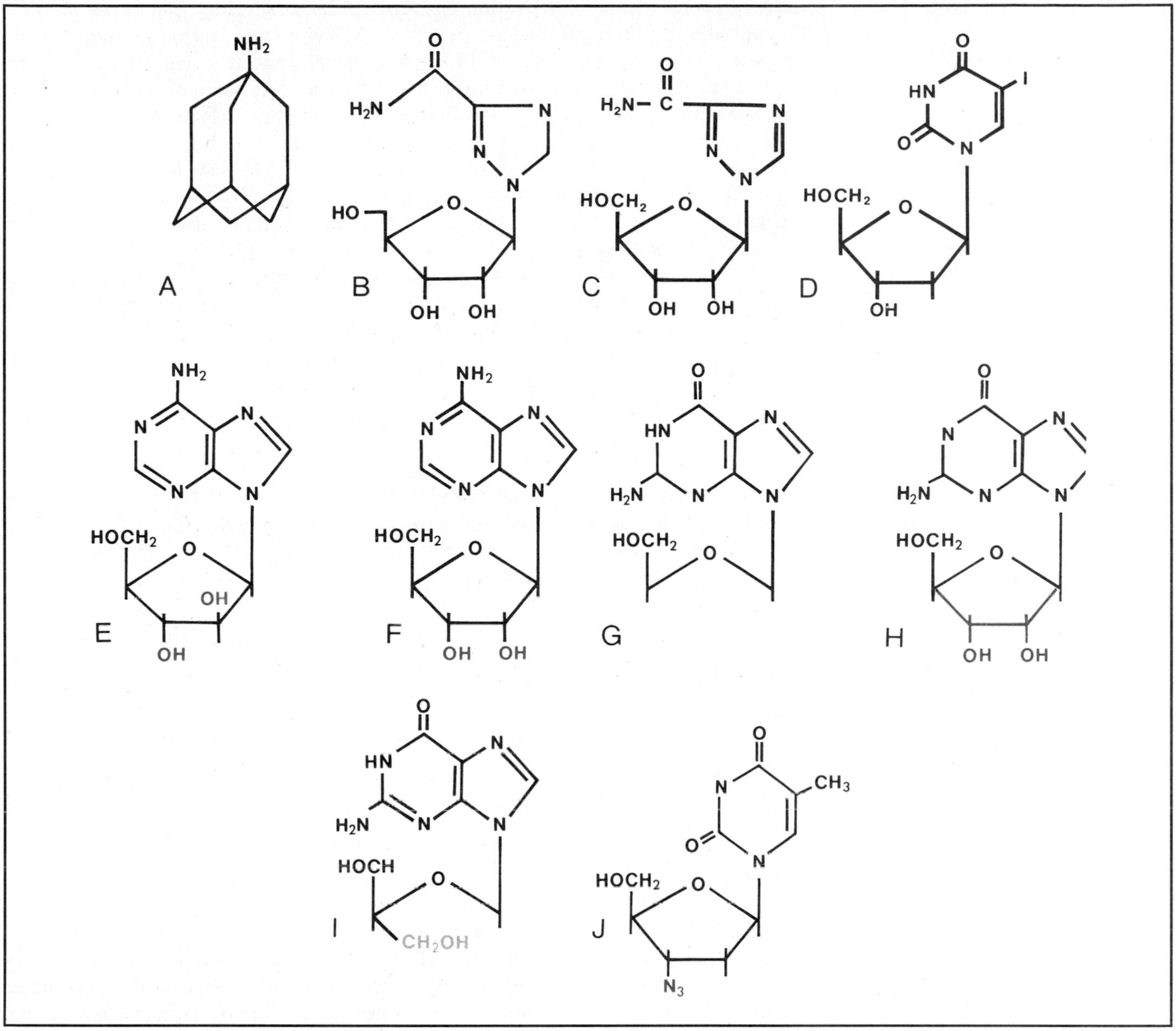

Figure 37.2. **A**, Amantidine. **B**, Rimantadine. **C**, Ribavirin. **D**, Idoxuridine. **E**, Vidarabine. **F**, Deoxyadenosine. **G**, Acyclovir. **H**, Deoxyguanosine. **I**, Ganciclovir. **J**, Azidothymidine.

AMANTADINE

Amantadine (1-adamantanamine hydrochloride) and its analog, rimantadine (a-methyl-1-adamantanamine hydrochloride) are primary symmetrical amines (Fig. 37.2**A**, **B**) whose chemical structures give no clues as to the basis for their antiviral activities. They resemble nothing else known to exist in biological systems. Both compounds are potent inhibitors of the replication of influenza A virus. Their precise mechanisms of action are still being debated. Some data indicate that these compounds block the primary transcription of viral messages. More compelling data suggest that the site of action is earlier and results in the inhibition of viral uncoating. Amantadine has been found to be selectively concentrated in lysosomes and at high concentrations raises intralysosomal pH. This may impair the lysosome-mediated activation of influenza hemagglutinin that is required for penetration of the viral nucleocapsid into the cytoplasm and its subsequent uncoating. However, the drug is effective at lower concentrations than those required to raise the intralysosomal pH. Thus its mode of action remains obscure.

The anti-influenzal activity of amantadine was first reported in 1961, but enthusiasm for its clinical activity was low. The compound was nearly abandoned but for the fortuitous observation that it is extremely beneficial for controlling the disordered motor activity in parkinsonism. This may be only a therapeutic coincidence and does not necessarily suggest an association between parkinsonism and viral infections.

Controlled studies of laboratory-induced or naturally occurring influenza A infections demonstrated that amantadine and rimantadine exert significant prophylactic and therapeutic effects. Optimum use of these drugs is when the encounter with influenza A can be predicted, such as during epidemics. When treatment is initiated prior to exposure to the virus these drugs prevent clinical disease in over three-fourths of cases. For patients whose treatment is begun shortly after the first signs of influenza A infection become apparent, the reduction in severity of symptoms is about 50%.

Both amantadine and rimantadine are well tolerated at the therapeutic dose level—the therapeutic to toxic ratio of these drugs is high. About 3% to 5% of amantadine recipients (but very few rimantadine recipients) report mild central nervous system reactions, including jitteriness, insomnia, and difficulty in concentrating. Recent work has shown both agents to be fundamentally similar in therapeutic and toxic potential, but rimantadine achieves lower peak blood levels.

Amantadine is recommended for the prophylaxis of individuals who are at increased risk of severe infection during suspected influenza A epidemics. These include the elderly and patients with chronic cardiopulmonary disease. It is also recommended that treatment be initiated in these groups at the first sign of influenza. Even taking into account the limited therapeutic value of amantadine and rimantadine, the medical community has been slow to use them widely for influenza.

RIBAVIRIN

This purine nucleoside analog (1-D-ribofuranosyl-1,2,4-triazole-3-carboxamide) is a relatively broad-spectrum antiviral agent (Fig. 37.2C). In cell culture it inhibits some DNA viruses, including herpes simplex and many RNA viruses, including influenza A and B, respiratory syncytial virus, parainfluenza virus, measles virus, and several arenaviruses. The mechanism of action of this drug is also controversial. Since it is an analog of guanosine its phosphorylated form may inhibit the synthesis of guanosine-5′-monophosphate, upon which DNA and RNA synthesis depends. As a more circumscribed mechanism, ribavirin has been found to impair "capping" of virus-specific messenger RNA (the addition of especially methylated guanine nucleotides to the 5′ end of RNA molecules).

Ribavirin is readily available in many developing countries for the oral treatment of human virus infections despite the lack of adequate data to recommend its use. Anecdotal reports suggested that, for example, ribavirin might be effective as an oral treatment in both influenza A and influenza B infections; but unfortunately, controlled studies showed some hematologic toxicity and no clear efficacy.

A novel method of administering the drug avoids its systemic toxicity and yet enhances its antiviral activity. It involves delivery of the drug directly and in high concentrations to the critical site of influenza infection, namely the lung. Inhalation of an aerosol of ribavirin was shown to limit significantly the severity and duration of influenza A and B infection. Recent studies have proven the efficacy of this delivery system for infection with respiratory syncytial virus which is associated with severe bronchiolitis and pneumonia in infants.

A remarkable property of ribavirin is its activity against several highly virulent arenaviruses associated with hemorrhagic fever syndromes. In monkeys infected with these agents, intravenous and oral ribavirin have proven useful. Recently an open trial of oral ribavirin in western Africa showed that it reduces the mortality rate from the dreaded Lassa fever.

INTERFERON

Interferons were the first and still are the most extensively studied of antiviral substances. They are not synthetic drugs, but rather proteins made by the body itself. The discovery of interferon by Isaacs and Lindenmann in 1957 involved a brilliant and fortuitous observation, somewhat analogous to Fleming's recognition of penicillin in moldy cultures. Isaacs was interested in studying viral interference, a phenomenon still poorly understood in which infection renders a cell resistant to subsequent infection with a different virus. This property of virus infected cells allowed, for example, the first laboratory detection of rubella virus; although this virus does not produce visible damage to cells in culture, it does render them refractory to secondary infection with other viruses that can produce cytopathic damage.

In studying viral interference Isaacs and Lindenmann noted that resistance to viral infection could be transferred to uninfected cultures by the addition of media from infected cell cultures. The cell-free factors that mediated the transferable resistance to virus infection were found to be proteins, which they termed interferons. Two properties of interferons were quickly appreciated and led to the hope that at last broad-spectrum antiviral therapy may become available. First, interferons released from cells in response to infection by one virus provide resistance to infection by many other viruses; thus, interferons are not virus-specific. Second, the proteins are present in extremely small amounts, indicating that they are very potent molecules. It was reasoned that if interferons could be purified in sufficient quantities, they would be potent therapeutic agents with a broad spectrum of activity. As natural substances, it seemed likely that they would be relatively nontoxic—though one might wonder why large amounts are not mobilized spontaneously during infections!

Today we know that earlier assumptions were largely naive and only partially correct. Large amounts of interferons can now be generated by sophisticated purification methods or by recombinant DNA technologies, and their mechanisms of action, biological properties, and therapeutic potencies are finally being adequately defined. It is now known that there are three classes of interferons, including nearly two dozen different proteins (Table 29.1). Antiviral activity varies with each type and class of interferon. In cell culture interferons exert their antiviral effects by inducing cells to synthesize a number of enzymes that regulate transcription and translation of viral proteins. Both in animals and humans, the impact of treatment with interferons is more complex than in cell cultures because these compounds not only inhibit viral replication but also modulate host immune responses to the infection.

Clinical trials have shown that interferons, despite their natural origin, are inherently toxic and cause fatigue, fever and myalgias, and occasionally bone marrow suppression and neurologic problems. In fact, the recipients of interferons complain so frequently of flu-like symptoms that it can be reasonably argued that many of the constitutional complaints that attend common viral infections may result from host responses mediated by interferon.

Interferon treatment ameliorates severe varicella or zoster infections in immunocompromised hosts, delays cytomegalovirus infections in transplant recipients, prevents reactivation of herpes simplex in patients undergoing trigeminal nerve root decompression, and transiently diminishes the level of circulating hepatitis B virus in patients with chronic hepatitis. These many and diverse activities attest to the broad specificity of interferons. Unfortunately their effectiveness in each of these conditions has been insufficient to warrant their licensing for treatment of viral infections.

Why do not interferons have more dramatic clinical activity? Inadequate dosage cannot explain their limitations since circulating levels of the newer recombinant interferon preparations can exceed those observed in untreated infections. Here are some possible reasons why interferons may not be the hoped for wonder drugs. First, the production of different interferons may vary in response to different viruses. In a given infection the antiviral activity achieved may depend on the relative amount of each interferon expressed at a particular site. This may not be precisely duplicated by exogenous administration. Second, interferons exhibit their most potent activity against a number of RNA viruses that do not cause serious human disease.

The current best hope for antiviral therapy with interferons is considered to be in infections by papillomaviruses (see Chapter 34). Recurring anogenital and laryngeal papillomas are annoying and destructive. Several trials of topical, intralesional, and systemic interferon are under way for these infections. Preliminary data suggest that interferons speed their resolution. It should also be recognized that interferons play other therapeutic roles with some effectiveness against certain animal parasites and particular types of cancer.

IDOXURIDINE

In the late 1950s a large effort was undertaken to synthesize and screen nucleoside analogs for use in cancer treatment. By-products of the program were novel compounds that were also tested for antiviral activity. Idoxuridine (5-iodo-2'-deoxyuridine) is one agent that emerged from that program and that demonstrates in vitro activity against herpes simplex virus at nontoxic concentrations (Fig. 37.2**D**). By the early 1960s topical application of this compound had been shown to speed the resolution of corneal herpes. Thus idoxuridine became the first antiviral drug to be widely used. There was great temptation to extend its indications to other herpes simplex infections. Studies of its effectiveness in oral and genital herpes and other more severe infections taught us much of what we know about these diseases and their management with antiviral drugs.

It soon became apparent in these studies that casual and uncontrolled trials can lead to inappropriately optimistic conclusions. For example, when idoxuridine was tried for life-threatening infections such as herpes simplex encephalitis, early anecdotes were optimistic and led to an increasing demand for its compassionate use. To clarify its true value a controlled trial was initiated in which idoxuridine was compared with placebo infusions for herpes encephalitis. It was found that the drug-treated patients did no better, and possibly worse, than the placebo recipients. Idoxuridine was simply too toxic for systemic use. This study proved the necessity for placebo-controlled trials for evaluation of antiviral drugs.

Early studies with topical idoxuridine also documented that the efficacy of treatment of cutaneous herpes is limited by the ability of a drug to penetrate the skin. Dissolution of idoxuridine in a vehicle such as dimethyl sulfoxide allowed better skin penetration and improved its activity in animal models, but in human studies the agent was still too weak to be of significant benefit.

VIDARABINE

Arabinosyl adenine (vidarabine, ara-A, 9-D-arabinofuranosyladenine) is less active against herpesviruses than idoxuridine in vitro (Fig. 37.2**E**). However, it is much less cytotoxic than idoxuridine and has a significantly greater therapeutic ratio. Thus effective doses can be given systemically with minimal toxicity.

Large, well-designed controlled clinical trials have found that topical vidarabine is too weak to ameliorate oral or genital herpes infections in otherwise normal persons. Intravenously, however, vidarabine was proven to decrease the mortality of herpes simplex encephalitis and neonatal herpes simplex infections, and to lessen the morbidity of severe varicella and zoster infections in immunocompromised children and adults. These observations proved that serious human viral infections are amenable to specific therapeutic intervention. The pessimism regarding prospects for antiviral drug development began to wane.

ACYCLOVIR

Acyclovir (acycloguanosine, 9-[2-hydroxyethoxymethyl] guanine) has already supplanted vidarabine for treatment of several human herpesvirus infections (Fig. 37.2**G**). It is the first agent approved for clinical use that results from a rational and directed search for antiviral compounds. This strategy is being increasingly exploited. Once we know that a compound has some activity, it can be further modified and its derivatives tested for increased activity and better pharmacologic properties such as stability, solubility, or gastrointestinal absorption.

The mechanism of action of acyclovir has been well studied. Like idoxuridine and vidarabine, acyclovir is an inhibitor of DNA polymerase. When its activity against the cellular and viral polymerases is compared, acyclovir exhibits a level of specificity that substantially exceeds that of either of the older drugs. The reason is interesting: in order for acyclovir to inhibit DNA polymerase it must be phosphorylated in vivo by thymidine kinase (Fig. 37.3). It turns out that the herpes

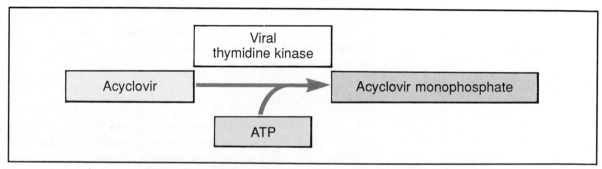

Figure 37.3. Phosphorylation of acyclovir by thymidine kinase.

Table 37.3
Typical concentrations of acyclovir required for 50% inhibition of herpesvirus replication in cell culture

Virus	μg/ml
Herpes simplex 1	0.1
Herpes simplex 2	0.3
Varicella-zoster virus	3
Epstein-Barr virus	3
Cytomegalovirus	>4.0

simplex virus encodes for a thymidine kinase that has the unique property of phosphorylating acyclovir far better than does the cell's own kinase. The resulting monophosphate is then further phosphorylated by cellular enzymes to generate acyclovir triphosphate. This moiety inhibits the DNA polymerases of some herpesviruses because its incorporation into nascent strands of DNA blocks further replication. Viral DNA polymerase is unable to attach bases beyond the point of addition of acyclovir because the drug lacks the 3′ carbon of the sugar ring at which phosphodiester bonds link nucleosides together.

How do these biochemical mechanisms translate into acyclovir's in vitro potency for each herpesvirus? Herpes simplex virus types 1 and 2 are effectively inhibited with submicromolar concentrations of acyclovir (Table 37.3). Epstein-Barr virus and varicella-zoster virus are less sensitive to the drug, while cytomegalovirus is not well inhibited. Why? We have only a partial answer to explain why all herpesviruses vary in their sensitivity to this compound. We know that the polymerase of each virus differs in the degree to which it substitutes acyclovir triphosphate for the natural substrate guanosine triphosphate. Cytomegalovirus does not encode its own thymidine kinase and inhibitory concentrations of acyclovir triphosphate cannot be generated in cytomegalovirus infected cells.

The clinical response to acyclovir therapy of patients has closely paralleled these in vitro results. The most significant benefits accrue in patients with herpes simplex virus infections. Clinical responses to acyclovir therapy are also seen in patients with varicella and zoster infections. Acyclovir has not reproducibly helped in alleviating cytomegalovirus infections.

The greatest benefit from acyclovir comes from treatment of prolonged or severe mucocutaneous herpes simplex virus infections. These include the first infections of normal patients or any infection of immune deficient hosts. Topical, oral, and intravenous formulations of acyclovir speed the clearing of virus, hasten the resolution of symptoms, and shorten the time for the lesions to heal (Fig. 37.4). Herpes infections in normal patients, which are inherently milder, are not helped by topical acyclovir treatment; these infections do not warrant intravenous therapy. A modest reduction in the severity of the milder forms of herpes infections can be achieved with prompt administration of oral acyclovir.

Acyclovir does not prevent or terminate latency of herpesviruses. In other words, the infection is as likely to recur whether or not acyclovir treatment was instituted promptly. Nevertheless, there is an effective way of circumventing this limitation. Long-term treatment with oral acyclovir suppresses most expected herpetic recurrences (Fig. 37.5). However, the suppressive effect of the drug is limited to the period of treatment. Even after 1 year of continuous treatment recurrences may develop promptly after its termination. This leads to an unusual dilemma for practitioners: Acyclovir, like nearly all drugs, is not free of toxic effects after long-term administration. An additional source of concern is that the virus may develop resistance to the drug. Thus, one needs to exercise restraint and judgment in selecting young patients for long-term, noncurative treatment for such a nonprogressive disorder.

GANCICLOVIR

The most serious gap in acyclovir's antiviral spectrum is its lack of activity against cytomegalovirus. A major cause of morbidity and mortality in transplant recipients and AIDS patients, cytomegalovirus has long been a major target for antiviral chemotherapy. The drugs mentioned above, alone or in various combinations, all fall short of ameliorating cytomegalovirus disease.

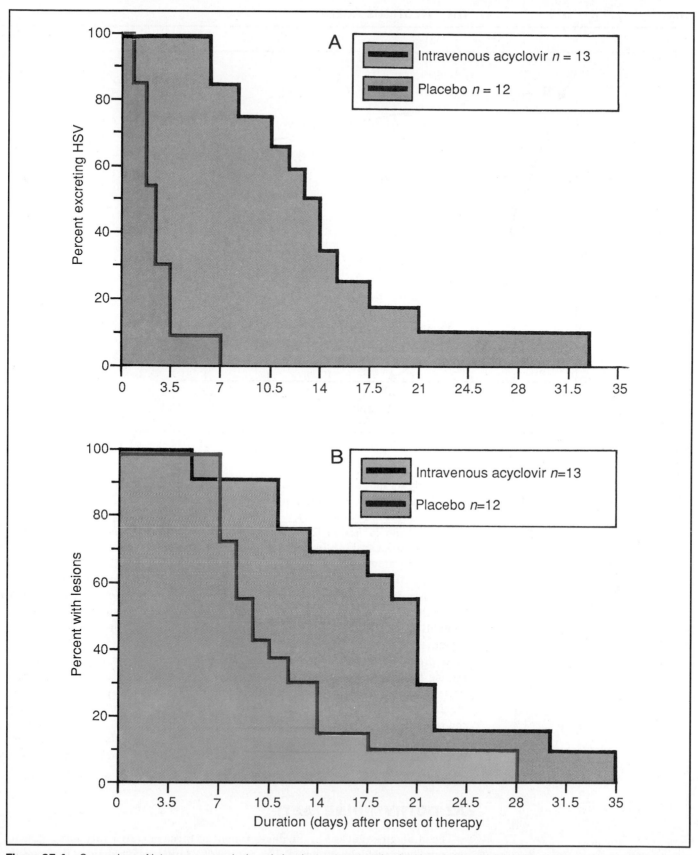

Figure 37.4. Comparison of intravenous acyclovir and placebo treatment on the duration of virus shedding (**A**) and time to healing (**B**) in normal patients with first episode genital herpes. (From Corey L, et al. Intravenous acyclovir for the treatment of primary genital herpes. *Ann Intern Med* 98:914–921, 1983).

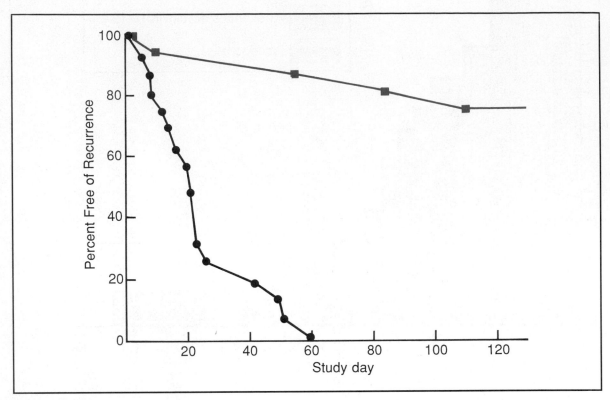

Figure 37.5. Patients with frequently recurring genital herpes were treated chronically with placebo (black) or acyclovir capsules (red). The likelihood of remaining free of recurrence is shown by study day. (From Straus S, et al: Suppression of recurrent genital herpes with oral acyclovir. *Trans Assoc Amer Phys* 97:278–283, 1984.)

In studying modifications of the acycloguanosine (acyclovir) molecule, one compound, ganciclovir (9-[1,3-dihydroxy-2-propoxymethyl] guanine) was found to have greatly improved activity against cytomegalovirus (Fig. 37.2). Its mechanism of action is similar to that of acyclovir, with preferential phosphorylation by viral kinases and inhibition of the viral DNA polymerase. The fact that it inhibits cytomegalovirus replication has led some to speculate that this virus may possess a still uncharacterized nucleotide kinase. It is more toxic than acyclovir, very possibly because cellular polymerases can utilize ganciclovir triphosphate better than acyclovir triphosphate. Furthermore, its free 3′ position permits chain elongation beyond the points of its incorporation, thus making the compound a potential mutagen.

In preliminary clinical trials ganciclovir has proved to be the first agent to reduce the amount of cytomegalvorius that can be recovered from an infected patient. Cytomegalovirus-induced retinitis in AIDS patients is stabilized by ganciclovir, but reactivation and progressive infection are seen in many patients once the treatment is stopped. DHPG has had less salutory effects in those bone marrow transplant recipients who rapidly develop fatal cytomegalovirus pneumonia. Even when the drug is used, the basic course of the infection remains unremitting and nearly always fatal.

AZIDOTHYMIDINE (AZT)

The strategies that led to the development of these effective anti-herpes agents are now being widely exploited. The synthesis of nucleoside analogs that can inhibit RNA and other DNA polymerases as well as other known viral enzymes, should, by the end of this century, lead to drugs with additional therapeutic indications. Nowhere is the need more urgent than for agents that inhibit reverse transcriptases. Screening compounds for their ability to inhibit the growth of AIDS viruses has identified several likely candidates for clinical testing. Some of these have already proven too toxic, but a few other candidates offer hope.

Particularly promising is azidothymidine (Fig. 37.2J). It inhibits AIDS virus replication at concentrations of 0.1 to 0.5 μg/ml, readily achieved via oral or parenteral routes but well below the cytotoxic level. Azidothymidine has proven to benefit patients with AIDS and opportunistic infections or with AIDS-related complex (ARC). Treatment improved the immune status, weight, and feeling of well-being, and prevented new opportunistic infections. Most important, azidothymidine treated patients lived longer. Unfortunately, this drug is toxic for the bone marrow, and its use over months and years necessitates repeated blood transfusions. Studies are under way to identify optimal treatment regimens with this drug.

DRUG RESISTANCE

The early days of antibacterial chemotherapy were marked by blissful naiveté about the impact of drug resistance. Those who study antiviral compounds are now forearmed with this knowledge and are careful to screen virus isolates from treated patients for evidence of drug resistance. Not surprisingly, resistant mutants can be readily prepared in the laboratory by growing viruses at subinhibitory drug concentrations.

Resistant strains have been recovered from patients as well but as yet have not proved to be especially troublesome. There may be two major reasons for optimism:

1. Most viral infections resolve spontaneously as a result of the successful efforts of the cellular immune defenses. The goal of antiviral therapy in most such instances is to *speed resolution*. Emergence of drug resistance may lead to delay in virus clearing, but in general the resistant viruses would present a problem mainly for individuals with impaired immune defenses.

2. Development of drug resistance may lead to a reduction of the inherent virulence of some viruses. Herpes simplex strains become resistant to acyclovir predominantly because of mutations in the gene for thymidine kinase. But thymidine kinase deficiency renders strains less virulent in animals and less likely to establish latent neural infection. In fact, patients with strains resistant to acyclovir do not suffer severe infections. Moreover, recurrences are associated with reactivation of the original drug-sensitive strains that remained unaltered in the nerve ganglia.

The current hopefulness about antiviral resistance could wane rapidly if virulent mutants were detected among the resistant ones. This prospect must be kept in mind, and new and available antiviral drugs must be used prudently.

SUGGESTED READINGS

Dolin R: Antiviral chemotherapy and chemoprophylaxis. *Science* 227:1296–1303, 1985.
Galasso GJ et al. (eds): *Antiviral Agents and Viral Diseases of Man.* New York, Raven Press, 1984.

Review of the Main Pathogenic Viruses

This chart is intended to review the main human viruses. Included are the agents of greatest medical relevance.

Many of the viruses that cause relatively uncommon diseases are not included. This chart may be completed to review material you have covered under this topic.

Virus	Group or Family	Nucleic Acid	Other Attributes	Disease(s) and Systems Involved	Relevant Chapter(s)
Smallpox					29
Adenovirus					29
Influenza					30, 45
Herpes simplex					31, 47, 53
Varicella-zoster Epstein-Barr					3
Hepatitis A					32
Hepatitis B					32
Other hepatitis					32
HIV					33
Warts					34
Polio					35
Coxsackie Other enteroviruses					35
Mumps					36
Measles					36
Rubella					53
Rhinovirus					45
Arbovirus encephalitis					55
Respiratory syncytial virus					45
Parvovirus					29
Rotavirus					46
Norwalk agent					46

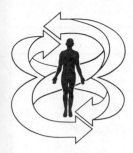

The Fungi and the Mycoses

38

G. Kobayashi
G. Medoff

WHAT ARE THE PATHOGENIC FUNGI

In most people's minds fungi conjure up the image of mildew and old shoes, moldy bread, or skin infections with graphic names like "athlete's foot" or "jock itch". In fact, fungi have a major influence on the health and livelihood of people throughout the world. They cause a wide spectrum of clinical disease, from simple cosmetic problems to potentially lethal systemic infections. They play an important role in degrading organic waste material in nature but are also economically destructive and cause widespread damage to food and fabrics. Fungi are used commercially in many fermentations, and produce steroid hormone derivatives and antibiotics such as penicillin.

Fungi are eucaryotes, with a defined nucleus enclosed by a nuclear membrane, a cell membrane that contains lipids, glycoproteins and sterols, mitochondria, Golgi apparatus, ribosomes bound to endoplasmic reticulum, and a cytoskeleton with microtubules, microfilaments and intermediate filaments (Chapter 2). Of course, this description applies to animal cells as well, a fact that constitutes a major problem in dealing with fungal infections. The infecting organisms are so similar to their host cells that it is difficult to devise therapeutic strategies specific for the parasite and nontoxic to the host.

Shapes and Structures

Pathogenic fungi have two forms: *filamentous*, the molds, or *unicellular*, the yeasts. Molds grow as microscopic, branching, thread-like filaments. These are

Figure 38.1. Somatic hyphae. **A,** Apical portion of nonseptate (coenocytic) hypha; the protoplasm is continuous and multinucleated **B,** Apical portion of septate hypha; protoplasm is interrupted by cross walls.

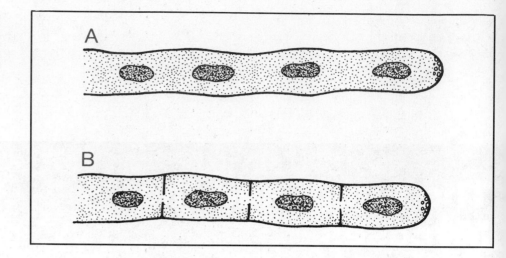

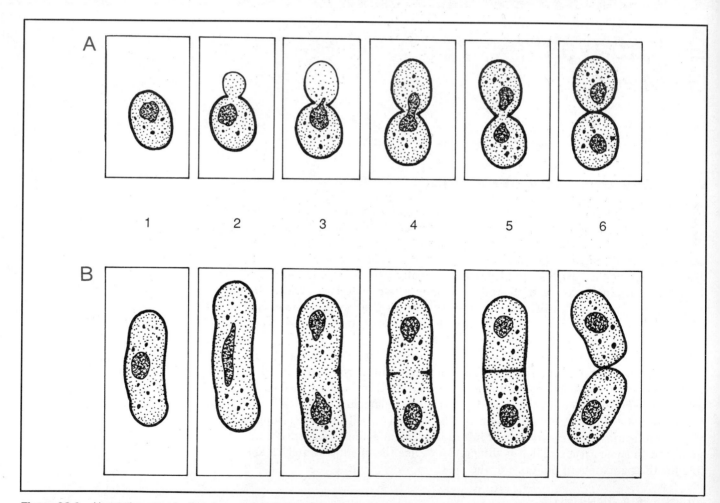

Figure 38.2. Vegetative reproduction of yeast. **A,** Cell reproducing by budding (blastospores formation). **B,** Cell reproducing by fission (cross-wall formation). *1* to *6* show successive steps in each form of reproduction.

called *hyphae* and are collectively referred to as the *mycelium*. A mycelium is what you see when you look at the white mat on moldy fruit. The hyphae are either septate (divided by partitions) or coenocytic (multinucleate without cross walls), a feature that is used in laboratory diagnosis (Fig. 38.1). On agar, hyphae grow outward from the point of inoculation by extension of the tips of filaments and then branch repeatedly.

Yeasts are single cells, ovoid or spherical, with a rigid cell wall and the same cellular complexity as the hyphae. Most yeasts divide by budding and a few divide by binary fission, such as bacteria (Fig. 38.2). On agar they form colonies that are similar to those of bacteria but usually become considerably larger. Some also produce a polysaccharide capsule, an important characteristic of the yeast that causes the disease cryptococcosis, *Cryptococcus neoformans*.

Dimorphism and Growth

Many important pathogenic fungi have two growth forms and can exist either as molds or as yeasts. For example, the agent of histoplasmosis, *Histoplasma capsulatum*, grows as yeast in some conditions and as mycelium in others (Fig. 38.3). This phenomenon is called *dimorphism*. In the laboratory, the transition between these two phases can be reversibly induced by changes in temperature, with the yeast phase being more typical of human body temperature.

The yeast-mycelium or mycelium-yeast shift is frequently associated with a change from a free living organism to a parasite. With most fungi that cause systemic infections, e.g., the agents of histoplasmosis and blastomycosis, the parasitic form is the yeast while the mold is the form found in the environment (soil). In a few unusual cases, such as *Candida*, this rule is reversed and the mycelial form is the one found in tissues.

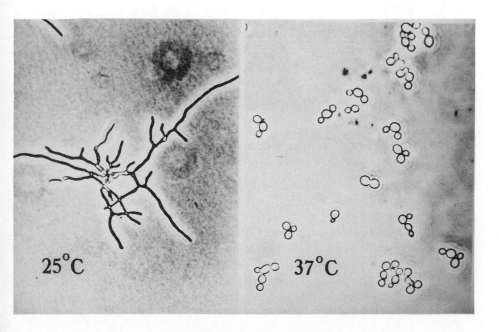

Figure 38.3. Temperature-induced morphogenesis in *Histoplasma capsulatum*. Cultures grow in the mycelial phase at 25°C and as yeasts at 37°C.

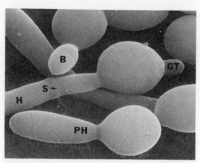

Figure 38.4. Electron photomicrograph of *Candida albicans* illustrating the following cellular morphological characters: pseudohypha (PH); hypha (H) with septum (S); germ tube (GT); blastospore (B). (From Cole GT, Nozawa Y: Dimorphism, in Cole GT, Kendrick B, (eds): *Biology of Conidial Fungi.* New York, Academic Press, 1981.)

Not all pathogenic fungi are dimorphic and undergo morphologic changes when they infect a host. Aspergilli, among the most common molds in the environment, are always filamentous, whereas *C. neoformans* is always a yeast. Certain yeasts, particularly species of *Candida*, carry out a modified form of budding in which newly budded cells remain attached to their parental cells. These aggregates are called *pseudohyphae* or in the aggregate, *pseudomycelium* (Fig. 38.4).

Most of the molecular biology and genetics of fungi has been studied using the common baker's or brewer's yeast, *Saccharomyces cerevisiae*; and to a lesser extent, the molds *Aspergillus nidulans* and *Neurospora crassa*. Less is known about pathogenic fungi, although active studies are being carried out on their virulence factors and dimorphic transitions. In the laboratory, most fungi are grown in media similar to those used for bacteria, though usually at a lower pH. All fungi are basically aerobic, but baker's yeast can grow for short periods without oxygen. In general, fungi prefer 25 to 30°C, although some of the organisms that cause deep mycoses grow well at 37°C and one thermophilic pathogen, *Aspergillus fumigatus*, grows well up to 50°C.

Fungi belong to a separate kingdom, the Eumycota, and are classified on the basis of their mode of sexual and asexual reproduction, morphology, life cycle, and to some extent, physiology. Until recently, the mode of sexual reproduction of most human fungal pathogens was not known. For this reason, they were dumped into a catch-all category, the *Fungi imperfecti*. Since the 1960s, the sexual reproductive states have been found for an increasing number of skin pathogenic fungi. Although the rules of nomenclature give preference to names of the perfect or sexual state (if known), the longer-established and more familiar names of the imperfect state are still used. Thus, the diagnostic laboratory will report the isolation of *C. neoformans* or *H. capsulatum* rather than the less familiar names of the sexual states.

THE MYCOSES

Fungal infections can be classified by areas of the body that are primarily affected.

- Superficial mycoses are infections limited to the outermost layers of skin and hair. Many are mild, readily diagnosed, and respond well to therapy.

- Slightly deeper in the epidermis are the sites of the *cutaneous mycoses*, like athlete's foot or ringworm. The fungi that cause these conditions are called the *dermatophytes*.

- The subcutaneous mycoses are a distinctive group of fungal disease that involve the dermis and the subcutaneous tissue.

- Systemic mycoses are infections with invasion of the internal organs of the body. It is convenient to differentiate between the systemic mycoses caused by *primary pathogens*, such as *H. capsulatum* or *Coccidioides immitis*, which can cause disease in healthy individuals, and those caused by *opportunistic fungi*, such as *Candida albicans*, which have only marginal pathogenicity and generally require a debilitated host for progressive infection to take place. In the systemic mycoses, most people affected usually have mild signs or subclinical manifestations. In contrast, opportunistic fungal infections almost always produce significant disease.

Encounter

With a handful of important exceptions, fungi implicated in human diseases are free living in nature. Most mycoses are acquired as a result of accidental encounters by inhalation or traumatic implantation from an exogenous source. *H. capsulatum* is found in soil contaminated by the excreta of bats, chickens, and starlings. *C. neoformans* is associated with pigeon roosts and soils contaminated by pigeon droppings.

Some of these fungi have distinct geographic preferences. Thus, *Coccidioides immitis* is found in the bioclimatic area known as the lower Sonoran life zone of the southwestern United States and similar geographic sites in Central and South America. This region has arid or semiarid climates, hot summers, few winter freezes, and alkaline soils. *Coccidioides immitis* has been found only in the New World (North, Central, and South America). On this same note, paracoccidioidomycosis, a disease caused by *Paracoccidioides brasiliensis*, is geographically limited to South and Central America. *Blastomyces dermatitidis*, once thought to exist only in the North American continent, has been found to have endemic foci in Africa. *Sporothrix schenckii* has been isolated frequently from rose and barberry thorns and decaying vegetation

In contrast to these environmental habitats, many of us carry *C. albicans* in the mouth, gastrointestinal tract and other mucous membrane linings as part of our normal flora. *Pityrosporum ovale* are yeasts found on the healthy human skin, particularly in the upper trunk, face and scalp, the areas that are rich in sebaceous glands which make lipids used by these organisms. Finally, dermatophytes that cause ringworm and athlete's foot are occasionally found on the skin and scalp of individuals in the absence of symptoms; they are thought to represent transient colonization or a carrier state.

Entry

The level of innate immunity in most humans is high, since fungal infections are usually mild and self-limiting. The intact skin or mucosal surfaces are the primary barriers to infection. Desiccation, epithelial cell turnover, the fatty acid content, and the low pH of the skin are believed to be important factors in host resistance. Also, the bacterial flora of the skin and mucous membranes compete with fungi and hinder their unrestricted growth. Alterations in the balance of the normal flora by use of antibiotics or changes in nutrition allow fungi such as *C. albicans* to proliferate and increase likelihood of entry and infection.

Spread and Multiplication

Within tissues, fungi are restrained by a variety of nonspecific mechanisms. In the case of *Candida*, for example, the fungistatic effect of serum has been shown to be due in part to transferrins, the human iron-binding proteins that deprive microbes of the iron they need for making respiratory enzymes. Serum also contains β-globulins, which cause a nonimmunological clumping of *Candida* and facilitate their elimination by inflammatory cells.

Tissue reaction to the presence of fungi varies with the species, the site of proliferation, and the duration of infection. Some mycoses are characterized by a low-grade inflammatory response that does not eliminate the fungi. Fungal cells can sometimes persist within macrophages or giant cells without being killed.

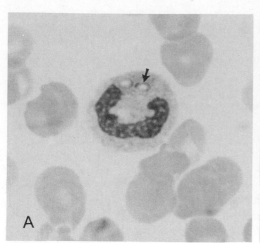

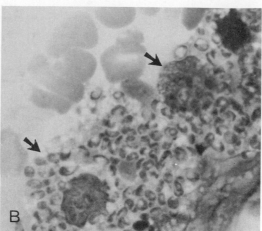

Figure 38.5. A, Peripheral blood smear showing neutrophil with phagocytized yeast cells (*arrow*) of *Histoplasma capsulatum*. **B**, Bone marrow aspirate showing histiocytes (*arrows*) filled with phagocytized yeast cells of *H. capsulatum*. (Courtesy of Laurel Krewson.)

For example, yeast cells of *H. capsulatum* can proliferate within the cytoplasm of macrophages and neutrophils and spread to other organs of the body within those cells (Fig. 38.5). Why they are able to survive within macrophages is unknown, but recent work suggests that they may be resistant to lysosomal enzymes. Most of the time, however, nonspecific inflammatory reactions are critically important in eliminating fungi. Phagocytosis by neutrophils is the earliest mechanism that prevents the establishment of fungal infections and is usually the most effective. Consistent with this, the frequency and virulence of disseminated *Candida* and *Aspergillus* infections are greater in patients with low numbers of neutrophils or with disorders of neutrophil functions, such as chronic granulomatous disease or myeloperoxidase deficiency. In the case of *Candida*, phagocytized cells are killed intracellularly by both the oxygen-dependent and independent mechanisms.

In some cases phagocytosis fails. For example, *C. neoformans* causes meningitis in people with normal phagocytic function. Just as with the encapsulated bacteria, these organisms escape phagocytosis because they are surrounded by a thick viscous capsule.

Fungi that are too big to be ingested can nevertheless be killed by immunological mechanisms. Fungal cells and their extracellular products are highly antigenic and evoke both cellular and humoral responses. There is evidence that antibodies play a role in the elimination of fungi from the body. Along with complement, antibodies participate in the extracellular killing of *Aspergillus fumigatus* and pseudohyphae of *C. albicans* by lymphocytes and phagocytic cells (Fig. 38.6). Instead of "ingesting" and "digesting" the fungi, phagocytic cells appear to secrete lethal lysosomal enzymes.

Resistance to fungal disease is due mainly to cellular or T lymphocyte–mediated immunity. This can be inferred from animal experiments and from the clinical observation that patients with depressed cellular immunity are especially prone to invasive and serious systemic fungal disease. For example, patients with AIDS commonly have mucocutaneous candidiasis and serious systemic infections with *C. neoformans*. As can be expected, patients with AIDS who live in endemic areas may acquire disseminated histoplasmosis or coccidioidomycosis.

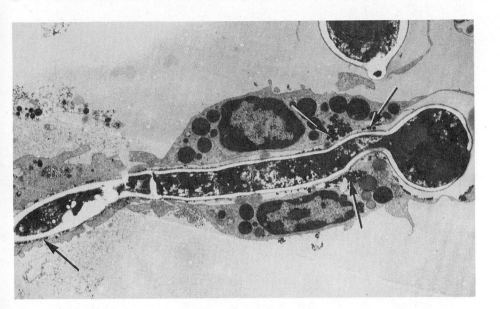

Figure 38.6. Electron photomicrograph of phagocytic cell ingesting a hypha of *Candida albicans*. (Courtesy of Dr. R. D. Diamond.)

Damage

As far as is known fungi that cause invasive disease do not secrete toxins that harm the host. Tissue damage most probably results from direct invasion with displacement, destruction of vital structures, and toxic effects of the inflammatory response. Fungi may also grow as masses of cells (fungus balls) that can occlude bronchi in the lung or tubules or even ureters in kidneys, leading to obstruction of outflow of biological fluids (sputum, urine) and secondary infection and tissue damage. *Aspergillus* or *Mucor* species have the propensity to grow in the walls of arteries or veins, leading to occlusion and ischemic tissue necrosis. Mats of fungi are formed as vegetation on heart valves in fungal endocarditis. Pieces can break off and travel through the blood to any organ in the body and cause arterial occlusion with resultant tissue necrosis.

Diagnosis

Fungal infections are diagnosed in the laboratory by direct microscopy, culture, and serology. Morphological characteristics of the organisms are valuable in the identification of all fungi, both in tissues and in culture. These are particularly useful in the diagnosis of serious systemic infections. Among the distinctive characteristics are the spherules of *Coccidioides immitis* in tissue (Fig. 38.7), the typical large budding yeasts of *Blastomyces dermatitidis* in pus (Fig. 38.8), the coenocytic hyphae of mucormycosis (Fig. 38.9), or the encapsulated yeast cells of *C. neoformans* in cerebrospinal fluid or brain tissue (Fig. 38.10). Their detection provides an immediate and reliable diagnosis in systemic infections. For opportunistic pathogens such as *Mucor*, *Candida*, and *Aspergillus*, microscopic examination of clinical specimens is particularly useful because culture alone may not be helpful (since these organisms are in the environment and can be part of the normal flora of the body). Here, histologic evidence of infection in tissue is usually the single most valuable diagnostic procedure, though a negative finding does not rule out infection.

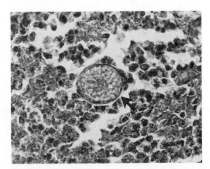

Figure 38.7. Surgical specimen of lung showing mature spherule (*arrow*) of *Coccidioides immitis* containing endospores.

Figure 38.8. Sputum sample containing yeast cells of *Blastomyces dermatitidis*. (Courtesy of Dr. B. H. Cooper.)

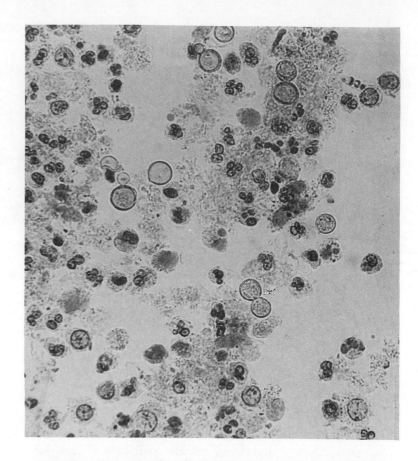

Figure 38.9. Section of lung showing ribbon-like nonseptate hyphae (*arrows*) characteristic of agents such as *Mucor* spp. that cause zygomycosis.

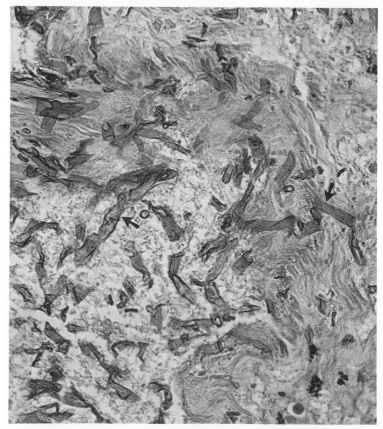

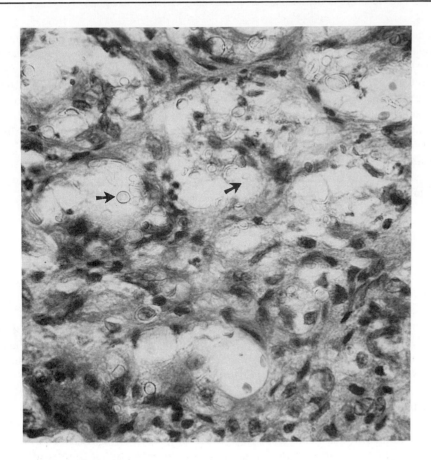

Figure 38.10. Tissue section of brain of patient with cryptococcosis. Note yeast cells (*arrows*) typical of *Cryptococcus neoformans* within spaces occupied by capsular material and general absence of cellular response.

Pathogenic fungi may also be recovered from infected tissues using culture procedures. When the organism isolated is a primary pathogen such as *H. capsulatum*, the diagnosis is unequivocal. Isolation of opportunistic organisms like *Candida* from superficial locations may have little clinical significance because it could represent colonization, but culturing them from blood is always significant.

Culturing clinical specimens does not always result in growth of the organisms. This is often true with invasive *Aspergillus* infections, which yield positive blood cultures in less than 10% of cases. We do not know why. Perhaps only a small portion of the mycelium is actively growing and capable of producing a positive culture, or possibly a large inoculum of these fungi is required for growth in vitro.

Fungi grow slowly and there is often considerable delay between the time the specimen is obtained and a positive culture. Relying on the results of the cultures may therefore cause a significant delay in starting therapy. Despite these limitations, cultures should always be done because "when they work, they work well."

Detection of antibodies specific for fungal antigens is sometimes helpful in diagnosis, particularly for the deep seated mycoses. Many serological and skin tests are available, but the results provide only presumptive evidence for infection and must be interpreted in light of clinical findings. It is particularly difficult to interpret the significance of positive skin tests to *H. capsulatum* in parts of the world where the disease is endemic. Almost everyone living in these areas has been exposed to this fungus and has developed a positive skin test indicative of delayed type hypersensitivity. The tests are further limited in usefulness because the antigens available are not specific enough. False-positive tests may also be due to symptomless colonization, previous subclinical infections, or anamnestic response due to previous skin tests. Delayed or false-negative responses, particularly in the immunosuppressed host, may also be a problem.

Recently, procedures for detecting circulating fungal antigens in body fluids have been developed. The most successful one detects soluble capsular polysaccharides of C. neoformans in cerebrospinal fluid. It is highly specific and sensitive. Similar tests for other fungi are not available at present but may well be developed.

Treatment

It is extremely important to realize that not all fungal infections require treatment. As we stated previously, humans have a high innate resistance to most of these agents. Most infections with fungi are subclinical, self-limiting, and do not result in disease. Some fungal infections respond to supportive measures, such as improving the nutritional status of the host or eliminating predisposing factors. Examples are Candida infections of the blood and urinary tract and Aspergillus infections of the lung. Predisposing causes of these diseases are the use of intravenous lines, catheters, and the administration of broad spectrum antibiotics. Management of these fungal infections is much easier when these causes are recognized and corrected.

Most antifungal agents in common use affect fungi more than host cells, but not by much (Chapter 2). Toxicity is a real problem in the treatment of these diseases. In addition, many antifungal compounds have limited therapeutic value because of problems with solubility, stability, and absorption. Compared with antibacterial agents, the number of effective antifungal agents is quite small (Chapter 3). With the increase in frequency of fungal infections, the search for additional effective agents has expanded.

Most useful antifungal antibiotics fall into one of two categories: those that affect fungal cell membranes, and those that are taken up by the cell and interrupt cellular processes (Chapter 3). Table 38.1 lists some of the useful antifungal agents and their most likely mechanisms of action.

Table 38.1
Antifungal antibiotics

Class	Compounds	Mechanism	Uses
Polyene	Amphotericin B, nystatin	Binds to sterols causing perturbations in cell membrane	Systemic disease Topical disease (candidiasis)
Imidazole	Clotrimazole miconazole ketoconazole	Inhibits ergosterol biosynthesis	Topical disease (ringworm) Systemic disease
Pyrimidine	5-fluorocytosine (5FC)	Inhibits DNA and RNA synthesis	Systemic disease
Grisans	Griseofulvin	Inhibits microtubule assembly	Topical disease

SYSTEMIC MYCOSES CAUSED BY PRIMARY PATHOGENS

Cases—An Outbreak

Thirty-five members of several families from the Midwest camped on a farm in northwestern Tennessee for 2 weeks. In return for the use of the site they helped the farmer clean out an old barn on the property. The barn had not been used for about 20 years and had become a gathering place for starlings. The walls and ground were caked with bird droppings and since the weather had been quite dry, considerable dust was stirred up when the ground was raked and the walls washed. The cleaning took several hours. Everyone then went home.

Over the next 6 to 12 days, eighteen members of the group got sick with chills, fever, cough and headache (Table 38.2). Several had substernal discomfort and others had painful red bumps on the front of their legs below the knee. Two patients had severe joint pains that shifted from the knees to the ankles and wrists.

In about 2 weeks, fourteen of the campers got well without treatment. Several of these patients had seen their physician and had chest x-rays. They showed infiltrates, which disappeared after several weeks. Repeat chest x-rays on these patients 1 year later showed calcified hilar lymph nodes and calcified nodules in the periphery of the lungs (Fig. 38.11). Over the next year one of these patients developed shortness of breath and progressive swelling of the lower extremities and the face. More x-rays showed a mass in his mediastinum that compressed several bronchi. A venogram showed compression of the

Table 38.2
Outcome of infection with *Histoplasma capsulatum* in 35 patients

No. patients	Clinical Course	Physical Findings	Chest X-rays	Laboratory Results
17	Asymptomatic	None	Some had abnormalities such as lung infiltrates or mild increase in lymph node size in the mediastinum. Months to years after the infection some had calcification of lymph nodes or calcified nodules (granulomas).	All developed a positive antibody reaction to antigens of *H. capsulatum*. All had positive skin tests with histoplasmin.
18	All developed chills, fever and cough. Some had muscle aches and pain in some joints. Some had substernal aching and a decreased appetite. Two patients developed painful red bumps on the front of their upper and lower legs. Biopsy showed erythema nodosum (an inflammatory skin and soft tissue reaction to the fungus). Fourteen of the 18 patients became asymptomatic within 3 weeks of the onset of the infections. One of the 14 noted shortness of breath and swelling of his face and legs 1 year after the infection. These symptoms progressed and he required surgery to strip thick fibrous tissue from his mediastinum.	Five of the 14 had enlarged lymph nodes in their necks. Four of the 18 had rales on auscultation of the chest. Two had the skin lesions already noted.	Eight of the 14 had patchy infiltrates. Some had enlarged hilar lymph nodes. Months to years after the infection, some developed calcified lymph nodes with calcified granulomas in the lung. The one patient who had difficulty had enlarged mediastinal lymph nodes that contracted and compressed major bronchi and the superior and inferior vena cava.	Most developed positive antibody tests. Most developed positive skin tests with histoplasmin antigen. Cultures of sputum of 7 of the 14 patients were positive for *H. capsulatum*.

Figure 38.11. Chest x-ray showing calcifications of the lung and mediastinal lymph nodes consistent with healed histoplasmosis.

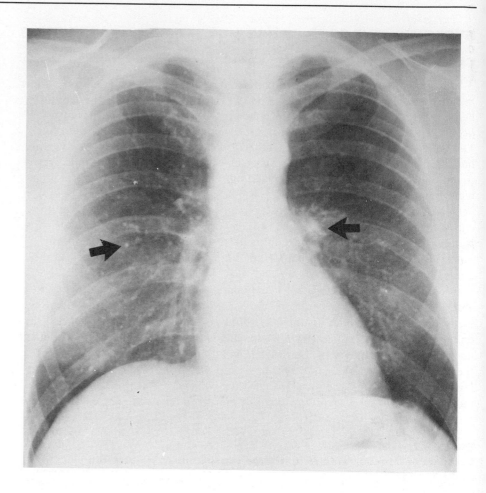

superior and inferior vena cava as well. Four of the other campers developed progressive histoplasmosis.

This is a description of a typical outbreak of histoplasmosis. Analysis of the case histories (Tables 38.2 and 38.3) will reveal the most important points of the pathophysiology of the disease.

Encounter

The outbreak occurred in the state of Tennessee, which is in the so-called histo belt, a geographic area in the southeastern portion of the United States bordering the Mississippi and Ohio river valleys. The outbreak described is typical because cases often occur in clusters after a common exposure. The endemic zone extends through many of the tropical countries of the world. A clinically distinct form of histoplasmosis occurs in Africa (caused by a variety known as *H. capsulatum* var. *duboisii*) and is characterized by involvement of subcutaneous tissue, the skin and bones, with little or no evidence of pulmonary disease.

H. capsulatum is a soil organism whose growth is enhanced by bird or bat excreta. Common sources of infection are old barns used as roosting sites by starlings, grackles or chickens. Bat-roosting sites such as trees or caves are also important sources of the organism, particularly in the tropics. In the outbreak described, the dry weather, coupled with the vigorous cleaning activities of the

Table 38.3
Outcome of infection with *Histoplasma capsulatum* in the four patients with clinically apparent disease

Patients	Clinical Course	Physical Findings	Chest X-rays	Laboratory Results
A	This patient had underlying emphysema. He never recovered completely from the original infection with *H. capsulatum* and he had continued weight loss and intermittent fever. He produced mucopurulent sputum that was occasionally bloody.	He looked chronically ill, was short of breath and had evidence of weight loss. He had a "barrel chest".	Emphysema, upper lobe infiltrates with cavitation.	High anti-histoplasma-antibody titers. Repetitive growth of *H. capsulatum* from sputum.
B	The patient also never recovered from the original infection with *H. capsulatum* Cough, chills and fever persisted. She had weight loss and night sweats. After 6 months she had extreme weakness and also had shallow ulcerations in her mouth.	There were three shallow ulcerations in her mouth.	Chronic upper lobe infiltrates. Calcification in lymph nodes in the mediastinum and in the adrenal glands.	High antibody titers. Positive culture of *H. capsulatum* from the bone marrow. She had laboratory evidence of insufficiency of the adrenal gland. Yeast cells were seen in macrophages on biopsy of one of the oral lesions. Culture of the biopsy grew *H. capsulatum*.
C	This patient became acutely ill 10 days after the original exposure to *H. capsulatum* She had chills, high spiking fevers, and shortness of breath.	She was short of breath and appeared acutely ill.	Miliary patterns of infiltrates in the lung and enlargement of hilar lymph nodes (compare with TB, Chapter 22).	Serological tests weakly positive. She had a positive culture of *H. capsulatum* from the sputum.
D	This patient is a male homosexual with AIDS. He became acutely ill 6 days after the exposure with chills, fever, and then went into shock and died.	He was close to death when seen initially. He had enlarged lymph nodes in his neck and evidence of weight loss.	Miliary pattern of infiltrates in the lung.	Negative serologic tests. Yeast cells seen in monocytes in peripheral blood and mononuclear cells in bone marrow. Positive cultures of *H. capsulatum* from blood, bone marrow, urine.

group, led to the aerosolization of spores and fragments of hyphae. These were inhaled, and their small size allowed them to evade the anatomic defense mechanisms of the respiratory tract and reach the alveoli of the lung (Chapter 45).

Entry

The events following entry of *H. capsulatum* into the alveoli are unknown, but based on the physiology of the organism and the relevant factors in host defense, we can construct the following scheme: when spores or mycelial fragments of *H.*

capsulatum are exposed to human body temperatures of 37°C, they transform into the yeast phase. Experiments with animals indicate that this transformation is required for pathogenicity. Also, only yeasts are seen in tissues of infected hosts. The virulence of different strains of *H. capsulatum* is related to their level of tolerance to the elevated temperature: low levels of virulence and tolerance to elevated temperatures are associated with a delayed transformation to the yeast phase and slower growth of the yeast.

Spread and Multiplication

In tissue, yeast cells of *H. capsulatum* are found within macrophages only. However, phagocytosis does not always lead to killing, and the intracellular habitat paradoxically results in protection of the fungus from other defenses of the host. What determines whether or not the macrophages will kill the yeast phase? Here again we lack factual information but the following factors are probably important:

• If the inoculum of organisms is very large, macrophages are simply overwhelmed by the sheer number of organisms they ingest.

• Macrophages have to be activated to kill the fungi efficiently. Activation of macrophages, which occurs rapidly in a host sensitized by previous infection, would limit the infection (see chapter 5).

• After ingestion, the organisms avoid being killed, perhaps by preventing the oxygen burst, or phagosome-lysosome fusion, or by resisting the degradative effects of lysosomes.

The outcome of the initial interaction between the host cells and the fungi is either death of the microbes or their multiplication and spread to local lymphatics and hence to other organs. After 1 to 2 weeks, cellular immunity is stimulated and host reticuloendothelial cells become more efficient in limiting growth and multiplication of the fungus. The infection is thus curtailed and eventually resolves. Yeast cells may remain viable within calcified lesions for years and may be a source for reactivation of infection when immunity wanes. This sequence of events is the same as in tuberculosis, and in fact the granulomas formed in response to *H. capsulatum* are very similar to those seen in tuberculosis (and for that matter all primary systemic mycoses).

Seventeen of the people exposed to *H. capsulatum* in the barn were asymptomatic. Perhaps they only inhaled a small number of organisms or had been sensitized by prior infection to deal efficiently with renewed exposure. About 80% to 90% of adults who have lived in the histo belt have positive skin tests to antigens of *H. capsulatum*, evidence of their cellular immunity.

Damage

Fourteen of the people developed a self limited disease that disappeared, presumably as cellular immunity developed. These people were left with the scars of the disease, seen on chest x-rays as calcified granulomas (Fig. 38.11). It is not known why calcifications occur, but macrophages in granulomas make a factor that elevates calcium levels in the blood. All these people had elevated antibody titers to fungal antigens. One person in this group developed a particularly intense immune response that resulted in a proliferative tissue reaction (mediastinal granulomatosis). Eventually, the advanced fibrosis actually impinged on vital structures in the chest (sclerosing mediastinitis). This process was not due to active infection but to the immune response gone awry. This is a rare complication of infection with *H. capsulatum*, and can only be treated surgically by removing the fibrotic tissue.

Each of the four people who developed progressive disease after the initial infection illustrates the failure of an important component of host defenses to limit infection:

Patient A had severe chronic obstructive pulmonary disease and emphysema. Because of the anatomic abnormalities and scarring in his lung, he could not clear the infection. An effective systemic response and the use of potent antifungal therapy limited the infection to the lung. Increasing damage to the lung by continued infection and local spread resulted in further destruction and a relentless downhill course until he died from pulmonary insufficiency 5 years after the onset of infection.

In patient B there was continued disease in the lungs and ultimately dissemination of the infection to other organs. Failure to limit and contain the infection may have been due to a particularly large inoculum inhaled at the time of exposure or to some subtle or transient defect in host defenses. In disseminated histoplasmosis, T cell function is defective but it is not known whether this is the cause or the result of the disease. One of the manifestations of the disease is ulcerations of the oral mucosa. It is not unusual to find mucosal lesions as the sole sign of disease. We do not understand why *H. capsulatum* has this unusual tropism for mucous membranes. It is not unique to this disease, but does help in the diagnosis. The fungus also spreads to many other organs, including the bone marrow and the adrenal glands, where it causes insufficiency of adrenal function (Addison's disease), a complication also seen in disseminated tuberculosis. This patient was treated with ketoconazole and did well. In general, when disseminated disease is diagnosed early in an otherwise apparently normal host, the prognosis is good.

Patient C suffered an acute overwhelming pulmonary infection, probably because she had been previously sensitized and on this occasion may have inhaled a very large inoculum. The damage to her lungs probably resulted from direct tissue damage by the fungi and from the inflammatory reaction made more severe by the previous sensitization. This patient was critically ill because her pulmonary function was severely compromised. After treatment with amphotericin B, the patient improved and the pulmonary infiltrates cleared rapidly.

Patient D had AIDS. Because he lacked a normal T cell response, he succumbed to an overwhelming infection that spread to every organ. He was unresponsive to intensive therapy with amphotericin B. This underlines the importance of the cooperation between host defenses and chemotherapy for a successful outcome. Disseminated histoplasmosis occurs in patients with AIDS either as the result of newly acquired infection or by reactivation of old disease. Like the tubercle bacillus, *H. capsulatum* may persist in a dormant state in cells of the reticuloendothelial system for many years after primary infection and may reactivate when host resistance becomes severely impaired.

Other Systemic Mycoses

The pathophysiology and clinical manifestations of histoplasmosis are very similar to those of the other primary systemic mycoses listed in Table 38.4, and all can be categorized along with tuberculosis as granulomatous infections.

Table 38.4
Systemic mycoses caused by primary pathogens

Disease	Etiologic Agent	Epidemiology	Clinical Disease	Histopathology	Therapy
Histoplasmosis	*Histoplasma capsulatum:* Dimorphic. Mycelia at 25°C. Typical tuber-culate macroconidia 8–14 μm in diameter and microconidia 2–4 μm in diameter. At 37°C and in tissue this organism is a budding yeast 2–3 × 3–4 μm in diameter.	Endemic in the United States in the Ohio and Mississippi River valleys. Endemic zone extends through Mexico, Central and South American, and parts of the Caribbean. Also found in Australia, the Far East, and Africa. It is a soil organism whose growth is enhanced in locations contaminated by bird or bat excreta. The organism is usually inhaled: cases occur in clusters and singly.	The percentage of patients with clinical symptoms varies depending on the degree of exposure and host response. About 90% of all primary cases are not clinically significant. Many individuals have x-ray signs consistent with past disease (i.e., calcifications) but cannot give a history of relevant symptoms. Less than 5% of infections will require treatment. Here there may be underlying conditions that make these individuals prone to progressive disease.	In acute disease numerous organisms (yeasts) are found in histiocytes. There are epithelioid granulomas that contain plasma cells, lymphocytes, macrophages, neutrophils and giant cells. In old disease, calcification may be prominent (known as "coin lesions").	Ketoconazole is the drug of choice. Amphotericin B is used in treatment of failures or rapidly progressive disease.
Blastomycosis	*Blastomyces dermatitidis:* Dimorphic. Mycelia at 25°C. Typical pear shaped conidia. At 37°C and in tissue this organism is a yeast 8–15 μm in diameter. Buds produced singly are attached to parent cell by broad base.	Isolated cases occur all over North America, although they are most frequently reported in the central and eastern United States and central provinces of Canada. Cases have been reported from Africa, Israel, Saudi Arabia, and eastern Europe. Clustering of cases occurs only occasionally.	Primary infection in lung is often inapparent although pulmonary infection may occur. Chronic skin and bone disease are the most common clinical presentations. Other forms are urogenital and disseminated disease involving multiple organs. Most infections cause disease and require therapy. The organism is rarely isolated from the environment but appears to be located in old buildings and soil. The organism is inhaled and invades via the lungs.	The tissue response varies from epithelioid granulomas to chronic suppuration, necrosis, and fibrosis. Cutaneous lesions are often characterized by an epithelial hyperplasia. Large budding yeast cells with broad bases are characteristic and seen in the microabscesses.	Same drugs as in histoplasmois.
Coccidiomycosis	*Coccidioides immitis:* Dimorphic. Mycelia at 25°C. As the culture ages, the septate filaments mature in such a manner that alternate cells develop into "arthroconidia" that have a "barrel shaped" appearance. In tissues at 37°C the organism develops into a sporangium ("spherule") 10–70 μm in diameter, filled with endospores.	Found in the south-western United States and parts of Central and South America. The organism is found in soil and infection occurs in persons who inhale the organism. Epidemics may be associated with dust storms.	Approximately 60% of these infections are asymptomatic. Forty percent are symptomatic with the spectrum of disease ranging from mild influenza-like complaints to frank pneumonia. The most common symptoms of primary disease are cough, fever, and chest pain. Night sweats and joint pain are not un-usual. An epidemiologic history should be taken to find out whether the patient has been in an endemic area. Other forms of the disease affect the meninges, bone, skin.	Three basic types of cellular reactions are seen in this disease: pyogenic, granulomat-ous, and mixed. Spherules and endospores may be numerous and can be seen. The histopathology of cutaneous lesions is similar to that seen in tuberculosis.	Ketoconazole is effective in nonmeningeal disease. Parenteral amphotericin B and direct instillation of the drug into the CNS is required to treat meningitis.

Table 38.4 (continued)

Disease	Etiologic Agent	Epidemiology	Clinical Disease	Histopathology	Therapy
Paracoccidiomycosis	*Paracoccidioides brasiliensis:* Dimorphic. Mycelia at 25°C. No typical pattern of sporulation. At 37°C and in tissues the organism is a yeast with several budding cells attached to its surface.	The infection is found in most countries of South America and in scattered areas of Central America. The infection is strikingly more common in males than females. The organism has only rarely been found in the natural environment, and the sources of exposure in human infections are unknown, but a number of factors imply infection by the respiratory route.	Primary pulmonary disease is often inapparent. Ulcerative granulomas of the buccal, nasal and occasionally the gastrointestinal mucosa are indicative of dissemination. The prevalence of positive skin tests in asymptomatic individuals indicates a low but consistent level of subclinical exposure.	Essentially identical to that seem in blastomycosis. Granulomatous reactions interspersed with pyogenic abscesses. Langhans' giant cells may contain the typical budding yeast cells.	Ketoconazole is the therapeutic agent of choice. Amphotericin B in treatment of failures.

SYSTEMATIC MYCOSES CAUSED BY OPPORTUNISTIC FUNGI

The more pathogenic the infecting microorganism, the less host susceptibility it needs to cause disease. The fungi we describe here are not very pathogenic, and in order to cause disease, need help, usually in the form of decreased host resistance. Understanding the underlying host defects in opportunistic fungal infections may allow us to reverse or to lessen the predisposing factors. If we cannot accomplish this, the prognosis is worse.

Patients at high risk are those with malignancies, burns, operations, trauma, or illnesses that require long-term use of intravenous or intra-arterial catheters. Also at risk are patients who have received broad-spectrum antibacterial therapy and whose normal intestinal bacterial flora has markedly decreased. In such cases, fungi like *C. albicans* proliferate unchecked and can take the place of the bacteria of the normal flora.

On the basis of clinical experience, a decrease in the number of functioning neutrophils is the most important host defect that affects the response to fungal infection. These infections are hard enough to treat in a normal host, but cure is almost impossible when there are few functioning white cells. Premature babies and the elderly also tend to do poorly when infected with fungi. Why do you think this is the case?

The weakly virulent fungi that cause opportunistic systemic mycoses are nearly ubiquitous. They may be part of our flora or they may be inhaled or ingested from the environment.

A Case of Endogenous Infection

A 19-year-old woman, Ms. J., was involved in a bicycle accident and sustained severe cervical spinal cord trauma resulting in quadriplegia. She required an indwelling urinary catheter, which led to multiple urinary tract infections. These were treated with a variety of broad-spectrum antibiotics. She has also had several episodes of Candida infections of her mouth, perineum, and vagina.

At the time of the present admission to the hospital there was again evidence of urinary tract infection manifested by cloudy urine and fever. On the 10th hospital day, urography revealed a large left kidney with delayed function and poor urine concentration.

Microscopic examination of sediment obtained by centrifuging urine samples and specimens of tissue obtained surgically showed budding yeast cells, pseudohyphae and hyphal elements; this permitted a rapid presumptive diagnosis of Candida infection. Further laboratory tests identified the organism as C. albicans. Blood cultures taken after a febrile episode grew the same organism.

C. albicans is the most frequent species that causes this type of infection, although infection may also be due to other species whose names can always be looked up. Careful examination of the retina with an ophthalmoscope revealed a "fluffy" cottony growth due to the organism. Ms. J.'s heart valve became infected and she developed a heart murmur. In addition, she developed weakness on the right side of her face.

Candida are carried in the posterior pharynx and the bowel of many healthy individuals. In the case of Ms. J., there was overgrowth of this organism because the normal flora was suppressed by the multiple courses of antibiotics. This yeast then contaminated the bladder and the infection spread into the urinary system. Candida appears to have a particular tropism for the kidney. From the kidney, the yeast probably spread through the blood to the several different organs described above. This was probably due to an organism-laden clot that traveled to her brain from her infected heart valve. Disseminated candidiasis often follows such a series of devastating events. Systemic infection is usually preceded by other superficial infections, like those involving the mouth, the pharynx, the esophagus, or other parts of the gastrointestinal tract or the vagina.

All forms of systemic Candida infections are potentially life threatening and require therapy. Consideration should always be given to the primary predisposing factors, and these should be minimized or reversed. In the case of Ms. J., the catheter and intravenous lines were probably infected at the time of the candidemia and had to be changed. Carefully monitored doses of amphotericin B and 5-fluorocytosine were used. Had the response not been adequate, Ms. J.'s infected heart valve would have had to be removed and replaced by a prosthesis.

This is an example of an opportunistic infection resulting from anatomic defects in the host. The white blood count and the immune responses were normal, yet successful management with antifungal drugs required repair of the anatomic defects. The prognosis is guarded.

A Case of Exogenous Infection

Mr. S., a 25-year-old man was hospitalized for treatment of acute lymphocytic leukemia. The initial diagnosis was made 20 months earlier, when he complained of general malaise and weakness. At the time his white blood cell count was greater than 100,000/mm³ with 93% lymphocytes and lymphoblasts, all values being abnormal. A bone marrow aspiration established the diagnosis of leukemia. He was treated with anticancer drugs that produced a complete remission.

One year later he had a relapse of leukemia. He was treated with large doses of anticancer agents, which resulted in leukopenia and thrombocytopenia. A

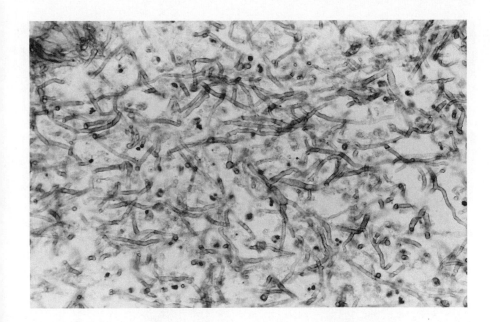

Figure 38.12. Tissue section infected with *Aspergillius fumigatus*. Septate hyphae and dichotomous branching are characteristic features of organisms belonging to this group of fungi.

chest x-ray showed nodular lesions in both lungs. Blood cultures were negative. Microscopic examination of sputum specimens and a skin biopsy of a purpuric lesion revealed septate branching hyphae 7 to 10 μm in diameter and several hundred micrometers in length (Fig. 38.12). Cultures resulted in colonies of a white mold that quickly developed a smoky-gray color. This, and the shape and arrangement of the asexual spores identified the organism as Aspergillus fumigatus.

Serological tests yielded an antibody titer of 1:4 to Aspergillus antigens, which is not conclusive. Nevertheless, a diagnosis of invasive aspergillosis was made, based on the clinical findings and the microscopic and culture results. Therapy with amphotericin B was initiated on Mr. S. without further delay. Often treatment for fungal infections in this kind of host has to start on the basis of clinical suspicion because diagnosis by culture of blood or other body fluids is inconclusive.

Aspergilli are a group of molds so ubiquitous that they may easily be cultured from the air, soil, or moldy vegetation. The major pathogenic species is *A. fumigatus*, but others may also cause disease. They are not part of the normal flora of humans and do not grow in normal tissue. They cause invasive disease only in profoundly immunocompromised subjects, particularly those with neutropenia, such as Mr. S. The initial site of invasion is usually the lung or the paranasal sinuses, and this was probably the case in this patient. The lesions seen in x-rays include focal consolidation, lobar pneumonia and lung cavities which contain "fungus balls" of the mold (Fig. 38.13). Patients with such invasive infections also have intracerebral abscesses, necrotic ulcers of skin, and lesions of bone, liver and the breast.

Aspergillus may also cause noninfectious disease, such as allergy or asthma following inhalation and growth of the fungus in the bronchial tree (*allergic bronchopulmonary aspergillosis*). They also elaborate toxic metabolic products, the aflatoxins, which are hepatotoxic or carcinogenic, although their role in cancers of humans has not been established.

Figure 38.13. A chest x-ray of primary *Aspergillus* pneumonia with "fungus balls."

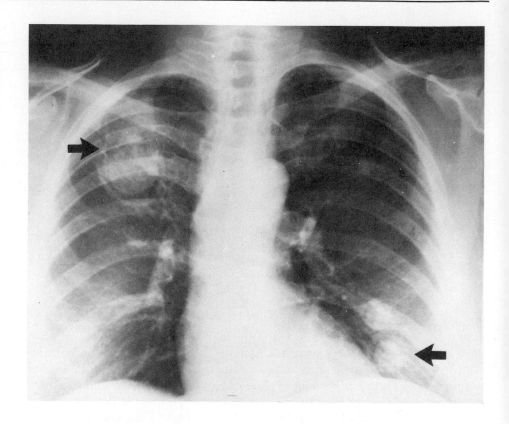

Other Mycoses Caused by Opportunistic Fungi

Severely immunocompromised hosts suffer from a large number of other opportunistic systemic fungal infections as well. The etiology of the most frequent ones is listed in Table 38.5. The so-called *zygomycoses* have two principal clinical presentations. The *rhinocerebral form* is unique to diabetics, particularly those with diabetic ketoacidosis. These patients often have sinus infections, periorbital cellulitis (infection of the connective tissue around the eye), and tissue necrosis that may extend to the central nervous system. It is not known why diabetes

Table 38.5
Mycoses Caused by Opportunistic Fungi

Disease	Fungus	Predisposing Factors	Involvement	Therapy
Cryptococcosis	*Cryptococcus neoformans*	Immunosuppression, none	Lung, most prominent in CNS, kidney, bone	Amphotericin B + 5FC
Candidiasis	*Candida albicans* and other species	Immunosuppression	Mucosal areas, GI tract, blood, kidney, other organs	Amphotericin B + 5FC
Aspergillosis	*Aspergillus fumigatus* and other species	Immunosuppression	Lungs, other organs	Amphotericin B
Zygomycosis	Several species	Diabetes, burns, immunosuppression	Blood vessels, eye, CNS nose, sinuses, lungs	Amphotericin B
Other	Many other species (each one infrequent)	Immunosuppression, trauma, or not known	Lungs, CNS, soft tissue, joints, eye, disseminated infection	Amphotericin B, miconazole

predisposes to this infection, but it has been postulated, on the basis of laboratory data, that the acidotic state of the diabetic patient stimulates growth of this fungus.

The second type, *disseminated zygomycosis*, has a clinical presentation almost identical to that of disseminated aspergillosis. In contrast to the hyphae of *Aspergillus* and *Candida* the fungal elements seen in pathologic specimens of mucormycosis are nonseptate, branch irregularly and produce bizarre balloon-shaped cells.

Cryptococcosis is usually listed among the opportunistic fungal infections, although it also occurs in normal persons. In fact, 50% of patients with cryptococcal meningitis in the United States have no known defect in host resistance. The etiologic agent is an encapsulated yeast, *Cryptococcus neoformans*, which is found in the excreta of birds, particularly pigeons. The organism is inhaled into the lungs, where it can cause pneumonia. However, the most frequent clinical presentation is meningitis. There is no explanation for the striking tropism of this organism for the central nervous system. Brain abscesses caused by *Cryptococcus* have a particularly interesting feature: They usually elicit little or no tissue response. Thus, damage is caused by displacement and pressure on brain tissue rather than by inflammation. The mechanism is also not known, but may have something to do with the properties of the capsule.

Diagnosis of cryptococcal meningitis is made by examining samples of cerebrospinal fluid for budding yeast cells with capsules outlined by India ink particles (Fig. 38.14). A serologic test can detect soluble capsular polysaccharide in the cerebrospinal fluid of more than 90% of patients with this disease. Both microscopic and serologic tests can be performed right after lumbar puncture and the diagnosis may be made before obtaining results from a culture, which takes several days. This allows early therapy with a combination of amphotericin B and 5-fluorocytosine.

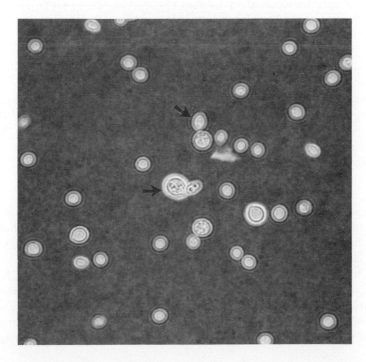

Figure 38.14. India ink preparation of spinal fluid containing encapsulated yeast cells of *Cryptococcus neoformans*.

Prognosis depends on the overall clinical status of the patient. A good prognostic sign is a falling antigen titer followed by the detection of circulating antibodies to the cryptococcal polysaccharide. If there is no underlying disease, 80% to 90% of patients respond to therapy. If patients are severely immunocompromised, less than 50% will survive.

SUBCUTANEOUS, CUTANEOUS, AND SUPERFICIAL MYCOSES

Subcutaneous Mycoses

A distinctive group of fungal disease involves the subcutaneous tissue, the dermis and the epidermis. These subcutaneous infections originate in the deeper tissue layers and eventually break out into the epidermis and adjacent structures. Spread through the bloodstream is unusual but the lymphatics may be involved as far as the draining lymph nodes. Most of these mycoses, along with other "jungle rots", are confined to tropical climates. Sporotrichosis is the only relatively common infection in temperate climates.

Subcutaneous infections are called *mycoses of implantation* because the organisms enter the skin via thorns or splinters. In addition to involving the subcutaneous tissue, the diseases of this group have several other features in common:

Encounter: The etiologic agents are ubiquitous and usually found in soil or decaying vegetation.

Entry: The patient can usually give a history of trauma preceding appearance of lesions. As a result the infections occur on the parts of the body that are most prone to be traumatized, e.g., feet, legs, hands, buttocks.

Spread: These infections are slow in onset and lesions evolve over many years. This persistence may be due to the noninvasive properties of this group of organisms and may be fostered by foreign material in the wounds. Malnutrition, which is common in the populations most frequently infected, may also be a contributing factor.

Diagnosis: Some of these organisms are commonly encountered in the laboratory, and single isolations must therefore be confirmed by repeated cultures. The presence of the fungi in tissue specimens is helpful in diagnosis.

Treatment: With few exceptions (sporotrichosis, chromoblastomycosis), the subcutaneous mycoses are difficult to treat and often require surgical intervention. The reason for the lack of response to drug therapy is unknown. Possibly, the organisms are only marginally sensitive to antifungal agents, but more likely, the chronic inflammatory reaction makes these fungi inaccessible both to drugs and to host defense mechanisms.

Subcutaneous sporotrichosis responds to potassium iodide, which is puzzling since this compound has no in vitro antifungal effect against the fungus. The reason for its therapeutic effect is not known, although some think that it may affect the host response to infection. It is interesting that only the subcutaneous form of sporotrichosis responds well to this compound.

Several bacterial infections, such as those caused by *Staphylococcus*, *Nocardia*, or *Actinomyces*, or by atypical mycobacteria, may mimic clinical and pathological manifestations of the subcutaneous fungal infections. Since most of these can be treated with antibacterial antibiotics, it is extremely important to determine the etiology of the infection. This is most effectively done by surgical biopsy. In the

Table 38.6
Subcutaneous mycoses

Disease	Etiologic Agent(s)	Clinical Disease	Therapy
Sporotrichosis	*Sporothrix schenkii*	Lymphocutaneous sporotrichosis is the disease most commonly associated with this fungus. The organism gains access to the deep layers of skin by traumatic implantation. A small hard painless nodule appears at the site of injury and it enlarges into a fluctuant mass that eventually breaks down and ulcerates. As the primary lesion enlarges, several other nodules begin to develop along lymphatics that drain that site. They also become fluctuant and ulcerate. The infection rarely extends beyond regional lymphatics.	Saturated solution of potassium iodide given orally is the drug of choice. Amphotericin B is used for diseases involving the lung and other organs.
Chromoblastomycosis	*Fonsecaea pedrosoi* many species	The most common form of chromoblastomycosis consists of warty, vegetative lesions that look like a cauliflower.	Surgical excision and cryosurgery. 5-Fluorocytosine has been used successfully, but response depends on the organism.
Other, e.g., rhinosporidiosis, lobomycosis	Many species	Many manifestations: deep subcutaneous masses, wart-like lesions, polyps, etc.	Surgical excision, antifungal drugs.

case of sporotrichosis, culture is more useful than histology, since the yeast-like organisms are difficult to find on histopathological examination. Table 38.6 summarizes the important features of the principal subcutaneous mycoses.

Cutaneous Mycoses or Dermatomycoses

The dermatomycoses of humans include a wide spectrum of infections of the skin and its appendages (hair and nails) by fungi known as dermatophytes. In the asexual state these fungi are classified in the genera *Microsporum*, *Trichophyton* and *Epidermophyton* on the basis of sporulation patterns and morphologic features of development. Some species are found worldwide, others are geographically restricted to certain parts of the world. These patterns are becoming disrupted by the increasing mobility of the world's population.

Cases

Two adult teaching volunteers in a school for mentally handicapped children were seen by their physicians because each had developed well-demarcated, scaly, itchy lesions on their skin (Fig. 38.15). Clinical history revealed that these

Figure 38.15. Clinical appearance of tinea corporis. Note the well-demarcated border of the lesions that suggest that a worm or larva is at the margin, hence the terms ringworm or ''tinea'' (worm) to describe the lesions.

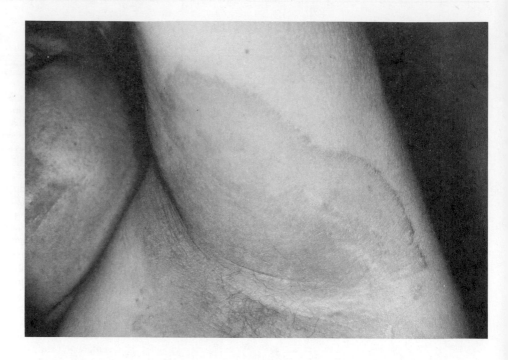

Figure 38.16. Specimen taken from skin of patient with tinea corporis, treated with 10% potassium hydroxide. A positive preparation is indicated by presence of hyphae (*arrows*).

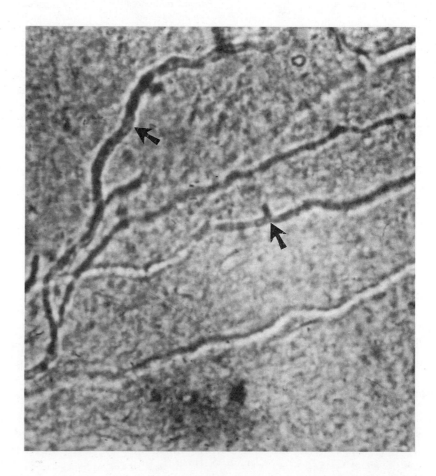

lesions had developed over a period of several weeks since they started their work. Both were childless and had no contact with domestic or wild animals. Microscopic examination of skin scales taken from the lesions showed the presence of fungal elements (Fig. 38.16) and cultures grew Trichophyton tonsurans.

An epidemiologic inquiry and clinical survey of seven students in the school revealed that two had hair loss. One of these had typical ringworm of the scalp and the other had highly inflammatory lesions associated with ringworm called kerion (Fig. 38.17). The five other students appeared asymptomatic except for mild dandruff. Cultures of scalp scrapings of two of these were positive for T. tonsurans.

The parents of the children were notified of these findings and asked to have their family physician examine the siblings of each student. The brother of one of the asymptomatic students who had a positive culture for T. tonsurans was found to have ringworm of the scalp. All of the children and the two adults were treated with griseofulvin and all responded well.

This example of an outbreak of dermatophytosis illustrates several points:

• In occupations where adults come into close contact with children, such as nursing and teaching of the handicapped, it is not uncommon to find ringworm of the body in adults during outbreaks of ringworm of the scalp in the children, both caused by the same organism.

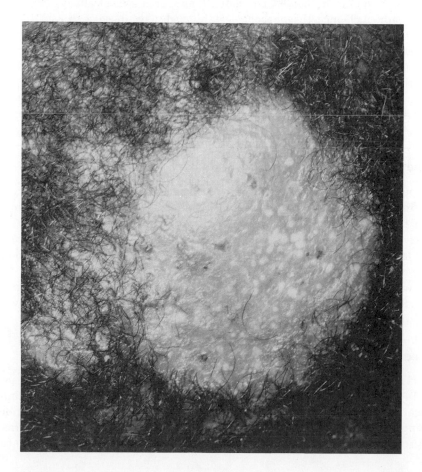

Figure 38.17. Clinical photograph of tinea capitis showing the inflammatory lesion called "kerion."

• The clinical manifestations of these infections are variable. Of the five students who had what appeared to be dandruff, two grew the fungus from the scalp. The two others had hair loss and distinct clinical diseases, regular ringworm and kerion.

• Ringworm of the scalp is a frequent problem in the pediatric population. At about puberty it spontaneously ceases to be a problem, treated or untreated. In the adult population ringworm of the scalp is rare. The patient usually has close association with infected children or animals that have clinical disease.

Encounter

Different species of dermatophytes have different ecological niches. Some species are most frequently isolated from the soil and are called *geophilic*. Other species, found most often in association with domestic and wild animals, are called *zoophilic*. A third group, the *anthropophilic* ones, are found almost exclusively in association with humans and their habitat.

It is important to identify the species in order to determine the possible source of infection. Identification even has some prognostic value. The anthropophilic dermatophytes tend to cause chronic infections and are more difficult to treat. The zoophilic and geophilic ones tend to cause inflammatory lesions that often heal spontaneously.

Dermatophytes are not members of the normal skin flora. Although they are occasionally found in people's toe clefts, these fungi almost always cause some minor pathology once they become established. The disease caused by these fungi is called *ringworm* or *tineas*. The term *tinea* comes from Latin (worm) and refers to the serpentine lesions that characterize these infections and which look as if a worm is burrowing at the margin. This term is used in conjunction with the part of the body that is affected to describe the disease, e.g., *tinea capitis* (head), *tinea pedis* (feet), *tinea corporis* (body), *tinea cruris* (crotch), etc. Other terms are often used by the layman to describe these diseases such as athlete's foot, jock itch, jungle rot, etc.

Entry

Experimental studies on dermatophyte infections have been useful for understanding their clinical manifestations. Volunteers who immersed their feet in water teeming with viable spores of the causative fungi did not get athlete's foot unless the skin was first traumatized. Continuous moist conditions were also important, and infections took place when the skin was occluded with nonporous materials. This increases hydration and temperature of the skin and interferes with the natural barrier function of the superficial layer, the stratum corneum. Such conditions are brought about by wearing nonporous shoes or covering the skin with occlusive bandages.

Spread and Multiplication

A classical ringworm lesion is characterized by the presence of fungal mycelium in the stratum corneum. Growth of the fungus sometimes results in minimal clinical signs of infection. In active disease there is an inflammatory reaction in the underlying epidermis and dermis. There is often scaling, indicating increased epidermal turnover. The hair follicles and hair shaft may be invaded. The fungi have a particular preference for keratinized tissues and do not invade living cells or the incompletely keratinized zone of the hair bulb. Although keratinases have been found in some dermatophytes, their role in the disease is unknown.

Damage

The clinical features of this disease are all related to the inflammation of the epidermis, dermis and the hair follicles. What sets this off is an immunologically mediated reaction to the fungal antigens that diffuse from the infected epidermis. You could call this a biological *contact dermatitis*. The extent of the inflammatory response and cellular infiltration correlates well with the degree of delayed hypersensitivity of the skin to extracts of *Trichophyton*. The term *kerion* is used to describe the highly inflammatory pustular form of infection in the scalp and beard areas. The pus results from secondary bacterial infections.

The ring-shape characteristics of dermatophyte lesions are the result of the organism growing outwardly in a centrifugal pattern. The area of the lesion that would yield viable fungal elements is at the inflamed margin. The central area generally has few or no viable fungi, and the healing tissue is refractory to infection. This pattern simulates the centrifugal growth of "fairy ring" mushrooms in a grassy field.

Systemic infections by dermatophytes are almost never known to occur, no matter how impaired the host. The most likely reasons are inability of dermatophytes to grow at body temperature and the presence of nonspecific serum factors (e.g., transferrin).

Environmental and cultural habits associated with types of clothing and shoes contribute to the incidence of dermatophytosis. Studies on institutionalized populations and families show that close and crowded living conditions are important in spreading the infections. Immunologic factors also contribute to their incidence and there is evidence that natural cell-mediated resistance to these infections is important.

The prevalence of dermatophytes and the incidence of disease are both difficult to determine since these diseases do not have to be reported to the U.S. Public Health Service. Fragmentary surveys from epidemiologic studies and case reports indicate that these are among the most common of human diseases. They are among the most common skin disorders in children under the age of 12 years and the second most common in older populations.

Different age groups manifest these diseases at different anatomic sites. In the pediatric population the most prevalent problem is ringworm of the scalp, which is most common in the 5- to 10-year-old children. At about puberty, this ceases to be a problem. On the other hand, athlete's foot, which is rarely a disease in childhood, gradually becomes the predominant infection and remains so throughout life. The reason for this shift is not well understood, but may be due to changes in the composition of sebum that occur at puberty, particularly in the even-numbered saturated fatty acids that have natural fungistatic activity. The fact that humans are generally shod is perhaps the major factor that leads to the high incidence of athlete's foot in adults. Subcutaneous fungal infections are more common in less well-developed countries, where many in the population do not wear shoes.

In the United States there is a disproportionate incidence of ringworm of the scalp in black children. We don't know why. Natives of India have higher incidence of this disease than resident Europeans. Studies from the Vietnam war revealed that athlete's foot in U.S. servicemen was mainly caused by *Trichophyton mentagrophytes*, whereas the native Vietnamese were more susceptible to *T. rubrum*.

The incidence of dermatophytosis is higher in males than females, with ratios of 3:1 for ringworm of the scalp and 6:1 for athlete's foot. Tinea cruris (jock itch) is also common in males and rare in females. Infection of the nails of the hands is more common in females, but nails of the feet are more often involved in males.

Diagnosis

When examined microscopically in scrapings of the skin surface in infected areas, dermatophytes all look alike. In culture, however, dermatophyte colonies have complex morphological characteristics that distinguish genus and species. Under the microscope, they differ in the morphology of specialized large multi-celled spores, the macroconidia.

Treatment

The dermatophytoses may be treated topically or systemically. Systemic treatment is necessary when hair or nails are infected since locally applied fungicides do not penetrate the tissue matrix where the fungus resides.

There are various local applications, creams, ointments, lotions, or paints which, when used regularly for 3 weeks or more, will clear many of the localized ringworm infections. Controlled trials have not demonstrated a clear leader among antiringworm drugs. In most cases, regular application is more important than the choice of agent.

Two antiringworm agents are given systemically by oral administration: the antibiotic griseofulvin and the synthetic imidazole ketoconazole.

Superficial Mycoses

Many of us harbor fungi on our skin and hairs without signs of disease. At times these fungal members of our normal flora cause very superficial infections that go no deeper than the stratum corneum. They are frequently mild and may go unnoticed. These conditions are often seen in warm and moist climates, but one, *tinea versicolor*, is frequently found in the temperate areas. Superficial mycoses are usually easy to treat with topical keratolytic agents.

SUGGESTED READINGS

Chandler FW, Kaplan W, Ajello L: *Histopathology of Mycotic Infections*. Chicago, Year Book, 1980.

Cole GT: Models of cell differentiation in conidial fungi. *Microbiol Rev* 50:95–132, 1986.

McGinnis MR: *Current Topics in Medical Mycology*, vols. 1 and 2. New York, Springer-Verlag, 1985, 1988.

Medoff G, Brajtburg J, Kobayashi GS, Bolard J: Antifungal agents useful in therapy of systemic fungal infections. *Ann Rev Pharmacol* 23:303–330, 1983.

Reiss E: *Molecular Immunology of Mycotic and Actinomycotic Infections*. New York, Elsevier, 1986.

Rippon JW: *Medical Mycology: The Pathogenic Fungi and Pathogenic Actinomycetes*, ed 3. Philadelphia, WB Saunders, 1988.

Szaniszlo PJ: *Fungal Dimorphism: With Emphasis on Fungi Pathogenic for Humans*. New York, Plenum Press, 1985.

Review of the Medically Important Fungi

This chart may be completed to review material covered under this topic

	Name of Disease or Fungus	Epidemiology	Main Symptoms
Systemic "true pathogens" 1.			
2.			
3.			
Systemic opportunistic 1.			
2.			
3.			
Subcutaneous 1.			
2.			
Superficial 1.			
2.			

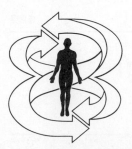

CHAPTER

Introduction to Parasitology

39

D.J. Krogstad

I
n developed countries parasitology suggests the strange and exotic—
"worms, wheezes, and weird diseases". *Parasitic diseases* occur most frequently in developing countries, but parasitic infections, often without clinical symptoms, are common even in the developed countries and are being
recognized with increasing frequency (Table 39.1). In North America and Europe
parasitic diseases are particularly prevalent among immunosuppressed patients.

Several parasitic diseases of humans are zoonoses—caused by agents that also
infect other mammals, birds, or reptiles (Chapter 55). In some instances, the
parasites require both humans and animals to complete their life cycle. For example, the developmental cycle of the beef tapeworm requires that both humans
and cattle become infected. In other instances, parasites of animals infect humans but cannot complete their biological development. An example is the blood
fluke (schistosome) of birds that causes "swimmer's itch". This parasite cannot
complete its developmental stages in people: Humans represent "dead-end hosts".

As with other infectious agents, here too we must distinguish between infection and disease. For example, a large proportion of the adults in the United
States have been infected with the protozoan *Toxoplasma gondii*, as shown by
the prevalence of antitoxoplasma antibodies. However, few people get sick from
this infection. Similarly, people with small numbers of intestinal worms are typically asymptomatic. This is well demonstrated in the case of hookworms, which
produce anemia by ingesting blood from vessels in the intestinal wall. Each
worm causes the loss of a small amount of blood (0.03 to 0.15 ml/day), thus the
severity of the disease is related to the number of worms present.

In contrast to the acute illnesses caused by many bacteria or viruses, parasitic
diseases are usually more chronic and are rarely lethal over a short period of

Table 39.1
Estimated worldwide prevalence of parasitic infections per year

Toxoplasmosis	1–2 billion
Ascariasis	1 billion
Hookworm disease	800–900 million
Amebiasis	200–400 million
Schistosomiasis	200–300 million
Malaria	200–300 million
Filariasis	250 million
Giardiasis	200 million
Pinworm infection	60–100 million
Strongyloidiasis	50–80 million
Guinea worm infection	20–40 million
Trypanosomiasis	15–20 million
Leishmaniasis	1–2 million

time, even if untreated. There are, however, important exceptions, such as malaria caused by *Plasmodium falciparum*, which may be rapidly fatal in normal non-immune persons. Other usually "mild" parasitic infections may cause disseminated disease and death in immunocompromised patients (e.g., toxoplasmosis).

DEFINITIONS

Protozoa

Protozoa are one-celled eucaryotes. Protozoan parasites of medical interest include the agents of amebiasis, giardiasis, malaria, cryptosporidiosis, leishmaniasis, and trypanosomiasis. Within the human host, some protozoa are intracellular (malaria parasites live within red cells; leishmanias live within macrophages), whereas others are extracellular (amebae and giardia reside in the gastrointestinal tract; pneumocystis is found free in the alveolus of the lung).

Protozoa that infect the blood and deep tissues are often intracellular and unable to withstand the external environment. Consequently, their life cycle does not usually include free environmental stages, and they are typically transmitted from one host to another by the bites of arthropods. For example, the plasmodia that cause malaria are transmitted by mosquitoes. Extracellular and intestinal protozoa, on the other hand, are transmitted most often by the fecal-oral route. These parasites typically have an active, or *trophozoite*, form that carries out vegetative growth, and a dormant cyst form that is resistant to drying and to acid in the stomach, thus allowing them to survive the transition between one host and another.

Helminths

Helminths, or worms, are multicellular animals (metazoa), considerably larger than the protozoa. Indeed, a human intestinal roundworm (*Ascaris lumbricoides*) bears a remarkable resemblance to an earthworm. Lots of different helminths cause human disease: tapeworms, hookworms, pinworms, whipworms, and so forth. Because of their large size, helminths are extracellular. They are sometimes found within tissues in a resting form called a *cyst*.

Most helminths infect the intestinal tract, but several important ones infect the internal organs. A few cause disease both in the intestine and in deep tissues, but most are quite specialized. Helminths may have complex life cycles that involve environmental or animal reservoirs. They may be transmitted by insect bites, oral ingestion, or penetration of unbroken skin.

Vectors

Vectors are living transmitters of disease. A well known example is the female *Anopheles* mosquito which transmits malaria. Other important vectors and the diseases they transmit include tsetse flies—sleeping sickness, black flies—river blindness, kissing bugs—Chagas' disease, and ticks—babesiosis. Most vectors are *arthropods*, such as mosquitoes, flies, and mites. Arthropods may transmit not only parasites but also bacteria (e.g., the agents of Lyme disease or Rocky Mountain spotted fever) and viruses (e.g., encephalitis viruses).

Reservoirs

Reservoirs are the sources of parasites in the environment. Reservoirs of parasitic infections may be other animals (pigs for trichinosis and pork tapeworm, cattle for beef tapeworm), but others are environmental (contaminated soil for roundworms and hookworms), or other humans (malarial plasmodia, amebae).

ENTRY

A striking aspect of animal parasites is the number of ways they have evolved to enter the host. The most common modes of entry are by oral ingestion or penetration through the skin. Transmission of parasitic disease is often due to contamination of food or water or to inadequate control of human wastes. This generalization is most applicable to diseases transmitted by the fecal-oral route or by larval penetration of the skin. Transmission of disease by the bite of the arthropods may be extraordinarily effective. For instance, malaria may be acquired by a single bite of an infected female mosquito during a stop at an airport in an endemic area.

SPREAD AND MULTIPLICATION

Although some parasitic diseases may be acquired by the ingestion or inoculation of only a few eggs or cysts, a sizable inoculum is often required. The size of the effective inoculum has been determined for a few parasites by experimental infections in human volunteers and animals, usually in conjunction with careful quantitative epidemiologic studies. Although a few eggs or cysts are usually capable of causing infections, large inocula are often necessary to produce diseases such as amebiasis in humans. In some instances, such as ascariasis, the larger the inoculum, the more severe the disease.

Species and Tissue Tropisms

The life cycle of a parasite is based on species and tissue tropisms, which determine in which organs and tissues of the host it can survive. Unfortunately, little is known about the basis of this important aspect of parasitism. For example, it is not known why the larvae of *Strongyloides* invade the bowel wall, whereas those of hookworms remain in the intestinal lumen. Nor is it known why the pork tapeworm can cause cysticercosis (a deep tissue infection) in humans, whereas the beef tapeworm does not. Studies indicate that tropisms may depend on specific receptors found on certain cell types but not on others. Thus, Duffy factor on the red blood cell surface is essential for the entry of one type of malaria parasite (*Plasmodium vivax*) into the red blood cell. Consequently, people lacking Duffy factor are resistant to *P. vivax* infection.

Temperature may also play an important role in the ability of parasites to infect and to cause disease. For example, *Leishmania donovani* replicates well at 37°C and causes visceral leishmaniasis or kala-azar, a disease of the bone marrow, liver, and spleen. In contrast, *L. tropica*, grows well at 25 to 30°C but poorly at 37°C, and causes an infection of the skin. Temperature changes alone induce particular stages in the life cycle of many parasites. For instance, leishmanias synthesize heat-shock proteins when they are transferred from the cooler insect into the warmer human body (from about 25 to 37°C). This process appears to play an essential role in the transformation of the parasite from the insect stage to the human stage (it is analogous to the mycelium-to-yeast transformation seen in dimorphic fungi).

DAMAGE AND HOST RESPONSE

As with other infectious agents, the manifestations of parasitic disease are due not only to activities of the parasite, but also to host responses. This is almost invariably true for the animal parasites that lodge in deep tissue, where they elicit an inflammatory response. Chronic inflammation is the hallmark of such diseases as schistosomiasis or lymphatic filariasis. Sometimes the inflammatory response may persist after the parasite dies, as in trichinosis.

Parasites stimulate the immune response and elicit both antibody production and cell-mediated immunity, like other microorganisms. They are, however, adept at circumventing these defense mechanisms. For instance, adult schistosomes (blood flukes) coat themselves with host plasma proteins and are thus not recognized as foreign. As a result, they are able to live within the circulatory system for decades without immune destruction. Intracellular parasites are often protected by their location and by special devices that they have evolved. For example, leishmanias, which live in the phagolysosomes of macrophages, secrete a superoxide dismutase that presumably protects them from killing by the phagocytes' superoxide production.

In worm infections, eosinophils appear in large numbers in the blood, probably in response to the parasites' surface glycoproteins and polysaccharides. Eosinophilia is often accompanied by increased production of IgE. Together, eosinophils and IgE appear to play a role in killing multicellular parasites. These responses are also useful in diagnosis, because they are typical of metazoan infections and are not seen in diseases caused by protozoa.

Certain parasites cause death of host tissue cells directly. Among the better studied examples is the ameba *Entamoeba histolytica* whose virulent strains destroy cells in culture. The process begins with the adherence of the amebae to the mammalian cells, mediated by lectins on the organisms and specific receptors on the surface of the cells. However, little is known of the subsequent steps that lead to cell death. Non-pathogenic amebae do not destroy mammalian cells in vitro.

Clinical Complications

The most important complications of many parasitic diseases occur years later. For instance, persons with schistosomiasis typically have chronic infection and bleeding from either the gastrointestinal tract (*S. mansoni*) or the urinary tract (*S. haematobium*). Years later, persons with heavy infections may develop, chronic complications, such as portal hypertension and esophageal varices (*S. mansoni*) or obstruction or cancer of the urinary tract (*S. haematobium*). Important clinical complications may also occur at sites distant from the original infection. Thus,

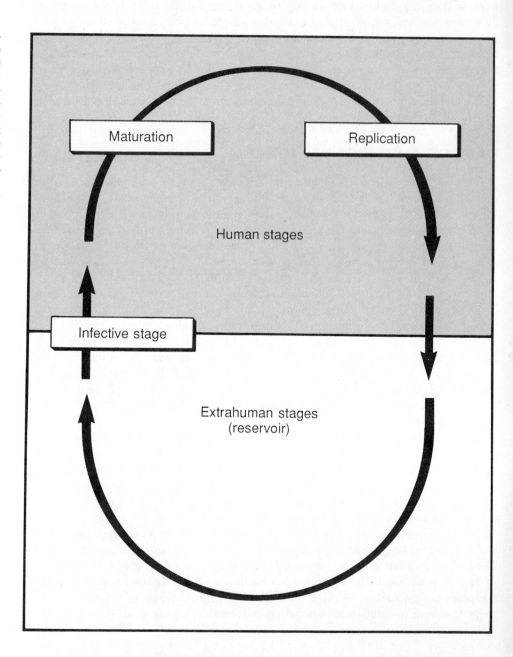

Figure 39.1. Idealized (model) parasite life cycle. The human stages of the life cycle are in the top half of these and subsequent diagrams. The extrahuman stages (in animate or inanimate reservoirs) are in the lower half. As the parasite matures (progressing clockwise through the *extrahuman stages*), it reaches the infective stage, invades the human host, matures, replicates and ultimately completes the life cycle by producing infective forms which are taken up by a vector or released into the environment.

infections due to the pork tapeworm (*Taenia solium*) are asymptomatic when the adult parasite remains in the intestine. Late complications result if the larval forms of the parasite hatch from the egg, cross the intestine to enter the bloodstream and encyst in deeper tissues. This cyst form of the parasite is called a cysticercus. These cysts are small (0.5 to 1.5 cm) and produce no major difficulties when they lodge in skeletal muscle. However, when they lodge in the central nervous system, they may produce hydrocephalus by blocking the flow of cerebrospinal fluid, or seizures by acting as a mass lesion in the brain.

Similarly, Chagas' disease (American trypanosomiasis) produces a relatively trivial skin lesion at the time of the initial infection. This may lead to a rapid acute infection or, many years later, to chronic infection. In patients with chronic infection, nerve damage may lead to failure of intestinal motility from massive distention of the esophagus or colon, or to heart block from damage to the cardiac conduction system. Fortunately, the majority of infected persons do not develop these complications. There are no clearly defined risk factors, however, that identify persons more likely to develop these later complications.

UNDERSTANDING THE LIFE CYCLE OF PARASITES MAY HELP IN DIAGNOSIS

The life cycles of parasites often suggest useful clues for diagnosis (Fig. 39.1). For instance, in the life cycle of hookworms, the adult female lives in the lumen of the human bowel. This predicts that she will release eggs into the stool, which is indeed the case. As a result, examination of stool for eggs is an effective and sensitive means of diagnosing hookworm infection. In contrast, stool examination is of little diagnostic value with another nematode, *Strongyloides*, where the female invades the bowel wall, and lays her eggs there rather than in the intestinal lumen. Because few if any *Strongyloides* eggs are released into the intestinal lumen, they are rarely seen on stool examination.

ENVIRONMENTAL CONSTRAINTS ON PARASITIC DISEASES

Understanding the life cycle often explains why a given parasitic disease is found in one area but not another (Table 39.2). For example, the transmission of schistosomiasis depends on the intermediate snail host, which is not present in North America or Europe. Viable eggs released from infected persons will not produce forms infective for humans if they cannot find a suitable snail host in which to mature. Thus, schistosomiasis is not endemic in the United States and will not be, no matter how many people with the disease enter this country. In contrast, *Anopheles* mosquitoes capable of transmitting malaria are found in the United States. Therefore, recent immigrants or travelers who acquired malaria in endemic areas may infect the indigenous mosquito pool. Transmission of malaria by this mechanism took place in the U.S. after World War II, the Korean war, and the Vietnam war. For this reason, ongoing malaria surveillance is particularly important when a large number of people from malaria-endemic areas enter the U.S. and settle in parts of the country where substantial numbers of anopheline mosquitoes are present.

Table 39.2
Geographic context of parasitic infection

Indigenous to the U.S. Mainland	Imported
Intestinal Helminths	
Ascaris lumbricoides (roundworm)	*Ancylostoma braziliense* (hookworm)
Enterobius vermicularis (pinworm)	*Schistosoma mansoni* (schistosomiasis)
Trichuris trichiura (whipworm)	*Schistosoma haematobium*
Strongyloides stercoralis (threadworm)	*Schistosoma japonicum*
Necator americanus (hookworm)	
Taenia saginata (beef tapeworm)	
Taenia solium (pork tapeworm)	
Diphyllobothrium latum (fish tapeworm)	
Hymenolepis nana (dwarf tapeworm)	
Toxocara canis, T. cati (visceral larva migrans)	
Trichinella spiralis (trichina)	
Echinococcus	
Echinococcus granulosus	*Echinococcus multilocularis*
Filarias	
Dirofilaria immitis (canine filariasis)	*Wuchereria bancrofti*
	Brugia malayi
	Onchocerca volvulus
	Loa loa
	Dracunculus medinensis
Flukes	*Paragonimus westermani* (lung fluke)
	Clonorchis sinensis (liver fluke)
Protozoa	
Entamoeba histolytica (amebiasis)	*Plasmodium vivax, P. falciparum, P.*
Giardia lamblia (giardiasis)	*ovale, P. malariae*
Toxoplasma gondii (toxoplasmosis)	*Leishmania donovani, L. tropica*
Babesia microti (babesiosis)	*Balantidium coli* (balantidiasis)
Pneumocystis carinii (pneumocystosis)	*Trypanosoma cruzi* (Chagas' disease)
Trichomonas vaginalis (trichomoniasis)	*Trypanosoma brucei* (African sleeping
Naegleria fowleri (meningoencephalitis)	sickness)
Cryptosporidium (cryptosporidiosis)	

STRATEGIES TO COMBAT PARASITIC INFECTIONS

"Good plumbing has done more for good health than good medicine."
—William Trager

The life cycles of parasites provide important clues for the control of transmission (Fig. 39.2, Table 39.3). For example, the infectious larvae of hookworms mature in human excrement and then penetrate human skin on contact. Therefore, sanitation and wearing of shoes are effective in reducing the incidence of hookworm infection. This disease was prevalent in the southern United States until these preventive measures were instituted on a large scale by the Rockefeller Commission in the 1930s. Sanitation is effective in preventing many parasitic diseases: ascariasis, strongyloidiasis, pinworm infection, beef and pork tapeworm infection, schistosomiasis, amebiasis, giardiasis, and cryptosporidiosis. An understanding of the parasite's life cycle is also helpful in the choice of antiparasitic

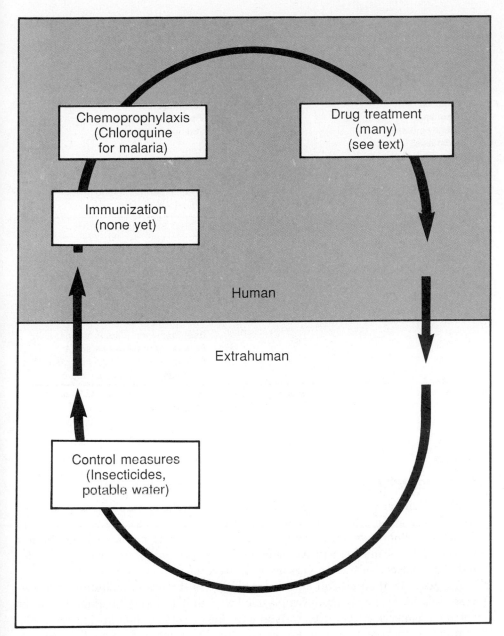

Figure 39.2. Points of potential intervention in the parasite life cycle. Control measures interfere with replication or survival of the extrahuman stages of the parasite. They prevent infection by reducing the number of infective stages to which humans are exposed. *Immunization (vaccination)* prevents infection by inhibiting or killing the parasite as it enters the human host. *Chemoprophylaxis* is used to inhibit parasite replication in order to prevent symptomatic infection. Neither immunization nor chemoprophylaxis prevents the initial entry of the parasite. *Drug treatment* is used to prevent death or severe morbidity in persons with established infections.

drugs. For example, different drugs are necessary for the intestinal and tissue stages of the pork tapeworm (*Taenia solium*): one drug, niclosamide, is effective against taeniasis (intestinal infection), but another, praziquantel, is useful for the treatment of the tissue stage of *T. solium* infection (cysticercosis).

Antiparasite strategies fall into three general categories: (*a*) drugs for chemoprophylaxis or treatment, (*b*) immunization, and (*c*) control measures in the field. Eradication programs have generally proven effective only when more than one of these strategies have been used simultaneously.

Table 39.3
Modes of spread of some parasitic diseases

Human to Human	Animal to Human
Fecal-Oral Spread	
Cryptosporidiosis	Cryptosporidiosis
Amebiasis	Toxoplasmosis
Giardiasis	Visceral larva migrans
Strongyloidiasis[a]	Echinococcosis
Ascariasis[b]	
Trichuris infection[b]	
Fecal-Cutaneous Contact—Without Ingestion	
Strongyloidiasis	Creeping eruption (dog or cat
Hookworm infection	hookworm)

Human Reservoir	Animal Reservoir
Vectorborne	
Lymphatic filariasis	Trypanosomiasis (sleeping sickness,
Onchocerciasis	Chagas' disease)
Malaria	Leishmaniasis
Leishmaniasis	
Inadequate Cooking	
	Beef tapeworm (*Taenia saginata*)
	Pork tapeworm (*Taenia solium*)
	Fish tapeworm (*Diphyllobothrium latum*)
	Toxoplasmosis (*Toxoplasma gondii*)

[a] Usually transmitted by fecal-cutaneous contact but may also be transmitted by the fecal-oral route.
[b] May require a period of time outside the human host in order to be infectious.

Drugs

Chemoprophylaxis

The requirements for a drug to be acceptable for chemoprophylaxis in healthy persons are substantially more stringent than those for use in the treatment of ill people. Minor side effects that are tolerable for short periods of time in sick persons (e.g., headache, nausea, or other GI disturbances) are unacceptable for indefinite periods of time in persons who are well.

An example of successful chemoprophylaxis is the use of chloroquine to prevent malaria. This drug produces plasma levels that suppress infection by all the agents of malaria, except drug-resistant strains of *Plasmodium falciparum*. Chloroquine taken once a week produces effective blood levels for about 1 week because it has a plasma half-life of about 4 days. The main disadvantage of this drug is that some strains of *P. falciparum* have become resistant to it. *Pneumocystis* pneumonia is another infection that may be prevented by drugs. Chemoprophylaxis with the antifolate trimethoprim-sulphamethoxazole combination sharply reduces the risk of this infection among children with acute lymphocytic leukemia and among persons with AIDS.

Treatment

Treatment is generally an inefficient means of disease control because there is often a long delay between infection and clinical presentation. If treatment is to be effective in reducing the transmission of a parasite, it must be given early, when the patients are infectious. However, many patients are asymptomatic when they are infectious and are no longer infectious by the time they show symptoms (as in cysticercosis).

Many of the treatment regimens used for parasitic disease are designed to prevent the systemic complications of chronic infection (such as portal hypertension in schistosomiasis or seizures in cysticercosis), which are often caused by host reactions. In contrast, many local manifestations (such as the passage of eggs in the stool in schistosomiasis or in the intestinal stage of tapeworm infection) are relatively tolerable. Other treatment regimens are designed to relieve acute complications: intravenous glucose for hypoglycemia in *P. falciparum* malaria or steroids for severe inflammation of the heart or brain in trichinosis.

In the last 5 to 10 years, several new drugs have appeared which constitute significant advances in the treatment of parasitic diseases: praziquantel for cysticercosis and schistosomiasis, ivermectin for onchocerciasis (Chapter 43), and possibly α-difluoromethyl ornithine (DFMO) for African trypanosomiasis (Chapter 40). In each case, the previously available drugs were toxic and often ineffective. Prior to praziquantel, there was no medical treatment for cysticercosis (the tissue invasive form of pork tapeworm infection).

Immunity and Immunization

A Major Problem: Evasion of the Host Immune Response

Many important parasites survive and produce disease because they are able to evade the host immune response. It is easy to see here that vaccines would not be helpful. Schistosomes masquerade as "self" by covering themselves with host antigens. Because of this protection, circulating antibodies (produced spontaneously or by vaccination) may not bind to their corresponding antigens and may thus be ineffective against these parasites. Trypanosomes evade the host immune response using another strategy, by altering their surface antigens (Chapter 40). When the host develops an effective immune response to one antigen, clones of trypanosomes emerge that express different antigens on their surface, leading to continued high-grade parasitemia. An effective vaccine against all these antigenic types seems impossible.

Stage-Specific Antigens and Antigenic Variation: Further Problems in Designing Vaccines

A parasite is likely to have different proteins or polysaccharides on its surface at different stages of its life cycle. Many of these components are antigenic, imparting different immunological characteristics to each stage of the parasite life cycle. For example, the form of the malaria parasite that is injected into humans by the mosquito is antigenically distinct from the form that infects red blood cells. Consequently, a person immunized with the insect form (the sporozoite) is susceptible to infection by the red blood cell stage of the parasite (the merozoite). Thus, an effective malaria vaccine will likely contain major antigens derived from several different stages of the parasite's life cycle.

The development of effective vaccines requires a thorough understanding of the immune response to parasitic infection. For instance, certain epitopes on the surface proteins on malarial parasites are repeated sequences that stimulate the greatest production of antibodies. Only in the last few years has it been realized that other epitopes of this protein may play an important role in cell-mediated immunity. Efforts to develop vaccines are under way for several important parasitic diseases besides malaria, namely schistosomiasis, onchocerciasis, lymphatic filariasis, and toxoplasmosis.

Control Measures

Effective control measures are potentially available for all parasitic diseases. The most effective measures are related to the mode of transmission and to the parasite's life cycle (Fig. 39.2). For example, mosquitoes that transmit malaria often bite at night, when people are sleeping. The mosquitoes rest under the eaves of houses before departing. Thus, insecticides such as DDT may reduce malaria transmission substantially when sprayed under the eaves. Unfortunately, this strategy is limited because some mosquitoes have developed resistance to DDT and because some bite outside the house during the day.

In areas such as North America and Europe, transmission of parasitic disease is often low, because sanitation interrupts the parasite's life cycle. Some of the most effective measures are beyond the means of many developing countries. Potable water, for example, is unavailable or too expensive in many parts of the world. During the dry season, the transmission of infection by the waterborne and fecal-oral routes increases in these regions because the small amounts of water available are used for both washing and drinking. Thus, control measures are often more difficult to implement in the developing countries where the major parasitic diseases are endemic.

CONCLUSIONS

The most striking difference between parasites and other infectious agents is the variety of host vectors and stages in their life cycles. Although at first bewildering, these life cycles provide important clues to understanding the parasitic diseases and help in diagnosis and in the development of public health strategies. In most cases we still do not know the biological basis for the ability of different stages of parasites to invade different hosts and different types of tissues.

Parasitic diseases are more prevalent in areas with inadequate sanitation, but are also important in regions with apparently high sanitary standards, such as Europe and North America. This is frequently due to the susceptibility of immunocompromised patients to these infections. In such patients, parasites escape their normal constraints and may multiply to high and dangerous numbers.

SUGGESTED READINGS

Brown HW, Neva FA: *Basic Clinical Parasitology,* ed 5. Norwalk, CT, Appleton-Centry Croft, 1983.

Cohen S, KS Warren: *Immunology of Parasitic Infections,* ed 2. London and Boston, Blackwell, 1986.

Desowitz, RS: *New Guinea Tapeworms and Jewish Grandmothers: Tales of Parasites and People.* New York, Norton, 1981.

Englund PT, Sher A (eds): *The Biology of Parasitism: A Molecular and Immunological Approach.* New York, Alan R Liss, 1988.

Kean BH, Mott KE, Russel AJ: *Tropical Medicine and Parasitology: Classical Investigations.* Ithaca, NY, Cornell Univ. Press, 1978.

Rose ME, McLaren JD (eds): *Pathophysiological Responses to Parasites.* London, British Society for Parasitology, 1986.

Trager W: *Living Together: The Biology of Animal Parasitism.* New York, Plenum Press, 1986.

Warren KS, Mahmoud AAF: *Tropical and Geographic Medicine.* New York, McGraw-Hill, 1984.

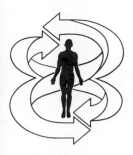

Blood and Tissue Protozoa

D.J. Krogstad

Protozoa that produce bloodstream infection typically cause anemia by destroying red blood cells (malaria and babesiosis). Protozoa that infect tissues may cause significant damage to the eyes, the brain, or the heart (toxoplasmosis), to the brain (African sleeping sickness), or to the heart and the gastrointestinal tract (Chagas' disease). The major blood and tissue protozoa are presented in Table 40.1.

PARASITES OF RED BLOOD CELLS

Malaria

Malaria is the most important of all protozoan diseases, and it is said to have caused "the greatest harm to the greatest number" of all infectious diseases. It occurs in many tropical and semitropical regions of the world (Table 39.1), with approximately 200 to 300 million cases annually. An estimated 2 to 3 million people die of malaria each year, especially malnourished African children. The reservoir of malaria is the infected human; transmission is via the bite of infected female anopheline mosquitoes.

Case

Mr. M. is a 54-year-old businessman from Liverpool who traveled to East Africa (Kenya and Tanzania) on a business trip and then went on a photographic safari. After 1 week in Nairobi, he took a 10-day trip through the wildlife preserves of Serengeti and Ngorogoro, with a final visit to Mombasa

Table 40.1

Comparison of major blood and tissue protozoa

	Organism	Reservoir	Mode of Transmission	Clinical Manifestations
Blood Protozoa	*Plasmodia* (malaria)	Infected humans	Vectorborne by the female *Anopheles* mosquito	Fever and chills with red cell lysis
	Babesia (babesiosis)	Rodents—voles, deer, mice	Vectorborne by the hard-bodied *Ixodes* tick	Fever and chills with red cell lysis
Tissue Protozoa	*Toxoplasma gondii* (toxoplasmosis)	Sheep, pigs, cattle, cats	Foodborne by the ingestion of inadequately cooked beef or lamb. Fecal-oral by the ingestion of infectious oocysts in cat feces	Intrauterine (congenital) infection may produce severe retardation. Mononucleosis-like illness most common. Infection of the brain (encephalitis) or heart (myocarditis) in severely immunocompromised patients
	Leishmania (leishmaniasis)	Infected humans, dogs, jackals, foxes, rats, ground squirrels, gerbils	Vectorborne by infected *Phlebotomus* sandflies	Trivial or mild (self-healing) skin lesions. Disfiguring mucocutaneous lesions. Systemic illness with involvement of liver, spleen, and bone marrow
	Pneumocystis carinii[a] (pneumocystosis)	Probably in infected humans and animals	Probably airborne for initial infection. Disease typically represents activation of previously quiescent infection with natural or iatrogenic immunosuppression	Pneumonia
	Trypanosoma cruzi (Chagas' disease, American trypanosomiasis)	Wildlife and domestic animals (zoonosis)	Vectorborne by reduviid bugs that rub infected feces in the bite wound	Gastrointestinal tract dysfunction from autonomic nerve damage (megacolon, megaesophagus). Cardiac dysfunction from damage to the conducting system (right bundle branch block)
	Trypanosoma brucei gambiense or rhodesiense (African trypanosomiasis sleeping sickness)	Infected humans. Wildlife and cattle	Vectorborne by the tsetse fly	Systemic illness with fever, headache, muscle, and joint pains. Progresses to central nervous system involvement with altered speech, gait, and reflexes (encephalitis)

[a] Recent evidence suggests that this may be a fungus.

on the Indian Ocean. During his flight home, 9 days after leaving the game parks, he developed a flu-like syndrome with headache, muscle aches, and a temperature of 38°C. After his return home, he saw a physician who diagnosed influenza (which can also cause headache, muscle aches, and fever). He had returned to England in February during an outbreak of influenza A.

Mr. M. was given acetaminophen, which initially reduced his fever and muscle aches. However, he felt worse the next day: he suddenly developed an intense chill that lasted for about 30 minutes and was followed by a fever to 40.2°C of 6 hours' duration. When the fever abated, Mr. M. became drenched in sweat and felt exhausted and drained. One and a half days later he had similar but more intense manifestations and was brought to the hospital unconscious. On examination, he had edema of the lungs. He showed no signs of endocarditis, and a lumbar puncture was negative for bacterial meningitis.

The attending physician, drawing on his experience while serving in the armed services abroad, recognized that the clinical manifestations of Mr. M. were typical of a malarial paroxysm. The recent history of travel to endemic areas helped sharpen his suspicion of the disease, and the diagnosis was confirmed when a Giemsa-stained smear of the patient's blood revealed large numbers of parasites within red blood cells. They were identified as Plasmodium falciparum by their characteristic ring shape. His hematocrit (packed red cell volume) was 18% (normal is 40% to 45%). Urinalysis revealed extensive hemolysis; his serum creatinine (a measure of renal function) was 5.4 mg/100 ml (normal is 1 mg or less per 100 ml).

Treatment was begun with intravenous quinidine, which is effective against P. falciparum strains resistant to the more commonly used antimalarial, chloroquine. Mr. M. was also given intravenous glucose as a precaution against hypoglycemia (which may produce coma in patients with severe P. falciparum malaria). Hypoglycemia may result both from consumption of glucose by large numbers of parasites and from the direct release of insulin from the pancreas produced by quinidine or quinine. For his pulmonary edema, Mr. M. required artificial ventilation with a respirator. He was given multiple transfusions for his anemia and was put on a dialysis machine because of his kidney failure. He recovered and was discharged after spending 10 days in the intensive care unit.

Encounter and Entry

Malaria may be transmitted 9 to 17 days after the female *Anopheles* mosquito ingests blood from a person infected with human species of *Plasmodium*. People typically develop symptoms of malaria 8 to 30 days later. Most cases of malaria in Europe and North America represent infections imported in persons who have traveled to endemic areas. However, mosquitoes that can serve as vectors exist in the United States (*Anopheles albimanus* in the East and *A. freeborni* in the West). When these mosquitoes bite travelers infected with plasmodia, malaria may be introduced into the United States, i.e., it may be transmitted to persons who have never traveled abroad. Introductions of malaria have occurred with the return of large numbers of infected veterans after several wars and more recently near San Diego, California, in association with infected Mexican migrant workers. Malaria may also be transmitted by blood transfusion or by the sharing of needles among intravenous drug users (induced malaria).

Spread and Multiplication

The life cycle of the malaria parasite is complex and rich in morphological detail (Fig. 40.1). In brief, the organisms are injected under the skin by infected mosquitoes as sporozoites. They travel through the blood and enter liver cells. After 8 to 14 days in the liver, they mature and are released once again into the bloodstream, in a form that can invade red blood cells (merozoites). After 2 or 3 days, the infected red blood cells burst, liberating more infective merozoites that infect previously unparasitized red blood cells. This part of the life cycle consists of asexual reproduction in the red blood cell. In the blood, some of the plasmodia may also develop into the sexual blood stage (gametocytes), which may be taken up by mosquitoes to carry out their sexual reproductive cycle. The parasites undergo further changes in the mosquito before once again becoming infective sporozoites. In each of these stages the plasmodial cells are recognizable morphologically (Fig. 40.1).

Human malaria is caused by four species of plasmodia that vary in their innate virulence. A major reason for this difference is that the various plasmodial species prefer red blood cells (RBCs) of different ages: P. falciparum invades erythrocytes of all ages, producing the highest parasitemias and the greatest risk of mortality;

Figure 40.1. Malaria life cycle. Sporozoites released from the salivary gland of the female Anopheles mosquito are injected under the skin when the mosquito bites a human (1). They then travel through the bloodstream and enter the liver (2). Within liver cells, the parasites mature to tissue *schizonts* (4). They are then released into the bloodstream as *merozoites* (5) and produce symptomatic infection as they invade and destroy red blood cells (RBCs). However, some parasites remain dormant in the liver as *hypnozoites* (2, *dashed lines* from 1–3). These parasites (in *Plasmodium vivax, P. ovale*) cause relapsing malaria. Once within the bloodstream, merozoites (5) invade RBCs (6), and mature to the *ring* (7,8), *trophozoite* (9), and *schizont* (10) asexual stages. Schizonts lyse their host RBCs as they complete their maturation and release the next generation of merozoites (II) which invades previously uninfected RBCs. Within RBCs some parasites differentiate to sexual forms (male and female *gametocytes*, 12). When these are taken up by a female Anopheles mosquito, the male gametocyte loses its flagellum to produce *male gametes* which fertilize the *female gamete* (13) to produce a *zygote* (14). The zygote invades the gut of the mosquito (15) and develops into an *oocyst* (16). Mature oocysts produce *sporozoites*, which migrate to the salivary gland of the mosquito (1) and repeat the cycle. *Dashed line* between 12 and 13 indicates that absence of the mosquito vector prevents natural transmission via this cycle. Note that infection by the injection of infected blood bypasses this constraint and permits transmission of malaria among intravenous drug addicts and to persons who receive blood transfusions from infected donors.

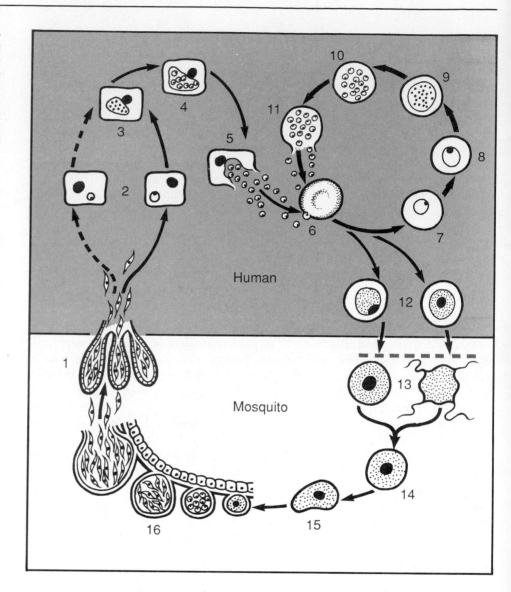

P. vivax prefers reticulocytes and young RBCs, *P. malariae*, older ones. Both *P. vivax* and *P. malariae* infect only 1% to 2% or less of RBCs, and thus produce less severe disease. The fourth species, *P. ovale* is virtually identical to *P. vivax* clinically and morphologically.

The intracellular location of the malaria parasite within the red blood cell has two important consequences:

• Red blood cells infected with *P. falciparum* develop special knobs on their surface as the result of parasite-induced changes in the RBC membrane. These knobs facilitate the adherence of infected RBCs to the endothelium of the venules and capillaries, and explain the localization of *P. falciparum*–infected cells in the deep vascular bed.

• The presence of the plasmodium makes red blood cells less deformable. The spleen removes older, more rigid red blood cells that are less able to bend and travel through capillaries. Thus, the spleen recognizes parasitized erythrocytes as less deformable, and plays an active role in removing them from the circulation. Not surprisingly, splenectomized people have higher degrees of parasitemia and more severe infections.

Damage

The main manifestations of malaria are fever, chills, and anemia. The typical malarial paroxysm (as in Mr. M.'s case) coincides with the simultaneous lysis of many red blood cells and the release of large numbers of merozoites. It is not clear what causes these manifestations or how the infection is synchronized. Although the infection may cause the release of a pyrogen, such a substance has not been demonstrated. The symptoms and signs observed in patients with malaria are often greater than can be accounted for by the degree of parasitemia. Thus, uninfected red blood cells may also be destroyed prematurely. Recent studies have suggested that tumor necrosis factor (cachectin) may be released in malaria and may be responsible for complications, such as edema of the lungs and shock (as seen in the case of Mr. M.).

The in vivo cycle of parasite replication can be quite synchronous and may produce a regular fever pattern—every 2 days with *P. vivax* or *P. ovale*, every 3 days with *P. malariae*. In contrast, the fever pattern is often irregular with *P. falciparum*, especially in nonimmune patients. Other frequent clinical presentations include an influenza-like syndrome (fever, muscle aches, and malaise) and gastroenteritis (nausea, diarrhea, vomiting). Patients with these signs and symptoms may be readily misdiagnosed, especially if the physician is not acquainted with malaria or fails to obtain a history of recent travel.

Human Genetics and Malaria

Genetic polymorphism of several human genes affects the entry, multiplication, and survival of malarial parasites and is important in determining the outcome of the infection. For example, entry of parasites into RBCs depends on their ability to bind to surface receptors. For *P. falciparum* and *P. vivax*, the receptors are glycophorin A and the Duffy blood group antigen, respectively. The variable susceptibility of American blacks to *P. vivax* infection is consistent with the distribution of Duffy antigen. African blacks are Duffy-negative and are resistant to *P. vivax* infection. Because malaria is such a devastating disease, it is likely that it has been a powerful selective force in human evolution.

Many epidemiological studies have shown that sickle cell hemoglobin (HbS) is common in areas of Africa with a high incidence of *P. falciparum*. Malaria is seldom found in carriers of the sickle cell trait, which suggests that this genetic determinant imparts a selective advantage to people living in areas where the parasite is common. Furthermore, in vitro studies have shown that at oxygen tensions similar to those in tissue, the parasites grow poorly in red blood cells with sickle cell hemoglobin, or HbS (Fig. 40.2). Thus, this population trades off the risk of a fatal disease, sickle cell anemia in the homozygous, for the protection of a larger group of the population, the heterozygous HbS carriers. This is an example of a balanced genetic polymorphism.

How does the sickle cell trait protect from malaria? *P. falciparum*–infected RBCs adhere to the walls of blood vessels via knobs that form as the parasites mature. This adherence to the peripheral microcirculation sequesters the parasitized RBCs in an area of reduced oxygen tension, which facilitates sickling and the killing of the parasites.

Figure 40.2. Effect of hypoxia on parasite growth in sickle hemoglobin red blood cells. In 18% oxygen, *P. falciparum* grow as well in sickle hemoglobin (SS) red blood cells (*filled circles*) as in either heterozygous (SA) red cells (*half-filled circles*) or normal (AA) RBCs (*open-circles* in 18% oxygen (*left panel*). In contrast, in 3% oxygen, *P. falciparum* parasites grow much less well in SS cells than in SA or AA cells (*right panel*). (From Friedman MJ: Erythrocytic mechanism of sickle cell resistance to malaria. *Proc Natl Acad Sci USA* 75: 1994, 1978).

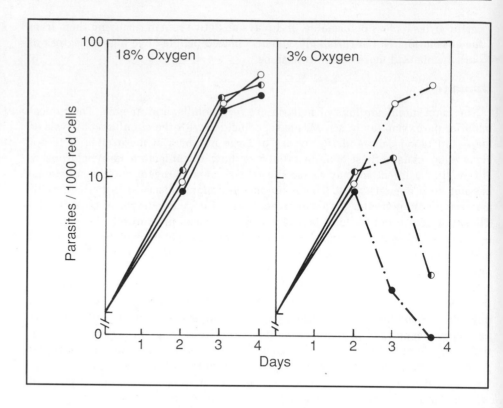

Other genetic abnormalities that restrict the growth of malarial parasites within RBCs are glucose-6-phosphate dehydrogenase (G6PD) deficiency and thalassemia. In the case of G6PD, it is thought that the reduced ability of the RBCs to produce NADPH via the pentose phosphate shunt results in an oxidative stress that inhibits parasite growth.

Diagnosis

The laboratory diagnosis of malaria is made by microscopic examination of a Giemsa-stained smear of peripheral blood using the oil immersion objective (Table 40.2). Wright's stain, which is used more often in the clinical hematology

Table 40.2
Morphologic diagnosis of malaria

	P. falciparum	*P. vivax*
Reliable Criteria		
Only rings on the peripheral smear	Yes	No
Enlargement of parasitized red blood cells	No	Yes
Schüffner's dots	No	Yes
Banana-shaped gametocytes	Yes[a]	No
Less Reliable Criteria		
Peripheral location of parasite within the red blood cell	Typical	Rare
Multiply infected red cells	Frequent	Rare

[a] Characteristic *P. falciparum* gametocytes may first appear days to a week after the patient first becomes ill and seeks medical attention.

laboratory, stains the parasites less well. If the parasitemia is low, a "thick smear" may be used to increase sensitivity. Because RBCs are lysed in the preparation of thick smears, this procedure provides no information about the effect of the parasite on the size of the RBCs or about the intracellular location of the parasite within the RBCs (central or peripheral). These morphological characteristics help a trained technologist differentiate among the species of plasmodia.

For practical purposes, the infecting species in acutely ill patients is either *P. falciparum* or *P. vivax*. This is because *P. malariae* most often causes subacute or chronic infections and *P. ovale* malaria is clinically so similar to *P. vivax* malaria that the distinction is usually insignificant. The morphological characteristics of the parasite allow one to distinguish *P. vivax* from *P. falciparum*. *P. vivax* causes infected RBCs to progressively enlarge as the parasite matures and produces eosinophilic "stippling" in the RBCs (Schüffner's dots). Neither red cell enlargement nor Schüffner's dots occur with *P. falciparum*. This distinction is important because *P. falciparum* infection poses a greater risk of death and is the only human malaria species that may be chloroquine resistant.

Serologic testing is of little value for the diagnosis of malaria in the acutely ill patient. This is because patients do not develop species-specific antibodies to the parasites for 3 to 5 weeks, but treatment must begin within 1 to 2 days of the onset of symptoms. Recent work has shown that hybridization with DNA probes may be useful in the diagnosis of malaria. The sensitivity of this technique is similar to that of the thick blood smear. However, the procedure presently requires the use of radioactive isotopes and is therefore not practical in the field in many developing countries.

Prevention and Treatment

Natural immunity to malaria is imperfect. Persons who have lived in malarious areas all their life and who have evidence of humoral and cellular responses to parasite antigens are nevertheless infected on a regular basis. Their infections tend, however, to be less severe than those of nonimmune persons, suggesting that the immune response plays a significant role. A number of workers have shown that antibodies directed against sporozoites, the form introduced by the insect (Fig. 40.1), are not sufficient to protect against the infection. For this reason, an effective vaccine will probably need to stimulate cell-mediated immunity and to include antigens derived from the various stages of the parasite. Unfortunately, studies of cell-mediated immunity are not as advanced as those of humoral immunity. The future will tell if such a vaccine is possible.

Chloroquine is the single most widely used drug for antimalarial chemoprophylaxis and treatment. It is effective against all strains of *Plasmodium*, except for resistant strains of *P. falciparum*. Such strains are now present in parts of Southeast Asia, South America, and Africa and complicate the prophylaxis and treatment of malaria. Thus, Mr. M. might well have acquired *P. falciparum* infection in East Africa even if he had been on chloroquine chemoprophylaxis. In contrast, he would have been protected in Haiti, where there is no chloroquine resistance. Updates on the prevalence of chloroquine-resistant *P. falciparum* and recommendations for antimalarial prophylaxis are published annually by the Centers for Disease Control and the World Health Organization.

Chloroquine is the only antimalarial considered to be safe in pregnancy. The chloroquine doses used for antimalarial chemoprophylaxis (5 mg base/kg/week) do not damage the retina, which is a risk when taking this drug at higher doses

(5 to 10 mg base/kg/day) for the treatment of rheumatoid arthritis and other rheumatoid diseases.

Patients infected with chloroquine-resistant *P. falciparum* can be treated with other agents, such as mefloquine, quinine, quinidine or Fansidar. Since quinine and Fansidar are potentially toxic, they are used more often for treatment than for chemoprophylaxis. Fansidar, for example, may produce generalized skin reactions with loss of epithelial integrity. Because persons with these complications are at significant risk of death from fluid and electrolyte loss and from infections, the indications for Fansidar in the chemoprophylaxis of malaria have been restricted. Amodiaquine, an analog of chloroquine, is effective in vitro and in vivo against many moderately chloroquine-resistant *P. falciparum*. However, recent studies indicate that this drug causes agranulocytosis and severe hepatitis. Therefore, it is not recommended for antimalarial chemoprophylaxis.

Chloroquine is not effective against the liver (hypnozoite) stages of *P. vivax* or *P. ovale*. Primaquine is effective against these stages and is used to prevent late relapses from maturation of the hypnozoite (to the tissue schizont stage and the subsequent release of infectious merozoites). However, primaquine is more toxic than chloroquine. It causes hemolysis in patients with G6PD deficiency, as well as nausea, vomiting, and diarrhea in patients with normal levels of the enzyme. Primaquine is not indicated for either *P. falciparum* or *P. malariae* infections because these parasites do not produce a dormant (hypnozoite) stage in the liver.

Mosquito control with insecticides and drainage of breeding sites has been the mainstay of malaria control in many countries, and has resulted in a dramatic decline in the incidence of the disease. Unfortunately, these measures are expensive and do not always work because mosquitoes may become resistant to some of the insecticides used. To some extent, individuals can try to protect themselves with mosquito netting, house screening, and insect repellants. The best hope for controlling malaria is the development of improved antimalarials and/or an effective vaccine.

Babesiosis

Like the plasmodia of malaria, *Babesia* are intraerythrocytic parasites and also produce illness by destroying the red blood cells they infect. Babesiosis, unlike malaria, is endemic in the United States, especially in the East Coast (notably on Nantucket and Martha's Vineyard). *Babesia microti*, the usual cause of human babesiosis in the United States, is rarely fatal. *B. bovis* and *B. argentina*, which have been reported more frequently from Europe, are fatal more often.

Clinical and Parasitological Features

Patients with babesiosis typically have a mild illness with fever, chills, sweats, muscle aches, and fatigue, which is difficult to diagnose. As in malaria, splenectomized patients are at risk of more severe disease. In persons with an intact spleen the percentage of infected RBCs is usually 0.2% or less; it can rise to more than 10% in splenectomized patients. In fact, the disease was first detected by postmortem studies of splenectomized patients. As in malaria, the spleen is thought to remove the less deformable babesia-infected RBCs from the circulation.

The life cycle of *Babesia* is shown in Figure 40.3. The natural reservoirs are small rodents such as field mice. The vector is the same tick that transmits Lyme disease and both infections may occasionally be transmitted at the same time.

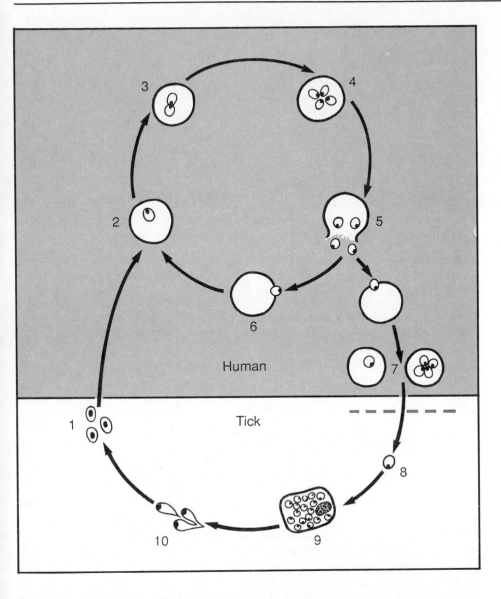

Figure 40.3. *Babesia* life cycle. Infectious merozoites are injected under the skin by the hard-bodied tick (*Ixodes*) vector (1). They invade RBCs directly (2). There is no intermediate liver stage in babesiosis as there is in malaria. Once within the RBCs, parasites replicate asexually by binary fission (3). *Babesia* characteristically form tetrads (4), lyse their host RBCs as they mature (5), and complete the cycle when parasitized RBCs are ingested by the tick vector (6). in the tick, trophozoites (8) multiply in the intestinal epithalium (9) and after further morphological changes (10), are able to infect humans. *Dashed line* between 7 and 8 indicates that natural transmission does not occur in areas without the hard-bodied tick.

Humans are infected accidentally in endemic areas and are not thought to contribute to the maintenance of the parasite's life cycle. The epidemiology of the disease is restricted by the presence of a suitable tick vector and wildlife reservoir, and by human contact with them.

The laboratory diagnosis of babesiosis requires finding the parasites in Giemsa-stained blood films using the oil immersion objective. They are seen as small rings, often in tetrads. These are the only forms found in peripheral blood and may be missed easily when the parasitemia is low. Their ring shape makes them easy to confuse with a similar form of *P. falciparum*. The distinction between the two is important because *Babesia* infections are treated with different chemotherapeutic agents than malaria: clindamycin plus quinine for babesiosis, versus a variety of drugs for malaria (see above).

Antibodies to *Babesia* can be detected in most infected persons; however, they often appear too late (3 to 4 weeks after the onset of infection) to be helpful in the diagnosis and treatment of acute babesiosis.

TISSUE PROTOZOA

Toxoplasmosis

The agent of toxoplasmosis, *Toxoplasma gondii,* is very common in humans: 35% to 40% of the adults in the United States have been infected by this organism as judged by positive antibody titers. However, fewer than 1% are ever diagnosed as having toxoplasmosis. In the few persons with signs and symptoms of active infection, the disease is varied and may be serious. It is particularly threatening to immunocompromised patients, such as those with AIDS, and to the developing fetus.

Toxoplasmosis is associated with three distinct syndromes:

- A "mononucleosis" syndrome that tests negative for the common viral agents of mononucleosis—Epstein-Barr virus and cytomegalovirus;

- A congenital infection that may have severe consequences if acquired in the first trimester of pregnancy (a clinical case description and a discussion of the effects of *T. gondii* on the developing fetus are presented in Chapter 53);

- Infections in immunocompromised hosts (especially those with AIDS), often involving the brain or the heart.

Encounter

People acquire toxoplasma infection by eating inadequately cooked meat or by ingesting food contaminated with infected cat feces. The more common of the two modes of transmission appears to be via the ingestion of inadequately cooked meat (lamb, mutton, or possibly beef) that contains the parasite's *tissue cyst* (produced by asexual reproduction; Fig. 40.4). Less frequently, humans become infected by ingesting cat feces containing fertile cysts called *oocysts.* The frequency with which this occurs is in dispute and is difficult to determine because a minority of toxoplasma-infected cats excrete oocysts in their stools and because we do not know how frequently humans ingest cat feces. The evidence that cats are important in the transmission of toxoplasma to humans comes from the observation that toxoplasmosis is absent from areas that do not have cats, such as isolated Pacific atolls. Once cats are introduced, humans become infected. Cats are necessary to complete the life cycle of the parasite because they harbor the sexual cycle of the organisms and produce environmentally resistant infective cysts in their stool.

After ingestion, the parasites are released from tissue cysts (oocysts) in the small intestine and penetrate the gut wall. They invade the bloodstream and disseminate throughout the body, including the brain and the heart. Over the first 4 to 6 weeks, normal hosts mount an immune response that controls the infection and leads to the formation of dormant tissue cysts in different parts of the body. Unless the person becomes immunosuppressed at some time in the future, the infection remains inactive.

Pathogenesis, Diagnosis, and Treatment

In the active phase of infection, toxoplasma are found within macrophages and can be observed with the high dry or oil immersion objectives. They survive intracellularly in part by preventing acidification of phagosomes and/or their fusion with lysosomes. However, when macrophages become activated they are

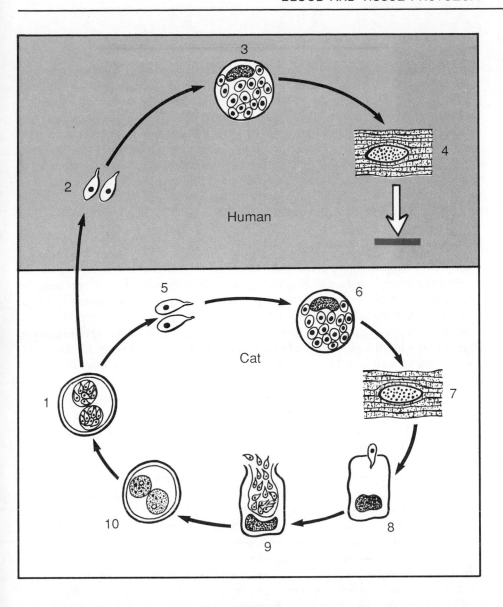

Figure 40.4. *Toxoplasma* life cycle. Humans and other mammals become infected with *Toxoplasma* by ingesting inadequately cooked meat containing tissue cysts or by ingesting infectious oocysts excreted in the feces of infected cats (1). Once in the human host, the oocyts mature to *tachyzoites* (2), enter the bloodstream and disseminate throughout the body (3). After the initial acute infection, most people mount a successful immune response that eliminates the active infectious (tachyzoite) form of the parasite and leaves only tissue cysts with dormant organisms (4). A similar progression is observed within the cat (steps 1 to 4), where the parasite also invades intestinal epithelial cells (6), but, in addition, establishes a sexual cycle (8,9), which results in the formation (10) and release (11) of infectious oocysts. *Red bar* below *open arrow* in step 4 in the upper half of the diagram indicates that human tissue infection is a dead end. Unless there is animal consumption of human remains or cannibalism, human tissue cysts disintegrate after the death of the host.

able to kill these parasites. In the absence of an adequate immune response, toxoplasma causes local inflammation that may result in severe necrosis and tissue damage. AIDS patients, if untreated, may die of toxoplasma infection of the brain.

In the immunologically competent host, the diagnosis of toxoplasmosis can be made by a rising antibody titer, especially of IgM antibodies. However, this measurement is often insensitive in the immunocompromised patient, who may be unable to produce a diagnostic rise in antibody titer. Toxoplasma tissue cysts may be recognized by their characteristic appearance in Giemsa-stained biopsy material. The trophozoites associated with acute infection may be difficult to detect morphologically; brain biopsy material should be stained with fluorescent or peroxidase-labeled antitoxoplasma antibodies to increase the sensitivity of detection.

Most otherwise healthy persons do not need treatment for this infection. In congenital infections it is often too late to begin treatment. For this reason many physicians screen women for anti-*Toxoplasma* antibody at the time of marriage. Women with pre-existing antibodies (prior to pregnancy) have virtually no risk of producing a congenitally infected child. With this screening strategy, one can concentrate on the women who sero-convert, offering them counseling, therapeutic abortion (if early in pregnancy), or treatment with experimental drugs, such as spiramycin. The risk of severe complications in the fetus is greatest for women who sero-convert in the first trimester of pregnancy. The frequency of congenital infection is greatest in the third trimester, but most of the children infected late in gestation have no detectable disease at the time of birth. If the diagnosis is made in time, immunocompromised patients may benefit from treatment with chemotherapeutic drugs (such as pyrimethamine plus sulfadoxine, or trimethoprim plus sulfamethoxazole).

Pneumocystis Infection

As with *Toxoplasma*, *Pneumocystis* infection is common, but overt disease is rare among normal persons. The widespread distribution of this organism is demonstrated by the proportion of people over the age of 4 who have antibodies to it, more than 70% in the United States. In fact, *Pneumocystis* qualifies as a member of the normal human flora. In contrast to toxoplasma, this organism causes only one disease—pneumonia. It has become the hallmark of the AIDS patient, for whom it is highly virulent. It also causes serious disease among malnourished children and other immunosuppressed persons.

Case

Ms. F., a 45-year-old woman, had been generally healthy before admission to the hospital. In the preceding 4 months her weight decreased from 58 to 47 kg and she reported night sweats and fatigue. Her history included the usual childhood diseases, two uneventful pregnancies, and two blood transfusions in Haiti 3 years ago, which she received for injuries sustained during an automobile accident.

On admission she had a fever of 38.4°C, nonproductive cough, bilateral pulmonary infiltrates on chest film and mild hypoxia. On the basis of her history of blood transfusion in Haiti, she was tested for HIV antibodies and found positive. An open lung biopsy revealed Pneumocystis carinii. She was treated with antibacterial chemotherapeutic agents that have proven effective against this agent, trimethoprim-sulfamethoxazole. However, her white blood cell count fell with this treatment and she was switched to pentamidine. Over the next 10 days, her white blood cell count rose and she recovered from the illness despite some renal insufficiency due to the pentamidine. She was discharged after 20 days in the hospital.

Pathogenesis, Diagnosis, and Treatment

The full life cycle of this parasite is not known. The organism is found frequently on careful examination of sections of lungs of people who have died from other causes. The epidemiological evidence for person-to-person or animal-to-human transmission is confusing and controversial. Active *P. carinii* infection may be elicited by giving steroids to normal rats, suggesting that they normally carry these organisms. It is not clear why *Pneumocystis* produce only pneumonia (perhaps it requires an increased oxygen tension). Rarely *Pneumocystis* organisms are seen at other sites, such as the spleen.

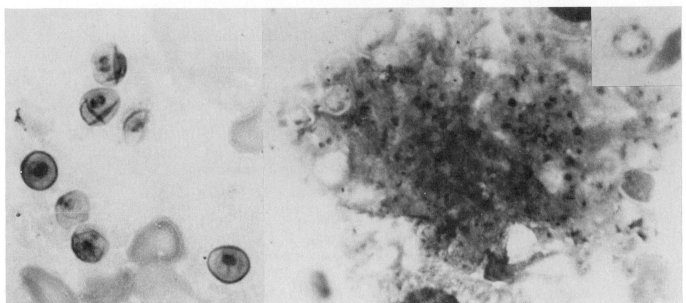

The diagnosis of *P. carinii* infection usually requires demonstration of the organism in open lung or transbronchial biopsies or bronchioalveolar lavage fluid using the high dry objective (Fig. 40.5). The organisms are seldom seen in sputum, except in patients with AIDS. Rapid microscopic staining techniques must be used because of the need for timely diagnosis. Serologic tests are of limited value because a diagnostic *rise* in antibody titer often takes 2 to 3 weeks after the onset of symptoms and may not occur in severely immunocompromised patients. With an acutely ill patient, one cannnot wait weeks to obtain a second specimen before beginning treatment. Also, a baseline earlier serum sample is often not available. Antigen detection tests are being developed but are not yet sufficiently sensitive or specific.

The two treatment regimens used in the case of Ms. F. are thought to be equally effective. Chemoprophylaxis with trimethoprim-sulfamethoxazole is useful for children who are at high risk, such as those with acute lymphocytic leukemia. According to a recent study, these drugs are also effective for chemoprophylaxis in patients with AIDS. Chronic use of these drugs may, however, be complicated by their potential bone marrow toxicity (leading to decreased counts of white and red blood cells and platelets). Other regimens under study include the use of trimetrexate or dapsone, or pentamidine which is aerosolized (rather than administered parenterally) to reduce its toxicity.

Figure 40.5. *Pneumocystis carinii. Left, Pneumocystis* carinii is usually identified by the staining of cysts with Gomori's methenamine silver nitrate (as in this figure). The cysts contain dark bodies which in some instances, as in the two upper organisms, may look like parentheses. The cyst wall often appears folded. *Right,* This figure is of a Giemsa-stained preparation showing *P. carinii* trophozoites, but not cysts. The large clump of cells is typical of that seen in AIDS patients. Giemsa does not stain the cysts, but these are recognized as round clear areas. *Inset* shows *P. carinii* cyst in which nuclei of the intracystic organism are arranged in clockface fashion. (Courtesy of Drs. M.S. Bartlett and J.W. Smith, Indiana University School of Medicine.)

Leishmaniasis

Leishmania species produce a spectrum of clinical syndromes, from superficial ulcers to serious lesions of the liver, spleen, and bone marrow, accompanied by systemic signs such as fever, weight loss, and anemia. Several species are pathogenic for humans. The reason for the great diversity in clinical disease is not well understood, but is due in part to the temperature preferences of the different species. Superficial lesions are produced by *Leishmania* species that grow better at lower temperatures (25 to 30°C) whereas those that invade the viscera grow better at 37°C.

Case

Mr. Q., a 26-year-old graduate student in anthropology, returned from a 6-month expedition to Peru with a nonhealing 2 x 5 cm lesion on his right shin. He reported that almost everyone in his group of 15 had similar lesions but that his was one of the few that had not healed. A smear of a biopsy from the edge of the lesion stained with Giemsa revealed Leishmania-containing macrophages. Mr. Q. was given the antiprotozoal drug pentostam for 4 weeks. The lesion began to heal slowly, and he was cured ultimately after treatment.

The Leishmania and Their Transmission

Leishmania are small protozoa that belong to the *flagellates* because they possess a prominent flagellum during part of their life cycle. In the cytoplasm, the flagellum is connected to an organelle called the kinetoplast which, like mitochondria, has its own DNA.

Leishmania are transmitted by the bite of sandflies—small, short-lived insects that feed on many mammals. These insects are generally found in tropical or subtropical parts of the world, which explains why this disease is rare in North America and Europe. However, sandflies are occasionally found in more temperate regions, and indigenous cases have been reported from the United States. Like malaria, leishmaniasis is seen mainly among travelers returning from tropical countries. Reservoirs of *Leishmania* include rodents, dogs, other animals, and infected humans.

Pathogenesis, Diagnosis, and Treatment

There are several species of *Leishmania*, each with different tissue tropisms and clinical manifestations. The diseases they cause include *localized skin ulcer* such as "chiclero disease" (after the harvesters of chewing gum, "chicle"), *mucocutaneous lesions* ("espundia"), *disseminated cutaneous leishmaniasis*, and *disseminated visceral leishmaniasis* ("kalaazar"). Mr. Q. had a form of cutaneous leishmaniasis that usually heals poorly and requires treatment.

The life cycle of *Leishmania* is shown in Figure 40.6. These parasites are well adapted to the human host: After entering the body through the bite of the sandfly, they differentiate into a form that, once phagocytized, elicits little production of hydrogen peroxide by macrophages. Thus, they rapidly become better able to survive in phagocytes. They also form their own superoxide dismutase, which protects them from superoxide made by macrophages during their oxidative burst. Finally, their uptake of nutrients, such as glucose and proline, is actually dependent on the acidic pH in the phagosome.

Leishmaniasis is best diagnosed by histologic examination of biopsy material using the high dry objective. However, this does not permit one to distinguish among the different species which, although they produce different clinical pictures, look alike under the microscope. *Leishmania* species can be distinguished by culture or by analyzing patterns of isoenzymes or of DNA restriction endonuclease fragments. A recently developed DNA hybridization technique allows one to distinguish parasite species in biopsy material without the need for culture. The increased sensitivity of this method takes advantage of repetitive DNA sequences (minicircles) in the kinetoplast.

A variety of drugs are used to treat leishmaniasis, especially for the invasive forms of the disease. Antimony-containing compounds are modestly successful.

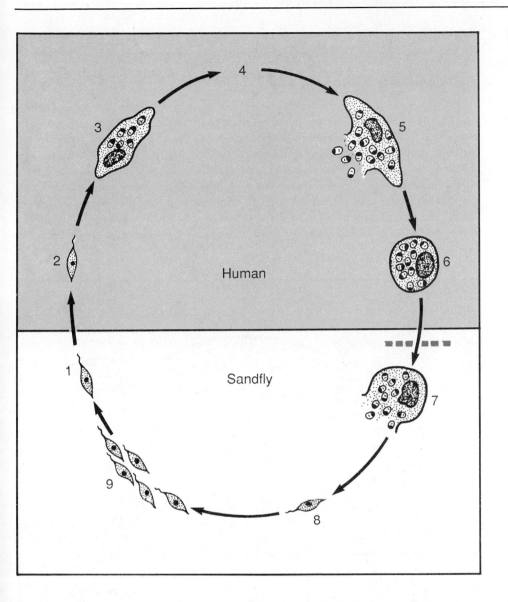

Figure 40.6. *Leishmania* life cycle. The flagellated (*promastigote*) insect form of the parasite (1) is injected under the skin by the sandfly (*Phlebotomus*) vector (2). Once within the human host, the parasite transforms to a nonflagellated (*amastigote*) form which is better prepared to evade the host immune response (it stimulates less release of H_2O_2 from mononuclear cells than the promastigote and produces its own superoxide dismutase). The parasite then invades reticuloendothelial cells (3), replicates (4), lyses those cells (5), and repeats the same sequence in other reticuloendothelial cells (6). In endemic areas, the cycle is completed when previously uninfected sandflies acquire infectious leishmanial amastigotes by biting infected humans (7). The amastigotes then transform to flagellated promastigotes (8) and replicate in the sandfly GI tract (9). Infective promastigotes are injected under the skin of another human when the parasitized sandfly takes a bloodmeal (1 and 2). *Dashed line* between 6 and 7 indicates that transmission is blocked at this point in nonendemic areas such as the United States because the sandfly (*Phlebotomus*) vector is not present.

However, disease of deep organs, such as the bone marrow, may produce fatal anemia and granulocytopenia, despite treatment.

American Trypanosomiasis (Chagas' disease)

Chagas' disease is caused by *Trypanosoma cruzi*. Infection with *T. cruzi* is common throughout Latin America. Overt disease is much less common, however, and the factors responsible for this difference are poorly understood.

Case

Senhor R., a 58-year-old Brazilian businessman, was admitted to a hospital in Sao Paulo for the evaluation of chronic constipation. Radiologic examination of his gastrointestinal tract revealed a large dilated colon (megacolon) and a somewhat less dilated esophagus (megaesophagus). A blood sample revealed *antibodies to T. cruzi. Because no drugs are effective after the onset of complications, Senhor R. was not given antiparasitic treatment.*

Pathogenesis, Diagnosis, and Treatment

The life cycle of *T. cruzi* is shown in Figure 40.7. In the endemic areas of South and Central America, most persons are infected by *T. cruzi* in childhood. The soft tissue and lymph node swelling around the eye produced by the bite of an infected reduviid bug (Romaña's sign) is so characteristic that it is virtually diagnostic. Although some persons develop serious (even fatal) illness, most develop a relatively mild disease, recover spontaneously, and remain asymptomatic. A small proportion of the people infected with *T. cruzi* develop complications 10-20 years later. The complications of Chagas' disease result from damage to nerves in the gastrointestinal tract (megaesophagus, megacolon) or to conducting tissue in

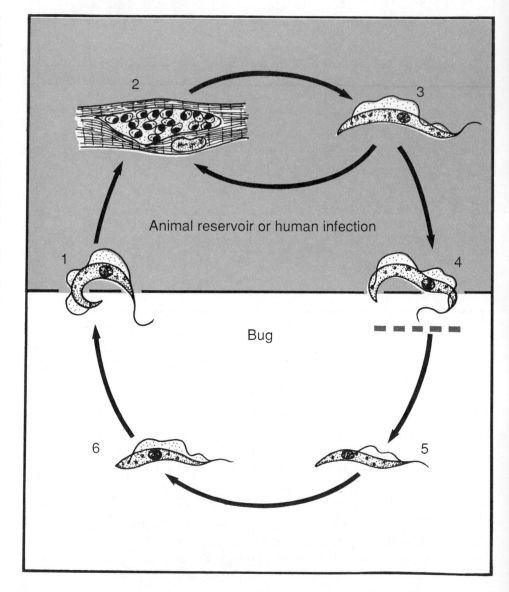

Figure 40.7. Chagas' disease (American trypanosomiasis). The reduviid bug vector deposits feces containing infectious *trypomastigotes* on the skin (1). People rub the itching bite wound, allowing the parasites to enter the bloodstream. In the human host, the trypomastigote transforms to an *amastigote* (analogous to the leishmanial amastigote) as it invades tissue such as muscle (2). Cells containing large numbers of amastigotes often rupture, liberating large numbers of trypomastigotes (3), which invade other host cells (*arrow* from 3 back to 2), or may be taken up by the vector to complete the cycle. In the vector (5), the parasite replicates as an *epimastigote* and produces additional infectious trypomastigotes (1). *Dashed line* below 4 indicates that natural transmission does not occur in areas without the reduviid bug vector. Although reduviid bugs are present in the Southern United States, indigenous cases are rare.

Animal reservoir or human infection

Bug

the heart (right bundle branch block). Infected reduviid bugs are present in the southern United States and are presumably responsible for the sporadic cases of Chagas' disease observed among lifelong residents of Florida, Louisiana, Mississippi, or California.

It is not clear why infection with *T. cruzi* produces autonomic nerve damage in the gastrointestinal tract (leading to megaesophagus or megacolon) or why it damages the cardiac conduction system. Usually, few organisms and a number of lymphocytes are seen in damaged tissue. Fibrosis is the hallmark of the pathology. Consequently, several investigators have postulated that autoimmune mechanisms may play a significant role in the pathogenesis of these complications.

The diagnosis of early infection is usually based on the appearance of the patient. Organisms may often be found in the blood if it is cultured in an appropriate medium or detected by the infection of reduviid bugs which have purposely been allowed to feed upon the patient. Antibodies appear within several weeks. Antibody titers usually remain positive for years. The diagnosis of chronic infection with complications is based on a positive antibody titer or history of exposure plus a known complication (such as megaesophagus, megacolon, or a cardiac conduction defect).

Patients with early acute Chagas' disease may respond to treatment with an experimental drug (benzimidazole, nitrofurazone). However, no treatment is known to be effective for patients with late complications. This may be because the critical damage has already taken place and is no longer reversible.

African Trypanosomiasis (Sleeping Sickness)

Sleeping sickness is caused by *Trypanosoma brucei* (Fig. 40.8). The infection is transmitted by the bite of infected tsetse flies in Africa. A remarkable feature of the parasite is its ability to change its predominant surface antigen repeatedly as the host develops immunity to the previous surface antigen. *T. brucei* and its vectors differ in several biological characteristics from *T. cruzi*, and the vectors of Chagas' disease. For example, *T. brucei* resides in the salivary glands of tsetse flies, and is transmitted directly by bites. *T. cruzi*, on the other hand, grows in the intestine of reduviid bugs, and is transmitted when feces deposited by the biting insect are introduced into the bite by scratching.

Case

The patient, Mr. S., was a 32-year-old student from Kenya living in Canada. He had fevers to 38°C and swollen lymph nodes at the back of his neck (occipital adenopathy or Winterbottom's sign) for 8 months. Two weeks ago, he developed a severe headache, stiff neck, and an aversion to light (photophobia). Trypanosomes were seen on Giemsa-stained specimens of blood and cerebrospinal fluid under the oil immersion objective. Mr. S. was treated with two drugs: suramin for hemolymphatic infection and an arsenical (tryparsamide) for central nervous system infection. He recovered after 4 weeks of treatment.

Pathogenesis, Diagnosis, and Treatment

The spread of African trypanosomiasis is restricted by the distribution of its tsetse fly vector (*Glossina*) and of the animal reservoirs. In East Africa the main reservoirs are wild game animals (such as impalas), in West Africa, the principal

Figure 40.8. Sleeping sickness (African trypanosomiasis). The tsetse fly vector inoculates infectious trypomastigotes under the skin (1) when it bites humans or other mammals. Once inside the new host (2), the parasite replicates in the bloodstream by binary fission as a trypomastigote (3). Unlike leishmania and the trypanosome that causes Chagas' disease, the trypanosomes that cause African sleeping sickness do not have promastigote or amastigote forms. The rate of movement of trypomastigotes from the bloodstream and lymph nodes to the central nervous system determines when the illness changes from a systemic (hemolymphatic) infection to an encephalitis. Circulating trypomastigotes (4) taken up anew by tsetse flies complete the cycle. Within the tsetse fly, the parasites replicate in the GI tract and transform to epimastigotes (5). *Dashed line* below 4 indicates that natural transmission does not occur in countries such as the United States where the tsetse fly vector is not present.

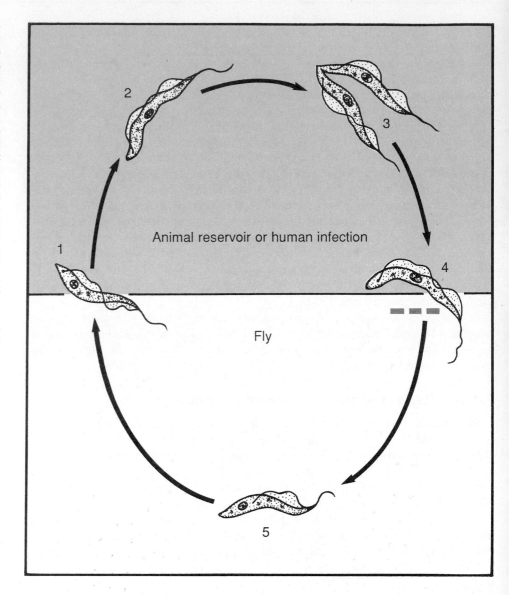

Animal reservoir or human infection

Fly

reservoirs are infected humans and domestic animals (such as cattle). Several weeks to months after the initial infection, patients develop a systemic illness with fever, swollen lymph nodes, and trypanosomes in the bloodstream. After several months (the East African form) or years (the West African form), the parasite crosses into the central nervous system and infects the brain and spinal fluid.

During months or years of chronic bloodstream infection, patients undergo bouts of parasitemia (Fig. 40.9). During each bout the parasite changes its dominant surface antigen (a glycoprotein), thus avoiding immune destruction by the host. The genetic basis for this variation has been studied in some detail. The genome of these parasites contains hundreds or thousands of genes for antigenically different surface glycoproteins, although only one is expressed at a time. Transcription of these genes is by a special mechanism: It requires that the gene be copied and that this copy be transposed into a special site in the genome, a

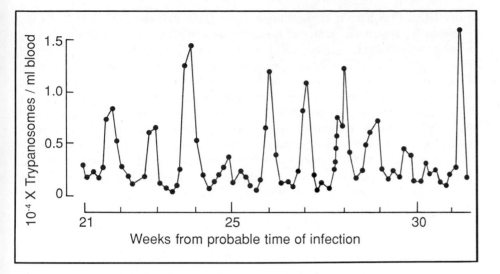

Figure 40.9. Periodic fluctuation in the number of *Trypanosoma brucei* in the blood of a patient with African trypanosomiasis. (Adapted from Ross R, Thompson D: *Proc Roy Soc London, B* 82: 411–415, 1910.)

"reading station". At their original site, these genes remain silent. The transposed gene is the one that is expressed.

Several drugs, including pentamidine and suramin, have some usefulness during the systemic stage of this infection. However, treatment is much more difficult after the infection has crossed into the central nervous system because toxic drugs, such as arsenicals, are required. Recent studies suggest that α-difluoromethyl ornithine (DFMO) may be effective for cases with CNS involvement. If this is the case, DFMO will substantially reduce the morbidity of treatment.

FREE LIVING AMEBAE

A number of protozoa, principally *Naegleria*, *Acanthamoeba*, and *Hartmannella*, have no known animal reservoir but produce serious systemic diseases, such as meningoencephalitis (inflammation of the meninges and the brain). These organisms may also cause infection of the eye, especially among persons wearing contact lenses.

Case

The patient was a 6-year-old girl living in Virginia. Three days ago, in the month of August, she swam in a nearby lake. Although she was well previously, within two days she developed a severe headache, neck stiffness, and eye pain on exposure to light (photophobia). A lumbar puncture revealed 300 mononucleated cells per mm³ and a few neutrophils. Many of these cells were actively motile in a wet mount, suggesting that they were not leukocytes but amebae. Despite treatment with antimicrobial drugs, the patient died 3 days later. Several other children who swam in the same lake also had headaches and mild neck stiffness, but recovered spontaneously.

Pathogenesis, Diagnosis, and Treatment

There are two types of amebic meningoencephalitis: (*a*) A usually fatal disease caused by *Naegleria fowleri*, as in this case, which typically occurs in young, previously healthy people, and is associated with extensive exposure to fresh water lakes that harbor these amebae, and (b) a disease caused by *Acantha-moeba* or *Hartmannella*, which is typically seen in older patients who are immunocompromised (such as those with lymphoma or diabetes). Both types of disease, once they become clinically apparent, tend to progress despite treatment. Although there are reports of recovery using multiple drugs (amphotericin B, miconazole, and rifampin), these regimens have not proven to be reproducibly effective.

In the meningoencephalitis caused by *Naegleria*, the parasite is thought to enter the central nervous system via the cribriform plate along the olfactory nerve tracts. Trauma or increased pressure, as may occur when diving into water, are believed to facilitate the entry of the organisms into the CNS. *Acanthamoeba* or *Hartmannella* are thought to spread to the central nervous system via the bloodstream. This is because patients with this disease often are found to have foci of infection at distant sites, such as the lung, on postmortem examination.

Infection of the cornea (keratitis) is produced by some of these free living amebae, and is an increasingly important (often undiagnosed) cause of visual loss among contact lens wearers or persons with other ocular trauma. It is important to recognize this infection (by morphologic examination of Giemsa-stained material using the high dry or oil immersion objectives), because treatment with topical or systemic imidazoles may save the patient's sight. These parasites may gain access to the eye from contaminated fluids used to clean contact lenses.

SUGGESTED READINGS

Malaria

Cranston HA, Boylan CW, Sutera SP, et al.: *Plasmodium falciparum* abolishes physiologic red cell deformability. *Science* 223:400–403, 1984.

Ferreira A, Schofield L, Ened V, et al.: Inhibition of development of exoerythrocytic forms of malaria parasites by gamma-interferon. *Science* 232:881–884, 1986.

Friedman MJ: Erythrocytic mechanism of sickle cell resistance of malaria. *Proc Nat Acad Sci USA* 75:1994–1997, 1978.

Hoffman SL, Oster CN, Plowe CV, et al.: Naturally acquired antibodies to sporozoites do not prevent malaria: vaccine development implications. *Science* 237:639–642, 1987.

Krogstad DJ, Gluzman IY, Kyle DE, et al.: Efflux of chloroquine from *Plasmodium falciparum*: mechanism of chloroquine resistance. *Science* 238:1283–1285, 1987.

Krogstad DJ, Schlessinger PH: Acid vesicle function, intracellular pathogens and the action of chloroquine against *Plasmodium falciparum*. *N Engl J Med* 317:542–549, 1987.

Miller LH, Howard RJ, Carter R, Good MF, Nussenzweig V, Nussenzweig RS: Research towards malaria vaccines. *Science* 234:1249–1256, 1986.

Babesiosis

Ruebush TK II, Juranek DD, Chisholm ES: Human babesiosis on Nantucket Island: Evidence for self-limited and subliminal infections. *N Engl J Med* 297:825–827, 1977.

Toxoplasmosis

Daffos F, Forester F, Capella-Pavlovsky M, Thulliez P, Aufrant C, Valenti D, Cox WL: Prenatal management of 746 pregnancies at risk for congenital toxoplasmosis. *N Eng J Med* 318:271–275, 1988.

Remington JS, Klein JO (eds): *Infectious Diseases of the Fetus and Newborn*, ed 2. Philadelphia, WB Saunders, 1983.

Shepp, DH, Hackman R C, Conley FK et al.: *Toxoplasma gondii* reactivation identified by detection of parasitemia in culture. *Ann Intern Med* 103:218–221, 1985.

Pneumocystis

Hughes WT, Rivera GK, Schell MJ, et al.: Successful intermittent chromoprophylaxis for *Pneumocystis carinii* pneumonitis. *N Engl J Med* 316:1627–1632, 1987.

Walzer PD, Perl DD, Krogstad DJ, et al.: *Pneumocystis carinii* pneumonia in the United States: epidemiologic, diagnostic and clinical features. *Ann Intern Med* 80:83–93, 1974.

Leishmanias

Chang KP, Bray RS (eds): *Leishmaniasis.* Amsterdam, Elsevier, 1985.

Zilberstein D, Dwyer DM: Protonmotive force-driven active transport of D-glucose and L-proline in the protozoan parasite *Leishmania donovani. Proc Nat Acad Sci USA* 83:1716–1720, 1988.

Trypanosomiasis

Englund PT, Hayduk SL, Marini JC: The molecular biology of trypanosomes. *Ann Rev Biochem* 51:695–726, 1982.

Hudson L (ed): *The Biology of Trypanosomes.* New York Springer-Verlag, 1985.

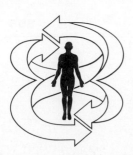

Intestinal and Vaginal Protozoa

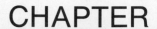

D.J. Krogstad

etween 5% and 10% of all people in the developing countries of the world harbor the pathogenic ameba *Entamoeba histolytica* in their stool. In the United States the figure is less than 1%. *Cryptosporidium* and *Giardia* are more frequent in the U.S. but their prevalence varies considerably among different regions. Table 41.1 shows a comparison of major intestinal protozoa.

Other protozoa also live in the lumen of organs besides the intestine. The main one is *Trichomonas vaginalis*, a common agent of vaginitis. It is usually transmitted sexually.

AMEBIASIS

The agent of amebiasis is *Entamoeba histolytica*. As its species name indicates, it may cause lysis of host tissue, especially in the colon. The lesions start as small ulcerations of the intestinal epithelium and spread laterally when they encounter the deeper layers of the colon, eventually producing flask-shaped ulcers. The organisms may also spread through the bloodstream to produce abscesses in the liver, the brain, and other organs. Despite their pathogenic potential, these organisms cause few or no symptoms in the majority of persons infected.

Case

The patient, Mr. A., is a 26-year-old who was discharged from the U.S. Army 2 years previously. He spent three of his six military years abroad, including

Table 41.1

Comparison of major intestinal protozoa

Organism	Reservoir	Mode of Transmission	Clinical Manifestations
Entamoeba histolytica (amebiasis)	Infected humans	Fecal-oral transmission by the ingestion of feces containing infectious cysts	Bloody diarrhea (dysentery) Distant abscesses (especially liver) Asymptomatic intestinal infection
Giardia lamblia (giardiasis)	Infected humans, and other mammals	Fecal-oral transmission by the ingestion of feces containing infectious cysts	Watery diarrhea, may also cause steatorrhea and malabsorption Asymptomatic intestinal infection
Cryptosporidium (cryptosporidiosis)	Infected humans, and a wide variety of other animal hosts (zoonosis)	Fecal-oral transmission by the ingestion of feces containing infectious cysts	Watery diarrhea

tours of duty in Korea, Panama, and Germany. During the last two years he developed intermittent diarrhea, with blood and mucus visible in the stool. Sigmoidoscopy (endoscopic examination of the colon) and an x-ray study of the intestine following a barium enema revealed pseudopolyps, consistent with inflammatory bowel disease. He was diagnosed as having ulcerative colitis, an inflammatory bowel disease of unknown cause, and was treated with steroids for that condition.

At the time of admission to the hospital, 4 months after beginning steroid therapy, Mr. A. reported the loss of about 11 kg of weight (down to 67 kg) and a recent increase in bloody stools and abdominal pain. He had no fever (probably because he was medicated with a large amount of steroids). Examination of his stool under the microscope showed many white and red blood cells but no amebae. However, a serological test for E. histolytica antibodies in serum (indirect hemagglutination) revealed a titer of 1:2000, which is high. A CT scan showed abscesses in the liver, lungs, and brain.

He had a stormy hospital stay with several episodes of bacteremia (secondary to disruption of the intestinal mucosa by the parasites) but recovered ultimately after the steroids were tapered and he was treated with the antiamebic agent, metronidazole.

Encounter

E. histolytica is transmitted from person to person via the fecal-oral route. It has a simple life cycle, with two forms: the actively growing, vegetative *trophozoite* and the dormant but highly resistant cyst (Fig. 41.1). The critical factors responsible for the transition from trophozoite to cyst are not understood. The transmission of *Entamoeba* and *Giardia* has a paradoxical aspect: patients with diarrhea pose a minor threat of transmission because they excrete the actively growing trophozoites which are labile—they are easily destroyed by drying in the environment or acid in the stomach. On the other hand, asymptomatic carriers excrete the tough cyst form of the parasite; they represent a greater danger of transmission because the cysts are resistant to drying and to gastric acid. This paradox illustrates the biological principle that successful parasites generally do not harm the host: When amebae are in balance with their host, they are excreted as cysts, which ensures the survival of the species.

Because the parasite is infectious in the cyst stage and does not require a period of differentiation in the environment, transmission of amebiasis is not

Figure 41.1. *Entamoeba histolytica* life cycle. Humans acquire amebic infection by oral ingestion of the cyst form of the parasite (1). Viable cysts may be ingested from the external environment (where they remain stable and infectious for prolonged periods after excretion), from the stool of other infected persons, or from the stools of the patients themselves (*arrow* from 7 to 2). In the upper GI tract, the parasite *excysts* after passing through the stomach (2), *replicates* asexually by binary fission (3) and *transforms* to the potentially pathogenic *trophozoite* form (4) which is typically found in the large intestine. Trophozoites die rapidly when they are shed into the external environment (5) (*solid line* below 5). When conditions in the GI tract are unfavorable, trophozoites transform into cysts (6 and 7) which can remain dormant for long periods of time in the host and the environment.

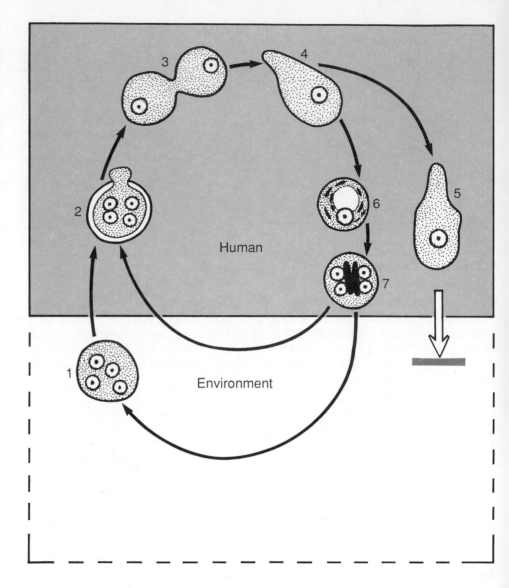

restricted to warm climates. In fact, E. *histolytica* may be transmitted in temperate and even polar regions. All that is necessary for transmission is that the feces of a carrier contaminate food or water. Sexual transmission (anal-oral or oral-genital) is also important, particularly among homosexual men.

The Pathogenesis of Amebiasis

E. *histolytica* is frequently found within the human colon in persons without symptoms of disease. In order to damage tissues, the amebae must adhere to specific receptors on host cells. The fact that this attachment is inhibited by intestinal mucus suggests that disruption of the mucus layer may be a critical event in the pathogenesis of amebiasis. Damage to host cells requires intimate cell-to-cell contact and takes place in three distinct steps: receptor-mediated attachment to the mammalian target cell, contact-dependent killing, and ingestion of the killed host cell by the ameba. Although certain strains of E. histolytica produce an enterotoxin, it is not yet clear whether enterotoxin production correlates with virulence.

White blood cells do not control amebic infection in the nonimmune host: pathogenic strains of amebae actually kill neutrophils and nonactivated macrophages. (Note the reversal of the usual "phagocyte-ingests-invader" theme.) The situation is different in the immune hosts in whom the most important line of defense appears to be cell-mediated immunity. This is suggested by finding that amebae can be killed in vitro by activated macrophages. Also, persons given steroids (which suppress cell-mediated immunity) tend to have disseminated infection despite high titers of antibodies, as was the case with Mr. A. Thus, circulating antibodies may not play a critical role in protection against amebic infection.

Diagnosis

The identification of E. histolytica in stools by microscopic examination is one of the most challenging diagnostic procedures in microbiology. The reason is that nonpathogenic amebae or even white blood cells in stool can be mistaken for amebae, resulting in false positive laboratory reports. Reliable results require examination by an experienced technologist using a high dry or oil immersion objective. False negative results are due frequently to the insensitivity of microscopic examination or to interfering substances, such as the barium given for x-rays. Thus, although a positive stool is helpful in diagnosis, a negative result does not prove that amebiasis is absent. For this reason, serological diagnosis is often attempted and is of considerable value. Serology is positive in more than 80% of people with invasion of the intestinal mucosa and in more than 96% to 100% of persons with systemic (metastatic) disease. In the United States, 1% or less of the general population has antibodies to E. histolytica. Among asymptomatic carriers the prevalence is approximately 10% to 15%. This is an instance in which circulating antibodies are of little protective value but are a good marker for the disease.

Treatment

The drug of choice for active amebic infection is metronidazole, the same antimicrobial used to treat infections caused by anaerobic bacteria. Pathogenic amebae carry out anaerobic metabolism and are able to partly reduce metronidazole and convert it into the active form in the same manner as Bacteroides (see Chapters 2 and 16). This drug is particularly suitable for infections of the nervous system because it crosses the blood-brain barrier well. Carriers with cysts in their stool and no evidence of active disease are treated with drugs such as diiodohydroxyquin or entamide furoate.

GIARDIASIS

The agent of giardiasis is an intestinal protozoan called Giardia lamblia, which is distributed all over the world. In the United States it is found in areas of poor sanitation or in day-care centers, where there is frequent opportunity for fecal-oral transmission. Giardia typically produces a mild but annoying diarrheal disease, often localized to the duodenum and jejunum.

Case

Ms. R. is a 36-year-old woman with an unremarkable medical history. Two months previous to seeing her physician she visited Colorado for 10 days of backpacking. One week after her return she developed diarrhea with three to five watery stools per day. These contained no pus or blood. She did not report fever or chills. She had a stool examination and was told that it was positive for G. lamblia. She was treated with an antiparasitic drug, Atabrine, and improved markedly over a 7-day period. Since then her symptoms recurred and the organisms have again been found in her stool.

Clinical Aspects

As with *E. histolytica,* giardiasis is acquired by ingestion of the cyst form of the parasite (Fig. 41.2). The acid in the stomach not only doesn't kill the cysts, but actually prepares them for change into the vegetative trophozoite form in the

Figure 41.2. *Giardia lamblia* life cycle. Humans acquire giardiasis by ingesting the cyst form of the parasite (1). As in amebiasis, the parasite excysts and transforms to a trophozoite in the upper gastrointestinal tract (2), where it replicates asexually by binary fission (3). Trophozoites cause disease by attaching to the epithelium of the small intestine via a ventral sucking disk (4). Trophozoites are not infectious for others because they are readily killed by drying in the external environment (*solid line* and *open arrow* below 6). As in amebiasis, humans acquire infection by ingesting cysts from the external environment (1), from the stools of other patients, or from their own stool (*arrow* from 5 to 2).

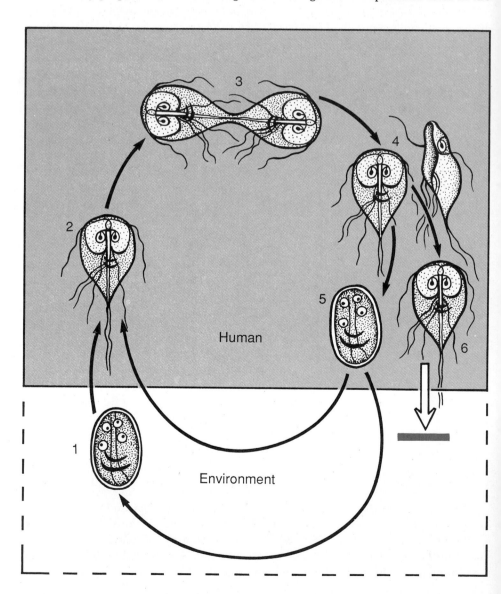

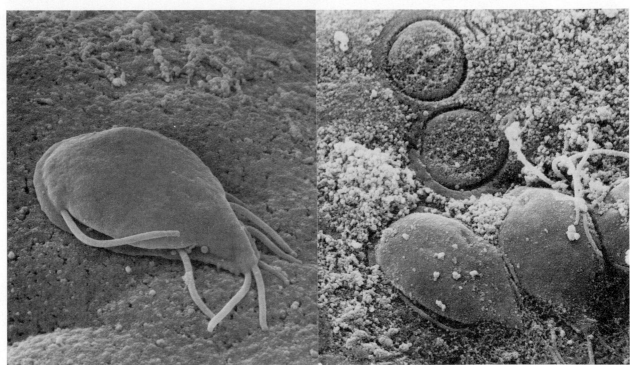

Figure 41.3. Scanning electron micrograph of *Giardia lamblia*. *Left*, Scanning electron micrograph of *G. lamblia* adhering to the gastrointestinal epithelium via its ventral sucking disk. Patients with giardiasis may have a significant reduction in the amount of absorptive surface available because of the large number of adhering parasites. *Right*, Upon detaching from the intestinal epithelium, the organisms often leave a clear impression on the microvillous surface (*upper circles*). (Courtesy of Dr. Stanley L. Erlandsen, Washington University School of Medicine.)

duodenum. *Giardia* trophozoites attach to the epithelium of the duodenum and jejunum using a ventral sucking disk. The vegetative forms have the characteristic appearance of a face adorned with mustache-like flagella visible under the high dry objective (Fig. 41.2). Cysts of *Giardia* are highly resistant in the environment and are found increasingly in ostensibly "pure" mountain streams contaminated by the feces of infected animals or humans. Giardiasis has been known as the "hiker's disease", but is also common in urban environments with poor sanitation, e.g., day-care centers. Like pathogenic amebae, these organisms may be transmitted in cold as well as in warm climates. Giardiasis is also an important infection among homosexual males.

Signs of malnutrition due to malabsorption may occur as a result of extensive infection, which may literally cover the mucosal surface of the small intestine (Fig. 41.3). Unlike *E. histolytica*, *Giardia* is not invasive and does not produce bloody diarrhea or metastatic infection. Giardiasis is treated with Atabrine, a drug previously used in malaria. As with Ms. R, relapses occur frequently. Although these relapses usually respond to retreatment, potential sources of reinfection (such as contaminated water and food, and infected sexual partners) must be considered. Metronidazole and a furan-type drug (furazolidone) have also been used. Hikers and campers may prevent unpleasant episodes of diarrhea by boiling their drinking water or treating it with iodine or chlorine.

CRYPTOSPORIDIOSIS

Cryptosporidiosis is a zoonosis, an animal disease that affects humans only accidentally. It was first discovered as a cause of diarrhea among veterinary students and animal handlers who acquired it from calves they were treating for diarrhea. It is now clear that cryptosporidiosis is an important diarrheal disease in both developed and developing countries.

Case

Mr. H. received a renal transplant 2 years ago. He was well until 6 weeks ago, although he had taken immunosuppressive drugs to prevent graft rejection. Six weeks ago he began to have watery stools 3 to 8 times a day. He reported no fever, nor did he see blood or pus in the stools. A microscopic examination of his stool (with the oil immersion objective) using an acid-fast stain revealed the presence of cryptosporidia (these organisms have the property, unusual among protozoa, of being acid fast).

Figure 41.4. *Cryptosporidium* life cycle. Humans acquire infection by ingesting infectious oocysts (1) that were excreted by themselves (4, 5), by other infected humans, or by animal hosts such as calves, birds, or reptiles (8, 9, 10, 11, 12). Once inside the human host (2), the parasite attaches to the epithelial surface of the GI tract and replicates (3), producing additional infectious oocysts (4). Unlike *Toxoplasma* (another coccidian parasite), cryptosporidia do not invade GI epithelial cells or disseminate through the bloodstream. In the immunologically normal host, cryptosporidia undergo only one cycle of asexual reproduction and produce a self-limited diarrhea. In the immunocompromised host, cryptosporidia undergo multiple cycles of asexual replication (5, 6, 7) and may produce watery diarrhea that continues indefinitely.

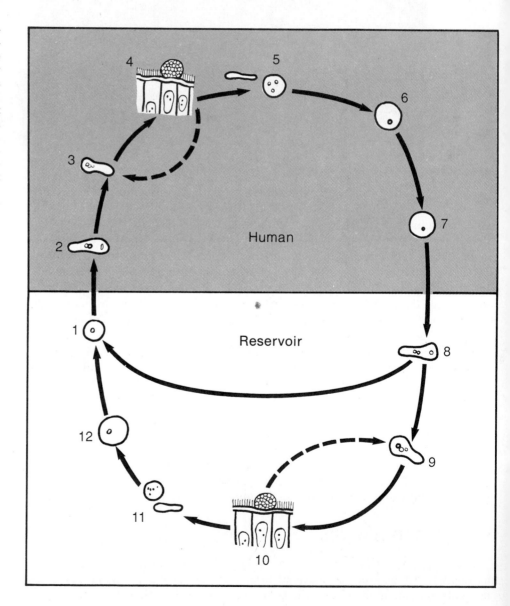

Clinical Aspects

Cryptosporidium resembles *Toxoplasma* in that infectious oocyst forms are produced in the intestine and spread to other animals. However, unlike *Toxoplasma*, cryptosporidia do not invade the intestinal epithelial cells, nor do they disseminate to produce systemic infection. They carry out their whole life cycle among the microvilli of the small intestine (Fig. 41.4). In immunocompetent people, the life cycle only takes place once or twice; it results in a single episode of diarrhea which usually lasts 2 weeks or less. In the immunocompromised patient, the life cycle of the organism is repeated many times and is associated with persistent watery diarrhea.

Cryptosporidiosis is often acquired in rural areas because of greater contact with animals. However, it may also spread from person to person in crowded urban environments such as day-care centers. It is now recognized as a frequent cause of diarrhea in Great Britain and the United States and it is particularly important among patients with AIDS or AIDS-related syndromes.

TRICHOMONIASIS

Trichomonas vaginalis is an extremely common inhabitant of the vagina; it is found in 15% or more of women, where it occasionally causes vaginitis. Less common and less pathogenic are species of *Trichomonas* found in the gastrointestinal tract (*Trichomonas hominis*) or the mouth (*Trichomonas tenax*).

Clinical Aspects

T. vaginalis infection is transmitted by sexual intercourse. However, the parasite cannot replicate in the acid environment of the normal vagina (pH $\leq$ 4.9). The vaginitis observed in infected woman is typically associated with a frothy creamy discharge. Symptomatic *T. vaginalis* infection is uncommon among men, although most partners of symptomatic woman become infected. On occasion, men develop symptomatic *T. vaginalis* infection of the urethra, epididymis, or prostate. Rarely penile ulcers are observed in infected men.

Treatment

Single-dose metronidazole treatment is recommended by most investigators. Alternatives include timidazole (another nitroimidazole that has been used extensively in Europe), when it is approved by the U.S. Food and Drug Administration. In pregnant woman (in whom there is particular concern about the potential carcinogenic effects of the nitromidazoles), douching with vinegar may suppress symptomatic infection by lowering vaginal pH.

SUGGESTED READINGS

Amebiasis

Allason-Jones E, Mindel A Sargeaunt P. Williams P: *Entamoeba histolytica* as a common intestinal parasite in homosexual men. *N Engl J Med* 315:353–356, 1986.

Martinez-Palomo A (ed): Amebiasis. Amsterdam, Elsevier, 1986.

Ravdin JI (ed): *Amebiasis: Human Infection by Entamoeba histolytica.* New York, Wiley, 1988.

Giardiasis

Erlandsen SL, Meyer EA (eds): *Giardia and Giardiasis: Biology, Pathogenesis, and Epidemiology.* New York, Plenum, 1984.

Gillin FD, Reiner DS, Gault MJ, et al.: Encystation and expression of cyst antigens by *Giardia lamblia* in vitro. *Science* 235:1040–1043, 1987.

Lev B, Ward H, Keusch GT, Pereira ME: Lectin activation in *Giardia lamblia* by host protease: a novel host-parasite interaction. *Science* 232:71–73, 1986.

Cryptosporidiosis

Jokipii L, Jokipii AM: Timing of symptoms and oocyst excretion in human cryptosporidiosis. *N Engl J Med* 315:1643–1647, 1986.

Soave R, Armstrong D: *Cryptosporidium* and cryptosporidiosis. *Rev Infect Dis* 8:1012–1023, 1986.

Wolfson JS, Richter JM, Waldron MA, et al: Cryptosporidiosis in immunocompetent patients. *N Engl J Med* 312:1278–1282, 1984.

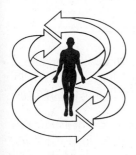

Intestinal Helminths

D.J. Krogstad

The helminths, or worms, are multicellular animals. They include many free living harmless species but also some pathogenic ones that infect a high proportion of all people on earth (Table 39.1). Helminthic diseases are sometimes mistakenly thought to be a problem peculiar to the tropics. In fact, people in the temperate zone (especially if immunocompromised) may become seriously afflicted by these diseases.

Helminths include the largest parasites that affect humans, ranging from 10 yard-long tapeworms down to pinworms, which are barely visible with the naked eye. Many are able to carry out their life cycle within the human body, but others have complex life cycles that include insect vectors and animal reservoirs. Helminths fall into three large groups, roundworms (*nematodes*), tapeworms (*cestodes*), and flukes (*trematodes*), generally distinguishable by their shape. They will be discussed briefly below; specialized parasitology textbooks should be consulted for details.

As we move from the world of unicellular microbes into that of multicellular animals, we must retain some of the main themes of host-parasite interaction. Thus, the most important factors that determine the severity of helminthic infections are the number of worms and the immune state of patient. Normal people can tolerate a sizable number of worms, especially in the intestine, with few if any clinical symptoms. Most frequently, worms are kept in check, and the infection does not progress significantly. However, in the immunocompromised patient, (whether suffering from malnutrition, therapeutic immunosuppression, or a disease such as AIDS) helminthic infections may well cause serious illness. Helminths produce disease by a variety of pathogenic mechanisms, the main ones

Table 42.1
Pathophysiologic mechanisms in helminthic diseases

Mechanism	Example
Mechanical Obstruction or Mass Effect	
Intestinal obstruction	*Ascaris* "worm ball"
Lymphatic obstruction	Lymphatic filariasis elephantiasis
Displacement of normal tissue	Echinococcosis ("hydatid disease") Cysticercosis
Facilitating Bacterial Invasion into Normally Sterile Spaces	
	Strongyloidiasis
Production of Anemia (Nutritional)	
Due to sucking blood	Hookworms
Due to vitamin B_{12} depletion	Fish tapeworm
Chronic inflammation	
	Schistosomiasis Onchocerciasis

being mechanical (including obstruction), tissue invasion, chronic inflammation, and nutritional (loss of blood or of vitamin B_{12}) (Table 42.1). The type of clinical manifestation produced usually depends on the organ or tissue where the damage occurs.

From the point of view of human disease, helminths can be divided into the intestinal helminths (this chapter) and the *blood* and *tissue helminths* (Chapter 43). Intestinal helminths tend to cause chronic infections that may contribute to the malnutrition of their host (Table 42.1). If present in large numbers, they may also occlude the intestinal lumen. Intestinal helminths can be divided into the roundworms, which enter the body by passage through the skin as well as through the mouth, and the tapeworms, which are acquired solely through the mouth.

INTESTINAL ROUNDWORMS USUALLY ACQUIRED BY PASSAGE THROUGH THE SKIN

The most important examples of this group of human roundworms are *Strongyloides* and hookworms (Table 42.2).

Table 42.2
The main intestinal helminths

Example	Reservoir	Clinical Manifestations
Acquired by Passage Through the Skin		
Roundworms		
Strongyloides stercoralis	Infected humans	GI manifestations that may mimic peptic ulcer or gallbladder disease Disseminated infection ("hyperinfection syndrome")
Hookworms *N. americanus* *A. duodenale*	Infected humans	Iron-deficiency anemia from chronic GI blood loss
Acquired by Ingestion		
Roundworms		
Ascaris lumbricoides	Infected humans	Often asymptomatic except for passage of 25 to 30-cm worms May produce GI or biliary obstruction, or peritonitis from intestinal perforation
Pinworm *Enterobius vermicularis*	Infected humans, especially children	Itching of the perianal or genital region
Whipworm *Trichuris trichiura*	Infected humans	Often asymptomatic; damage to intestinal mucosa, malnutrition and anemia if severe
Tapeworms		
Taenia solium	Pigs	Intestinal infection (taeniasis) is typically asymptomatic; for cysticercosis, see Table 43.1
Taenia saginata	Cattle	Intestinal infection (taeniasis) is typically asymptomatic.
Diphyllobothrium latum	Fish	Intestinal infection is typically asymptomatic, but may lead to vitamin B_{12} deficiency

Strongyloidiasis

We will use strongyloidiasis as a paradigm of intestinal parasitic disease. This disease is prevalent in tropical areas of the globe but may also be found elsewhere. If the infecting worms are present in large numbers, they may cause intestinal malfunction. They may perforate the intestinal wall, resulting in serious bacterial septicemias. In addition, they may re-infect the same host, especially if immunocompromised, to produce a lethal systemic disease.

Case

Simone, a 3-year-old girl living in a Caribbean island, appeared malnourished (her height and weight placed her below the third percentile for her age), but had otherwise been well. Two weeks before admission, she developed abdominal pain and diarrhea, which became bloody 1 week later. When she was admitted to the hospital her abdomen was rigid on palpation (consistent with peritonitis). Stool examination revealed larvae of Strongyloides stercoralis, although they were originally misidentified as those of hookworms. Simone was taken to the operating room and found to have multiple perforations of the small and large intestine, with diffuse peritonitis. Despite antibiotic treatment for her bacteremia (secondary to peritonitis), she died 3 days after surgery.

Encounter and Entry

The life cycle of *Strongyloides* does not require an external soil phase (Fig. 42.1). In areas of poor sanitation, this worm is transmitted via human feces, regardless of climate. Thus, strongyloidiasis outbreaks have been reported from institutions for the mentally retarded in temperate zones, from Eskimo settlements north of the Arctic circle, and from the tropics.

Strongyloides penetrate human skin as *filariform larvae* (perhaps best remembered by thinking of them as "filing" their way through the skin). Thus, transmission of these parasites does not require the ingestion of contaminated feces; transmission is typically fecal-cutaneous, not fecal-oral. People become infected with *Strongyloides* by contact with infected human stool or with soil that has been contaminated by human stool containing filariform larvae. After they penetrate the skin, filariform larvae enter the bloodstream and lymphatics and become trapped in the lungs. Here they break through the alveolar wall into the alveolar lumen, are coughed up, and then are swallowed into the gastrointestinal tract where they continue their life cycle (Fig. 42.1), primarily in the duodenum and jejunum.

Pathobiology

Many people infected with *Strongyloides* carry a small number of the worms in the intestine and few exhibit clinical manifestations. Like other intestinal roundworms, *Strongyloides* has three opportunities to cause damage during its life cycle:

- While passing through the skin. *Strongyloides* does not usually cause damage at this step, but other worms (e.g., hookworms) may produce itching and a rash, neither of which tend to be severe.

Figure 42.1. The general *Strongyloides* and human hookworm life cycle. The invasive *filariform* larvae of these parasites penetrate unbroken human skin (I). Once inside the host, *Strongyloides* and human hookworm larvae migrate through the subcutaneous tissues to the bloodstream (2), enter the lung by crossing into the alveoli (3), travel up the trachea, and are coughed up and swallowed into the gastrointestinal tract (4). In contrast to *Strongyloides* and hookworm, the filariform larvae that cause creeping eruption (the larvae of dog or cat hookworms) are unable to enter the bloodstream and migrate to the lung. Instead, they wander through the subcutaneous tissues causing cutaneous larva migrans. *Solid line* and *open arrow* (above and to the left of 1) indicate that the larvae of this parasite are unable to complete their normal life cycle in a human host. The larvae of *Strongyloides* and hookworm mature (5) within the upper gastrointestinal tract. As shown on the right side of the diagram, female hookworm larvae remain within the lumen of the gastrointestinal tract, releasing their eggs into the stool (6), which then pass into the environment (9). Because the female *Strongyloides* larvae enter the bowel wall, their eggs do not appear in the stool (left side of 6) and only the larvae (7) are normally found in the stool. On occasion, these larvae mature to the filariform stage in the gastrointestinal tract (8) to produce endogeneous reinfection (autoinfection). Because hookworm larvae require maturation in the environment to become infectious (bottom half of the diagram), autoinfection cannot occur in this disease.

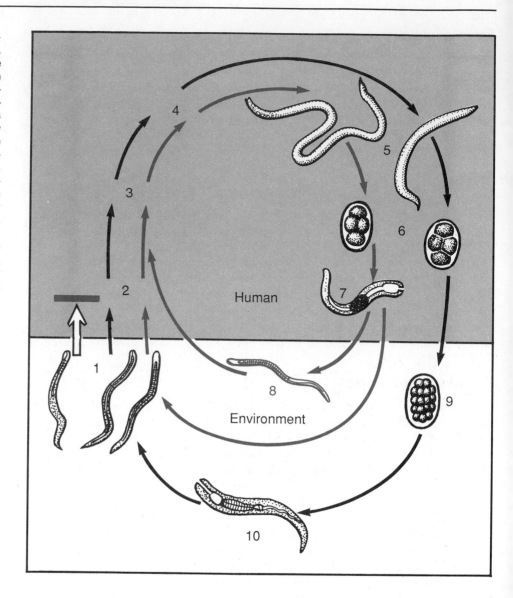

- During passage through the lungs. *Strongyloides* may elicit a transient response characterized by cough, wheezing, and fever.

- In the intestine. Although *Strongyloides* infection is usually asymptomatic, it may cause pain, vomiting, and diarrhea when the number of worms becomes large.

Unlike the other intestinal roundworms, *Strongyloides* has yet another opportunity for causing damage: Female *Strongyloides* have the unusual ability to invade the bowel wall to lay their eggs. This may cause severe disease because rhabditiform larvae hatching from these eggs can cross the intestinal wall into the peritoneum, causing intestinal perforations which permit intestinal bacteria to follow and produce peritonitis. Strongyloidiasis may produce acute clinical syndromes (such as the peritonitis in the case described), or may mimic more chronic abdominal problems such as peptic ulcer or gallbladder disease.

There is another feature that distinguishes *Strongyloides* from the other intestinal roundworms: Because the female *Strongyloides* lay their eggs in the bowel wall, instead of the intestinal lumen, the larvae may hatch and mature while still in the body. Thus, they are often infectious within the intestinal mucosa or by the time they reach the anal or perirectal area. Reinfection may then occur from larval invasion of the perianal skin even if the patient has not been exposed to new external sources of infection. *Strongyloides* reinfection produces a characteristic snake-like (serpiginous) urticarial rash ("larva currens"), which is typically located near the anus. As in the case of Simone, the process of endogenous reinfection may produce a fatal hyperinfection syndrome. Patients immunosuppressed by malnutrition (as was Simone) or by drugs have a much greater risk of dissemination and of the hyperinfection syndrome. In fact, in the tropics, strongyloidiasis is a major cause of death in kidney transplant recipients. Presumably, these patients can control the infection before transplantation, but become unable to do so when their cell-mediated immunity is compromised by the immunosuppressive drugs used to avoid rejection of the transplanted kidney.

Because the hyperinfection syndrome is often seen in patients with impaired cell-mediated immunity, it seems likely that this kind of immunity is the critical factor in the control of strongyloidiasis. The relative role of mononuclear cells and eosinophils has not been elucidated, nor is it known if these worms coat themselves with host proteins.

Strongyloides infections may become chronic and produce symptoms for decades. Persistent infections lasting more than 35 to 40 years have been described among former prisoners of war (from World War II). These persons often have chronic syndromes that are misdiagnosed as peptic ulcer or gallbladder disease and fail to respond to medical or surgical treatments for those conditions. Patients in whom autoinfection has been controlled may develop urticarial skin lesions from the migration of larvae at the surface of the skin.

Diagnosis and Treatment

Strongyloidiasis is often difficult to diagnose because the worms lay their eggs in the bowel wall and the eggs are rarely found in the stool. In addition, *Strongyloides* larvae are easily confused with hookworm larvae (as in our case). Both are readily detected with low power (100×) magnification.

Patients with strongyloidiasis may have marked eosinophilia (10% to 20% of white blood cells, more than 10,000 to 20,000 eosinophils per microliter of blood). However, if eosinophilia is not reported in a severely ill patient, it does not exclude the disease. The reason is that the outpouring of neutrophils resulting from secondary bacterial infection may obscure the eosinophilia (note the difference between determining the *percentage* of eosinophils among all white blood cells and their *absolute number* per microliter). Patients thought to have strongyloidiasis should be studied first by stool examination. Even if three or more stool examinations reveal no larvae, examination of the duodenal contents or duodenal biopsy may be positive.

Thiabendazole is the drug of choice for strongyloidiasis although it may produce vomiting and has other side effects. Thiabendazole is thought to act by binding to β-tubulin of the parasite.

OTHER INTESTINAL HELMINTHS ACQUIRED THROUGH THE SKIN (THE HOOKWORMS)

Hookworm disease is caused by two species of roundworms: *Necator americanus* or *Ancylostoma duodenale*. Human hookworms carry out the same general life cycle as *Strongyloides*, but differ from it in several ways:

• After being shed in the stool, hookworm eggs require a period of maturation in a warm environment to produce infective filariform larvae (unlike *Strongyloides*). Consequently, hookworm infection is restricted to warm climates. Transmission of hookworm infection requires contamination of the soil with untreated human feces and subsequent exposure of unprotected human skin to the infected feces. Hookworm infection may be prevented by sanitation (using indoor or outdoor toilets or treating feces used for fertilizer), or by wearing shoes. Hookworm infection was common in the southern United States up to the early part of this century.

• Hookworms cannot complete their life cycle in the human host (unlike *Strongyloides*). Thus, hookworm infection cannot produce a hyperinfection syndrome.

• Unlike *Strongyloides*, hookworms do not invade the bowel wall and thus do not produce severe bacterial superinfections.

• Hookworms produce chronic anemia by hanging on to the intestinal mucosa with their teeth, secreting an anticoagulant, and sucking the patient's blood. This results in a slow steady blood loss (0.03 ml per worm per day for *Necator americanus*, 0.15 ml for *Ancylostoma duodenale*). Hookworms affect some 800 to 900 million people throughout the globe; it has been estimated that the total loss of human blood to these little vampires is at least 1 million liters daily. The severity of the anemia is proportional to the worm burden. Severe infections in children may produce chronic anemia that may lead to developmental retardation.

• As they penetrate the skin at the time of initial infection, hookworm larvae may also cause local manifestations, namely itching and irritation ("ground itch"). People may also become infected with the cat and dog hookworms; this condition is known as creeping eruption (or cutaneous larva migrans). Unlike *Strongyloides* or human hookworm, the filariform larvae of dog or cat hookworms cannot make their way from the skin into the circulation. As a result, the filariform larvae crawl randomly in the skin and die after several days to a week.

Diagnosis and Treatment

The adult female hookworm releases 10,000 to 20,000 eggs per day into the bowel lumen, which makes it easy to diagnose significant hookworm infections by stool examination using low-power (100 ×) magnification. In fact, it is possible to estimate the number of worms present and the average daily blood loss by quantitating the number of eggs in the stool.

Mebendazole, pyrantel pamoate and several other drugs can be effectively used to treat hookworm infection. Mebendazole, like thiabendazole, binds to the β-tubulin of the parasite. Emergency treatment is not required because hookworms produce chronic, but not acute or invasive disease. Patients with hookworm disease may require dietary supplementation with iron and folic acid to produce sufficient numbers of red blood cells to correct their anemia.

INTESTINAL HELMINTHS ACQUIRED BY INGESTION

Another large group of intestinal helminths are acquired by ingestion rather than by penetration through the skin. Helminths in this group belong to widely separate taxonomic groups, roundworms (the human and animal *Ascaris*, pinworms and whipworms) and tapeworms. These parasites infect large numbers of people and cause infections that range from asymptomatic to very severe.

Ascariasis

Ascaris is one of the largest of the human parasites, up to 30 cm in length, and one of the most frequently encountered worldwide. It affects perhaps one quarter of the human population, including a substantial number of people in the southern United States. A few *Ascaris* are generally well tolerated, but a large worm load may cause serious illness.

Case

A 4-year-old boy who lived in the southern United States had been well until 3 weeks previously, although he had always been small for his age (height and weight at the 10th percentile). His parents reported that he passed "earthworms" with his stool. For the last 2–3 weeks he had vague abdominal pain with nausea. He had been unable to eat, his abdomen was distended, and he had no bowel movements for 5 days. X-rays of his abdomen were consistent with intestinal obstruction. Stool examination revealed large numbers of Ascaris eggs. He was given mebendazole and placed on intravenous fluids. One day after beginning treatment, he passed large numbers of Ascaris. Three days later, his abdomen was no longer distended, he was able to eat and drink, and had a normal bowel movement.

Encounter and Pathobiology

After excretion in the stool, *Ascaris* eggs require several weeks in a warm environment to mature to the infective stage (Fig. 42.2). For this reason, ascariasis, like hookworm disease, is restricted to warm climates and to areas where the soil is contaminated by untreated human feces. Unlike hookworms and *Strongyloides, Ascaris* larvae cannot penetrate the skin and are acquired exclusively via the fecal-oral route. The eggs must be ingested to complete the cycle. Generally speaking, the other phases of the *Ascaris* life cycle inside the human host resemble those of hookworms. Once ingested, the larvae hatch in the small intestine, penetrate the mucosa and submucosa, and enter venules or lymphatics. They travel to the lung, and migrate up the trachea to the pharynx, where they are swallowed and regain access to the gastrointestinal tract. The worms mature in the intestinal lumen and the females release their eggs into the stool.

Large numbers of larvae (from a large number of ingested eggs) may produce pneumonia as they cross from the bloodstream into the lungs. This reaction may be particularly severe if the patient has been sensitized by previous *Ascaris* infection. Later, if adult worms are present in large numbers in the intestine, they may form a large mass (worm ball) and produce intestinal obstruction, as in the case presented. On occasion, individual worms may produce biliary obstruction (by migrating up the bile duct and occluding it) or peritonitis (by perforating the

Figure 42.2. *Ascaris* life cycle. *Ascaris lumbricoides* (human roundworm) and dog or cat roundworm (visceral larva migrans). Humans acquire these infections by ingesting embryonated roundworm eggs from the environment (1). After ingestion, the parasites hatch in the upper intestine (2), cross the bowel wall (3) and enter the bloodstream. The human *Ascaris* (innermost set of *arrows* in the top half of the diagram) enters the lung by crossing into the alveolus (4), travels up the trachea, is swallowed and reenters the GI tract to develop to a mature adult (6). *Open arrow* and *solid line* on the diagram indicate that neither dog nor cat *Ascaris* are able to enter the lung from the bloodstream. As a result, these parasites wander aimlessly through deep tissues and are unable to return to the gastrointestinal tract (5). Thus, stool examinations are negative in patients with visceral larva migrans and positive in patients with human *Ascaris* infection (7). In the environment, fertilized *Ascaris* eggs (8) germinate and divide (9, 10) and produce embryonated eggs (1) that are infectious if orally ingested. This process takes several weeks and requires a warm moist climate. In visceral larva migrans, the infectious eggs are shed by infected dogs or cats, rather than humans.

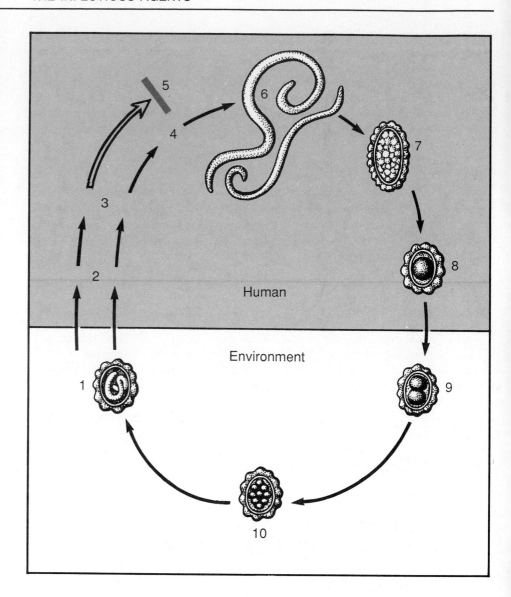

intestinal wall). Moderate intestinal worm burdens, on the other hand, may be totally asymptomatic.

Humans may also be infected by ingesting dog or cat *Ascaris*, also by fecal-oral transmission. The resulting infection is known as *visceral larva migrans*. These worms (like the animal hookworms that cause creeping eruption) are unable to complete their cycle in humans, who are dead-end hosts. The abortive nature of human infection by parasites of other primary hosts (dog or cat *Ascaris*—visceral larva migrans; dog or cat hookworms—creeping eruption) is a vivid reminder of the specificity of host-parasite interactions. After leaving the intestine, dog or cat *Ascaris* wander randomly through the tissues rather than crossing the lung to the trachea. Enlargement of the liver and spleen (hepatosplenomegaly) may result from the inflammatory response to the worms. Eosinophilia is usually marked because the worms invade the deep tissues.

Diagnosis and Treatment

Ascariasis is diagnosed readily by stool examination using low-power (100×) magnification, since each adult female worm releases approximately 200,000 eggs per day into the intestinal lumen. As with hookworm, one can estimate the number of worms present by the numbers of eggs in the stool.

Mebendazole, pyrantel pamoate, piperazine and a number of other agents treat *Ascaris* infection of the gastrointestinal tract effectively. Medical treatment with these agents typically relieves intestinal obstruction without surgical intervention.

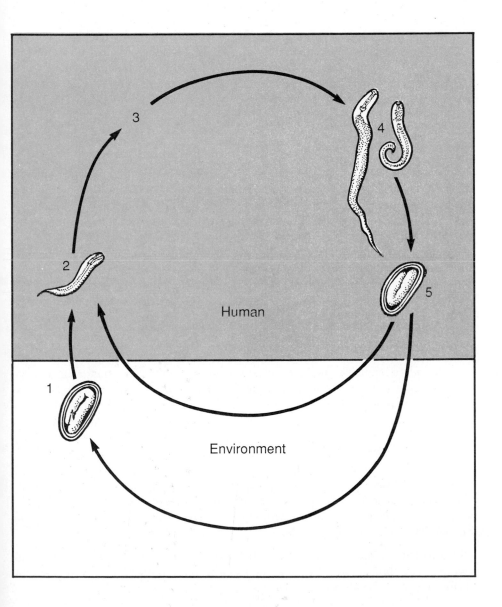

Figure 42.3. Pinworm life cycle—*Enterobius vermicularis*. Humans acquire pinworm infection by the ingestion of embryonated eggs (1). After ingestion, these eggs hatch in the small intestine (2), mature to adults in the large intestine (3, 4) and produce eggs (5). Because the gravid female lays her eggs in the perianal area, the eggs may be shed into the environment (*lower half of diagram*) or inadvertently ingested by the patient or their close contacts when fingers which scratched the perianal area are licked or used to prepare food.

Pinworm

Pinworm infection is common in both temperate and tropical regions, affecting at least 200 million people. It is most prevalent among small children, who typically infect their siblings and parents, and among institutionalized persons. Pinworms seldom produce serious disease, but may cause considerable discomfort. A typical case would be that of a healthy 3-year-old girl who is brought to the pediatrician because she has developed what the mother thinks to be "unacceptable behavior": She frequently scratches herself in the anal and vaginal areas.

Pinworms do not require an extrinsic incubation period, thus the infection is transmitted readily in any area with fecal-oral contamination (Fig. 42.3). The eggs resist drying and may be transmitted to other members of the household from bed clothes or dust. After oral ingestion, the eggs hatch in the duodenum and jejunum. After maturation and fertilization, the larvae mature in the ileum and large intestine. Gravid females migrate out of the rectum to the perianal skin to lay eggs. Perianal itching (the most typical presentation) results from the deposition of eggs by the gravid female in that area and may be caused by dermal sensitivity to parasite antigens. Scratching facilitates the spread of the infection because infective eggs may be picked up and spread to the same person or to others. Other moist areas, such as the vagina, may also be affected. On occasion, the parasite may be found in the lumen of the appendix, although this is rarely thought to produce appendicitis.

Diagnosis and Treatment

Pinworm infection is easy to diagnose using a microscope slide covered with Scotch tape (adhesive side out) or its commercially prepared paddle version. The buttocks are gently separated and the slide (or paddle) is placed between them before the patient arises in the morning. Pinworm eggs are large enough to be identified under the microscope using low-power (100×) magnification.

A number of anthelminthics, including mebendazole, pyrantel pamoate and other drugs, treat pinworm infection effectively. The major concern is to assure that the entire family is treated (including relatives who live with or visit the infected child, babysitters, and other children at the day-care center), because one untreated person may reinfect others.

Intestinal Tapeworms

As the name suggests, tapeworms are long and ribbon-like, made up of rectangular segments in a chain. An individual tapeworm is an animal colony, since each segment (known as a *proglottid*) is a self-contained unit capable of reproduction, metabolism, and food uptake (tapeworms have no gut). Tapeworms attach to the intestinal wall by a head (*scolex*) that has sucking discs or grooves (Fig. 42.4). In their intermediate animal host, these worms penetrate into deep tissues and develop into infective larval forms.

The most common human tapeworms are acquired by eating uncooked or inadequately cooked beef (*Taenia saginata*), pork (*Taenia solium*), fish (*Diphyllobothrium latum*), or by contact with rodent feces (*Hymenolepis nana*). Some tapeworms cause two types of disease:

• Intestinal infection (*taeniasis*), caused by the pork, beef, fish, or rodent tapeworms. The clinical picture of intestinal infection is generally mild, and is essentially the same for all four tapeworms.

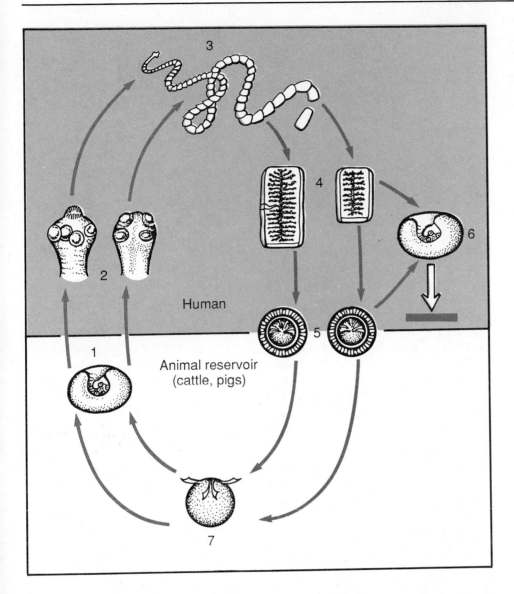

Figure 42.4. Intestinal tapeworm life cycle—*Taenia solium* (pork tapeworm) and *Taenia saginata* (beef tapeworm). Humans acquire these infections by ingesting the tissue stage of the parasite (cysticercus) in inadequately cooked meat (1). The parasite then hatches in the intestine (2) and matures to an intestinal tapeworm 10 m or more in length (3). The pork tapeworm (*outside of diagram*) has a crown of spines on its head and also has fewer pairs of lateral uterine branches in its proglottids (segments) than the beef tapeworm (4). The eggs of these two parasites (5) are identical morphologically. As shown in the diagram, only the pork tapeworm (*Taenia solium*) produces human cysticercosis (6). When human feces containing viable eggs are ingested by either pigs or cattle, the eggs hatch (7) and produce the tissue (cysticercal) stage of the infection in those animals (1) to complete the cycle.

- Deep tissue infection, produced by the pork tapeworm (*cysticercosis*) or the carnivore tapeworm (*echinococcosis*, or *hydatid disease*).

These two types of diseases are very different and must be distinguished. Unfortunately, confusion is possible because one tapeworm (pork tapeworm) may produce both taeniasis and deep tissue infection in the same patient.

Case

The wife of a high-ranking government official accompanied her husband on a trip to the Near East. During a diplomatic reception they were served steak tartare (raw beef), a traditional dish in that region. Three months later she noticed thin white rectangular segments in her stool (approximately 1 × 2 × 0.2 cm). She experienced nausea, apparently brought about by seeing the worms in her stool. Laboratory studies revealed that the segments were proglottids of Taenia saginata. Her stool also contained eggs of this worm.

She was reassured by her physician, who told her that this infection is unlikely to have clinical consequences in a healthy person. On the other hand, he could understand her revulsion at seeing the worm segments in her stool and visualizing the rest of the worm inside her. The physician prescribed niclosamide, which led to the elimination of the rest of the tapeworm.

Encounter

The life cycle of beef tapeworm requires both humans and cattle (Fig. 42.4). Cattle become infected by ingesting human feces containing the parasite's eggs; humans become infected by eating beef that contains larvae (cysticerci). The eggs hatch in the intestine of cattle and enter their bloodstream to lodge in peripheral tissues, where they develop into cysticerci (Chapter 43). Beef tapeworm infection can only exist in areas where infected humans defecate near cattle. These areas, however, are found in most of countries of the world.

All human intestinal tapeworm infections correlate with gastronomic preferences: they are found mainly among people who consume their meat undercooked or raw (as in the case described). This is not the only factor involved, since transmission clearly depends on a lack of sanitation. These diseases are common in many parts of the world, but are infrequent in Western Europe and the United States, with the exception of fish tapeworms, which may have a resurgence thanks to the increased consumption of sushi (raw fish á la Japonais). Cooking effectively destroys the larvae, but cooks have been known to become infected by tasting raw food during preparation: fish tapeworm infection is said to be an occupational hazard of Jewish or Scandinavian cooks making "gefilte fish" or "lutefisk".

Pathobiology

The infectious tissue larvae from the intermediate host (beef, pork, fish) hatch in the human small intestine and mature into adult tapeworms. The worms may live in the human intestine for several decades and attain lengths of up to 10 meters, which has given rise to the popular but mistaken notion that they increase a person's appetite by consuming a significant amount of their food intake.

Most patients are asymptomatic, but some have nausea, diarrhea, and weight loss. The infection is usually noted only because of the presence of proglottids in the stool. In the case of fish tapeworm infection, almost half the cases have low levels of vitamin B_{12}, leading to serious so-called megaloblastic anemia. This deficiency appears to be due to competition between the host and the parasite for this vitamin in the diet. Note that the intestinal disease caused by tapeworm is very different from that in the tissues (Chapter 43).

Diagnosis and Treatment

Most tapeworm infections are readily diagnosed by stool examination. The proglottids are macroscopic and can be seen by the naked eye. The eggs are large enough (31 to 43 μm in diameter) to be seen using low-power magnification (100 ×). Although the eggs of pork and beef tapeworms are identical, their proglottids may be distinguished by the experienced observer (those of T. *solium* have uteri with fewer pairs of lateral branches).

Most patients (>90%) are cured with a single dose of niclosamide. Those who are not cured often had nausea or vomiting with their first treatment, and typically respond to a second treatment with the drug.

SUGGESTED READINGS

Ettling J: *The Germ of Laziness: Rockefeller Philanthropy and Public Health in the New South.* Cambridge, MA, Harvard Univ. Press, 1981.

Genta RM, Weesner R, Douce RW Huitger-O'Connor T, Walzer PD: Strongyloidiasis in U.S. veterans of the Vietnam and other wars. *JAMA* 258:49–52, 1987.

Maxwell C, Hussain R, Nutman TB, Poindexter RW, Little MD, Schad GA, Ottesen EA: The clinical and immunological responses of normal human volunteers to low dose hookworm (*Necator americanus*) infection. *Am J Trop Med Hyg* 37:126–134, 1087.

Neva FA: Biology and immunology of human strongyloidiasis. *J Infect Dis* 153:397–406, 1986.

Phillis JA, Harrold AJ Whiteman GV, et al.: Pulmonary infiltrates, asthma and eosinophilia due to *Ascaris suum* infestation in man. *N Engl J Med* 286:965–970, 1972. (An account of a fraternity stunt in which unsuspecting students were given pig ascaris.)

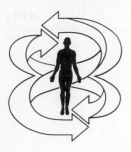

Tissue and Blood Helminths

D.J. Krogstad

Helminths cause a variety of diseases by establishing residence in deep tissues. As with the intestinal helminths, some are acquired by ingestion and others by penetration through the skin—either by direct entry of the parasites or by insect bites. The diseases they produce almost invariably involve chronic inflammation, and thus are due in part to the host immune response to the parasite. As with the intestinal helminths, when the worm burden is low, infections are almost always asymptomatic. Since many worms are long-lived in humans, a large number may gradually accumulate as the consequence of repeated encounters. When present in large numbers in sensitive target organs, helminths may produce severe disease and even death. Helminths that cause deep tissue infections include members of all three groups: roundworms, tapeworms, and flukes (Table 43.1).

TISSUE HELMINTHS ACQUIRED BY INGESTION

The main helminths in this group are the roundworm *Trichinella* and the tapeworms that invade deep tissues.

Trichinosis

Trichinosis is caused by the presence of *Trichinella spiralis* larvae in the heart, skeletal muscle, brain, gastrointestinal tract. Most infected people are asympto-

Table 43.1
The main tissue and blood helminths

Examples	Reservoir	Mode of Transmission	Clinical Manifestations
Acquired by Ingestion			
Tapeworms			
Hydatid disease			
Echinococcus granulosus	Sheep, cattle, horses	Fecal-oral (eggs)	Tissue-displacing and invasive lesions, most common in liver but seen in lung, CNS, and elsewhere
Cysticercosis	Pigs	Foodborne (cysticerci)	Tissue-displacing lesions, most critical in CNS
Taenia solium			
Roundworms			
Visceral larva migrans			
Toxocara canis	Dogs	Fecal-oral (eggs)	Systemic illness with malaise, eosinophilia, often enlarged liver and spleen
Toxocara cati	Cats		
Trichinosis	Pigs (also bears)	Foodborne (larvae)	Mild infection produces malaise, mild diarrhea and periorbital edema. Severe infection may be life threatening with CNS and heart involvement
Trichinella spiralis			
Guinea worm	Infected humans	Waterborne-oral (larvae)	Malaise, fever, other systemic symptoms when the adult worm emerges 1 year after initial infection
Dracunculus medinensis			
Flukes			
Lung fluke	Animals, humans?	Foodborne (metacercariae in crabs)	Cysts rupture in lung, leading to secondary bacterial infection, chronic bronchitis, and a tuberculosis-like picture
Paragonimus westermani			
Liver fluke	Fish, animals, humans	Foodborne (metacercariae in fresh-water fish)	Often asymptomatic. If worm load is high, can lead to biliary stones, chronic inflammation, liver cancer.
Clonorchis sinensis			
Acquired by Passage Through the Skin			
Blood Flukes			
Schistosomes	Infected humans	Water-cutaneous (cercariae)	Symptoms vary with the intensity of infection, from asymptomatic to hematuria and bladder cancer (*S. haematobium*), and blood in stool and portal hypertension (*S. mansoni* and *S. japonicum*)
S. mansoni			
S. haematobium			
S. japonicum			
Roundworms			
Cutaneous larva migrans (dog, cat hookworms)	Dogs, cats	Fecal-cutaneous (filariform larvae)	Superficial skin lesions progressing at a rate of ≤2 cm/day
Filaria			
Lymphatic filariasis	Infected humans (larvae)	Mosquito bite	Vary from asymptomatic to massive enlargement of the legs, scrotum, and breasts with recurrent filarial fevers
Wuchereria bancrofti,			
Brugia malayi			
River blindness	Infected humans	Black fly bite (larvae)	Multiple subcutaneous nodules. Blindness from reaction to microfilariae crossing the eye
Onchocerca volvulus			

matic and are not seriously ill. Paradoxically, trichinosis is more common in the United States than in a number of developing countries. This is because many other countries are more careful to ensure that pigs are not fed uncooked garbage contaminated with viable trichinella larvae. Fortunately, there are only a few hundred clinically significant cases in the United States each year.

Case

A 45-year-old immigrant from Laos living in California had been well until 3 days after celebrating with relatives at a feast which featured a highly seasoned but undercooked pork dish. Two days after the celebration, he developed diarrhea and abdominal pain. Two days later, he developed severe muscle pain, swelling around the eyes, and headache. Physical examination revealed "splinter" hemorrhages in his fingernails. Laboratory studies demonstrated a marked eosinophilia (12,000/μl). Biopsies of his tender muscles and of the splinter hemorrhages revealed Trichinella larvae.

Encounter and Pathobiology

The life cycle of *Trichinella* is illustrated in Figure 43.1. After the ingestion of meat containing viable encysted *Trichinella* (usually in undercooked pork), the infective larvae hatch and mature in the small intestine of pigs or humans. The adult worms release larvae that cross the mucosa to enter the intestinal lymphatics and the bloodstream (producing diarrhea and pain in the process). These larvae are then carried to all parts of the body via the bloodstream. The larvae *encyst* in striated and cardiac muscle fibers, and produce a marked initial inflammatory response. The cysts usually calcify, although the worms may remain viable for up to 30 years. The cycle is completed when meat containing viable larvae is eaten.

In recent years, the incidence of trichinosis has diminished, as judged by the prevalence of *Trichinella* cysts at autopsy. The figure has decreased from 16% to less than 1% over the last 30 to 40 years, partly because of legislation prohibiting the use of uncooked garbage for feeding pigs, and partly because of increased public awareness about the danger of eating undercooked pork. *Trichinella* is also found in other animals such as wild pigs and bears, including polar bears, and has caused several outbreaks among hunters and in Eskimo communities.

The manifestations of this disease correlate with the load of worms in tissues and range from asymptomatic to fatal. Several studies suggest that larger inocula (ingestion of many viable larvae) result in more severe disease with a shorter incubation period (2 to 3 days vs. 10 days or more). Patients with 1000 to 5000 larvae per gram of tissue may die from involvement of the heart or central nervous system. Studies in experimental animals suggest that cell-mediated immunity is important in the control of *Trichinella* infection. For instance, the marked eosinophilia seen with repeated infection requires intact cell-mediated immunity (previously sensitized T cells).

Diagnosis and Treatment

Rises in antibody titer are diagnostic. However, they typically occur 3 to 4 weeks or more after the initial infection and are thus useless for the management of severely ill patients (in whom the incubation period may be as short as 2 to 3 days). In severely ill patients (as in the case presented), muscle biopsy often reveals *Trichinella* larvae under low-power (100×) magnification and permits a definitive diagnosis long before serologic testing.

Both steroids and thiabendazole have been used in severely ill patients (with myocarditis and/or encephalitis). However, no drugs have been shown to be effec-

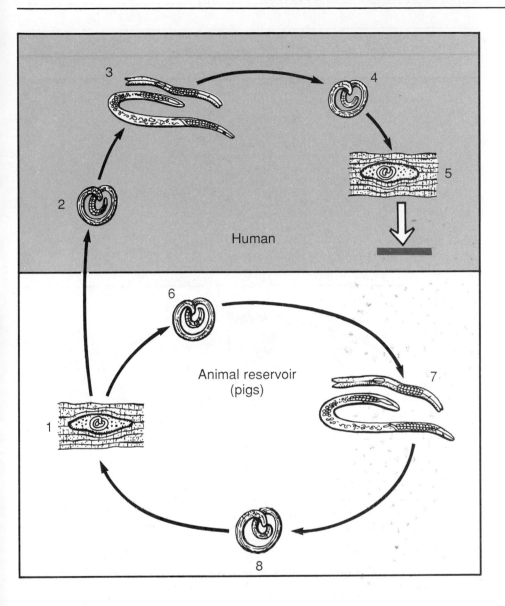

Figure 43.1. *Trichinella* life cycle—*Trichinella spiralis*. Humans acquire trichinosis by the ingestion of undercooked pork containing viable encysted *Trichinella* larvae (1). After ingestion, these larvae hatch in the intestine (2), mature to adults (3), and release larvae that invade the intestinal wall and enter the bloodstream (4), encysting in striated or cardiac muscle (5). Human infection is normally a dead end in terms of the natural transmission of trichinosis (*open arrow* and *solid line* below 5. Similar phenomena are observed in the pig reservoir, and in bears, which may also harbor *Trichinella* larvae (6–8 on lower half of diagram).

tive in controlled clinical trials. Although thiabendazole and mebendazole have been used for their anthelmintic activity, they also have anti-inflammatory activity and may produce symptomatic improvement by that mechanism.

Tissue Forms of Tapeworm Infection

The larvae (cysticerci) of a few species of tapeworms infect deep tissues of humans and cause diseases that may have severe manifestations. Their life cycle is illustrated in Figure 43.2. Illness caused by the tissue form of the pork tapeworm is known as cysticercosis; that due to tapeworms of carnivores is known as echinococcosis.

Figure 43.2. *Echinococcus* life cycle. This tapeworm has a tissue stage, but not a tapeworm stage in humans. Humans acquire the infection by ingesting eggs in the feces of infected carnivores (1), such as dogs or wolves. After ingestion, the eggs hatch in the intestine (2) and the larvae cross from the GI tract to the tissues (3), where they develop into cysts containing daughter cysts (4). As indicated by the *open arrow* and *solid line* below 4, this is a dead-end infection in humans. In the extra-human carnivore reservoirs, echinoccal tapeworm infection is acquired by ingesting the contaminated remains of herbivores infected with the tissue cyst stage of the parasite. Herbivores acquire the tissue cyst stage by ingesting eggs in the stool of infected carnivores (1). These eggs are identical morphologically to those produced by *Taenia solium* and *Taenia saginata*. After ingestion by an herbivore, the eggs hatch, cross the GI tract and produce tissue cysts like those seen in humans [especially in the liver (6)]. When ingested by carnivores, they also produce scolices (7) which mature (8) to tapeworms (9) that release infective eggs in the stool (1) to complete the cycle.

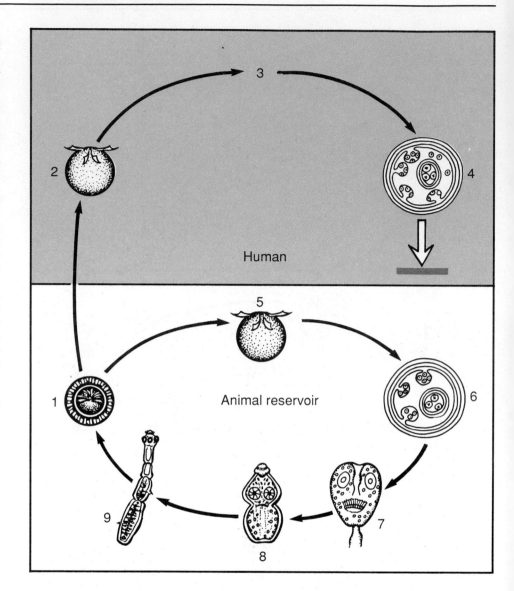

Cases

Cysticercosis

A 33-year-old nurse had been a Peace Corps volunteer in Thailand 10 years earlier. After her return, she found proglottids of the pork tapeworm Taenia solium in her stool. Two years previously (eight years after her return) she noticed multiple subcutaneous nodules across her chest and on her arms. She now had headaches and two generalized seizures and was brought to the emergency room. A CT scan of her brain revealed 42 lesions consistent with cysticerci. Her headaches worsened during treatment with praziquantel. However, with steroids to reduce brain swelling and antiepileptic drugs to control her seizures, she was able to complete the praziquantel treatment. She was withdrawn from the antiepileptics 1 year later and has had no additional seizures.

Echinococcosis

A 39-year-old Navajo woman was examined for abdominal pain. Two years previously she had first noticed a sensation of fullness in the right upper quadrant of her abdomen. Since that time, this sensation has increased and there is now an obvious swelling (8 × 10 cm) in the area of the liver. Stool examination revealed no tapeworm eggs. A CT scan of the liver demonstrated a large (12-cm diameter) encapsulated lesion consistent with tapeworm cysts. Serologic testing revealed antibodies against Echinococcus. Because of the size of the liver lesion, the mass was removed surgically, using liquid nitrogen to prevent spillage of its contents into the peritoneum.

Encounter

Echinococcus infections are acquired by ingesting infective eggs, rather than tissue cysticerci. The usual source of *Echinococcus granulosus* is the stool of dogs or other carnivores (wolves, coyotes). Thus, transmission is by the fecal-oral route, not by eating contaminated meat. The infectious forms of the parasite hatch in the small intestine but do not reside there. Rather, they penetrate the intestinal wall and form cysticerci in many organs.

Echinococcosis or hydatid disease is found in most areas of the world, including the United States. The cycle is maintained between sheep and sheep dogs in the southwestern United States. Native Americans who keep sheep in that region are often victims of the disease. There is also a "sylvatic" cycle in the northern United States and Alaska, with wolves as the carnivores, and elk and other large game as the herbivores. *Echinococcus multilocularis* is an analogous parasite, for which foxes and cats are the carnivore hosts and mice and voles are the herbivores.

Human cysticercosis is believed to be acquired by ingesting *T. solium* eggs (from feces-containing infective eggs). However, some workers believe that cysticercosis may also result endogenously from taeniasis (intestinal infection by the tapeworm form of the parasite). The life cycle of *T. solium* requires that pigs become infected by ingesting the eggs of this parasite and that humans eat inadequately cooked pork (this is analogous to the beef tapeworm life cycle). These conditions exist in many areas of the developing world. In Mexico, as many as 10% to 15% of persons hospitalized for neurologic problems have evidence of central nervous system cysticercosis at autopsy.

Pathobiology

The sequence of events in echinococcosis and in cysticercosis is generally similar. The parasites lodge under the skin or within internal organs, such as the brain or liver, and develop a cyst wall surrounded by a fibrous capsule of host origin. In echinococcosis, the cysts enlarge over time to form daughter cysts (each of which has an embryonic tapeworm). Echinococcal cysts in the liver usually produce a few symptoms until they reach 8 to 10 cm or more in diameter. They then may leak or rupture, and pose a significant risk of death from anaphylaxis.

On the other hand, in cysticercosis, the cyst remains constant in size at 1 to 2 cm, until it dies, when its effect on the surrounding host tissue may increase due to the host's inflammatory response. Peripheral cysticerci outside the central nervous system are usually asymptomatic. However, within the central nervous system, even small cysticerci may cause cerebral dysfunction, including seizures and blindness. This is a good example of the correlation between the location and the severity of a disease. Cysticerci may cause symptoms when the parasites die and displacement of normal tissue is magnified by the host's inflammatory response. This typically occurs 5 to 10 years after infection, but may occur as much as 50 years later.

Diagnosis and Treatment

Because cysticerci may be present in patients without evidence of intestinal infection, *T. solium* cysticercosis is usually diagnosed by its deep tissue manifestations (including lesions visible by CT scan or by "soft" x-ray technique in the long axes of skeletal muscles). A positive serologic test for antibodies to *T. solium* is helpful, especially among persons who live in Europe, the United States, or other areas of low incidence. This test is typically negative in persons with intestinal *T. solium* infection only.

Praziquantel is effective in the treatment of cysticercosis and is thought to act as a calcium agonist. It kills the organism and decreases the size of the lesions because the fluid-filled cyst collapses and most of the parasite is ultimately resorbed by the host. However, central nervous system symptoms may transiently worsen during treatment because of the inflammatory response to dying cysticerci. As indicated in the case presentation, the concomitant use of steroids typically alleviates the headaches and seizures that may be caused by this treatment. Treatment is an inefficient means of disease control because of the delay between intestinal infection (when patients are asymptomatic, although their stool is infectious for pigs) and clinical presentation (when their stool is no longer infectious for pigs). If treatment is to be effective in reducing transmission of the parasites, it must be given early, when the patients are infectious. Prior to praziquantel, there was no medical treatment for cysticercosis. At best, individual cysticerci at critical locations, such as the aqueduct of Sylvius in the brain, could be excised surgically.

No drugs have been shown to be safe and effective for echinococcosis. Although mebendazole has been used, most reports are anecdotal and the drug has been associated with several sudden (otherwise unexplained) deaths. Surgical removal can cure the infection although there is risk of spillage and dissemination of the infection. A number of special techniques have been tried in an effort to prevent spillage or to kill organisms that are released during surgery (instillation of formalin or silver nitrate, cryosurgery with liquid nitrogen).

TISSUE HELMINTHS THAT PENETRATE THE SKIN

This group includes worms that can cross the skin directly, the *schistosomes* (blood flukes) and those that penetrate via insect bites, the *filariae* (roundworms).

Schistosomiasis

Schistosomiasis is an important and frequent disease in tropical regions. It is estimated that about 200 to 300 million people are affected worldwide. Schistosomiasis produces a variety of clinical syndromes, depending on the anatomic loca-

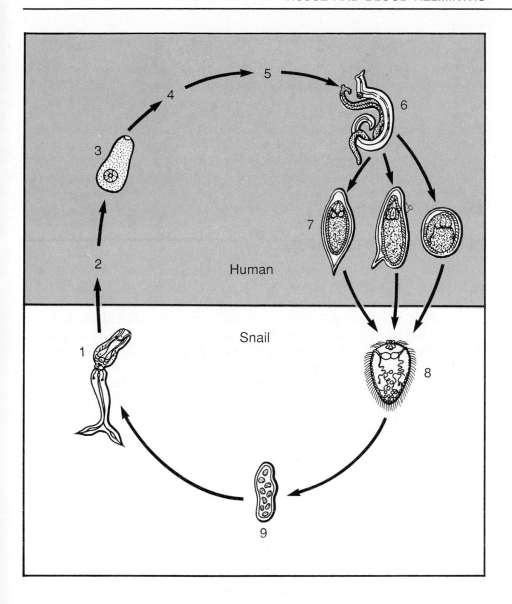

Figure 43.3. Schistosomal life cycle. Humans acquire schistosomiasis by the exposure of unprotected skin to water containing infectious cercariae (1). The cercariae penetrate unbroken skin (2), lose their tails, and become schistosomulae (3). They then travel through the bloodstream, cross the lungs (4) and mature (5) in the venous system of the liver to adult worms (6). After a period of 6–8 weeks, pairs of adult worms travel to the venous plexuses of the bladder (*S. haematobium*), the large intestine (*S. mansoni*), or the small intestine (*S. japonicum*), where they remain for decades releasing their characteristic eggs (left to right for *S. hematobium, S. mansoni, and S. japonicum* at 7). Eggs released into fresh water hatch to miracidia (8), which invade the snail intermediate host where they mature to sporocysts (9). They then release cercariae (1) to complete the cycle.

tion of the adult worms and the eggs they release. There are three main pathogenic species with different geographic distributions, found largely in warm climates: *Schistosoma haematobium, S. mansoni,* and *S. japonicum.* Their distribution depends on the presence of the snail intermediate host. The schistosomal life cycle is illustrated in Figure 43.3.

Cases

Case 1. Intestinal Schistosomiasis

A 48-year-old woman from Egypt had noticed for many years that her stool was dark. During the last year, she also had two episodes of vomiting blood. Examination of her esophagus and stomach with a fiberoptic gastroscope revealed dilated veins in the esophagus which were oozing large amounts of blood.

Because viable eggs of S. mansoni *were still being excreted in her stool, she was treated with praziquantel.*

Case 2. Schistosomiasis of the Bladder

A 38-year-old European man had worked in West Africa for 10 years on a rice-growing irrigation scheme. During the past year, he noticed blood in his urine. Examination of his urine showed the presence of S. haematobium eggs. At cystoscopy, his bladder had a cobblestone pattern, consistent with the granulomatous changes seen in schistosomiasis. Typical eggs were seen in the bladder biopsies taken during cystoscopy. He was treated with a single dose of praziquantel (40 mg/kg).

Encounter and Pathobiology

The life cycle of schistosomes requires development in certain species of fresh water snails which are their intermediate hosts. The infective stage of the parasite emerges from the snails and swims in water until it finds a suitable host. Because these snails are not present in the United States, schistosomiasis cannot be transmitted in the United States, despite the migration of infected persons from Africa and the Middle East. Suitable snails are present in parts of the Caribbean.

The infective forms released from the snails are called cercariae. They are capable of burrowing through the skin of people standing, swimming, or walking through infected water, as in rice paddies (case 2). In the body, the cercariae lose their tails and change into forms called *schistosomulae*, which can enter the bloodstream. The parasites then pass through the pulmonary circulation to the portal venous system, where they mature. After several weeks, pairs of male and female adults move to the venous plexuses of the large intestine (*S. mansoni*), small intestine (*S. japonicum*), or bladder (*S. haematobium*). The mating worms remain locked together, copulating in the venous system for 10 years or more. The eggs they release may be excreted via the stool (*S. mansoni, S. japonicum*) or the urine (*S. haematobium*). The life cycle is completed when the eggs are released into fresh water, where they hatch and penetrate the appropriate snail intermediate host.

S. mansoni and *S. japonicum* adult worms reside in the venous plexuses of the intestine. There they release eggs which travel to the intestine and the liver. The host immune response to the eggs produces the pathological changes of schistosomiasis, such as granulomatous reactions in the liver, which may lead to portal hypertension and thus to dilated collateral veins in the esophagus (esophageal varices, as in case 1). *S. haematobium* adults live in the venous plexus of the urinary bladder and produce blood in the urine (hematuria), granulomatous inflammatory changes in the bladder, and bladder carcinoma. Changes in the bladder and ureters (ureterovesical obstruction) produced by the host immune response to these schistosomes may cause secondary bacterial infections of the bladder, leading occasionally to Gram negative septicemia.

The pathological changes in schistosomiasis are due primarily to the host's inflammatory immune response to the eggs. Adult worms are not recognized as foreign, although they may live in the bloodstream for decades. Two important anomalous host-parasite interactions are central to the pathogenesis of schistosomiasis:

• The profound granulomatous reaction to schistosome eggs, which produces the important pathology of the disease and its long-term complications. The reasons for this excessive immune response are not clear, but appear to include enhanced reactivity of the regulatory (T_4) subsets of T lymphocytes to schistosome egg antigen.

• Lack of an effective immune response to male and female adult worms, which reside in the vascular system for decades without being eliminated by the host. Studies have shown that adult worms have adsorbed host proteins (including serum albumin and HLA antigens) on their surface. These findings suggest that the parasite disguises itself with these host proteins in order to evade the host's immune response.

Cercariae often produce itching as they penetrate the skin. The cercariae of nonhuman schistosomes (of birds and fish) also cause itching as they penetrate the skin (swimmers' itch, clam diggers' itch), but do not enter the bloodstream or mature within the human body.

Diagnosis and Treatment

Most schistosome infections are diagnosed readily by microscopic examination of stool (*S. mansoni, S. japonicum*) or urine (*S. haematobium*) or by biopsy of a rectal valve (*S. mansoni*). Schistosome eggs (150 × 60 μm) are large enough to be identified easily under the microscope with low-power (100 ×) magnification. Unfortunately, it can be difficult to find schistosome eggs in the stool or urine of patients who are chronically infected and at risk of developing long-term complications. In such patients, serologic testing for antischistosome antibodies may be of value. However, a positive serologic test does not distinguish between recent vs. old or light vs. severe infections. Serologic testing is most useful in people who have had single defined exposures in endemic areas. It is of little use for lifelong residents of endemic areas, since most are seropositive but may or may not experience complications.

Praziquantel is the treatment of choice for schistosomiasis. Oxamniquine is an alternative for *S. mansoni* and may also be given as a single oral dose. Both these drugs have permitted oral mass treatment programs, which were impossible with the prolonged intravenous protocols necessary with the antimonial drugs used previously. Antischistosome antimonials were often toxic. They produced hepatitis, myalgias, fever and frequently failed to eradicate the adult worms.

Filariasis

The main filarial infections in humans are lymphatic filariasis (*elephantiasis*) and onchocerciasis (*river blindness*). The adult filarial worms live in the lymphatics in lymphatic filariasis and in subcutaneous tissue in onchocerciasis. Their offspring, known as *microfilariae*, travel through the subcutaneous tissue or circulate in the blood. Lymphatic filariasis affects some 200 million people in tropical regions, especially in Asia. This disease leads to tissue swelling, some of elephantine proportions (hence the name elephantiasis). Some 50 million persons in Africa, Asia, and tropical Latin America have onchocerciasis; about 10% of them will become blind from the disease and some 30% will have visual impairments. There are West African villages where most people become blind from this disease by the time they reach adulthood. None of these diseases are endemic in the United States. The life cycle of filariae is illustrated in Figure 43.4.

Figure 43.4. Filarial life cycle—onchocerciasis, lymphatic filariasis. Humans acquire infection with the filariae that cause onchocerciasis or elephantiasis by the bite of black flies or mosquitoes, respectively. After third-stage larvae (1) are injected under the skin by the vector, the larvae mature (2) to adult worms (3) that release microfilariae in the subcutaneous tissue (onchocerciasis) or in lymphatics (lymphatic filariasis) (4). Microfilariae ingested by the insect vector during feeding mature through a series of stages (5–8) to infectious third-stage larvae (1) within approximately 2 weeks. Natural transmission of onchocerciasis does not occur in countries such as the United States because the black flies necessary to complete the life cycle are not present. Although the mosquitoes that transmit lymphatic filariasis are present in the United States, transmission does not occur because there is no reservoir of infected humans.

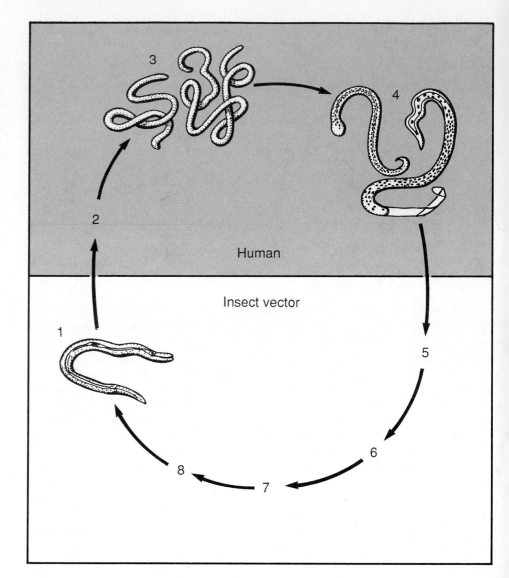

Cases

Elephantiasis

A 48-year-old native of a Philippine island lived in a village where many men and women had elephantiasis. He first noticed swelling of his right leg when he was twenty years old. Since that time he has had intermittent fevers of 38.5 to 39.9°C associated with red streaks from his groin to the foot on both legs. Both feet and his scrotum are now chronically swollen. Typical microfilariae consistent with *Wuchereria bancrofti* were seen in a Giemsa-stained blood smear taken at 2 AM. His recurrent episodes of lymphangitis were treated with an antimicrobial effective against streptococci. The antifilarial drug diethylcarbamazine was given, but discontinued when it produced shock and hypotension.

Onchocerciasis

A 32-year-old man from Nigeria was seen for an evaluation in a hospital of a nearby town. His village was situated near a rapidly running stream where the men fish and hunt. Like many of his neighbors, he began to lose vision in his late 20s. Three nodules (2 × 3 × 2 cm) are present on his trunk. Skin snips reveal microfilariae of Onchocerca volvulus. He was treated with a single oral dose of ivermectin.

Encounter and Pathobiology

Infective filarial larvae are injected into the skin by biting insects. The distribution of the diseases is limited primarily by that of their vectors and of infected persons. Onchocerciasis, which is transmitted by *Simulium* black flies is not found in the United States, where it would not be possible to transmit the disease (because these black flies are not present), even if infected persons were found in large numbers. In contrast, lymphatic filariasis is transmitted by species of mosquitoes that are present in the United States. This disease is not endemic in the United States because there is no reservoir of infected persons.

The typical manifestations of lymphatic filariasis are low-grade fever and inflammation of lymphatics and lymph nodes. With repeated episodes, the lymphatics become occluded and fluids leak into tissues, and produce severe swelling. As the disease progresses, patients with adult worms frequently experience repeated episodes of acute inflammation. The lower limbs and the scrotum may become swollen to gigantic size. The diurnal cycle observed in lymphatic filariasis facilitates transmission because the microfilariae are more prevalent in the bloodstream at night, when mosquitoes bite more frequently. Onchocerciasis is manifested by subcutaneous nodules, primarily on the head and neck in Central America, on the trunk and pelvis in Africa. Nodule formation is not as serious as the inflammatory response which may cause blindness and dermatitis.

The inflammatory response is directed against the microfilariae in onchocerciasis and against the adult worms in lymphatic filariasis. Adult filarial worms are tolerated for years in the lymphatics and the subcutaneous tissues (like adult schistosomes). The mechanisms responsible for this immunological unresponsiveness are not well understood, but include increased activity of specific subsets (T_8) of suppressor T cells.

Diagnosis and Treatment

Infections which release microfilariae into the bloodstream (lymphatic filariasis) may be diagnosed by examining smears of peripheral blood. The microfilariae may be scarce and difficult to find. The sensitivity of the method can be increased by lysing red blood cells with a detergent and using a filter to trap the remaining white cells and microfilariae, and by sampling the blood at night for microfilariae with nocturnal periodicity (*W. bancrofti*). Filarial infections that release microfilariae into the skin are diagnosed by examining a skin snip. In all these specimens, microfilariae are identified with Giemsa stain under the high dry or oil immersion objectives. Recent studies suggest that antigen detection using anti-filarial antibodies may be a more sensitive and convenient method.

The treatment available for lymphatic filariasis is unsatisfactory. The drugs diethylcarbamazine and ivermectin reduce the number of circulating microfilariae but do not eliminate the adult worms. Diethylcarbamazine in particular may produce severe systemic reactions (as in the elephantiasis case). These reactions may be caused by the sudden release of large amounts of antigen, allowing the formation of damaging antigen-antibody complexes (type III hypersensitivity reaction, Chapter 5). Diethylcarbamazine treatment may exacerbate the pathology of onchocerciasis, and should not be used for onchocerciasis. Several drugs (e.g., suramin) have been used to kill the adult worms but are rarely employed because of their toxicity. In onchocerciasis, recent studies indicate that a single oral dose of ivermectin reduces microfilarial counts in the skin for up to six months with relatively few side effects. These studies suggest that ivermectin is likely to become the drug of choice for the treatment of onchocerciasis. Surgical resection of subcutaneous nodules in onchocerciasis removes the source of microfilariae and may thus decrease the risk of blindness. However, it is impossible to be sure that all nodules have been removed because they are often in deep tissue and are not palpable.

Prevention of these diseases relies mainly on vector control. Unfortunately, the flies that transmit onchocerciasis breed in clean, fast-running streams and rivers. Although they can be controlled readily with insecticides, effective spraying may be difficult in these areas.

SUGGESTED READINGS

Trichinella

Campbell WC: *Trichinella and Trichinosis*. New York, Plenum Press, 1983.

Tapeworms

Palacios E, Rodriguez CJ, Taveras JM: *Cysticercosis of the Central Nervous System*. Springfield, IL, C Thomas, 1983.

Smith JD, Thompson RCA: *The Biology of Echinococcus and Hydatid Disease*. London, Allen Unwin, 1986.

Sotelo J, Escobedo F, Rodriguez-Carbajal J, Torres B, Rubio-Donnadieu F: Therapy of parenchymal brain cysticercosis with praziquantel. *Am J Trop Med Hyg* 38:380–385, 1984.

Schistosomes

Capron A, Dessaint JP, Caprom M, Ouma JH, Butterworth AE: Immunity to schistosomes: progress towards a vaccine. *Science* 238:1065–1072, 1987.

MacInnis AJ (ed): *Upjohn-UCLA Symposium on Molecular Paradigms for Eradicating Helminthic Parasites*. New York, Alan R Liss, 1987.

Filariasis

Cupp EW, Bernardo MJ, Kiszewski AE, Collins RC, Taylor HR, Aziz MA, Greene BM: The effects of ivermectin on transmission of *Onchocerca volvulus*. *Science* 259:740–742, 1986.

Evered D, Clark S (ed): *Symposium on Filariasis*. Ciba Foundation Symp. 127. New York, Wiley, 1987.

Kumarasawami V, Ottesen EA, Vijayasekaran V, Devi U, Swaminathan M, Aziz MA, Savina GR, Prabhakar R. Tripathy SP: Ivermectin for the treatment of *Wuchereria bancrofti* filariasis: efficacy and adverse reactions. *JAMA* 259:3150–3153, 1988.

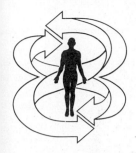

Ectoparasites (Scabies)

44

E.N. Robinson, Jr.
Z. McGee

Scabies is caused by mites, and "crabs" is caused by lice. These and other ectoparasites live in the skin and do not enter the deep tissues (Table 44.1). Most of us are also bitten, at least on occasion, by mosquitoes, biting flies, fleas, ticks, and chiggers, chiefly for the purpose of sucking our blood. When these arthropods reside on our skin for long periods of time, it is called an *infestation*. Scabies and pediculosis (crabs) are treatable common infestations. Because the mode of transmission of scabies is not only sexual, other close (nonsexual) contacts should also be treated.

Table 44.1
Some ectoparasites of humans

Type of Ectoparasite	Name	Infestation
Mites	*Sarcoptes*	Scabies
Lice	*Pediculus phthirus*	Body or head lice, pubic lice (crabs)
Maggots	*Dermatobia*	Botfly myiasis (maggot infestation)

CASE

Mr. S., a 25-year-old, had been plagued for several weeks by an intensely pruritic (itchy) rash consisting of reddened bumps (papules) located in his groin and on his elbows and hands. He had not slept well for 2 days because of constant itching and scratching. The severity of the itching was evidenced by *the excoriations (scratch marks) on his skin and by the blood on his bed-clothes from scratching each night. He lived with his wife and two children who had no such symptoms, and a dog with the mange.*

LIFE CYCLE

What is scabies? It is a disease caused by *Sarcoptes scabiei*, a 400-μm-long mite with no distinct head, two pairs of front legs or suckers and two pairs of hind bristles. Scabies mites look rather like catchers' mitts with legs. In the realm of parasites, sarcoptes are true travelers: They can move up to an inch per minute and can travel from the neck to the wrist in a few hours. Once on the surface of an unsuspecting human, they speed to those areas of the body where they like to live: the hands (especially finger webs and the sides of fingers), parts of the wrists, elbows, axillae, breasts, and around the umbilicus, groin, and buttock. Scabies is rarely found on the skin above the neck.

Scabies mites do not survive long on inanimate objects (fomites). They are readily killed at elevated temperatures (10 minutes at 50°C) and are paralyzed by cool temperatures (16°C). The natural reservoir of *Sarcoptes scabiei* is the human skin.

Scabies mites burrow into the superficial layers of skin at 0.5 to 5 mm/day (Fig. 44.1). Their life span is 30 days. Each mite spends its existence burrowing, ingesting, munching on skin and occasionally coming to the surface to search for a mate. After mating, the female lays two to three eggs per day within the burrow (Fig. 44.2).

Figure 44.1. Scabietic burrow in the stratum corneum of the skin (arrow), partially opened by sectioning parallel to the skin surface. At the extreme right is a mite egg. In the middle is a larval mite with the front half hidden under the ledge. (From Shelley WB, Shelley ED: Scanning electron microscopy of the scabies burrow and its contents, with special reference to the *Sarcoptes scabiei* egg. *J. Am Acad Dermatol* 9:673–679, 1983.)

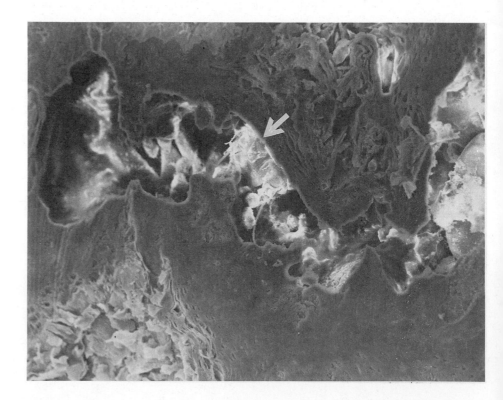

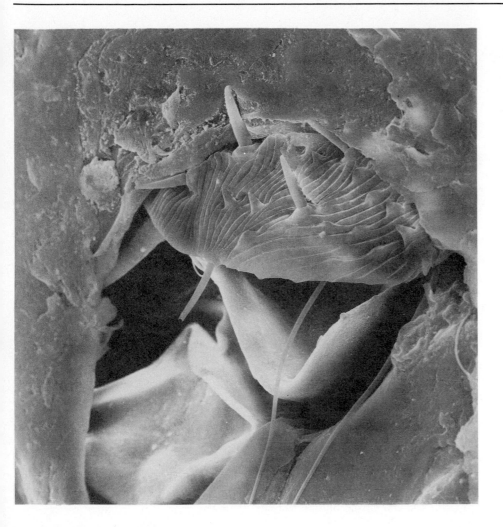

Figure 44.2. Scanning electron micrograph of a scabies mite and two eggs within a burrow in a patient's skin. The two bright structures beneath the mite are eggs collapsed by drying in preparation of the specimen. (From Shelley WB, Shelley ED: Itch mite on the way to work. *JAMA* 249:1353, 1983.)

OTHER ECTOPARASITES

Other *Sarcoptes* mites are among the etiologic agents of dog mange (itching and hair loss) and may be transmitted from dogs to humans. However, dog scabies do not find humans very palatable and this infestation is limited both in location (arms and legs of the dog owner) and time.

Scabies may be differentiated on clinical and morphological grounds from the other common cause of genital infestation, *Phthirus pubis*, also known as lice or "crabs" (Table 44.1). Pubic lice are surface dwellers and do not burrow into the skin. They possess three pairs of legs containing hook-like claws with which they hang onto hair shafts. The adults feed by anchoring their mouths to the skin, stabbing an opening, pouring saliva into the wound to prevent clotting, and sucking blood. The female pubic louse glues her eggs ("nits") to the base of hair shafts or to the adult lice sitting on the surface of the skin. Most eggs are found within 5 mm of the base of the hair because the eggs hatch within 5 to 10 days and the hair shaft grows at a millimeter or less per day. The eggs are cemented on the hair and will not slide along the hair shaft like dandruff. Frequently when small "scabs" are removed from an infested groin and examined under the light microscope, they will get up and walk away, i.e., they are adult lice.

ENCOUNTER

For many years it was thought that scabies was only found in the unwashed and poor and was predominantly transmitted through "social adventures" such as sexual promiscuity. However the misconception that scabetic infestation is only a disease of misfits and the unfortunate was eliminated in a delightfully written paper by John H. Stokes (*JAMA* 106:674, 1936). He wrote:

Scabies is a disease of herding, promiscuity and travel, of family, school and vacation life. A plague of armies, tenements and slums. It may with equal force invade a pedigreed school, Camp Wawa Wawa or the baronial castle on the hill. An ever present differential consideration, wholly without social boundaries, the possible explanation of the itches of the tycoon, the socialite and the university professor equally with the mechanic's daughter on relief.

Indeed, Napoleon Bonaparte may have struck his famous pose while scratching at periumbilical scabies.

Roughly 5% to 30% of any population may be found to be harboring scabies mites depending on the culture, extent of crowding, and state of hygiene of the population studied. During the first part of this century, scabies pandemics occurred in 30-year cycles and were attributed partially to the waning of herd immunity. However, these cycles coincided with two world wars that impacted drastically on culture, crowding, and cleanliness. The absence of a pandemic during the last two decades has been attributed to the lack of world war, rather than any appreciable change in herd immunity toward scabies.

Scabies have become labeled as sexually transmitted even though the majority of scabetic infestations are not transmitted from groin to groin. Infestations are transmitted more readily by close physical contact (e.g., by holding hands or sleeping in the same bed with an infested partner) than by brief sexual encounters. The majority of scabetic infestations are introduced into households by friends or relatives. Schoolchildren who hold hands are excellent vectors for spreading scabies from one household to another.

PATHOBIOLOGY

Two host defenses limit the number of scabetic mites on any individual: the immune response and hygiene. As the mites burrow through the uppermost layers of skin, they leave trails of feces and eggs in their wake (Fig. 44.1). This detritus consists of foreign proteins and antigens to which the host eventually responds with hypersensitivity. It may take weeks or months before an immune response is mounted. However, once hypersensitivity is established, intense inflammation ensues in the areas of infestation. Indeed the serpiginous (snake-like) tracts or burrows of the mite are frequently outlined by inflammation. This inflammation causes the itching of scabies. The scabies mites themselves are not felt. The inflammation reduces, but does not eliminate scabies mites from the host. Once an inflammatory response occurs, the scabies mites tend to move elsewhere on the body, as if the inflamed area were no longer habitable.

The second aspect of host defense is mechanical debridement and hygiene. The act of scratching removes skin containing eggs and tunneling mites. Mites wandering on the surface of the skin are washed away during bathing.

The importance of host responses in controlling scabies is illustrated by a rare entity known as "Norwegian scabies". This occurs in individuals who do not itch or cannot scratch. They may not be able to mount a hypersensitivity response because of nutritional deficiencies, cancer or steroids, or may have diseases that block the ability to perceive the pain of inflammation (leprosy, spinal cord injuries, or tabes dorsalis/neurosyphilis). In these individuals the scabies mites reproduce unopposed. Such debilitated persons may harbor three million mites in their thickly crusted skin. Because people with Norwegian scabies are typically unaware of their infestation, it is generally discovered only when people who have come in contact with them develop symptomatic scabies.

DIAGNOSIS

Several historical clues should raise the suspicion of scabies. Few other dermatologic conditions produce nocturnal itching that result in bloody sheets and pajamas. Few other dermatologic conditions spread to sexual partners or to other members of a household or an institution.

Once suspicion is aroused, the finding of scabetic burrows or the actual mites in the skin is diagnostic. Burrows can frequently be hard to see with the unaided eye. Shining a light tangentially to the skin and using a hand-held magnifying glass may help visualize burrows that are otherwise hard to see. Alternatively, liquid tetracycline may be placed on the surface of involved skin and allowed to seep into the burrow. When ultraviolet light is shined on the lesion, tetracycline fluoresces and outlines the burrow. Similar results can be obtained using blue or black ink. A word of caution: When wiping the affected area with alcohol to remove the excess tetracycline or ink, it is best to warn the patient that alcohol on an excoriated scabetic papule may be quite uncomfortable.

TREATMENT

Several effective creams and lotions kill scabies mites as well as pubic lice. Each of the creams must be applied to the entire body from the neck down with special attention to the areas preferred by the parasite. Clothes and bed linens should be washed in the hot cycle of a washing machine (there is no need to boil them). Furniture can generally be considered safe. All members of the household, whether symptomatic or not, should receive similar treatment to eradicate the infestation from the household.

The most important point to stress with any individual being treated with scabicides is that the itching and rash result from the immune response to the detritus of the scabies mites—live or dead. Resistance of the mites to scabicides has not been documented. Thus, even though all mites are killed with one or two applications of the scabicide, the patient still has intense itching due to the presence of dead but antigenic mites. These symptoms may persist for weeks until residual scabetic antigens are shed with the skin. The natural tendency of most patients is to assume that they are still infested because they are still itching. This leads to the repetitive application of creams and lotions. The scabicides most frequently prescribed will cause dry skin when used repeatedly. Dry skin itches, and a vicious cycle is established.

There are a few readily identifiable causes for failure of scabicides to remove the infestations: (a) inappropriate application of the lotion (were there areas of skin that were missed?); (b) reinfestation (were all members of the household and sexual partners treated?); (c) reemergence of scabies from ova that were not killed during a single application of lotion.

Given this wealth of information regarding *Sarcoptes scabiei*, how do we counsel Mr. S.? The fact that he had scabies may or may not be related to any extramarital misadventures on his part. Scabies is transmitted socially and only occasionally sexually. The most likely persons to introduce scabies into any household are generally children who acquire it at school.

Mr. S may be the only one who has symptoms, but the chances are that several members of his household are infested. Therefore each member of the household should receive therapy in order to interrupt incubating (asymptomatic) scabies and to prevent reinfestations. It is unlikely that the dog was the source of Mr. S's problems. If its mange is due to canine scabies, the dog can be treated with a chlordane dip.

SUGGESTED READINGS

Friedman R: *The Story of Scabies*. New York, Froben Press, 1947.
Orkin M (ed): *Scabies and Pediculosis*. Philadelphia, JB Lippincott, 1977.

Review of the Main Pathogenic Animal Parasites

These charts are intended to help you review the main animal parasites only. Included are the parasites of greatest medical relevance

Many of the animal parasites that cause relatively uncommon diseases are not included. These charts may be completed to review the material covered under this topic.

PROTOZOA

	Reservoir	Mode of Transmission	Location in Body	Disease and Main Attributes	Chapter(s)
Blood					
Malaria (*Plasmodium vivax, malariae. falciparum*)					40
Babesia					40
Deep tissue					
Toxoplasma					40, 53
Pneumocystis					40, 54
Leishmania					40
Trypanosomes (Sleeping sickness and Chagas' disease)					40
Intestinal					
Entamoeba histolytica					41
Giardia lamblia					41
Cryptosporidium					41

HELMINTHS (WORMS)
(Try to *recognize* Latin names. You need not memorize them)

	Reservoir	Mode of Transmission	Location in Body	Disease and Main Attributes	Chapters
Intestinal					
Tapeworms (*Taenia*, several)					42
Hookworms (*Ancylostoma, Necator*)					42
Ascaris (*A. lumbricoides*) (+visceral larva migrans)					42
Pinworms (*Enterobius vermicularis*)					42
Whipworms (*Trichuris trichiura*)					42
Blood and deep tissue					
Cysticercus (*Taenia solium*) and Echinococcus					43
Trichina (*Trichinella spiralis*)					43
Schistosomes (*S. haematobium, S. mansoni, S. japonicum*)					43
Filaria (*Wuchereria, Brugia, Loa loa*)					43

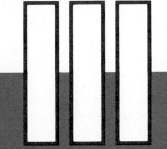

SECTION III

Pathophysiology of Infectious Diseases

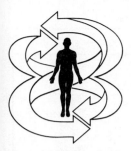

Respiratory System

45

G.A. Storch

The respiratory tract is the most common site for infection by pathogenic microorganisms. Perhaps because they occur so often and are usually mild, respiratory infections are frequently taken for granted. In fact, they represent an immense disease burden on our society and thus have a major economic impact. Upper respiratory infections (URIs) account for more visits to physicians than any other diagnosis. It has been estimated that in the United States, influenza-like illnesses are responsible for more than 400 million days of restricted activity each year. In addition, some respiratory infections have severe consequences, especially in individuals compromised by other diseases. Pneumonia, the most severe form of respiratory infection, is frequently life threatening and still accounts for a large number of deaths in the U.S. population.

That the respiratory tract becomes infected frequently is not surprising when we consider that it is in direct contact with the environment and is continuously exposed to microorganisms suspended in the air we breathe. Some are highly virulent and may infect a normal person even in small numbers, but most of these organisms do not cause infection unless other factors interfere with host defenses. The warm, moist environment of the respiratory tract seems an ideal place for the growth of microorganisms. One of the questions that this chapter will address is why these frequent infections are not even more frequent.

Infection may be localized at any level of the respiratory tract, and the location is a major determinant of the clinical manifestations. The clinical syndromes associated with infection at different locations are shown in Figure 45.1. Infections of the conjunctivae, the middle ear, and the paranasal sinuses are included

Figure 45.1. Clinical syndromes associated with infection at different locations within the respiratory tract.

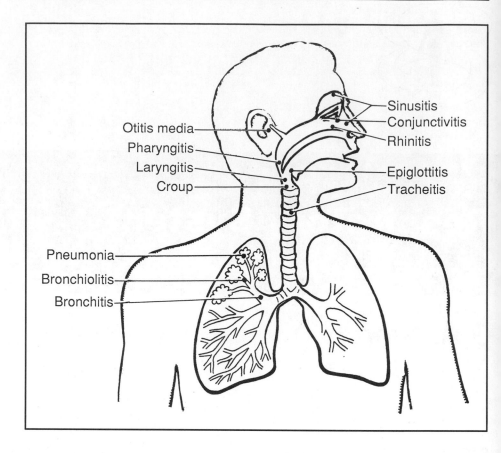

because these areas are continuous with the respiratory tract and lined by respiratory epithelium. Several important diseases of this system are discussed in other chapters (pneumococcal pneumonia, Chapter 13; whooping cough, Chapter 20; pulmonary tuberculosis, Chapter 22; chlamydial pneumonitis, Chapter 24; mycoplasma pneumonia, Chapter 27; influenza, Chapter 30; infections of the sinuses and middle ear, Chapter 52).

The clinical manifestations of respiratory tract infection also depend on the causative agent. Thus, viruses are particularly important in the upper respiratory tract and account for most cases of pharyngitis. Bacteria are the most important causes of otitis media, sinusitis, pharyngitis, epiglottitis, bronchitis, and pneumonia. Fungi and protozoa rarely cause serious respiratory tract infection in normal individuals but are important causes of pneumonia in the immunocompromised host. Some of the common pathogens that produce infection at different locations in this system are listed in Table 45.1. Their relative contribution to respiratory tract disease is shown in Figure 45.2.

Although the casual observer may think that there is a constant background of respiratory tract infections in the population, close observation coupled with laboratory studies reveal that there are large and small epidemics due to specific agents. The results of careful viral surveillance carried out in Houston, Texas over a period of several years are shown in Figure 45.3.

Some microorganisms have a strong predilection for certain sites in the respiratory tract, either because of specific tropism or selective survival (Chapters 1 and 29). The reason the common cold occurs in the nose and not further down the

Table 45.1

Pathogens producing disease at different levels of the respiratory tract

Location	Common Pathogens
Nasopharynx	Rhinovirus, *Coronavirus*, other respiratory viruses, *Staphylococcus aureus*
Oropharynx	Group A streptococcus (*Streptococcus pyogenes*), *Corynebacterium diphtheriae*, Epstein-Barr virus, adenovirus, enteroviruses
Conjunctiva	*Streptococcus pneumoniae, Haemophilus influenzae, Neisseria gonorrhoeae, Chlamydia trachomatis*, adenovirus
Middle ear and paranasal sinuses	*Streptococcus pneumoniae, Haemophilus influenzae, Branhamella catarrhalis*, Group A streptococcus (*Streptococcus pyogenes*)
Epiglottitis	*Haemophilus influenzae*
Larynx-trachea	Parainfluenza viruses, *Staphylococcus aureus*
Bronchi	*Streptococcus pneumoniae, Haemophilus influenzae, Mycoplasma pneumoniae*, influenza viruses, measles virus
Bronchioles	Respiratory syncytial virus
Lungs	(See Table 45.5)

respiratory tract is that the cold viruses grow best at 33°C—a temperature found in the nose and not in the lungs.

This chapter divides the respiratory system into three major anatomic regions:

• The nose and throat;

• The airways;

• The lungs.

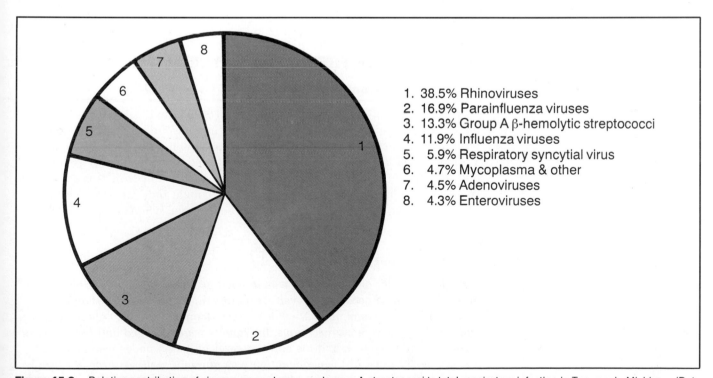

1. 38.5% Rhinoviruses
2. 16.9% Parainfluenza viruses
3. 13.3% Group A β-hemolytic streptococci
4. 11.9% Influenza viruses
5. 5.9% Respiratory syncytial virus
6. 4.7% Mycoplasma & other
7. 4.5% Adenoviruses
8. 4.3% Enteroviruses

Figure 45.2. Relative contribution of viruses, mycoplasma, and group A streptococci to total respiratory infection in Tecumseh, Michigan. (Data from Monto AS, Ullman BM: *JAMA*, 227:164–169, 1974.)

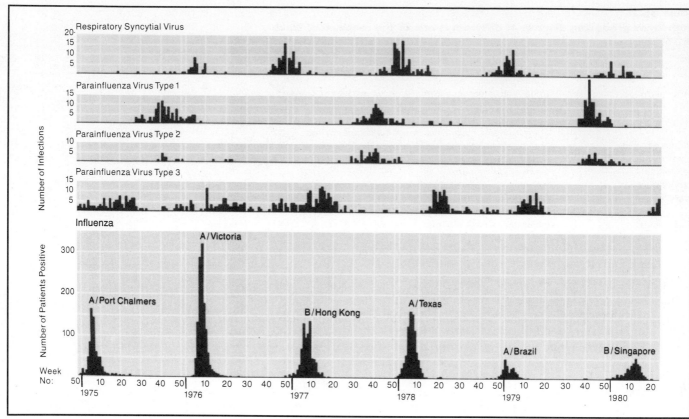

Figure 45.3. Patterns of occurrence of respiratory syncytial, parainfluenza, and influenza virus infections in Houston, Texas. (Data from Glezen WP, et al., *N Engl J Med* 288:498–505, 1973. Reprinted with permission from *Virology*, The Upjohn Co., 1983.)

INFECTIONS OF THE NOSE AND THROAT

A Case of the Common Cold

Ms. C., a 28-year-old woman, realized she was getting a cold when she noticed a scratchy feeling in the throat, sneezing, nasal discharge, low-grade fever, and malaise. The symptoms worsened, reaching a peak after 48 hours. Within several days her nasal discharge thickened and was slightly yellowish, and then subsided over the next several days. All her other symptoms resolved completely within about 7 days of onset. She thought that she acquired the illness from her 7-year-old child, who had had similar symptoms a few days earlier.

A Case of Pharyngitis

Freddy, a 5-year-old child who was in good general health, was brought to the pediatrician because of fever, irritability, and a sore throat that began 1 day earlier. On examination, he had a 102°F temperature, his conjunctivae and oropharynx were erythematous, his tonsils were enlarged and coated with a patchy white exudate, and his anterior cervical lymph nodes were enlarged and tender. The rest of the examination was unremarkable. A throat culture was negative for group A streptococcus. The symptoms worsened slightly over the next day and then resolved without treatment over a 5-day period.

Although the posterior nasopharynx merges with the oropharynx, there are important differences between infections of the nose and throat. Some are illustrated in the above cases. Most infections of the nasopharynx are caused by viruses and give rise to the signs and symptoms that are known collectively as the common cold. Approximately 40% to 50% of colds are caused by the *rhinovirus* group. *Coronaviruses* are the next most common group of agents, accounting for approximately 10% of colds. The remainder are caused by a variety of respiratory viruses listed in Table 45.2. Although the patient with a cold may experience a scratchy feeling in the throat, nasal symptoms are usually more prominent. Bacterial infection of the nose occurs occasionally, but this is not a common clinical problem.

Infection of the oropharynx, *pharyngitis*, is associated with discomfort in the throat, especially during swallowing. Sometimes nasal symptoms are also present. Viruses lead bacteria as the most common etiological agents (Table 45.3). It is difficult to differentiate between viral and bacterial pharyngitis on the basis of clinical findings; in practice the distinction is made by performing a throat culture to detect group A streptococci, which is by far the most important *bacterial* cause of pharyngitis. Other streptococci account for a small proportion of cases, as do gonococci in sexually active individuals. In the past, oropharyngeal diphtheria caused an important form of pharyngitis, but this disease is rarely seen in the United States today. Among the viruses, the adenovirus group is particularly prominent and may be suspected if conjunctivitis is also present (pharyngoconjunctival fever). In adolescents and young adults, Epstein-Barr virus is a common cause of pharyngitis, which is one of the manifestations of infectious mononucleosis. The enteroviruses, especially the group A coxsackieviruses, sometimes produce small vesicles on the mucous membrane of the throat. This clinical picture is known as *herpangina*.

Human Rhinoviruses and the Common Cold

The human rhinovirus remains the pathogen most closely linked to the common cold. Along with the enteroviruses (poliovirus, coxsackie A and B viruses, echoviruses, and hepatitis A virus), the rhinoviruses comprise the Picornaviridae family (Chapter 35). Unlike other respiratory viruses such as influenza, parainfluenza, or respiratory syncytial virus, rhinoviruses have no lipid envelope surrounding the viral nucleocapsid. Antigenic diversity is a striking characteristic of the rhinoviruses, with at least 89 serotypes recognized to date. (Any two rhinovirus isolates are considered to be of different serotypes if their infectivity is not neutralized by the same antiserum.) Although there is some cross-reactivity among different serotypes, the extent of antigenic diversity has caused pessimism about the prospects for a rhinovirus vaccine.

Encounter

Rhinovirus infections are very common. The average person experiences approximately one such infection per year, and schoolchildren and those in contact with them may experience many more. These infections occur most commonly in the fall and spring. Multiple serotypes circulate simultaneously, but over time different serotypes predominate.

Infected humans (particularly children) are the only known reservoir for these viruses. The mode of transmission has been the subject of intense experimental study. One series of experiments demonstrated that transmission may occur if

Table 45.2
Causes of the common cold

Agent	Relative importance
Rhinovirus	+ + + +
Coronavirus	+ +
Parainfluenza virus	+[a]
Respiratory syncytial virus	+[a]
Influenza virus	+
Adenovirus	+
Other viruses	+ +
Unknown	+ + + +

[a] + + or more in children

Table 45.3
Causes of pharyngitis

Agent	Relative Importance
Streptococcus pyogenes (Group A β-hemolytic)	+ + + +
Rhinovirus	+ +
Adenovirus	+ +
Coronavirus	+ +
Epstein-Barr virus	+ +
Herpes simplex virus	+
Parainfluenza virus	+
Influenza virus	+
Coxsackievirus	+
Mixed anaerobic bacteria	+
Neisseria gonorrhoeae	+
Corynebacterium diphtheriae	+
Corynebacterium haemolyticum	+
Mycoplasma pneumoniae	+
Francisella tularensis	+
Unknown	+ + + +

Figure 45.4. Participant in an experiment designed to study the mode of transmission of rhinoviruses. The arm braces worn by the subject allowed normal poker playing but prevented the wearer from touching any part of his head or face. (From Dick EC, et al: Aerosol transmission of rhinovirus colds. *J Infect Dis* 156:442–448, 1987.)

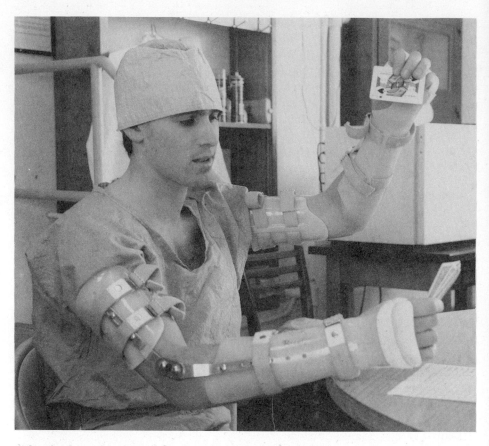

individuals touch their nose or eyes after their hands become contaminated with rhinovirus (either from contaminated nasal secretions or environmental objects). In recent experiments, susceptible volunteers played poker with persons who had symptomatic rhinovirus infection, and became infected even if they were restrained from touching their face (Fig. 45.4). This suggests that rhinovirus infection may be transmitted by aerosols, as well as by direct inoculation. The effective production and dispersal of aerosol droplets during a sneeze is shown in Figure. 45.5.

Figure 45.5. Droplet dispersal following a sneeze by a patient with a cold; note strings of mucus. (From Jennison: *Aerobiology* 17:106, 1947.)

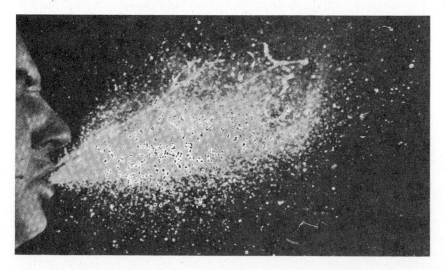

Entry, Spread, and Multiplication

In experimental studies, even a small inoculum of rhinovirus suffices to initiate an infection. The first step in infection is the binding of the virus to specific receptors on respiratory epithelial cells. The receptor has not yet been fully characterized, but recent studies have shown that there is a single one for most rhinovirus serotypes. This is an exciting finding, because the existence of a common early stage for all rhinovirus infections suggests possibilities for a generalized prevention. Detailed structural studies of rhinoviruses have revealed that the part of the virus that binds to the cellular receptor is located within a cleft or "canyon" on the surface of the virion. Neutralizing antibodies are thought to prevent infection by binding to the virions at sites near the canyon, making it impossible for the binding site on the virus to come in contact with the cellular receptor.

Rhinoviruses are thought to spread in respiratory epithelium by local extension. In experimental colds, the posterior nasopharynx is the site of the most intense infection. Neither viremia nor infection at sites outside of the respiratory tract are known to occur in these infections.

Damage

The nose of a patient with a cold becomes engorged with blood (hyperemic) and edematous. The thin nasal discharge contains large amounts of serum proteins. As the cold progresses, the discharge becomes mucopurulent and contains many cells, especially neutrophils. Respiratory epithelial cells are also present, some of which contain rhinovirus antigens, indicating that they are infected by the virus. If a biopsy of the mucosa were to be performed early in the course of a cold, it would reveal edema of subepithelial connective tissue with relatively small numbers of inflammatory cells. In contrast to some other viral respiratory infections, particularly influenza, only minimal histopathologic changes would be observed, even in areas where viral antigens are present.

How does rhinovirus infection produce its characteristic disease manifestations? In general, there is a correlation between the severity of the cold and the amount of rhinovirus that can be recovered. Large amounts of virus are found without tissue destruction, however, indicating that disease manifestations must be produced by other mechanisms than viral-induced cytopathology. Further support for this notion comes from finding that nasal secretions of persons with a cold contain large amounts of the vasoactive substance bradykinin. In addition, it is thought that direct stimulation of nerve endings in the nasal mucosa produces some of the manifestations of the cold.

Despite the discomfort resulting from the events occurring in the nose, most rhinovirus infections are mild and have few other consequences. The most common complications are sinusitis, otitis media, and exacerbation of chronic bronchitis or asthma. Sinusitis or otitis media complicating a cold are usually due to bacterial infections that develop because the normal draining of the sinuses or the middle ear is blocked.

Prevention and Treatment

Some degree of immunity to rhinovirus infection does develop. Infected people generate immunity effective against viruses of the same serotype. This immunity may be due at least in part to antibodies found in nasal secretions. It is reasonable to speculate that antirhinovirus antibody, particularly of the IgA class, might exert a protective effect by blocking the binding of the virus to the cell receptor.

A vaccine to prevent the common cold does not yet appear feasible, not only because of the serologic diversity of these viruses but also because they account for no more than 50% of colds. Nevertheless, several novel approaches to prophylaxis are currently being explored. One is the use of recombinant α-interferon administered by nasal spray. In recent studies this was effective in preventing colds if used just after the first cold occurred in a family. An earlier approach of using interferon nasal sprays throughout the cold season was not successful because the nasal symptoms produced by long-term interferon administration were as bothersome as those of a cold (Chapter 37). Other chemotherapeutic agents are also under study. New approaches of this kind may finally led to progress in controlling the widely experienced miseries of the common cold.

INFECTIONS OF THE EPIGLOTTIS

A Case of Epiglottitis

A 3-year-old girl was put to bed with a low-grade temperature. In the middle of the night she awoke and her parents found that her fever was higher and that she had trouble breathing. The family pediatrician told the parents to take the child immediately to the local hospital. On examination, the child was sitting upright and drooling. A presumptive diagnosis of epiglottitis was made and the child taken to the operating room, where an endotracheal tube was inserted. An x-ray of the lateral neck was taken en route to the operating room and revealed swelling of the epiglottis (Fig. 45.6). When her throat was examined as she was being intubated, her epiglottis was seen to be very red and swollen. She was treated with antibiotics effective against Haemophilus influenzae type b. The next day the laboratory reported that blood and epiglottis cultures grew H. influenzae. She responded promptly to treatment and made a complete recovery.

Acute epiglottitis is probably the most serious form of URI. This distinct clinical syndrome can be rapidly fatal because the airway may become completely obstructed from swelling of the epiglottis and surrounding structures. Acute epiglottitis occurs most often in young children, with the cause almost invariably H. influenzae type b (see Chapter 15). It is fortunately relatively uncommon, encountered less than once a year in a busy pediatric practice; but the practitioner must always be vigilant since early recognition of acute epiglottitis is extremely important to prevent airway obstruction.

Pathobiology of Epiglottitis

This disease probably becomes established by direct extension of infection from the nasopharynx. Bacteremia is almost always present and is secondary to infection of the epiglottis. We do not know what determines who among the many individuals colonized with H. influenzae type b develops this disease. Nor do we understand the marked tropism of this organism for the epiglottis nor why other bacteria or viruses rarely cause epiglottitis.

Epiglottitis is an acute inflammation, with edema and infiltration with neutrophils. Microabscesses containing H. influenzae type b may be present. Metastatic complications are less common in epiglottitis than in H. influenzae meningitis,

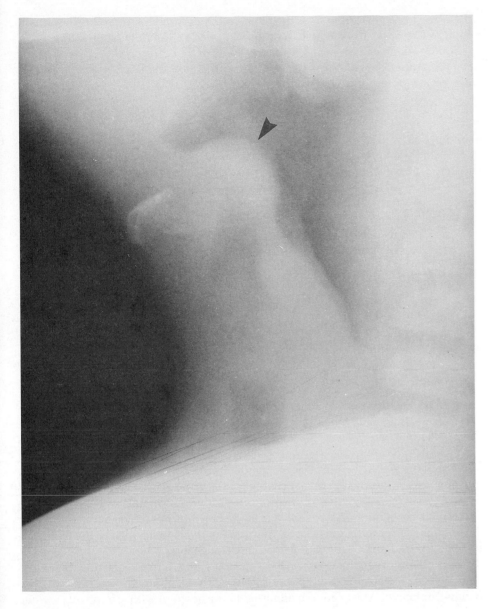

Figure 45.6. X-ray of the neck, taken in a lateral projection, reveals marked swelling of the epiglottis (*arrow*). (Courtesy of Dr. G. Shackleford.)

possibly because patients with epiglottitis seek medical attention earlier in the course of their illness. Fortunately, epiglottitis responds readily to treatment with antibiotics, and the outcome is good provided early recognition allows the airway to be protected, as illustrated in this case.

INFECTIONS OF THE LARYNX AND TRACHEA

A Case of Croup

A 19-month-old boy developed a runny nose, hoarseness, cough, and a low-grade temperature. His pediatrician diagnosed a viral URI and prescribed no specific treatment. That night the child suffered from a barking cough. His breathing was forced and noisy, especially with inspiration. Alarmed, the parents called the pediatrician, who told them that the child undoubtedly had *croup. He advised them to take the child in the bathroom steamed up by running the hot water in the shower, and to call back 15 minutes later if the respiratory difficulty worsened. It in fact subsided and the child fell back to sleep. A similar but milder episode occurred the next night. Over the next few days all symptoms gradually resolved.*

Infection of the larynx and upper airway in young children is often associated with the clinical syndrome of *croup*, as in this case. Croup (the obstruction of the upper airway) has a characteristically sudden onset, barking cough, difficulty with respiration, and often sudden resolution. Almost all cases are caused by viruses, especially the *parainfluenza viruses*. Infection with parainfluenza virus types 1 to 3 is very common in young children, and repeated infections may occur. Rarely, bacteria—particularly *Staphylococcus aureus*—cause clinical findings similar to those of viral croup. Typically, mild upper respiratory symptoms such as nasal discharge and dry cough are present 1 to 3 days before the signs of airway obstruction become evident. In most cases the illness is self-limited and resolves after 3 to 7 days.

In adults, the major clinical manifestation of infections of the larynx is hoarseness. Most acute laryngeal infection in adults is caused by respiratory viruses. Although these infections may be annoying, they are generally mild and self-limited. Other less common causes of laryngeal infection include tubercle bacilli and yeast such as *Candida albicans*, especially in immunocompromised patients.

Pathobiology of Croup

Infection begins at or near the site of original inoculation in the upper airway and spreads downward by direct extension. Viremia and spread to sites outside the airway have no known clinical consequences. The upper airway obstruction characteristic of croup results from swelling of the tracheal mucous membrane. Because the tracheal wall has nonexpandable rings of cartilage, swelling of the mucous membrane results in narrowing of the tracheal lumen, which worsens during inspiration, resulting in inspiratory stridor. Histamine and IgE antibody specific for parainfluenza virus have been detected in nasopharyngeal secretions of children with croup, suggesting that immunologic mechanisms involving inflammatory mediators may be involved in pathogenesis.

Some children experience recurrent episodes of croup, suggesting that they may have a predisposition to airway hyperreactivity, although the basis for this remains unknown. Most children admitted to the hospital with croup have greater reduction in the oxygen content of their blood than can be explained by the degree of obstruction to airflow. This suggests that the lungs as well as the airways may be involved in the infectious process. No specific drug treatment for parainfluenza virus infection is available at this time, and management consists of providing oxygen and support of the airway if needed.

INFECTIONS OF THE LARGE BRONCHI

A Case of Influenza

A 28-year-old physician developed symptoms of cough, myalgias (aches and pains in the muscles), headache made worse by the coughing, substernal chest pain, and high fever. She suspected influenza because an outbreak was in progress and she had recently taken care of several patients with similar symptoms. During the next 3 days she felt awful and was bedridden because of weakness and a persistent temperature of 103°F. The symptoms gradually resolved over the next few days without specific treatment, and after 7 to 10 days she was able to resume her usual activities. A throat culture she took on the first day of illness confirmed the diagnosis of viral influenza.

Many different organisms cause infections of the large bronchi. Among viruses, the prototype is influenza, illustrated here and more fully discussed in Chapter 30. Bronchitis is also caused by other viruses, mycoplasmas, chlamydiae, pneumococci, and *H. influenzae.*

INFECTIONS OF THE BRONCHIOLES

A Case of Bronchiolitis

A 4-month-old infant boy developed a nasal discharge and low-grade fever and was fussy. The next day the parents called the pediatrician because he was having difficulty breathing. On examination he had an obvious nasal discharge, was breathing 60 times per minute, and had mild nasal flaring and rib retractions. Auscultation of the lungs revealed scattered rales (crackles) and wheezes. A chest x-ray revealed hyperexpansion of the lungs and patchy infiltrates in the lungs. The baby was admitted to the hospital, where treatment consisted of oxygen, humidified air delivered via a mist tent, fluids, and suctioning of secretions. He began to improve after 48 hours and was discharged home, where the symptoms gradually resolved over the next 7 days. A fluorescent antibody stain of nasal secretions performed on the day of admission was positive for respiratory syncytial virus antigen, and 3 days later a culture was reported as positive for that virus.

Respiratory Syncytial Virus

Respiratory syncytial virus (RSV) is often described as the most dangerous cause of respiratory infection in young children. In addition to bronchiolitis, it also causes pneumonia and URI. Like the influenza and parainfluenza viruses, RSV is a member of the negative-stranded RNA paramyxovirus family. It is enveloped, with two virally specified glycoproteins as part of the structure. One of them, the *large glycoprotein*, or G, is responsible for the initial binding of the virus to the host cell; the other, the *fusion protein*, or F, permits fusion of the viral envelope with the host cell membrane, leading to entry of the virus. The F protein also induces the fusion of the membranes of infected cells. RSV gets its name from the resulting formation of syncytia or multinucleated masses of fused cells (see Figure 36.3 for a similar syncytium produced by measles virus). In contrast to the rhinoviruses or the influenza viruses, isolates of RSV do not display much antigenic heterogeneity. Recent studies have defined two subtypes and variants within each, but it is not yet known if the subtypes vary clinically or epidemiologically.

Encounter and Entry

The epidemiology of RSV infection has been extensively studied. The virus has been found in every part of the world where it has been sought. In temperate areas it causes a highly seasonal disease, with epidemics every winter and essentially disease-free summers. Infection is almost universal in early childhood.

Table 45.4
Transmission of respiratory syncytial virus

Volunteers	Cuddlers[a]	Touchers[b]	Sitters[c]
Exposed	7	10	14
Infected	5	4	0
Incubation time	4 days	5.5 days	

[a] Close contact with infected infant.
[b] Self-inoculation after touching surfaces contaminated with infants' secretions.
[c] Sitting more than 6 ft from infected infant.
Adapted from Hall CB, Douglas RG: Mode of transmission of respiratory syncytial virus. *J Pediatr* 99:100, 1981.

Most infections lead to symptomatic illness, but no more than 1% are severe enough to require hospitalization. The mortality rate for hospitalized cases is less than 5%, but is higher in patients at risk, especially those with congenital heart disease, bronchopulmonary dysplasia related to prematurity, neuromuscular disease, or immunodeficiency.

The only known source of RSV is infected humans who shed the virus in nasal secretions. As in the case of the rhinoviruses, transmission is thought to occur when secretions containing virus contaminate the hands of individuals. Small-particle airborne transmission plays at most a minor role in transmission: In a classical experiment, volunteers in close physical contact with RSV-infected infants were more readily infected than those who remained 6 feet away (Table 45.4).

Spread, Multiplication, and Damage

Infection proceeds downward along the respiratory mucosa, starting from the initial site of inoculation. Cell-to-cell transmission of virus may be important in this process. It is possible that aspiration of virus-contaminated secretions accelerates the process. There is no clinically significant spread to distant sites.

Severe RSV infection results in one of two somewhat overlapping clinical syndromes: bronchiolitis and pneumonia. The child with bronchiolitis has difficulty breathing and there is functional evidence of airway obstruction resembling asthma. Breathing is very noisy, with wheezing. As illustrated in the case history, the chest x-ray reveals hyperexpansion of the lungs, resulting from trapped air, and may also show streaky infiltrates, usually in both lungs. In the child with pneumonia, pulmonary infiltrates are more prominent. Wheezing and hyperexpansion may also occur, but less prominently than in bronchiolitis. In either syndrome, the airways are inflamed and edematous.

Tissue sections from fatal cases show necrosis of the epithelial cells that line the small bronchioles. There is also infiltration of lymphocytes between the mucosal epithelial cells and evidence of increased mucous secretion. The underlying elastic and muscle fibers are not affected. In cases of pneumonia, alveolar involvement consisting of swelling of the alveolar lining cells and interstitial inflammation accompanies bronchiolar involvement.

Bronchiolitis can be distinguished from asthma because bronchiolitis usually occurs in infants 2 to 8 months of age in whom bronchial smooth muscle is incompletely developed. Thus smooth muscle contraction may be less important in bronchiolitis than in asthma. If an individual bronchiole is completely obstructed, the portion of the lung ventilated by it may collapse. If obstruction is incomplete, a ball-valve effect may occur, leading to hyperexpansion of the distal lung. The entire process is associated with mismatches in ventilation and perfusion of the lung, and results in decreased oxygenation, along with the increased work of breathing.

In most cases, the infection is self-limited and recovery begins after several days. However, in the severe cases that occur in children compromised by other diseases, there may be respiratory failure and the child may die unless mechanical ventilation is provided. There is considerable concern that severe bronchiolitis in infancy may be associated with chronic lung disease in later life. Infants with bronchiolitis are more likely to have episodes of wheezing as they grow older, but any relationship between bronchiolitis in infancy and chronic lung disease in adulthood remains conjectural.

Doubts have been raised about the role of the immune system in protecting against RSV infections. First, most individuals experience multiple infections with RSV, indicating that immunity is incomplete. Second, infants are often infected at a time when they still have serum neutralizing antibody from their mothers. Despite these negative findings, there is now evidence that the immune system provides protection, since children with both congenital and acquired immune deficiencies suffer prolonged and severe RSV infection. Infants with high levels of serum antibody against RSV are less likely to develop lower respiratory tract involvement than infants with lower levels. Finally, in experimental animals, the administration of monoclonal antibodies to RSV glycoproteins or inoculation with vaccinia virus genetically engineered to express these antigens prevents lower respiratory tract involvement (although not usually nasal infection).

Do immune mechanisms contribute to the clinical manifestations of RSV infection? This is hinted by its resemblance to asthma, a process that involves the immune mediated release of broncho-constricting inflammatory mediators. Increased levels of histamine and IgE antibody directed against RSV have been found in nasal secretions from children with RSV bronchiolitis. Another hint that the immune system might contribute to RSV disease derives from an experience in the 1960s with an experimental killed RSV vaccine. Children given this vaccine not only were unprotected against RSV infection, but actually developed more severe disease following natural exposure to RSV!

Prevention and Treatment

Because RSV infection is so prevalent and accounts for considerable morbidity, this virus is an important candidate for vaccine development. For a number of years there was understandably little activity in this area, for fear of repeating the experience with the earlier vaccine. Recently, interest in an RSV vaccine has been renewed, and promising results have been reported by cloning DNA copies of the viral genes. In the area of treatment, a new era began recently with the introduction of the antiviral drug ribavirin to treat severe RSV infection (Chapter 37). The usefulness of this drug in clinical practice is currently being determined.

INFECTIONS OF THE LUNGS

Pneumonia, infection of the lung parenchyma, may be caused by many different pathogens, sometimes with distinctive clinical manifestations. Thus, pneumonia is not one disease but many different ones that share a common anatomic location. Pneumonias can be classified in various ways. We will use a clinical and epidemiologic classification (Table 45.5), based on the perspective of the clinician encountering patients with pneumonia. This classification is important because it can form the basis for managing the patient's illness even before a specific etiology has been proven.

In this classification, the first important distinction is between *acute pneumonia* (fairly sudden onset with progression of symptoms over a very few days), and *subacute and chronic pneumonia*. Among the acute pneumonias, a second very important distinction is made between *cases acquired in the community* and *cases acquired by patients in hospitals* (when hospitalized for conditions other than pneumonia). The latter are referred to as *hospital acquired* or *nosocomial* and are classified separately because the responsible pathogens are frequently different from those that produce pneumonia in nonhospitalized individuals.

Most of the common forms of acute community-acquired pneumonia are caused by pathogens that are *transmitted from person to person* (for example, pneumococci). A second group, encountered less frequently under ordinary circumstances, includes pneumonias caused by pathogens that *have an animal or environmental reservoir*. In many cases, the diagnosis of pneumonias of this group is difficult unless the physician seeks out the circumstances of exposures (for example, exposure to a parrot leading to psittacosis). *Pneumonias in infants and young children* are placed in a third group because they have a distinctive etiological spectrum.

Table 45.5
Classification of pneumonia syndromes

Acute	
Community-acquired	
Person-to-person transmission	*Streptococcus pneumoniae, Mycoplasma pneumoniae, Haemophilus influenzae, Staphylococcus aureus Streptococcus pyogenes, Klebsiella pneumoniae, Neisseria meningitidis, Branhamella catarrhalis*, Influenza virus
Animal or environmental exposure	*Legionella pneumophila, Francisella tularensis, Coxiella burnetii, Chlamydia psittaci, Yersinia pestis* (plague), *Bacillus anthracis* (anthrax), *Pseudomonas pseudomallei* (melioidosis), *Pasteurella multocida* (pasteurellosis)
Pneumonia in the infant and young child	*Chlamydia trachomatis*, respiratory syncytial virus and other respiratory viruses, *Staphylococcus aureus*, Group B streptococci, Cytomegalovirus, *Ureaplasma urealyticum* (?), *Pneumocystis carinii* (?) *Streptococcus pneumoniae, Haemophilus influenzae* type b.
Nosocomial pneumonia	Enterobacteriaceae, *Pseudomonas aeruginosa, Acinetobacter calcoaceticus, Staphylococcus aureus*
Subacute or Chronic	
Pulmonary Tuberculosis	*Mycobacterium tuberculosis*
Fungal	*Histoplasma capsulatum, Blastomyces dermatitidis, Coccidioides immitis, Cryptococcus neoformans,*
Aspiration pneumonia and lung abscess	Mixed anaerobic and aerobic bacterial organisms
Pneumonia in the immunocompromised patient	*Pneumocystis carinii*, cytomegalovirus, atypical mycobacteria, *Nocardia, Aspergillus, Phycomycetes, Candida*

In contrast with patients with acute pneumonia are those with lung infections that have been present for weeks or months. Several forms of subacute and chronic pneumonias can be distinguished. They are tuberculosis, fungal pneumonia, and anaerobic lung abscesses. It is important to realize that this classification is based on the common clinical patterns of disease, but that exceptions occur. For example, occasionally patients with tuberculosis, histoplasmosis, or lung abscesses may experience acute, rapidly progressing disease.

A Case of Community-Acquired Pneumonia in a Child

Paul, an 8-month-old Native American boy who had been previously in good health, was brought to a physician because of fever and rapid breathing. On examination, he was noted to look acutely ill, to have a temperature of 104.4°F, and to have a respiratory rate of 70 per minute. A chest x-ray revealed consolidation of the right middle and lower lobes (Fig. 45.7). His white cell count was 26,000/μl, which is markedly elevated over the normal. Since sputum samples cannot usually be obtained from young children, a rapid latex agglutination test for Haemophilus influenzae type b antigen was performed on the boy's urine. The result was positive, suggesting that this organism was responsible for the pneumonia. (Antigen detection tests such as latex agglutination are convenient because they give rapid answers. They are

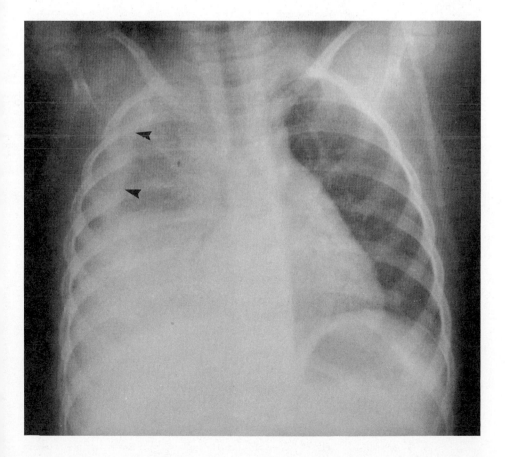

Figure 45.7. Chest x-ray of patient with *Haemophilus influenzae* type b pneumonia reveals consolidation of the middle and lower lobes. A pleural effusion is also present (*arrows*). (Courtesy of Dr. G. Shackleford.)

especially useful when the patient has been treated with antibiotics, rendering cultures negative. In this case, antigen was still detectable.) Paul was treated with antibiotics effective against that organism and recovered uneventfully. Blood cultures drawn before antibiotics were given were positive for H. influenzae type b.

A Case of Pneumonia in a Chronic Alcoholic

Mr. L., a 52-year-old man with severe chronic alcoholism, was brought to an emergency room by a policeman who had found him lying on a street. Physical examination revealed a lethargic, disheveled, middle-aged male with a temperature of 102°F and a respiratory rate of 36 per minute. During respiration, the left side of the chest moved much less than the right side (splinting). On auscultation, there was evidence of consolidation of the upper lobe of the left lung. A sample of bloody sputum was obtained by tracheal suction, and a Gram stain revealed many neutrophils and Gram negative rods. A chest x-ray confirmed the consolidation of the left lower lobe (Fig. 45.8).

Mr. L. was treated with broad-spectrum antibiotics. The sputum culture was reported to have a heavy growth of Klebsiella pneumoniae, one of the

Figure 45.8. Pneumonia caused by *Klebsiella pneumoniae*. Chest x-ray reveals extensive consolidation of the left lower lobe. Cavity formation is apparent within the involved area (*arrow*). (Courtesy of Dr. S.S. Sagel.)

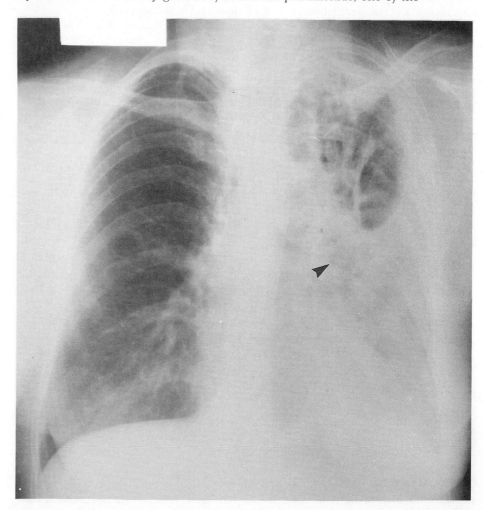

Enterobacteriaceae. Mr. L's hospital course was stormy and he required mechanical ventilation for 4 days. Eventually he recovered and was discharged to a chronic care hospital after 3 weeks.

Comments

What are the complaints of the patients and the findings on examination that lead physicians to make the diagnosis of pneumonia? Most patients with the disease have fever and feel sick. Many also present with clues, often very obvious, that point to the chest as the location of disease. Some clues are chest pain, frequently "pleuritic" (exacerbated by respiratory motion), and a cough that may or may not be productive of sputum. Those with extensive involvement of the lungs may have shortness of breath, rapid respiration, and poor color, even cyanosis. If breathing is painful, expansion of the chest may be limited (splinting). Auscultation may reveal rales, which are usually indicative of alveolar disease. The most important diagnostic finding of all is a chest x-ray. Pneumonia is usually visible as a shadow or "infiltrate", the pattern of which may be a clue to the identity of the pathogen causing pneumonia. Skilled interpretation is important, because other processes, tumors, pulmonary edema, or pulmonary hemorrhage, may produce radiographic changes very similar to those of pneumonia.

In general, the most common forms of acute community-acquired pneumonias are those caused by the pneumococcus and *Mycoplasma pneumoniae*, described in Chapters 13 and 27, respectively. The clinical features of Paul, the 8-month-old baby (his ill appearance, high temperature, elevated white blood cell count, and chest x-ray), all would lead the physician to suspect an acute bacterial pneumonia. These manifestations are characteristic of pneumococcal pneumonia, which is common in all age groups (see Fig. 13.1 for a chest x-ray of a case of pneumococcal pneumonia). However, the astute physician may be tipped off to *Haemophilus* as the etiology by the age and ethnic background of the child. *H. influenzae* type b accounts for a high proportion of serious systemic bacterial infections in children in the first year of life. Although it affects children in all socioeconomic groups, the incidence is higher in non-whites and is particularly high among Native Americans and Alaskan Eskimos. It is important to recognize this etiologic agent, first because of its tendency to cause meningitis and other forms of invasive infection and second, because it is frequently resistant to antibiotics that may be used to treat pneumococcal pneumonia.

A particular aspect of acute childhood pneumonias is that they are more often caused by viruses than by bacteria. Illness caused by respiratory syncytial virus, influenza and parainfluenza viruses, or adenoviruses tends to be milder, and spontaneous recovery is the rule unless the child is compromised in some other way. This is a unique situation, since viruses are infrequent causes of pneumonia in the other age groups, except during influenza epidemics. Children who develop pneumonia in the first few months of life are often infected with organisms acquired from the mother, including chlamydiae and cytomegalovirus.

Mr. L.'s case illustrates another form of acute community-acquired pneumonia, that caused by aerobic Gram negative bacilli. The factors that place such an individual at risk for this disease, chronic alcoholism and exposure, also predispose him to pneumonia by the pneumococcus, by *Legionella pneumophila*, and by anaerobic bacteria (aspiration pneumonia). The clinical features of this case, including the involvement of the right upper lobe, bulging at an interlobar fissure (indicative of the expansive nature of the inflammatory process), and bloody sputum, are characteristic of pneumonia due to *K. pneumoniae*. However, these characteristics are not unique, and similar illness may be caused by many other bacteria. Laboratory testing is required to make the specific etiological diagnosis. In current medical practice, most cases of pneumonia caused by members of the Enterobacteriaceae occur in hospital patients or residents of nursing home.

Encounter

Encounter with the agents that cause pneumonia takes place in different ways:

• Pneumonias may be caused by *colonization-infection*, where the causative organism is transmitted from person to person usually without environmental reservoirs. Transmission is typically airborne over short distances, or by contaminated secretions or fomites. In the case of some pathogens such as the pneumococcus, *H. influenzae*, and *Staphylococcus aureus*, most individuals who encounter the organism become colonized, but only a few develop disease, directly or after a variable period of colonization.

• Pneumonias also may be caused by organisms *associated with the environment or with animals*. Most of these are transmitted by the airborne route, although some have insect vectors. Organisms that follow this pattern are shown in Table 45.6. An example is Legionnaires' disease, discussed in detail in Chapter 26.

• *Aspiration pneumonias* are usually caused by entry into the lungs of the normal microbial contents of the upper respiratory tract. Typical cases lead to lung abscess and other anaerobic lung infections. The causative agents are part of the normal oral flora, which may cause disease when translocated in large numbers to an abnormal location.

Entry and Spread

Pathogens may reach the lungs by one of five routes: (*a*) direct inhalation, (*b*) aspiration of upper airway contents, (*c*) spread along the mucous membrane surface, (*d*) hematogenous spread, and rarely (*e*) direct penetration. Of these, inhalation and aspiration are the most common.

Inhalation and aspiration. Obviously the respiratory tract is exposed to potential pathogens suspended in the inhaled air. Less obvious is that it is also exposed to potential pathogens by aspiration of oropharyngeal contents. Studies with radioactive tracers have shown that in normal individuals, aspiration is not uncommon during deep sleep. In addition, intoxication or unconsciousness may cause an individual to aspirate large amounts of oropharyngeal material or even material from the stomach and upper small intestine (see chapter 46 on gastrointestinal infections). Defenses that protect against aspiration include the epiglottis, which physically protects the airway; the laryngeal spasm reflex, which also prevents material from entering it; and the cough reflex, which expels material from the airway. Aspiration of oropharyngeal contents is the most important mode of entry for organisms that exhibit the colonization-infection pattern.

Direct spread. Respiratory viruses such as influenza and respiratory syncytial virus initiate infection in the upper airway and spread to the lower respiratory tract by spreading directly along the respiratory epithelium, a route possibly facilitated by aspiration.

Hematogenous spread. In hematogenous spread the lung is a secondary site of infection. This mechanism is unusual but clearly implicated in cases of staphylococcal pneumonia in intravenous drug abusers. In many of these cases the tricuspid heart valve is infected, and pulmonary infection results when infectious material from the valve embolizes to the lungs. Hematogenous spread has also been implicated in pneumonia caused by *Escherichia coli* and other Gram negative rods.

Defense Mechanisms of the Lungs

The defense of the lungs (Fig. 45.9) begins in the nose, where specialized hairs, known as vibrissae, filter out large particles suspended in inhaled air. Large particles (more than 10 μm in diameter) tend to settle at points of abrupt changes in direction of airflow, such as the posterior nasopharynx. Smaller particles, less than 3 μm in diameter, are likely to elude these barriers and reach the terminal bronchioles and alveoli. The importance of the upper airway structures in defending the lungs is illustrated in patients in whom these structures are bypassed. Endotracheal tubes used in anesthesia and mechanical ventilation provide a conduit from the outside environment to the lower airway; patients with these tubes in place are markedly predisposed to pneumonia.

Figure 45.9. The defense mechanisms of the respiratory tract. Aerodynamic factors include the presence of vibrissae in the nasal passage and abrupt changes in the direction of flow of the air column. The epiglottis and cough reflex prevent introduction of particulate matter into the lower airway. The ciliated respiratory epithelium propels the overlying mucus layer (red) upwards toward the mouth. In the alveoli, macrophages, humoral factors (including immunoglobulins and complement), and neutrophils (when inflammation is present) all assist in preventing or clearing infection.

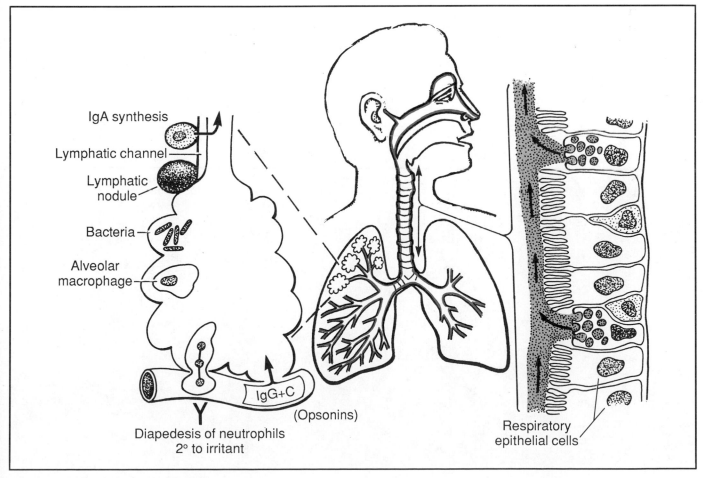

IgA synthesis

Lymphatic channel

Lymphatic nodule

Bacteria

Alveolar macrophage

IgG+C

(Opsonins)

Diapedesis of neutrophils 2° to irritant

Respiratory epithelial cells

The respiratory epithelium itself has specialized defenses against infection. The tight junctions between cells prevent direct penetration. Epithelial cells from the nose to the terminal bronchioles are covered with cilia that beat coordinately. Overlying them is a covering of mucus containing antimicrobial compounds such as lysozyme, lactoferrin, and secretory IgA antibodies. Each ciliated cell has approximately 200 cilia, which beat at speeds up to 500 times per minute, serving to move the overlying mucus layer upwards towards the larynx at a rate as high as 4 to 6 mm/minute. The cilia and mucus are called the *mucociliary escalator.* Certain patients with impaired ciliary function have frequent respiratory infections. An example is a condition known as Kartagener's syndrome, in which patients have structurally and functionally altered cilia (these patients also exhibit the dramatic condition called dextrocardia, or right-sided heart). Ciliary function may also be impaired by viral or mycoplasma infections and is at risk of damage by smoking (Fig. 45.10).

The final lung defenses are found in the alveoli: IgA antibodies, complement components, possibly surfactant itself, and most important, the alveolar macrophages. These phagocytic cells function as active scavengers, ingesting, and killing invading pathogens. When they cannot contain infection by themselves, they are helped by other phagocytic cells that do not normally reside

Figure 45.10. Electron micrograph of nasal epithelium from a healthy child (**A**) and a child with adenovirus infection (**B**). The nasal epithelium in **A** is characteristic of the pseudostratified ciliated columnar epithelium lining the large conducting airways. Normal ciliated cells are seen on either side of a mucous cell that is filled and distended with secretory material. **B** shows the altered ultrastructure and loss of ciliated cells that may accompany viral infection.

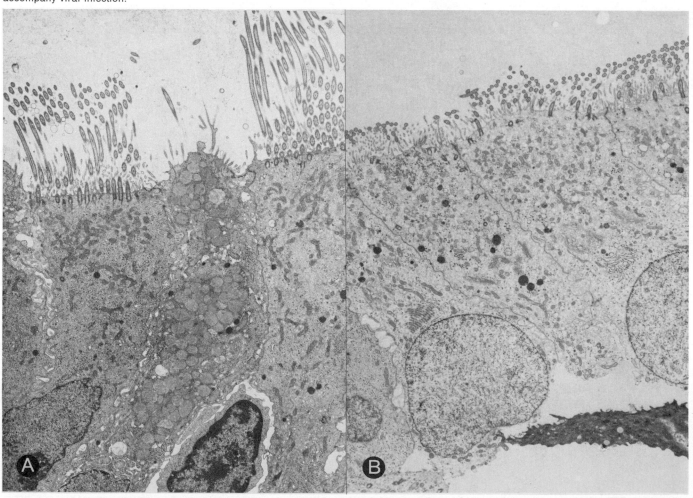

in the lungs, especially neutrophils. Encapsulated bacteria can effectively evade phagocytosis, while others not only survive but can multiply within phagocytic cells. Thus, tubercle bacilli, *Histoplasma capsulatum*, and legionella find a haven within macrophages, resist killing, and multiply in large numbers. If macrophages become activated through nonspecific or specific immune mechanisms, they can limit the multiplication of such intracellular invaders.

In the case of viral infection, the cells invaded are often not normally phagocytic and lack obvious means to kill the invader. Histopathologic studies of the lungs (or other affected tissues) of patients with viral infection show infiltration by large numbers of lymphocytes and plasma cells, suggesting that viral infection stimulates the recruitment of lymphoid cells rather than neutrophils. These lymphocytes contribute to host defense by antibody production and by attacking infected cells via cytotoxic T lymphocytes, natural killer cells, and antibody-dependent cell-mediated cytotoxicity.

Damage

The deleterious effects of pneumonia on the host fall into two categories:

- Systemic effects that result from infection any place in the body, including fever, shock (particularly with Gram negative bacilli), and wasting (for example, in chronic tuberculosis).

- Interference with the ability of the lungs to carry out air exchange. This may result from marked thickening of the membrane that separates erythrocytes from inspired air in the alveoli. In bronchopneumonia, difficulty in gas exchange probably results from regional mismatches in the ventilation and perfusion of the lungs.

There are marked differences in the amount of permanent lung damage in the various types of pneumonia. It is remarkable that in severe pneumococcal pneumonia, the lung often heals completely without any scar formation (Fig. 13.4). The reason is that although there is an exuberant inflammatory response within the alveoli, there is no necrosis of the underlying lung skeleton that could provoke scar formation and permanent loss of functional lung tissue. In contrast, lung infections caused by Gram negative rods and anaerobic bacteria frequently result in permanent lung tissue destruction. The fibrotic healing of a necrotizing pneumonia is referred to as *healing by organization*.

The specific manifestations of pneumonia vary widely and fall into several patterns. The commonly used terminology is confusing because it derives in part from gross pathology, microscopic histopathology, and chest x-ray. Adding to the confusion is the custom of using terms differently in different settings. Nevertheless, these terms are in widespread use and we will attempt to define them:

- *Lobar pneumonia* refers to a homogeneous involvement of a distinct region of the lung. Most of the involvement is within the alveoli, and the bronchioles and the interstitium are relatively spared. The infection spreads between alveoli until it is contained by the anatomic barriers that separate one segment from another. Thus an entire segment or even an entire lobe becomes involved (Figs. 13.1, 45.11). The most frequent agents of lobar pneumonia in adults are the pneumococcus, *H. influenzae*, and legionella.

- In *bronchopneumonia* the pathologic process originates in the small airways and extends to nearby areas of the lung. The process is much more patchy than

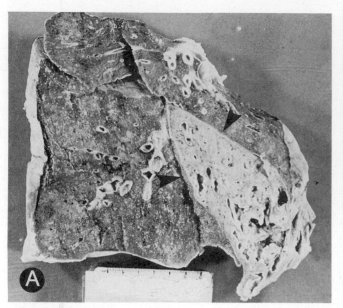

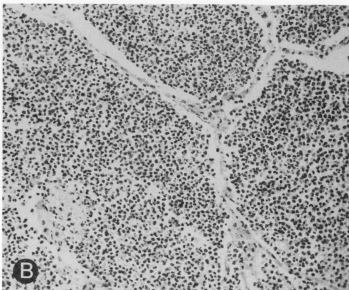

Figure 45.11. Lobar pneumonia. **A,** An autopsy specimen in which homogeneous consolidation of the right middle lobe is evident (*arrow*). **B,** A microscopic view showing lung alveoli filled with an infiltrate of inflammatory cells including both neutrophils and mononuclear cells. Note the lack of involvement of the interstitium. (Courtesy of Dr. C. Kuhn.)

lobar pneumonia, often occurring in more than one area of the lung and not confined by the anatomic barriers (Fig. 45.12). Typical causes of bronchopneumonia include *Mycoplasma pneumoniae* and respiratory viruses.

- *Interstitial pneumonia* refers to involvement of the lung interstitium. When viral infections such as influenza involve the lung, they tend to produce an interstitial pneumonia (Figs. 27.1 and 45.13). One of the most common causes is cytomegalovirus, which usually infects patients with severe suppression of the

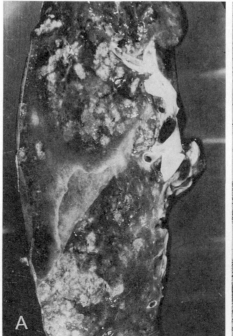

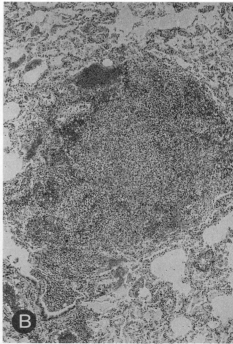

Figure 45.12. Bronchopneumonia. **A,** An autopsy specimen showing multiple areas of bronchopneumonia. Each area represents inflammation centered around an airway. **B,** A microscopic view showing an area of inflammation in a region distal to a respiratory bronchiole. (Courtesy of Dr. C. Kuhn.)

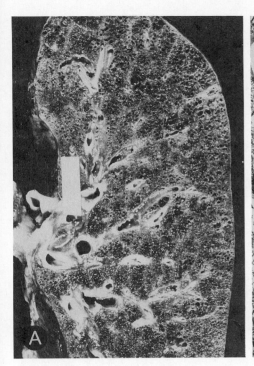 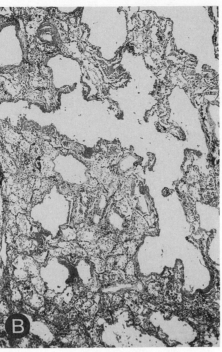

Figure 45.13. Interstitial pneumonia. **A,** An autopsy specimen showing diffuse interstitial involvement of the lung from a patient who died with influenza pneumonia. Characteristic features are the uniform panlobar involvement with no predictable relationship to microscopic air passages and the accentuation of air-spaces. **B,** A microscopic view of the same lung revealing involvement of both the interstitium and the alveoli. A uniformly dilated alveolar duct is present lined in areas by hyaline membrane, which would appear eosinophilic and refractile when viewed microscopically. The interstitium is widened and sparsely infiltrated by mononuclear cells. (Courtesy of Dr. C. Kuhn.)

immune system. *Pneumocystis carinii* pneumonia in an AIDS patient falls in this category.

• A fourth pattern of involvement is the *lung abscess*. Here, one or more areas of lung parenchyma are replaced by cavities filled with debris generated by the infectious process. Many bacteria and fungi are capable of producing lung abscesses, but currently a large proportion of cases are caused by anaerobic bacteria.

Infections may spread from the lung beyond the respiratory tract, for example into the pleural space, creating a condition called *empyema*. More rarely, the process may extend to involve mediastinal structures such as the pericardium. Microorganisms may spread outside the chest via the lymphatic drainage of the lung, reaching the bloodstream via the thoracic duct. Brain abscess, pyogenic arthritis, and endocarditis are all unusual but well-known complications of bacterial pneumonia.

Some Examples of Other Pneumonias

Aspiration Pneumonias

A Case of Aspiration Pneumonia Leading to a Lung Abscess

Mr. A., a 46-year-old man with a poorly controlled seizure disorder, was brought to a physician because of cough, fever, and weight loss occurring over a 2-week period. A physical examination revealed an ill appearing male with a temperature of 101°F and a foul-smelling breath. He had "amphoric" breath sounds (resembling those produced by blowing across the mouth of a bottle), suggestive of a lung cavity. A chest x-ray showed a large cavity in the left

Figure 45.14. Lung abscess. X-ray showing a cavitary lesion (*arrow*) with surrounding infiltrate. (Courtesy of Dr. S. S. Sagel.)

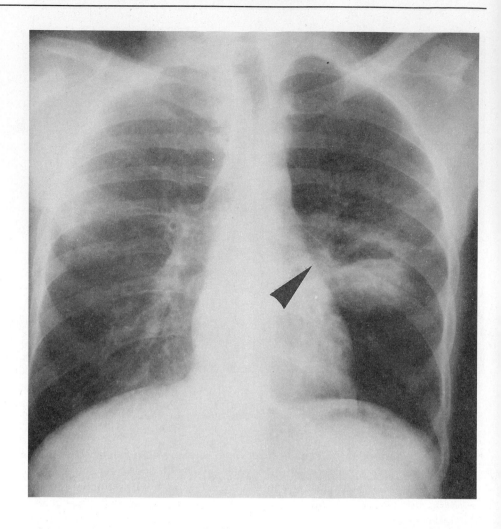

mid-lung with extensive surrounding inflammation (Fig. 45.14). He was admitted to the hospital and treated with high-dose intravenous penicillin. He began to feel better almost immediately and his fever disappeared over the course of a week. After 3 months on oral penicillin, he was judged to be cured.

Lung abscesses such as those of Mr. A. are usually a consequence of gross aspiration of oropharyngeal or gastric contents. The resulting infection has a number of distinguishing features:

- The clinical course tends to be less acute than that of most other forms of bacterial pneumonia. Mr. A may have been ill for several weeks or even months before seeking medical attention.

- The typical lung abscess represents a polymicrobial infection with multiple species of bacteria. The bacteria most commonly involved are anaerobes and microaerophilic organisms from the normal flora of the mouth. Lung abscesses can also result from infection with other organisms that can also destroy lung tissue, including *S. aureus, K. pneumoniae,* mycobacteria, and others.

Although the definitive diagnosis is usually made on the basis of the chest x-ray, there may be clues that may lead the astute physician to suspect a lung abscess. Cough, malaise, and fever of several weeks duration, sometimes ac-

companied by unexplained weight loss, should make the physician think of subacute processes in the chest, both infectious and noninfectious. Risk factors, if
present, are an important clue pointing toward lung abscess. Finally, as in the
case of Mr. A., the patient's breath and sputum may have a putrid odor that
is highly suggestive of anaerobic infection. In some cases, this odor is so strong
that the diagnosis can be suspected as soon as the physician enters the patient's
room.

Lung abscesses typically occur following the aspiration of a larger quantity of
oropharyngeal contents than can be disposed of by the normal defense mechanisms of the lung. Thus, the disease occurs most often in individuals who are
prone to aspirate. The most important risk factor is alteration of consciousness
for any reason, including anesthesia, sedation, intoxication, drug overdose, injuries, and seizures. Lung abscess may also be caused by fragments of teeth
aspirated during dental procedures.

In some cases of severe aspiration, gastric contents may enter the lungs. Probably because of their low pH and proteolytic enzymes, gastric contents induce
an intense chemical pneumonitis that is not in itself an infection; but secondary
infection of the injured lung may occur.

If not treated promptly, lung abscess may spread to involve the pleural space,
resulting in empyema. An unusual distant complication of lung abscess is brain
abscess, resulting from spread of the infection via the bloodstream. It is notable
that infections at distant sites other than the brain are extremely infrequent as
a complication of lung abscesses.

Pneumonias in Immunocompromised Patients

Pneumonia is a common occurrence in immunocompromised individuals, including those who undergo cancer chemotherapy, those with AIDS, and those
with congenital immunodeficiencies (Chapter 54). Most cases are caused by opportunistic pathogens that rarely cause infections in normal individuals. Examples include *Pneumocystis carinii*, the fungus *Aspergillus fumigatus*, and the
virus cytomegalovirus. Many of these infections can be diagnosed only by carrying
out invasive procedures such as bronchoscopy or lung biopsy. Some patients,
especially those with more severe forms of immunodeficiency, may be infected
with more than one pathogen at a time. At the extreme, patients with AIDS are
not uncommonly infected simultaneously with *P. carinii*, cytomegalovirus, and
others.

Pneumonias Resulting from Unusual Exposures

A number of pneumonias not commonly encountered in day-to-day practice
result from agents found in animals or in the environment (Table 45.6). These
infections occur when people's activities bring them into contact with these organisms. For example, *Chlamydia psittaci* is a common cause of disease in birds,
and *psittacosis*, or parrot fever, may be acquired by inhalation (Chapter 24). This
illness is unlikely to be diagnosed correctly unless the physician obtains the history of contact with birds.

Another example is *Q fever*, caused by the rickettsia *Coxiella burnetii* and
usually acquired from sheep, goats, and cattle. The organism is stable in the environment, and infection can occur after exposure to contaminated material from
infected animals. Here too, the diagnosis is difficult unless the physician elicits
the history of exposure to animals or their environment. Several fungal infections

Table 45.6
Pneumonia resulting from unusual exposure

Disease	Causative Organism	Source
Psittacosis (parrot fever)	*Chlamydia psittaci*	Infected birds
Q fever	*Coxiella burnetii*	Infected animals
Histoplasmosis	*Histoplasma capsulatum*	Infected soil, bats
Coccidioidomycosis	*Coccidioides immitis*	Soil
Cryptococcosis	*Cryptococcus neoformans*	Soil, pigeons
Plague	*Yersinia pestis*	Infected insect vectors, animals
Melioidiosis	*Pseudomonas pseudomallei*	Soil
Tularemia	*Francisella tularensis*	Infected animals, ticks

also affect the lungs (Chapter 38), e.g., *histoplasmosis*, especially in the Mississippi and Ohio river valleys, particularly where the soil has been enriched by bird droppings; *coccidioidomycosis* in the deserts of the southwestern United States; and cryptococcosis, in areas frequented by pigeons. The latter is frequently but not exclusively found in individuals who are immunocompromised.

Diagnosis

There is considerable overlap in the clinical manifestations of pneumonia but the astute physician may be able to use some refined clinical and epidemiologic indicators to arrive at a specific diagnosis. For instance, pneumococcal pneumonia may occur at any age, but has a predilection for the very young and the elderly. It usually has a rapid onset and an acute course. *H. influenzae* is suspected in children under age 4 and in adults with chronic lung disease. Lobar involvement is less common with staphylococci than with pneumococci, and progression is even more rapid. Patients with staphylococcal pneumonia are more likely to belong to several risk groups: debilitated nursing home residents, individuals who have recently had influenza, intravenous drug users, or children under 1 year of age. Patients with cystic fibrosis may also suffer from staphylococcal pneumonia, although it is most frequently caused by *Pseudomonas aeruginosa*. Pneumonia caused by *K. pneumoniae* occurs in hospital or nursing home residents, but is also seen in the community, usually in debilitated individuals. Since *K. pneumonia* is also a necrotizing process, the sputum is often bloody, resembling currant jelly.

A markedly elevated neutrophil count is generally indicative of bacterial infection, especially when accompanied by an increased proportion of immature cells. The examination of sputum is often quite revealing. For example, thick yellow or greenish sputum is suggestive of bacterial infection. The presence of squamous epithelial cells in large numbers indicates contamination by oropharyngeal contents, and a culture of such a specimen may yield misleading information. Large numbers of neutrophils indicate bacterial infection—although their absence does not rule it out, especially if the patient is neutropenic. Finding a predominant organism in the Gram stain may point towards the etiologic agent. Thus, lancet-shaped Gram positive diplococci suggest pneumococci; large round Gram positive cocci in clusters, staphylococci; small pleomorphic Gram negative rods, H. flu; and larger and thicker Gram negative rods, enterics such as *K. pneumoniae*. Unfortunately, the microscopic examination of sputum has limitations: Some patients cannot produce sputum, and the agents of Legionnaires' disease and mycoplasma pneumonia are not visible by routine microscopy.

Sputum culture has other limitations. First, mycobacteria, mycoplasma, and viruses require specialized culture methods. Second, many of the bacteria that frequently cause pneumonia are also common colonizers of the upper airway, so that culturing these organisms is not proof that they are causing illness. This particular problem may be circumvented, though with difficulty, by bypassing the contaminated upper airways and obtaining the specimen directly from the site of infection in the lower airways. This can be done in several ways. One is transtracheal aspiration, a procedure in which a large bore needle is inserted through the cricoid membrane of the trachea and used to aspirate secretions. This technique is not widely used because of its potential complications. A second method, used only occasionally, is transthoracic needle aspiration, usually under fluoroscopic or computed tomographic guidance. The most widely employed method for obtaining a specimen from the lower airways is by bronchoscopy, or passage of an endoscope into the bronchial tree. This allows visualization of the airway as well as aspiration of material for specimens. Bronchoscopy, however, is also too impractical and invasive to be performed on all patients with pneumonia before beginning therapy.

Treatment

The importance of making a specific etiological diagnosis in pneumonia is that treatment differs markedly depending on the causative agent. For example, penicillin is highly effective for pneumococcal pneumonia but would be ineffective in most cases of *Mycoplasma*, staphylococcal, or *Haemophilus* pneumonia. It would certainly not be effective for tuberculosis or histoplasmosis.

The tremendous diversity of potential etiologies makes it impractical to discuss the coverage for all possible agents. What should be remembered is that careful consideration of clinical and epidemiological factors often allows the physician to institute a rational and effective plan while efforts are under way to establish a specific microbiological diagnosis.

SUGGESTED READINGS

Brain JD, Proctor DF, Reid LM, (eds): *Respiratory Defense Mechanisms.* New York, Marcel Dekker, 1977.

Denny FW, Clyde WA, Jr: Acute lower respiratory infections in non-hospitalized children. *J Pediatr* 108:635, 1986.

Dick EC, Jennings LC, Mink KA, Wartgow CD, Inhorn SL: Aerosal transmission of rhinovirus colds. *J Infect Dis* 156:442–448, 1987.

Green GM: In defense of the lung. *Am Rev Respirat Dis* 102s:691–705, 1970.

Huxley EJ, Viroslav J, Gray WR, Pierce AK: Pharyngeal aspiration in normal adults and patients with depressed consciousness. *Am J Med* 64:564–568, 1978.

Pennington JE (ed): *Respiratory Infections: Diagnosis and Management.* New York, Raven Press, 1983.

Sande MA, Hudson LD, Root RK, (eds): *Respiratory Infections.* New York, Churchill Livingstone, 1986.

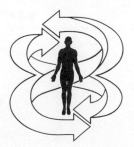

Digestive System

46

D.M. Thea
G. Keusch

The digestive system is a microbiologist's paradise. In health or disease, it is a microbial garden of unsurpassed variety and complexity. It varies in degrees of colonization from the "buggiest" parts of the body, at both ends, to the nearly sterile environment of the small intestine and accessory glands (Fig. 46.1). The pathway through the alimentary tract is open, except for the stomach, an effective sterilization chamber that limits entry of microorganisms to the small bowel and beyond.

A community of perhaps 400 distinct species of bacteria, fungi and protozoa form the resident flora of the normal gastrointestinal tract. Bacteria in the colon are present at approximately one tenth their theoretical density limit ($\sim 10^{12}$/g) and, amazingly, produce no intestinal dysfunction. On the contrary, they form a symbiotic relationship with the host (Chapter 9). This is achieved with remarkable stability and constancy of the microbial population. While we merely furnish it with foodstuff, it provides a number of essential services for us. Among these are accessory digestive functions such as converting unabsorbable carbohydrates to absorbable organic acids, supplying essential vitamin K, and aiding in the reabsorption and conservation of estrogens and androgens excreted in the bile. The mere presence of the normal organisms helps us resist colonization by invading pathogens.

The frequency of infections of the digestive system varies from the most prevalent human infectious disease, dental caries, to fairly common diarrheas and food poisoning, to unusual opportunistic infections of immune compromised pa-

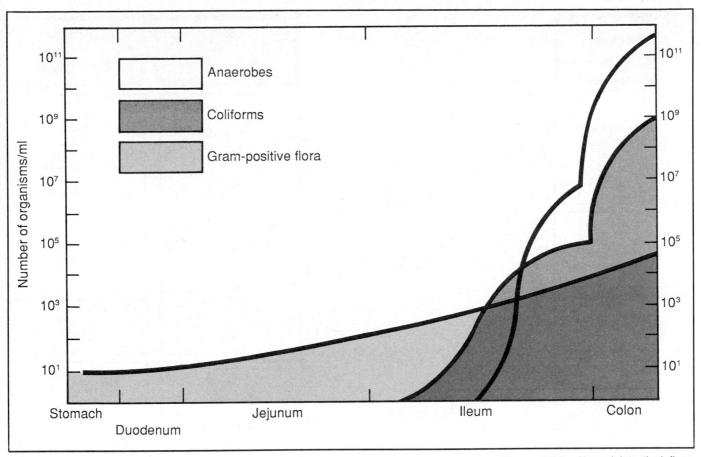

Figure 46.1. Normal intestinal flora. The GI tract and typical numbers of bacteria at the main sites.

tients. Worldwide, diarrheal diseases are a far greater cause of morbidity and mortality than are the more familiar diseases of the industrialized nations (heart disease, cancer and strokes). Unfortunately, infants and small children are disproportionately affected, especially in the parts of the world that have poor sanitation and nutrition. Despite a significant decline in the mortality associated with diarrheal disease in the United States, it remains among the most common complaints of people seen in general medical practice. Along with middle ear infections, it is the bane of day-care centers ("ears and rears").

Infections of this system range in severity from asymptomatic or silent infections (e.g., polio) through mild diarrhea (e.g., "staph" food poisoning) to life-threatening loss of fluid and electrolytes (e.g., cholera) or severe mucosal ulceration complicated by intestinal perforation (e.g., bacillary dysentery). Likewise, the nature and clinical manifestations of these infections are variable. This is not surprising when one considers the striking local differentiation along the alimentary tract and in the associated hepatobiliary tree and pancreas (Fig. 46.2).

ENTRY

Each portion of the alimentary tract has special anatomic, physiological, and biochemical barriers to infection (Fig. 46.2). The most general impediment to infective agents is an unbroken mucosal epithelium covering all parts of this system

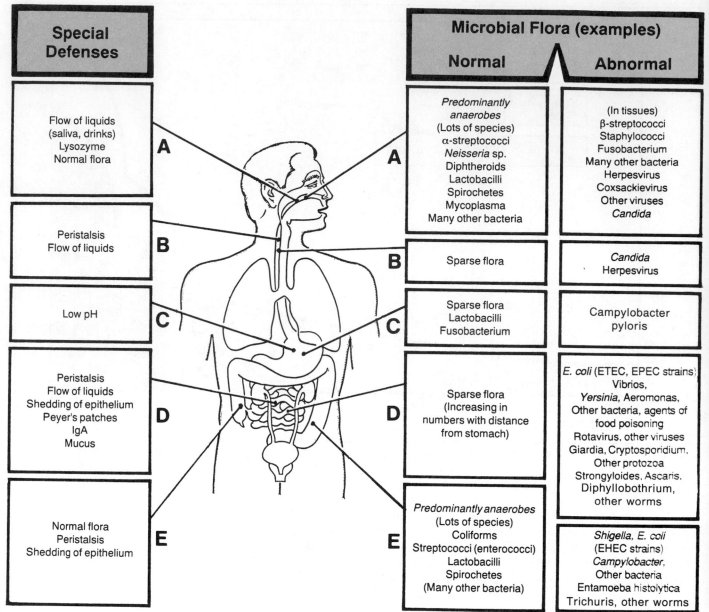

Figure 46.2. A microbiological overview of the digestive system.

(Fig. 46.3). Its importance is illustrated when people receive ionizing radiation or cytotoxic cancer chemotherapy, which interferes with the normal replacement of sloughed epithelial cells. One of the earliest manifestations of damage is nausea, vomiting and mucositis, superficial ulcerations of the mucosa of the entire gastrointestinal tract. Members of the normal flora can now reach deep tissues and may even disseminate through the bloodstream to other organs.

Some defense mechanisms, such as *mucus formation* and *gut motility*, hinder the adherence of microorganisms to the epithelial wall. In the intestine, the mucus layer functions as a mechanical obstacle to protect the epithelium; it also coats bacteria which makes it easier to pass them along by peristalsis. *Glycocalyx*, the glycoprotein and polysaccharide layer that covers the surface of cells, is many

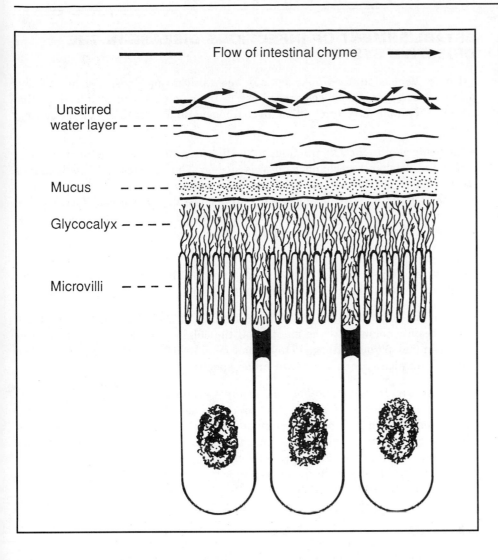

Flow of intestinal chyme ⟶

Unstirred
water layer – – – –

Mucus – – – –

Glycocalyx – – – –

Microvilli – – – –

Figure 46.3. Schematic representation of host barriers faced by intestinal pathogens. (From Cawley JF: Infectious diarrhea. *Am J Med* 78 (Suppl 6B):65–71, 1985.)

"bacterial body lengths" in depth and has "decoy" binding sites which entrap certain invading organisms. *Bile* plays an important role in selecting which bacteria and viruses are able to colonize the intestines. As expected, both organisms of the normal flora and common intestinal pathogens are resistant to the detergent action of bile salts. Most enteric viruses, polio or hepatitis A for example, lack a lipid-containing envelope that could make them sensitive to bile. Certain bacteria, e.g., the typhoid bacilli, are so highly bile resistant that they can even grow in the gallbladder.

A number of cellular and soluble factors have less well understood defensive functions. For instance, there is evidence that secretory IgA immunoglobulins and the protein lactoferrin in mother's milk help prevent colonization of the infant by certain bacteria. While it is likely that IgA has a similar function in adults, it has been difficult to prove its role. The intestinal tract is also the final stopping point for white blood cells, especially neutrophils. It is not known if exit of these cells into the lumen of the gut plays a role in controlling pathogens or in maintaining the balance with the normal flora. Could this be a reason why the gut is so often the source of systemic infections in granulocytopenic patients?

ESTABLISHMENT OF INFECTIOUS DISEASE IN THE DIGESTIVE SYSTEM

Under what conditions do infectious agents overcome these defense mechanisms? Several circumstances predispose to the establishment of infectious disease in the alimentary tract either by pathogens or by members of the normal flora:

- *Anatomic alterations.* Obstructions to the flow of liquids remove one of the most powerful defensive mechanisms of this system. Thus, stones in the gallbladder that impede the flow of bile predispose the biliary tree to infections. The presence of large diverticuli (intestinal outpouches) or the surgical formation of intestinal "blind loops" creates sites with reduced flow of intestinal contents, leading to bacterial overgrowth and metabolic derangements.

- *Changes in stomach acidity.* Alteration of the acid barrier of the stomach by disease, surgery, or drugs increases the survival of pathogens across this organ and may lead to bacterial infection downstream.

- *Alterations in the normal flora.* In the regions of the digestive tract that are most heavily colonized—the mouth and the colon—changes in the density of the flora may permit pathogens to become established. The most frequent cause of such an alteration is the use of broad-spectrum antibiotics.

- *Encounter with specific pathogenic agents.* Certain bacteria, viruses, protozoa, and helminths cause disease even in the absence of predisposing factors. Note that at each site, pathogens must be able to resist the specific local defenses. In general, they all resist stomach acid and have certain virulence factors (e.g., pili for adhesion, toxin production). However, microorganisms face different survival problems in the mouth, the small intestine or the colon and possess different specific attributes.

DAMAGE

The signs and symptoms of infections related to the digestive system are produced in several general ways:

- *Pharmacological action.* Some bacteria produce toxins that alter normal intestinal function without causing lasting damage to their target cells. Typical examples are the enterotoxins made by *Vibrio cholerae* or by some strains of *Escherichia coli*, which provoke copious watery diarrhea. Because the small bowel is primarily responsible for absorbing most of the 9 to 10 liters of fluid that pass through the gut each day, small reductions in its absorptive capacity result in arrival of large amounts of fluid to the colon, overwhelming its relatively modest absorptive capacity. "Overflow" diarrhea results; it may rapidly lead to profound dehydration and electrolyte loss, as seen in cholera.

- *Local inflammation.* Any site of the alimentary tract may become inflamed as the consequence of microbial invasion. In many instances the invasion is limited to the epithelial layer but may spread to contiguous tissue and beyond. The mouth is often affected, usually in the gums, by infections caused by bacteria that normally reside in the gingival pocket (periodontitis). In the intestine infections causing inflammation can result in dysentery.

- *Deep tissue invasion.* This takes place because certain organisms have the ability to spread to adjacent tissues and to enter the blood or lymph. Examples are the worm *Strongyloides* and the protozoan *Entamoeba*, which are capable of burrowing through the intestinal wall, or *Salmonella*, which penetrates the lymphatics and may eventually reach the bloodstream. Interestingly, *Strongyloides* itself is often colonized by gut bacteria, as a result invasion with this worm can result in polymicrobial septicemia.

- *Perforation.* When the mucosal epithelia are perforated, the normal flora spills into sterile areas and invades deep tissue, often with serious consequences. Thus, rupture of an inflamed appendix may lead to peritonitis, and traumatic perforation of the esophagus to mediastinitis.

The variety of infectious diseases of this system is staggering. Your task will be simplified by keeping in mind the pathophysiological steps involved in establishing an infectious disease. Because they differ greatly in their clinical manifestations, we divide this chapter into infectious diseases of the principal sites of infection, the mouth, stomach, biliary tree, and intestines.

THE MOUTH

Virtually all the pathogens of the alimentary tract enter through the mouth. It is the portal that allows microorganisms to enter the body aboard food, fluids, or fingers. What are the specific defenses of the mouth?

- The *nonpathogenic resident flora*, including bacteria, fungi (e.g., *Candida*), and protozoa (e.g., the ameba *Entamoeba gingivalis*). These organisms resist the establishment of newcomers both by the occupancy of suitable sites and by the production of acids and other metabolic inhibitors.

- *The mechanical action of saliva and the tongue.* We produce more than a liter of saliva per day which, with assistance from the tongue, mechanically dislodges and flushes microorganisms from mucosal surfaces. Should salivary flow be reduced, as with dehydration or during fasting, the bacterial content of saliva increases markedly.

Table 46.1
Composition of the Intestinal Flora of Adult Humans

Bacterial Species	Bacterial Concentration (log number $_{10}$/ml or g)			
	Stomach	Jejunum	Ileum	Colon
Total Viable Count	$0-10^3$	$0-10^5$	10^2-10^7	$10^{10}-10^{12}$
Aerobes or facultative anaerobes				
Enterobacteria	$0-10^2$	$0-10^3$	10^2-10^7	10^4-10^{10}
Streptococci	$0-10^2$	$0-10^4$	10^2-10^6	10^5-10^{10}
Staphylococci	$0-10^2$	$0-10^3$	10^2-10^5	10^4-10^9
Lactobacilli	$0-10^3$	$0-10^4$	10^2-10^5	10^4-10^{10}
Fungi	$0-10^2$	$0-10^2$	10^2-10^4	10^4-10^6
Anaerobes				
Bacteroides	Rare	$0-10^3$	10^3-10^7	$10^{10}-10^{12}$
Bifidobacteria	Rare	$0-10^4$	10^3-10^9	10^8-10^{12}
Streptococci	Rare	$0-10^3$	10^2-10^6	$10^{10}-10^{12}$
Clostridia	Rare	Rare	10^2-10^6	10^6-10^{11}
Eubacteria	Rare	Rare	Rare	10^9-10^{12}

From Keusch GT, Gorbach SL: Ecology of the gastrointestinal tract. In Berkse et al (eds): *Gastroenterology*, ed 4. Philadelphia, WB Saunders, 1985.

- *Antimicrobial constituents of saliva*, notably lysozyme and secreted antibodies. As mentioned above, secretory IgA selectively inhibits the adherence of certain bacteria to mucosal cells. Lysozyme is effective mainly against Gram positive bacteria.

Several properties allow bacteria to evade these host defenses. Some are able to stick to teeth or mucosal surfaces. Attachment to teeth is not direct, but rather to a coating of sticky macromolecules, mainly proteins, the *dental pellicle*. The bacteria themselves produce polysaccharides that help in adherence. For example, *Streptococcus mutans* transforms sucrose into polysaccharides (dextrans and levans), which are particularly sticky. They are layered on the pellicle to form a matrix that allows further adherence of other organisms. The result is *dental plaque*, one of the densest collections of bacteria in the body—and perhaps the first human microbial flora to be seen under a microscope by van Leeuwenhoek in the 17th century. Microbial metabolism in plaque transforms dietary sugar into acids, mainly lactic acid, that are responsible for dental caries (cavities). Other bacteria, especially strict anaerobes, reside in the gingival crevices between the tooth and gum, where they evade the washing effects of the saliva and of normal tooth brushing.

The bacteria of the indigenous oral flora are not highly virulent, but when there is a break in the mucosal barrier, such as with advanced gingivitis (*periodontal disease*), they may invade surrounding healthy tissue. This is also a likely portal of entry of α-hemolytic streptococci that cause subacute bacterial endocarditis in patients with rheumatic heart disease. A synergistic cooperation among several different types of bacteria, both aerobic and strictly anaerobic, leads to a severe and rapidly advancing mixed infection of the soft tissues about the oral cavity. *Ludwig's angina*, a polymicrobial infection of the sublingual and submandibular spaces that arises from a tooth (often the second and third mandibular molars), is a cellulitis—an infection of submucosal or subcutaneous connective tissue, which may at times progress rapidly, compromise the airway, and threaten the patient with asphyxiation.

A Case of Thrush

Cynthia, a 7-month-old girl, was treated by her pediatrician for a middle ear infection. She was given a 7-day course of a penicillin, amoxicillin, which cleared the infection within 4 days. Antibiotics were continued, but on the sixth day of therapy the mother noticed that the child was irritable and feeding poorly. During a follow-up visit at the clinic, her pediatrician noted several creamy white, curd-like patches on the tongue and buccal mucosa. When scraped, they were clearly painful and left a raw, bleeding surface. Microscopic examination showed filamentous elements typical of fungi. This permitted the diagnosis of thrush, or oral candidiasis. Antibiotics were stopped, a topical antifungal solution was administered, and the patches disappeared within two days.

Pathobiology

The white patches adherent to the oral mucosa consisted of *pseudomembranes* made up of the yeast *Candida*, mixed with desquamated epithelial cells, leukocytes, oral bacteria, necrotic tissue, and food debris. *Candida albicans* and related species are yeasts found in the environment which establish themselves in the alimentary tract early in life (Chapter 38). The adult vagina is commonly colonized with these organisms, and they may be acquired by the baby during delivery. Small numbers of *Candida* live harmlessly in the alimentary tract until the balance between indigenous bacterial flora and host defenses is upset. In the case of Cynthia, this occurred with the administration of antibiotics, which killed many of the normal oral bacteria and allowed *Candida* to proliferate.

Candida exploits changes in the normal host flora, breaks in the mucous membrane, decreased number or function of neutrophils, or defects in complement, humoral or cellular immunity. Predisposing conditions for oral and other forms of candidiasis include endocrine disturbances, malnutrition, malignancy, immunosuppressive drugs or infections, and genetic abnormalities of the immune system. Normal individuals are also frequently affected. *Candida* vaginitis is commonly encountered in postpubertal women who are taking broad-spectrum antibiotics, often because of urinary tract infections. The prolonged use of inhaled steroids for asthmatics may also predispose to candidal overgrowth in the mouth. In the more pronounced forms of immunodeficiency, the organism may disseminate through the bloodstream and infect virtually any organ system.

Candida may also invade the esophagus, an organ little prone to infection. Candidal esophagitis is seen in patients with specific T cell abnormalities, such as chronic mucocutaneous candidiasis or AIDS. The differential diagnosis of esophagitis in immune compromised patients includes infection by herpes simplex type 1 virus (HSV). This is the second most common infection of the esophagus and has clinical manifestations similar to those caused by *Candida*.

Diagnosis

Thrush is characteristic in appearance and the diagnosis can usually be made on inspection. It is confirmed by examination of scraped material under a microscope and detection of characteristic pseudohyphae. Culture is not necessary and often misleading, since *Candida* is a commensal and can be cultured from the mouths of many normal people.

Prevention and Treatment

Because candidal colonization of the gastrointestinal tract is frequent, prevention and treatment consist primarily of correcting predisposing factors and avoiding the unnecessary use of antibiotics. Candidiasis of the mouth is usually superficial and responds to the topical application of antifungal agents such as nystatin. If the infection reaches deeper than the mucosa, it may be necessary to use a systemic antifungal agent, such as intravenous amphotericin B.

THE STOMACH

Until recently, the stomach has received little attention as a locus of infections of the alimentary tract. It was not considered to be infected often, although it was always appreciated that it plays an important role in protecting the gut further downstream by its secretion of acid. The vast majority of oral or food-borne bacteria, washed with saliva into the stomach, are destroyed under these conditions.

In some individuals the stomach is indeed sterile, and in most others the concentration of bacteria is very low, generally less than 10^3 bacteria/ml. Among the bacteria that are found in the stomach, the predominant ones are Gram positives, e.g., *Streptococcus, Staphylococcus, Lactobacillus,* and *Peptostreptococcus.* In the normal stomach there are very few enteric Gram negative rods, *Bacteroides* or *Clostridium*—organisms typically associated with the lower gastrointestinal tract.

It is now believed that gastric infections nevertheless occur and much more commonly than was previously thought. A newly identified bacterial species, *Campylobacter pyloris,* is associated with and may be involved in the production of gastritis and perhaps peptic ulcers. It has yet to be determined conclusively whether this is a true pathogen or merely a commensal organism on a previously altered mucosa. However, suggestive evidence is mounting: It has been isolated from the gastric mucosa of 95% of patients with peptic ulcer disease and virtually all those with active chronic gastritis. This organism is rarely found in healthy people. A volunteer inoculated with *C. pyloris* developed gastritis, which cleared after being given antibiotics. Will gastric ulcers enter the ranks of infectious diseases?

Some bacteria, including pathogens, if introduced into the stomach with food, will survive and enter the small intestine alive. This depends largely on the buffering effects of food, especially in patients who do not produce normal amounts of gastric hydrochloric acid because of disease, partial or total gastrectomy, drug therapy (e.g., H_2-blockers), or antacids consumption. The infective dose of cholera bacilli or salmonellae in human volunteers, for example, was 10,000-fold lower when the organisms were administered together with 2 g of sodium bicarbonate.

When gastric acidity is chronically decreased, a condition known as achlorhydria, the stomach usually becomes colonized by enteric Gram negative rods. This could have two important consequences:

• Increase in the number of enteric bacteria in the small bowel, which contributes to the development of a disease called the bacterial overgrowth syndrome (see below).

• Regurgitation of the abnormal gastric flora, which becomes a source of nosocomial (hospital acquired) aspiration pneumonia (Chapter 57).

THE BILIARY TREE AND THE LIVER

Infections of the gallbladder (*cholecystitis*) are a frequent complication of obstruction to the flow of bile due, for example, to gallstones. The clinical presentation is often sudden and dramatic. The hallmark is pain, which may build to a crescendo and then subside, only to soon recur. This pattern is called *biliary colic.* Nausea and vomiting are usual accompaniments and may be intractable. The majority of cases have shaking chills, high spiking fever, and jaundice due to obstruction of the duct. These manifestations may become more severe if the obstruction also involves the common bile duct. In these cases, the infection and inflammation may ascend to the intrahepatic bile ducts, a condition known as *ascending cholangitis.*

The ascending spread of a bacterial infection to the liver parenchyma may result in abscess formation. Given the large amount of blood filtered by the liver, seeding may also occur in cases of bacteremia. Among the bacteria that cause liver infections are those derived from the bowel, which are carried to the liver by the portal system. Primary bacterial infections of the liver parenchyma itself are not common, perhaps contravened by the enormous defensive capacity of the Kupffer cells. Bacteria that infect the liver tend to be intracellular pathogens that survive life in macrophages to cause granulomatous infections. Examples are the agents of typhoid fever, Q fever, brucellosis, and tuberculosis. In most instances, the lesions characteristic of these diseases are not found primarily in the liver.

Infectious diseases of the liver will not be discussed in detail here. The most important ones are due to hepatitis viruses (Chapter 32). The liver is also the site of parasitic infections such as amebiasis (Chapter 41), schistosomiasis (Chapter 42), leishmaniasis (Chapter 40), and others. An important though clinically silent part of the life cycle of the malarial parasites takes place here.

Case

Ms. F., an obese 48-year-old mother of eight with a vague history of intermittent "stomach problems", awoke with moderate midepigastric pain. Approximately 2 hours before going to bed she had eaten a large meal of fried chicken and vegetables. The pain soon shifted to her right upper quadrant and was occasionally felt in the area of the right scapula. She vomited several times and then improved but had residual pain for several days with numerous similar but less intense attacks. By the sixth day she felt again sick and developed jaundice and a shaking chill. In the emergency room she was in obvious pain and had a temperature of 40°C. Her skin was slightly yellowish. There was marked tenderness to palpation of the right upper quadrant of her abdomen. An 8 cm tubular mass was felt under the margin of the right ribs. Her white blood cell count was elevated (14,000/μl), suggesting a bacterial infection. Her liver function tests were abnormal—in particular serum bilirubin and alkaline phosphatase were elevated—suggesting biliary obstruction.

Blood was drawn for culturing and antibiotic therapy was begun. An ultrasound examination showed that her gallbladder was markedly distended and contained several stones. Other tests showed that the gallbladder was not emptying properly. The diagnosis of acute cholecystitis was made. Within 36 hours of admission the pain improved and the fever resolved. The blood cultures grew E. coli. The patient was scheduled for surgery to remove the affected gallbladder and stones.

Pathobiology

Both infections of the gallbladder, *cholecystitis*, and of the bile duct, *cholangitis*, are secondary consequences of obstruction. Usually, the process begins not with infection but with obstruction and distention. Under these conditions, bile constituents become concentrated, which may initiate a cycle of inflammation and damage in the gallbladder wall. The disease may not progress, but the process increases the probability that infection may develop. It is common to obtain from patients with these diseases a history of recurrent attacks of biliary colic, resulting from obstruction of the biliary outlet. It is possible that Ms. F.'s vague "stomach problems" of the past were episodes of mild biliary colic caused by transient and/or partial obstructions of the duct by her gallstones. In time her gallbladder became infected and the character of her illness changed.

Once bacterial infection becomes established, tissue damage may be accelerated by the resulting inflammatory response. Healing is unlikely to occur without relief of the obstruction, spontaneous or surgical, and specific antimicrobial therapy.

A particularly rapid and severe form of gallbladder infection is seen in patients with compromised arterial blood supply to the gallbladder wall, such as diabetics or the elderly. If the infecting organisms invade the gallbladder wall, they may produce a condition called *emphysematous cholecystitis*. It is distinguished by rapid clinical onset, extensive gangrene, presence of gas in the gallbladder (when caused by gas forming species such as *Clostridia*), and high mortality. Surgical removal of the gallbladder (cholecystectomy) is indicated because of the frequent occurrence of gangrene, high risk of perforation, and extensive peritonitis.

The typical clinical presentation of cholangitis is similar to cholecystitis, as in Ms. F's case, but is more consistently accompanied by fever, chills, jaundice, and pain with ascent into the liver. The most common obstructing causes are stones, strictures, and neoplasms. Considerable pressure built up within the duct seems to be a prerequisite for infection. Experiments in dogs have shown that the normal common ductal pressure of 70 mm H_2O must be raised to 250 mm H_2O before *E. coli* injected into the bloodstream produce infection in the gallbladder. It is not known why the resulting distention facilitates bacterial invasion of the duct wall, but microscopic tears are an obvious possibility.

Organisms that infect the gallbladder and bile duct are usually derived from the gastrointestinal tract, *E. coli* being the single most frequent one. Approximately 40% of these infections are caused by a mixed facultative and strictly anaerobic flora. They ascend from the duodenum, which normally contains few microorganisms but becomes colonized where there is bacterial overgrowth in the stomach (achlorhydria) or the small bowel (blind loops, diverticula, obstruction).

Typhoid bacilli have an unusual predilection for the gallbladder (Chapter 18). These organisms may persist for long times within or on the surface of the gallstones. They produce little or no inflammation, and the person may not be aware of being a carrier. All carriers, cognizant or not, shed bacteria into the environment and may infect other people.

Diagnosis

When the clinical presentation of cholecystitis is typical, as in the example of Ms. F., a tentative diagnosis of cholecystitis can be made on clinical grounds. Unfortunately, this disease is especially prone to misdiagnosis, since it often presents itself in a less typical form. Probably the most helpful test is an imaging technique that can reliably visualize obstruction or distention in the biliary system, such as ultrasound or radionuclide scanning. Direct culture of the infected bile is rarely performed, because of the difficulty in obtaining a specimen. Instead, microbiological diagnosis depends on growing bacteria from the blood.

Prevention and Treatment

Treatment should be individualized for each patient, but antibiotics should be started fast, without waiting for the blood culture results, if symptoms of the disease are severe. The drugs should be chosen for their activity against the usual intestinal facultative anaerobic flora and strict anaerobes, and should of course be started after blood cultures have been drawn. In any case, to effect a definitive cure, the underlying obstruction must be relieved. This may occur spontaneously or require surgery. The timing and need for surgery to remove stones and an inflamed gallbladder are controversial. There are sound arguments for both early and late cholecystectomy, although there is no disagreement on the need for surgery when there is threat of impending perforation or of emphysematous cholecystitis.

THE SMALL AND LARGE INTESTINES

We will now discuss diseases that illustrate the diversity of infectious problems of the gut, based on host factors and on virulence attributes of the organisms. Examples of other classic infections of the intestines caused by bacteria are discussed in Chapters 17 and 18, and by animal parasites in Chapters 41 and 43.

Bacterial Overgrowth Syndrome

The anatomy and physiology of our alimentary tract ensure that we have first crack at the food we eat (Fig. 46.2). Thanks to the sterilizing power of the stomach and the defenses of the small intestine, we absorb most of our nutrients without microbial competition. The human intestinal contents rich in unabsorbed sugars, fats, and other nutrients do not normally come in contact with large numbers of bacteria.

The presence of a large microbial biomass in the absorptive small intestine leads to competition for certain vitamins and malabsorption of fats. It produces a disease known as *bacterial overgrowth syndrome*. The study of bacterial overgrowth in the small intestine has helped us understand the normal relationship of the gut flora to gut function.

Case

Two years before the current illness, Mr. O., a 65-year-old male, had an operation for removal of a tumor that obstructed his stomach outlet. The surgeon removed part of the stomach and duodenum and connected the remainder of the stomach with the jejunum (gastrojejunostomy), bypassing the unresected duodenum. He subsequently developed chronic diarrhea and his weight dropped from 63 to 44 kg. His nutritional history indicated that his food intake was adequate and could not account for the weight loss. The diarrhea had recently become bulky, smelly, and greasy. He felt fatigued, was short of breath on exertion, and had numbness and tingling in the hands and feet. On examination he was extremely thin and appeared ill with a pale complexion.

Laboratory tests showed a severe anemia with large red blood cells ("megaloblastic" anemia) and leukopenia with many hypersegmented neutrophils. The serum level of fat soluble vitamins was depressed and that of vitamin B_{12} undetectable, although intrinsic factor was present in his gastric juice. Several tests of gastrointestinal function revealed malabsorption. He was diagnosed as suffering from bacterial overgrowth syndrome. (Although not done in this case, intubation of the small bowel might well have revealed about 10^9 B. fragilis and 10^6 E. coli per milliliter of bowel content). Fat-soluble vitamins and vitamin B_{12} were replaced, and Mr. O. was placed on a course of tetracycline. The diarrhea resolved and the tests of absorptive function improved. He continued on antibiotic therapy and over the next 2 months, he returned to his normal weight and felt entirely well.

Pathobiology

Prior surgery left this patient with a loop of small bowel removed from the main flow of intestinal contents. The result of this "blind loop" was stasis of the contents without the normal and continuous flushing action of the intestinal segment. The resulting bacterial proliferation led to impaired absorption of fats and fat-soluble vitamins (see below).

Bacterial overgrowth in the small intestine may also arise from a number of abnormalities that produce blind loops, other than surgical procedures or diverticuli. Motor abnormalities may severely depress peristalsis (diabetic neuropathy, scleroderma, gastric atony), or gastric achlorhydria may permit large bacterial inocula to reach the proximal small bowel. Under these conditions, bacterial overgrowth occurs very rapidly, another testimony to the sterilizing power of the stomach and the small intestine. As stagnation progresses, the small number of bacteria normally present increases dramatically. Careful anaerobic sampling of the small intestine in these conditions has revealed counts as high as 10^{10} bacteria/ml, levels comparable to those in the colon. By far, the most numerous bacteria and those most likely to be responsible for the physiological derangement are strict anaerobes, mainly *Bacteroides*.

Bacterial overgrowth in the small intestine may have the following effects:

- Increased fecal fat, *steatorrhea*, which is due primarily to malabsorption of fat as consequence of depletion of the bile acid pool. Why this depletion? Because bile acids such as cholic acid are normally conjugated with glycine or taurine in the liver, secreted in the bile and reabsorbed in the terminal ileum in the conjugated form. Bacterial overgrowth can deconjugate these compounds, making them unavailable for reabsorption.

- *Deficiency of vitamin B_{12}.* Normally, vitamin B_{12} or cobalamin is complexed with intrinsic factor from the stomach and absorbed in this form from the terminal ileum. With bacterial overgrowth, it is utilized by bacteria, making it unavailable for uptake by the host. With prolonged B_{12} malabsorption (longer than 1 year), endogenous stores are depleted, and cellular systems with a high rate of turnover and DNA synthesis (bone marrow, CNS, gut epithelium) are severely impaired. The results are megaloblastic anemia and structural gut abnormalities. The epithelial villi are shortened due to decreased turnover and atrophy of enterocytes, decreasing the absorptive area. Thus, bacterial overgrowth sets off a cascade of malabsorptive events. Vitamin B_{12} is also required for myelin synthesis, and its deficiency results in degeneration of the spinal cord, producing a classical neurological syndrome.

- *Diarrhea*, the excess of fecal water and electrolyte excretion. This is not seen in all patients with this condition, but usually results from the degradation of unabsorbed carbohydrates in the colon by the normal flora, resulting in an increased concentration of osmotically active solutes. Diarrhea then results from this osmotic load since water will move across the mucosa into the lumen.

- *Malabsorption of vitamins A and D.* Malabsorption of fat-soluble vitamins, particularly A and D, causes severe visual disturbance (night blindness) and softening of the bones (osteomalacia). Interestingly, vitamin K deficiency does not usually occur. The reduced absorption of this other fat-soluble vitamin is offset by the markedly increased vitamin production by the plentiful bacteria— ordinarily our main source of vitamin K.

Diagnosis and Treatment

This condition is usually diagnosed when malabsorption and nutritional deficiencies are present together with predisposing anatomic or physiological conditions, such as blind intestinal loops. Treatment requires correction of the surgical or medical predisposing condition in conjunction with careful nutritional repletion and, most importantly, broad-spectrum antibiotic therapy. This condition has a tendency to relapse and repeated courses of therapy may be necessary.

Diarrhea and Dysentery

Diarrhea is not easy to define: It is caused by some infections but is also seen in a large number of noninfectious conditions. It may be caused by different mechanisms and manifest itself in different forms. Dysentery is a more circumscribed term used for inflammatory disorders, mainly of the colon.

Diarrhea can be considered an adaptive mechanism, developed by the body to rid itself of noxious material (or by the microorganisms to ensure their transfer from one host to another). There is an obvious if teleological analogy with vomiting, which is used to rid the stomach of noxious material. In the "old days", both events were elicited enthusiastically in households by giving the children either tincture of ipecac or castor oil for any number of reasons. It used to be part of growing up.

The cases presented here illustrate distinctive ecological features of the pathogens or of their interactions with the host.

Case 1. Vibrio cholerae

Approximately 2 days after returning from Mardi Gras in New Orleans, Mr. V., a 24-year-old student who was the runner up in the raw oyster eating contest, abruptly started to vomit. Within hours he was restricted to the bathroom with voluminous and nearly continuous but painless watery diarrhea. Soon thereafter he became lightheaded, with a rapid pulse and was prostrate. Later that evening his roommate brought him to the emergency room, where he was found to be afebrile but profoundly dehydrated, with severely altered levels of serum electrolytes.

In the hospital, it was noticed that his stool had the appearance of "rice water" (so called because of the numerous flecks of mucus in a slightly yellow fluid), without blood or bile. Microscopic examination revealed no white blood cells. Curiously, the stool had a sweetish smell, very different from that of normal. Intravenous rehydration was administered initially and then switched to an oral rehydration solution. The physician requested that the laboratory look for Vibrio cholerae and stool was cultured on a special medium called TCBS agar. A stool culture became positive for V. cholerae on the second hospital day and he was diagnosed as suffering from cholera. Stool volume had diminished somewhat by this time but because it was still brisk, he was given tetracycline for 2 days. By the end of the fourth hospital day he was discharged with all symptoms and abnormalities resolved.

Case 2. Shigella sonnei

Tommy, a 4-year-old attending a community day-care center, became irritable and developed watery diarrhea. His mother noted a low-grade fever and put him to bed. About 24 hours later he was worse, with a fever of 40.0°C and complained of abdominal pain, mostly in the left lower quadrant. His diarrhea decreased in volume but increased in frequency and was obviously painful. Because his stool contained blood, mucus and pus, his mother brought Tommy to the pediatrician, who noted that the child was mildly dehydrated and had many white blood cells when his stool was examined microscopically. Tommy was the fifth child with similar complaints from the same day-care center seen by the pediatrician that day. Shigella sonnei was cultured from the stool of each of them, permitting the diagnosis of an outbreak of bacillary dysentery. Since these isolates were all resistant to ampicillin, Tommy was given trimethoprim and sulfamethoxazole for 5 days. All symptoms resolved 4 days later.

Case 3. Rotavirus

Mary Ann, a 7-month-old, was recently switched from breast to bottle feeding. Usually a satisfied and happy child, she became irritable, began to vomit, and had a low-grade fever. Mild upper respiratory symptoms also developed, with cough, nasal discharge, and pharyngitis. The gastrointestinal symptoms persisted for 2 days and she was brought to the pediatrician who made the diagnosis of rotavirus gastroenteritis by detecting viral antigen in the stool with an ELISA (enzyme-linked immunosorbent assay). Oral rehydration solution was given at home and Mary Ann made an uneventful recovery by the sixth day.

Case 4. Yersinia enterocolitica

Mr. C. took his family to southern Sweden to visit his parents who were dairy farmers outside Malmö. Sven, 5 years old, and Ingrid, 12 years old, enjoyed helping to care for the numerous domestic animals on the farm. They were also fond of eating home-cured meat and raw milk. Between 7 and 10 days of arrival all members of the C. family became ill. Sven developed watery, mucoid diarrhea with occasional flecks of blood, low-grade fever, and diffuse abdominal pain, all of which resolved spontaneously after 4 days. Ingrid's episode began similarly, but worsened after 3 days, when her pain localized to the right lower quadrant, associated with high fever and leucocytosis. At the hospital where she was brought, Ingrid's signs and symptoms suggested appendicitis. On surgery, her appendix was found to be normal, however the terminal ileum was inflamed, with many enlarged mesenteric lymph nodes.

Stool cultures done on admission were specially cultured at 25°C and grew Yersinia enterocolitica. By that time Ingrid had made a nearly complete recovery. Mr. C., like Sven, developed an acute mucoid diarrhea, abdominal pain, and fever which remitted by the fourth day. Three weeks later he developed painful swelling of several joints and a painful raised rash over his shins (erythema nodosum). In spite of lack of symptoms of ongoing gastrointestinal disease, his stool tested positive for Yersinia and he was treated with trimethoprim-sulfamethoxazole. The rash and arthritis slowly resolved but returned several months later and then spontaneously remitted for good.

As these cases illustrate, the gut reacts to infecting organisms in a number of ways: diarrhea, characterized by increased fluid and electrolyte loss in the stool, and dysentery, a bloody and often purulent enteric discharge accompanied by pain, fever, and cramps. These diseases are also distinguished by their anatomic site. Diarrhea is usually a disease of the small bowel and dysentery of the large bowel. They are generally caused by different agents, but some (e.g., Shigella) may cause either diarrhea or dysentery. The same organism may cause distinct clinical manifestations in people that differ only in age (e.g., Y. enterocolitica).

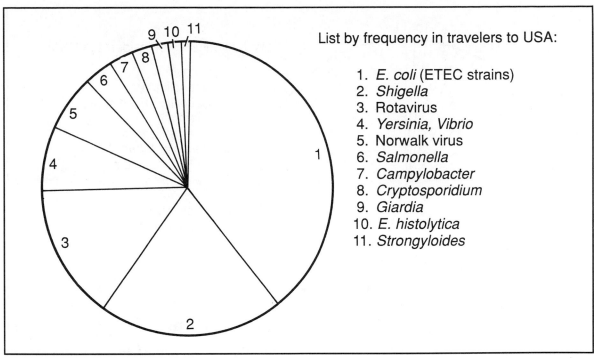

List by frequency in travelers to USA:

1. *E. coli* (ETEC strains)
2. *Shigella*
3. Rotavirus
4. *Yersinia, Vibrio*
5. Norwalk virus
6. *Salmonella*
7. *Campylobacter*
8. *Cryptosporidium*
9. *Giardia*
10. *E. histolytica*
11. *Strongyloides*

Figure 46.4. Distribution of agents of diarrhea in travelers to the United States.

Encounter

The list of intestinal pathogens keeps expanding as well-known organisms appear in unexpected frequency and in new settings, and as new ones are recognized (Figs. 46.4 and 46.5, Table 46.2). In previous chapters we discussed some of the more common agents of intestinal infections (Chapters 17, enteric bacteria in general; 18, *Salmonella*; 42, amebiasis; 41 and 43, intestinal worms; food poisoning is discussed in Chapter 58). To this list we should add a few more. *Campylobacter jejuni*, formerly thought to be a rare cause of diarrhea, is now known to be one of the most common intestinal pathogens throughout the world. Within the last several years, *Aeromonas hydrophila* and *Plesiomonas* sp. have become established as important agents of waterborne or shellfish-associated outbreaks. Likewise, the protozoan *Cryptosporidium* (Chapter 41) has emerged as one of the most common agents of childhood diarrhea here and abroad, whereas it was formerly thought to affect mainly animals (and occasionally animal handlers, or severely immunocompromised people). Diarrhea may be caused in large numbers of patients either by new viruses in normal hosts (calicivirus, astrovirus, enteric adenovirus), or by well-known viruses in immunocompromised patients (cytomegalovirus, herpes simplex virus). As the list of enteric pathogens lengthens and we begin to understand how they produce disease, the practical challenge of diagnosis and treatment increases.

The cases described illustrate some points of microbial ecology and how people encounter certain microorganisms. *V. cholerae* is normally found in brackish tidal waters. In the United States, it is endemic in the Gulf of Mexico near New Orleans and in the Pacific Ocean near Southern California. Shellfish can concentrate bacteria present in the water. Mr. V., the cholera patient, was no doubt infected by eating an enormous helping of oysters. He may have been susceptible due to

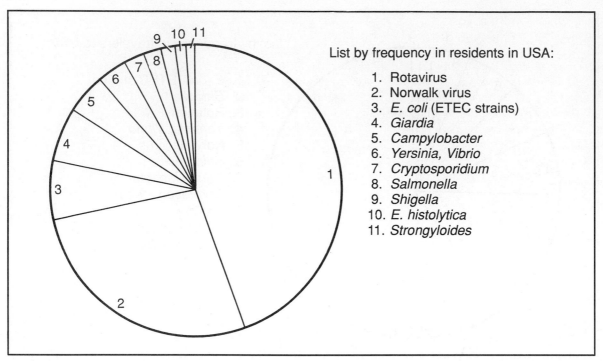

List by frequency in residents in USA:

1. Rotavirus
2. Norwalk virus
3. *E. coli* (ETEC strains)
4. *Giardia*
5. *Campylobacter*
6. *Yersinia, Vibrio*
7. *Cryptosporidium*
8. *Salmonella*
9. *Shigella*
10. *E. histolytica*
11. *Strongyloides*

Figure 46.5. Distribution of agents of diarrhea in residents of the United States.

achlorhydria (which was not evaluated) or he may have ingested an unfortunately high concentration of the organisms along with his plate of bivalves.

Unlike the cholera bacilli, which are environmental organisms, *Shigella* is found only in close association with humans. It takes relatively few organisms to cause shigellosis (also known as bacillary dysentery), one reason why the disease readily spreads between persons in close contact. The outbreak in a day-care center is typical of transmission between individuals sharing close quarters and often encountering fecal material. Thus, in the United States it is seen most frequently where hygiene breaks down, as in day-care centers or mental institutions. *Yersinia enterocolitica* has yet another ecological characteristic: It is often zoonotic (acquired from infected animals, see Chapter 55) and may be transmitted by drinking raw milk.

Table 46.2
Some Etiologic Agents of Diarrhea

Organism	Source
Escherichia coli	Human feces–contaminated foods
Salmonella	Contaminated foods, especially poultry products
Shigella	Fecal-oral
Campylobacter	Farm animals, contaminated food (e.g., raw eggs)
Yersinia enterocolitica	Animal products
Vibrio cholerae	Water and shellfish
Vibrio parahaemolyticus	Seafood (e.g., sardines, shellfish)
Bacillus cereus	Contaminated foods (e.g., recooked rice)
Clostridium perfringens	Contaminated foods (e.g., reheated meat)
Entamoeba histolytica	Human feces–contaminated foods
Giardia lamblia	Human feces–contaminated foods
Cryptosporidium	Fecal-oral and water

Diarrhea affecting infants aged 6 to about 24 months old is most likely of viral etiology, with rotavirus by far the most common. In temperate regions this is seasonal and produces "winter vomiting disease"; in tropical zones it occurs the year around. Adults may be silent carriers and introduce the virus into the family. In areas of the world where malnutrition is prevalent, severe diarrhea is associated with measles, which is highly contagious and kills large numbers of infants. The use of the measles vaccine in these populations may reduce the incidence of this life-threatening diarrhea.

A distinct group of enteric infections is seen in male homosexuals. The special conditions of anal intercourse permit the distal bowel to become infected by pathogens typically associated with sexually transmitted diseases. Proctocolitis due to *Neisseria gonorrhoeae*, *Chlamydia trachomatis*, herpes simplex virus, or *Treponema pallidum* has been recognized as the "gay bowel syndrome." The modifications of sexual practices among homosexual men initiated by the AIDS epidemic has diminished the frequency of these infections. More usual enteric pathogens, such as *Campylobacter*, *Shigella*, and *Entamoeba histolytica*, may be transmitted sexually on occasion.

Damage

With certain exceptions and overlaps, enteric infections can be distinguished by their anatomic location (Table 46.3) or the ability of the causative agents to invade tissues or produce a toxin or both. For this reason we will consider the small and large intestines separately.

Small Intestine

The mechanisms involved in diarrhea arising in the small intestine differ according to the type of pathogenic agent:

- Toxigenic bacteria which colonize in the intestine, e.g., *V. cholerae*, *E. coli*, and *C. perfringens*. Diarrhea is secondary to their production of toxins that may

Table 46.3
Clinical features of diarrheal disease

	Small Bowel	Large Bowel
Pathogens	*V. cholerae*	*Shigella*
	E. coli (LT/ST strains)	*E. coli* (EIEC, or invasive)
	Rotavirus	*Campylobacter*
	Norwalk agent (virus)	*Entamoeba histolytica*
	Giardia lamblia	
	Cryptosporidium	
Location of pain	Midabdomen	Lower abdomen, rectum
Volume of stool	Large	Small
Type of stool	Watery	Mucoid
Blood in stool	Rare	Common
WBCs in stool	Rare	Common (except in amebiasis)
Proctoscopy	Normal	Mucosal ulcers; hemorrhagic friable mucosa

Adapted from Gorbach SL: Infectious diarrhea, In Sleisenger WH, Fordtran SS (eds): *Gastrointestinal Disease. Pathophysiology, Diagnosis, Management.* Philadelphia, WB Saunders, 1983, Chapt. 57, p. 956.

cause the accumulation of cyclic nucleotides (cAMP, cGTP) which in turn stimulate net chloride secretion, and/or inhibit sodium uptake resulting in fluid loss. These mechanisms are discussed in detail in Chapter 7.

• Viruses that cause death of intestinal epithelial cells. The main agents are the rotaviruses (case 3), the so-called Norwalk agent, and enteroviruses. These viruses cause diarrhea by destroying enterocytes at the villi and not affecting those in the crypts. Normally the villus cells absorb electrolyte from the gut lumen, whereas crypt cells secrete chloride ions. Destroying the villus cells leads to decreased fluid absorption, which results in net secretion of fluid into the lumen. In addition, the microvillar membrane of the villus cells has a rich supply of disaccharidases. When the membrane is destroyed, disaccharides are not broken down or absorbed but pass into the colon, where they are metabolized by the bacterial flora to osmotically more active compounds. Thus, fluid is drawn into the lumen, which worsens the diarrhea and is partly responsible for a postenteritic syndrome seen in children in whom mild diarrhea persists for considerable time after the infection is resolved.

• Protozoa, *Giardia* and *Cryptosporidium*, which infect the small bowel (Chapter 41). It is not yet known if a toxin is involved or how these organisms colonize or invade the gut epithelium.

• Bacteria that cause true food poisoning. This form of diarrhea occurs when toxigenic bacteria (e.g., *Staphylococcus aureus, B. cereus*) are allowed to proliferate in food some time before it is eaten. This results in the accumulation of toxins which are ingested along with the food. Because bacterial multiplication in the body is not necessary, the effects are often felt within a few hours after the tainted meal is eaten. Examples are discussed in Chapter 58.

Clearly, not all infections of the small intestine produce a secretory diarrhea. Some organisms such as *Campylobacter jejuni* or *Yersinia enterocolitica* (as illustrated by the C. family, case 4) may infect the terminal ileum, producing a watery, sometimes bloody stool. The varied presentations of illness in the C. family also illustrate the age-related differences in disease caused by the same organism. *Y. enterocolitica* is somewhat unique in this respect. Little is known about the reasons for this. It infects primarily the terminal ileum and colon in all patients, but in infants less than 5 years of age it manifests itself as watery diarrhea. In older children, such as Sven, diarrhea may be minimal or absent and the mesenteric adenitis may mimic an acute appendicitis. Many of the adults get arthritis within weeks after the onset of diarrhea. This is probably an immunological phenomenon, as organisms are not found in the joint fluid. Interestingly, those affected by arthritis often possess the histocompatibility antigen HLA-B27.

Large Intestine

Bacterial pathogens that affect the large intestine tend to produce epithelial damage, mucosal inflammation, and dysentery. The major large bowel invasive pathogens causing dysentery are *Shigella, Salmonella, Campylobacter, Yersinia*, certain strains of *E. coli*, and *Entamoeba*. Because inflammation is prominent and usually located in the distal large bowel, pain often worsens with bowel movements (tenesmus). The mucosa is easily damaged and looks ulcerated when examined by proctoscopy (Fig. 46.6). The fecal effluent may initially be watery and substantial, and it decreases in volume and soon consists of blood, mucus, and

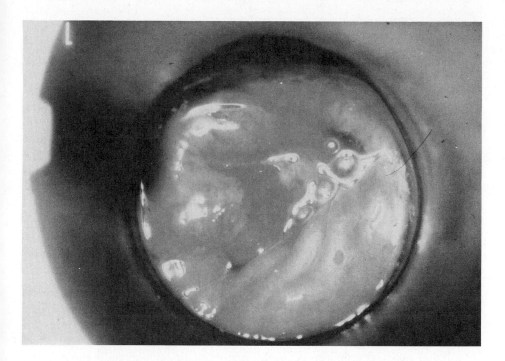

Figure 46.6. Proctoscopic view of the rectum of a patient with shigella dysentery. The inflamed bloody mucosa and the excessive mucus secretions are readily seen.

pus (Fig. 17.1). White blood cells are typically scarce in amebic dysentery because they are lysed by the amebic trophozoites present in the lesions. Certain bacteria (*Campylobacter*, *Salmonella*, and *Yersinia*) comprise an overlap group that produces a dysentery-like illness in the terminal ileum with occasional extension to the colon. A different disease is caused by *Clostridium difficile* and its toxins, usually arising after administration of certain antibiotics that wipe out much of the other resident flora. It is manifested by an adherent pseudomembrane with considerable mucosal inflammation and damage but without tissue invasion (Chapter 21).

Serious complications arise occasionally from infection of the colon by invasive organisms. Shigellosis may be associated with severe malnutrition, leading to a protein deficiency syndrome in children known as "kwashiorkor" (see Fig. 61.5). Shigellosis sometimes results in rectal prolapse or in a distention of the colon known as toxic megacolon, with a complete cessation of colonic peristalsis. Systemic complication may also occur, leading to clinical manifestations known as the hemolytic uremic syndrome, leukemoid reactions with very high white blood cell counts, encephalopathy, and others. Amebiasis may lead to perforation or obstruction, or the organisms may spread to produce abscesses in other organs, especially the liver.

Gut-Associated Lymph Tissue

A third type of enteric infection is exemplified by typhoid fever (Chapter 18) and is occasionally seen with *Yersinia* species and *Campylobacter fetus*. It is characterized by invasion of the gut-associated lymph tissue of the small bowel. From there, the organisms disseminate to the liver and bloodstream (*enteric fever*) or regional lymph system (*mesenteric adenitis*). Diarrhea may be absent or transient, and if fecal leucocytes are present, they tend to be mononuclear, attesting to the chronic nature of these infections. Ingrid C. suffered from this type of disease.

Surgical Complications of Intestinal Infections

Perforation of the wall of either the small or the large intestine may be caused by trauma or by intestinal infections. Either way, it results in spillage of intestinal contents into the normally sterile peritoneal cavity. Infections may lead to perforation in one of two ways: (a) direct damage to the gut wall by the inflammatory response (edema and cellular infiltration), or (b) bursting due to increase in pressure due to altered peristalsis or inflammatory obstruction. The severity of the resulting peritonitis is generally related to the volume of the inoculum, its pattern of spread in the abdomen, and the ability of the omentum to wall off the abscess. A small amount of fecal contents may be handled by the defenses in the peritoneum, but a large inoculum can easily overwhelm them. These infections tend to be severe, and if untreated are often life threatening. They are caused by a mixed strictly anaerobic-facultative anaerobic bacterial flora and represent a classical therapeutic challenge. Pathogenic mechanisms are discussed in Chapter 16.

Diagnosis

Most of the patients with acute diarrhea have a mild and self-limited course and never seek medical attention. It is not practical to search for enteric pathogens in all patients with diarrhea. Nor, in a large proportion of cases, is it warranted to do more than to give replenishing fluids and electrolytes, usually by mouth and not intravenously. A careful history of the symptoms is the most important part of the investigation and often narrows the diagnostic possibilities. The clues that suggest a treatable form of disease include fever, tenesmus, persistent or severe abdominal pain, weight loss, blood in the stool, recent travel, antibiotic use or raw seafood meals, male homosexual practices, or prolonged duration of symptoms.

Culturing of stool samples for "enteric pathogens," which is often and reflexively requested by many physicians, is primarily intended to isolate species of *Salmonella* and *Shigella*. Isolation or identification of the other enteric pathogens requires special culture techniques, evaluation of serotype, or tests for toxin production (Chapter 60). Animal parasites, protozoa, or helminths may require special concentration or staining procedures. It is therefore important to narrow the list of possible organisms that are sought and to inform the laboratory in order to avoid overburdening it with mountains of stool. Note how this can be of help: If laboratory personnel know that you suspect *Yersinia enterocolitica*, they would incubate cultures at 25°C; at this temperature the organisms are motile and readily distinguishable from other similar pathogens. Because of the newly recognized high prevalence of *Campylobacter jejuni* it is appropriate to request that this organism be specially looked for, especially in cases with fever and tenesmus, or if leucocytes are present in the stool. In this instance, the laboratory would use special selective media and an incubation temperature higher than 37°C. V. *cholerae* was isolated from Mr. V.'s stool because the laboratory had been alerted to this possibility and used a nonroutine selective medium, TCBS agar.

If nonbloody diarrhea persists or remains unexplained, a sample of upper small bowel contents may be examined for *G. lamblia* or *S. stercoralis* by use of a string that has been swallowed, allowed to pass into the duodenum and then retrieved. Cryptosporidium infection is diagnosed in stool or in biopsy specimens because these organisms are acid fast, an unusual feature among protozoa.

It should be kept in mind that the clinical value of a particular test is determined by whether or not the results will meaningfully affect the management of the patient. Sometimes the information is used not for treatment of the individual patient, but to determine if special isolation measures are warranted. Thus, the presence of rotavirus in Mary Ann's stool did not materially change the treatment plan: Antibacterial antibiotics were not indicated anyway, and rehydration would have been administered in any event. However, the positive ELISA test for rotaviruses suggested that if she were hospitalized or near to other susceptible infants, she would have to be isolated from them.

Treatment

Most acute infectious diarrheas are mild, self-limited, and best treated with oral fluid replacement and continued feeding. When to resort to specific antimicrobial or more aggressive intravenous replacement therapy is determined by the severity or duration of diarrhea or the presence of shock or dysenteric symptoms. In general, infections caused by toxigenic and invasive *E. coli*, *Campylobacter fetus*, and *Shigella* are improved with antibiotics. The disadvantage is that these organisms may develop drug resistance. Also, antibiotic treatment may not alter the course and may increase the risk of developing a carrier state, with the potential of increased spread of the infection, as with *Salmonella*. Other specific antimicrobials are prescribed for helminths, *G. lamblia*, *E. histolytica*, or gonococcal proctitis.

Antidiarrheal agents may reduce the frequency of stools, but there is no evidence to suggest that these drugs shorten the course of the illness. In fact, by increasing gut transit time, antimotility agents may impair the clearance of the original pathogen and thus prolong the infection and, very possibly, enhance the risk of invasiveness and septicemia. In addition, anticholinergics or opiates may produce a life-threatening condition of intestinal stasis known as the "toxic megalocolon".

An important medical breakthrough has been the development of oral rehydration therapy for mild to moderate diarrhea. Following the discovery that sodium and glucose transport are coupled in the small intestine, it was observed that the oral administration of glucose with essential electrolytes dramatically accelerates absorption of sodium, with water following to maintain osmolality. Moderate dehydration associated with cholera or other small bowel enteric diarrheas can now be corrected with oral replacement. Even in severe dehydration that requires rapid intravenous fluids to correct or prevent shock, oral rehydration may later be used alone for maintenance of adequate hydration. The impact of this simple concept on worldwide mortality from dehydration cannot be overstated, especially in the poorest corners of the globe where the disease is prevalent and severe. In these areas, the use of intravenous therapy is too expensive and trained personnel too scarce to provide it to more than a small proportion of patients. Technically uneducated people can be trained to mix the proper ingredients (sometime using bottle caps as measuring devices) or to dissolve prepackaged mixtures. The recipe for oral rehydration is remarkably simple:

To 1 liter of water add:

$\frac{1}{2}$ teaspoon salt (3 g)

$\frac{1}{4}$ teaspoon bicarbonate (1.5 g)

$\frac{1}{4}$ teaspoon KCl (1.5 g)

4 tablespoons sugar (20 g)

SUGGESTED READINGS

Esophagitis

Goff JS: Infectious causes of esophagitis. *Ann Rev Med* 39:163–169, 1988.

Odds FC: Candida infections: an overview. *CRC Crit Rev Microbiol* 15:1–5, 1987.

Gastritis

Graham DY, Klein PD: *Campylobacter pyloridis*: the past, the present, and speculations about the future. *Am J Gastroenterol* 82:283–286, 1987.

Waghorn DJ: *Campylobacter pyloridis*: a new organism to explain an old problem? *Postgrad Med J* 63:533–537, 1987.

Bacterial Overgrowth Syndrome

Marthias JR, Clench MH: Review: pathophysiology of diarrhea caused by bacterial overgrowth of the small intestine. *Am J Med Sci* 289:243–248, 1985.

Sherman P, Lichtman S: Small bowel bacterial overgrowth syndrome. *Digest Dis* 5:157–171, 1987.

Intestinal Infections

Bacterial diarrhea. *Clin Gastroenterol* 15:21–37, 1986.

Cantley JR: Infectious diarrhea: pathogenesis and risk factors. *J Med* 78:165–244, 1985.

Formal SB, Hale TL, Sansonetti P: Invasive enteric pathogens. *Rev Infect Dis* 5 (Suppl 14): S702–707, 1983.

Infectious diarrhea. Which culprit? Which strategy? *Postgrad Med* 73:175–182, 1983.

Levine MM: Antimicrobial therapy in infectious diarrhea. *Rev Infec Dis* (Suppl 2):S207–216, 1986.

Nelson JD: Epidemiology of diarrheal diseases in the United States. *Am J Med* 78 (Suppl 6B):91–97, 1985.

Quin TC, Bender BS, Bartlett JG: Antimicrobial therapy for infectious diarrhea. *Disease-A-Month* 32:165–244, 1986.

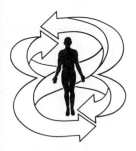

Central Nervous System

A.L. Smith

I nfections of the central nervous system (CNS) are relatively infrequent but
tend to have extremely serious consequences. Untreated bacterial meningitis, for example, is fatal in more than 70% of cases. Antibiotics have
reduced mortality in these diseases to less than 10%, but this is still unacceptably high. In addition, some CNS infections in childhood leave serious neurological sequelae that impair mental development and produce sensory deficits.

From a microbiological point of view, the brain and the spinal cord have
distinctive attributes: at the same time they are well protected and highly vulnerable. Thus, the CNS is anatomically protected by bones and membranes that
shield it from the exterior. However, in a limited space, the effects of infections
tend to be magnified: Even minor swelling and inflammation cause significant
damage. This is especially true in view of the essential functions of the CNS.
These two sides of the coin are also apparent on the physiological level: The
blood-brain barrier inhibits passage of microorganisms and toxic substances into
the brain and cerebrospinal fluid (CSF). Yet the same barrier impedes the passage of humoral and cellular defensive elements from the blood. It also hinders
the passage of many antimicrobial drugs, sometimes narrowing the therapeutic
options.

To understand the pathogenesis and outcome of infections in this distinctive
part of the body, you will need to recollect general aspects of neuroanatomy and
neurophysiology. The brain and spinal cord are suspended in the CSF and are
surrounded by three layers of meninges: the pia mater and arachnoid, which
constitute the leptomeninges, and the dura mater or pachymeninges (Fig. 47.1).
Infections of the CNS can be grouped by their anatomic location into infection
of the brain parenchyma, *encephalitis*; infection of the meninges, *meningitis*; and

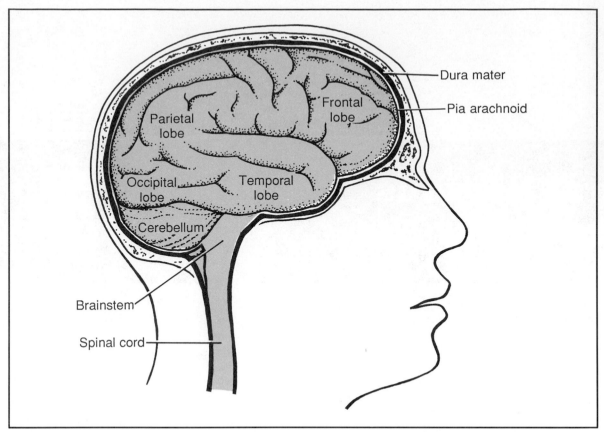

Figure 47.1. Gross anatomy of the cranium. The brain is within a closed space, surrounded by the meninges (dura mater and pia arachnoid) in close approximation to mucosal surfaces containing commensal flora (the nasopharynx).

infection of spinal cord tissue, *myelitis*. This anatomic separation of CNS infections is somewhat artificial, since all of these areas are connected and may be infected at the same time. In many cases, therefore, it is correct to speak of meningoencephalitis or even meningomyeloencephalitis.

Infections of the CNS may be caused by bacteria, viruses, fungi, or animal parasites that are either encountered in the environment or are members of the normal flora on body surfaces. In almost all CNS infections the causative agents were previously introduced into peripheral tissues of the host and made their way to the CNS either *via the systemic circulation* or *via neural pathways*. For instance, pathogens may have colonized the respiratory epithelium, penetrated it, and then entered the circulation (e.g., the meningococcus), or entered the bloodstream via the bite of an arthropod (e.g., Eastern equine encephalitis virus), of a dog (e.g., rabies virus), or through the placenta (e.g., rubella virus). A third way that microorganisms may enter the CNS is *by direct inoculation*, usually associated with trauma. In certain infections, the organisms are lodged within the CNS in a latent state and then manifest active disease sometime in the future (e.g., tuberculosis). The main types of infections and the most common etiologies are listed in Table 47.1.

ENCOUNTER

Infections of the CNS are caused by a small percentage of the pathogens that infect humans. Thus, these organisms must possess special characteristics that permit them to localize in the CNS. The most frequent agents and the types of disease they cause tend to fall into distinct categories: certain bacteria (pneumococci, *Haemophilus influenzae*, meningococci) classically cause meningitis but rarely infections of brain parenchyma, whereas others (staphylococci, anaerobic streptococci) cause brain abscesses but seldom meningitis. Some viruses cause encephalitis (herpes simplex); others cause meningitis (enteroviruses).

Once inside the CNS, viruses sometimes localize in specific regions. Certain viruses show an extreme tropism for certain neural cell types, e.g., polio, for the motor neurons of the spinal cord and medulla, and mumps virus for the cells of the ependyma of the fetus. The basis for such tropism is probably the distribution of viral receptors on specific cells. Some clues regarding this point come from experiments with reoviruses (see Chapter 8 for a detailed study). Depending on their type of surface hemagglutinin, reoviruses cause different kinds of severe infections of the CNS when injected into laboratory animals. Two types of hemagglutinin differ in their ability to bind to receptors on distinct neural cells. Viruses with type 1 hemagglutinin bind to ependymal cells, replicate, and cause inflammation at that site. Damage to the ependymal cells leads to occlusion of the ventricular aqueduct and to hydrocephalus (i.e., dilation of the ventricular system due to obstruction of CSF flow). In contrast, type 3 viruses bind to neurons and cause a fatal encephalitis (without ependymal cell infection). Thus, the anatomic location of these viruses depends, at least in part, on the specificity of their surface proteins for host cell receptors. This, in turn, determines the type of disease produced.

Localization is also believed to be favored by differences in blood flow. Does this explain why polio virus commonly infects the anterior horn cells of the spinal cord on the side of the dominant hand? Right-handed people are indeed more often affected on their right side.

Bacteria that cause CNS infections tend to differ in patients of different ages. Thus, in the newborn, bacterial meningitis is most commonly caused by *Escherichia coli* and group B β-hemolytic streptococci. Both are encapsulated strains. Over one half of the *E. coli* strains have a capsule made up of *K1 antigen*, suggesting that neuropathogenic strains have been specifically selected from the plethora of antigenically distinct *E. coli* strains. In contrast to other *E. coli* capsular antigens, K1 is a polysaccharide *rich in sialic acid*. So are capsular polysaccharides of group B streptococci. Why sialic acid? Apparently, polysaccharides containing this compound aid in bacterial adherence (and growth) on the meninges. K1 antigen also has antiphagocytic properties and inhibits the alternative pathway of complement activation.

Who, Where, and When

The foremost epidemiological features of infections of the CNS are age, geographic location, and the time of the year. For example, encephalitis in infants is more likely to be due to enteroviruses, because enteroviruses are spread by the fecal-oral route and children are more prone to come in contact with contaminated feces (Chapter 35). In adults encephalitis is more likely to be due to arboviruses (Table 47.2). Spread of arboviruses by arthropods also has seasonal variations, which follow the life cycle of the vectors (Chapter 55). The geographic distribution of some of these viruses is well illustrated by the name given to the diseases caused by arboviruses (Eastern, Western, Japanese encephalitis, etc.) This is sometimes misleading because St. Louis encephalitis, for example, was first studied

Table 47.1
Type of infection and frequent causative agents

Acute meningitis
 Bacteria
  Neisseria meningitidis
  Haemophilus influenzae, type b
  Streptococcus pneumoniae
  Group B streptococci
  E. coli
 Viruses
  Mumps virus
  Enteroviruses
Chronic meningitis
 M. tuberculosis
 Cryptococcus neoformans
 Other fungi
Acute encephalitis
 Viruses
  Arboviruses
  Herpesviruses
  Enteroviruses
  Mumps virus
Acute abscesses
 Bacteria
  Staphylococci
  Mixed anaerobe/aerobe flora
  Group A or D streptococci
Chronic abscesses
 Bacteria
  Mycobacterium tuberculosis
 Fungi
  Cryptococcus neoformans
 Animal parasites
  Cysticercus (*Tenia*)

Table 47.2
Viruses causing encephalitis

Virus	Geograhic Location	Major Age Group	Predominant Season	Notable Feature
Herpes simplex	All	All	None	Focal symptoms
St. Louis encephalitis	All	Older adults	Summer/fall	Mortality increases with age
Eastern equine encephalitis	East Coast and Texas	Children	Summer/fall	Disabling sequelae
Western equine encephalitis	West of Mississippi	Infants and children	Summer/fall	Most cases mild
La Crosse encephalitis	Upper Midwest	Children	Summer/fall	Most cases mild
Enteroviruses	All	Infants and children	Summer	Severity inverse to age
Rabies	All	All	All	Animal bite uniformly fatal
Varicella	All	Children	Winter	Rare
HIV	All	Adults	All	Dementia in AIDS patients

in that city, but is the arbovirus disease most commonly encountered throughout the United States.

ENTRY

The Hematogenous Route

Most cases of CNS infection are caused by entry of the organisms from the circulation (Fig. 47.2). The precise mechanism that permits them to penetrate the blood-brain barrier is not known. It is presumed that the choroid plexus, the site of greatest formation of the CSF, provides the most common site of entry. These are highly vascular structures, and inflammation on the blood side may result in the spillage of microorganisms into the CNS side. The likelihood of CNS infection is generally correlated with the microbial load of the blood (see Chapter 15 on *H. influenzae*).

The Neural Route

Most neurotropic viruses also reach the CNS by the circulation, but a few utilize special neural pathways (Fig. 47.2). The best known case of neural transmission is rabies, where the virus travels to the anterior horns of the spinal cord via peripheral nerves. Rabies virus enters the axon of a peripheral nerve and travels to neuronal perikaryon in retrograde fashion, presumably on a microtubular filament. Another well-known example of neural transmission is herpes simplex, where the virus ascends via the trigeminal nerve root (Chapter 31). As mentioned above, experimental studies with reoviruses showed that the choice of the hematogenous or the neural route depends on genetic differences in the viral hemagglutin (Chapter 8).

We should also mention the speculative but intriguing notion that viruses and other infectious agents may penetrate the body via the olfactory nerve endings, which are the only elements of the nervous system in direct contact with the exterior. Experimental studies suggest that herpes viruses may reach the brain

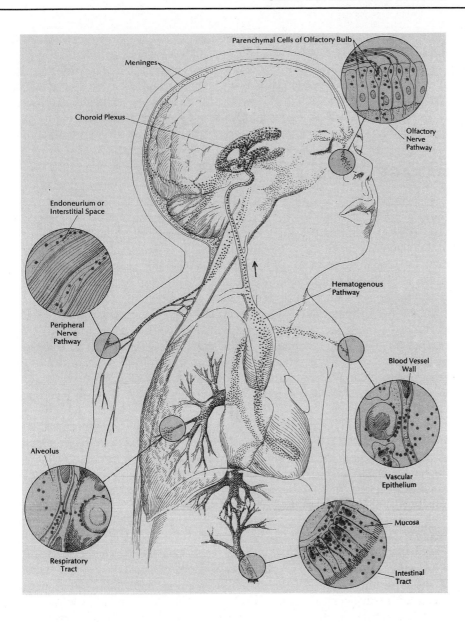

Figure 47.2. Pathways of entry of agents that cause CNS infections. In bloodborne infections, agents from the respiratory tract, gut, or vascular epithelium enter via the choroid plexus. Inside the CNS, they spread either by contiguity or through extracellular spaces. Some neurotropic viruses reach the brain via peripheral nerves or via the olfactory nerve endings. (From Menkes JH: Viral neurological infections in children. *Hospital Practice* 12:100–109, 1977.)

by this route. The ameba *Naegleria*, which causes a rare but lethal meningoencephalitis, is also thought to penetrate the CNS by trauma to the cribiform plate, as might happen when a person dives into water containing these amebae.

SPREAD AND MULTIPLICATION

Once a pathogen has reached the CNS, it finds itself in a relatively sequestered compartment that does not have as ready a recourse to defense mechanisms as most other regions of the body. For example, complement levels are very low in the CSF, apparently due to poor penetration from the blood, and also because the CSF contains a substance that partially inactivates complement. Therefore, lysis or phagocytosis of bacteria do not readily occur in the brain, the meninges, and the CSF. However, the CNS is not as immunologically restricted as was once supposed. It possesses an intrinsic immunologic surveillance mechanism in the microglia. In addition, it is now believed that the CNS has a lymph-like system consisting of the Virchow-Robin spaces (the perivascular sheaths surrounding the blood vessels as they enter the brain). These spaces contain macrophages and lymphocytes, and are thought to be the site where these cells enter into the CSF. Does the existence of these mechanisms suggest that infections of the CNS are more frequent than is believed, but are often kept in check by host defenses?

DAMAGE

Tissue dysfunction in CNS infections is caused in a variety of ways. Death of host cells may be due directly to the action of bacterial toxins, to lytic cycles of viral replication, or as the result of intracellular growth of bacteria and fungi. In most infections, however, cell death and tissue destruction result from the host's own inflammatory response. The multiplication and spread of microorganisms in the CNS elicits an inflammatory response similar to, but generally less intense, than that seen in other areas of the body. Characteristic of inflammation of the CNS are infiltration of microglia and proliferation of astrocytes. As in other parts of the body, the inflammatory response of the CNS has a humoral and a cellular component. The humoral component develops first and consists of edema caused by increased capillary permeability. Neutrophils and macrophages infiltrate the area, phagocytizing microorganisms as well as dead cells. Neutrophils often lyse in the process, releasing lysosomal enzymes that digest cells and tissue material in the immediate area.

Swelling of the brain due to inflammation within the closed cranial vault (cerebral edema) may by itself produce cerebral cortical symptoms from decreased capillary perfusion. More severe forms of cerebral edema can cause herniation of the temporal lobe through the falx, or of the brainstem into the foramen magnum, producing severe brain damage or death. Thus, neurologic symptoms during infection of the CNS may be due to *focal tissue lesions*, which produce specific functional deficits, or due to cerebral edema that leads to *global loss of higher cerebral cortical function*.

The functional characteristics of the CNS often help diagnose specific kinds of infections and identify the areas involved. For example, psychosis, impairment of memory, and seizures suggest herpes simplex encephalitis (because of the preferred involvement of the temporal lobe); stiffness of the neck without impairment of cerebral function is characteristic of meningitis; flaccid paralysis of the lower extremities suggests poliovirus infection of motor neurons of the spinal cord. Figure 47.3 depicts focal symptoms produced by certain CNS infections.

The following case histories and discussion describe characteristic infections of the CNS and how they are diagnosed. They include cases of meningitis, encephalitis, and brain abscess.

MENINGITIS

The majority of cases of meningitis can be classified in simple ways:

• By clinical presentation: acute, subacute, or chronic;

• By etiology: bacterial, fungal, or viral;

• By epidemiology: sporadic or epidemic.

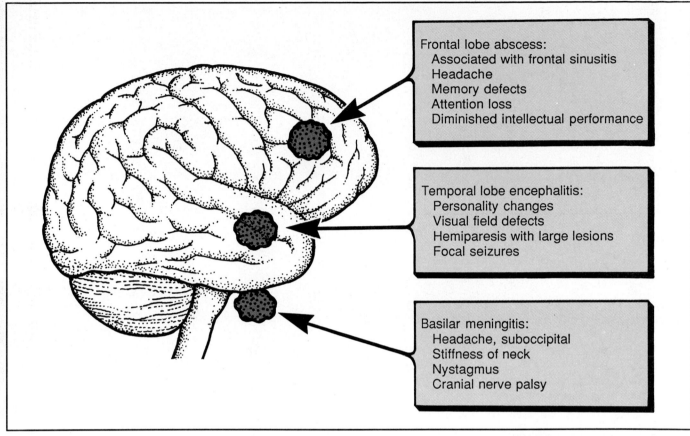

Frontal lobe abscess:
  Associated with frontal sinusitis
  Headache
  Memory defects
  Attention loss
  Diminished intellectual performance

Temporal lobe encephalitis:
  Personality changes
  Visual field defects
  Hemiparesis with large lesions
  Focal seizures

Basilar meningitis:
  Headache, suboccipital
  Stiffness of neck
  Nystagmus
  Cranial nerve palsy

Figure 47.3. Anatomic basis of localization of symptoms in CNS infections. Focal involvement of cerebral cortex produces specific signs and symptoms depending on the primary function of that part of the brain. In contrast, pyogenic meningitis produces global cerebral cortical dysfunction due to diffuse cerebral edema.

Acute meningitis is often caused by bacteria, chiefly *E. coli* and group B streptococci in young infants; meningococci, *H. influenzae*, and pneumococci in children; and pneumococci in adults (see Table 15.2). Overall, *H. influenzae* is the most common cause of meningitis, even though it infects mainly children between the ages of 6 and 60 months (Chapter 15). Subacute or chronic meningitis tends to be caused by fungi (mainly *Cryptococcus*) or by tubercle bacilli (all organisms that cause chronic inflammatory, granulomatous tissue reactions). Below we discuss an outbreak of meningococcal meningitis, an event that is known to occur when young adults are placed together.

Acute Meningitis

Case

One week after arriving at the Army recruit camp at Fort Ord (California), Pvt. T. A. had become the first of three cases of meningitis. He had a precipitous onset of fever and headache and within hours felt a pain in his neck when he moved his head. On lumbar puncture, his pressure was slightly elevated, 220 mm H_2O (the normal range is 70 to 200 mm H_2O). A smear of the CSF revealed small Gram negative coccobacilli and numerous leukocytes (Fig. 47.4). A culture grew the meningococcus, Neisseria meningitidis. Two weeks after intravenous administration of penicillin G, Pvt. T. A. nearly completely recovered, when Pvt. F. H. developed the same symptoms and was

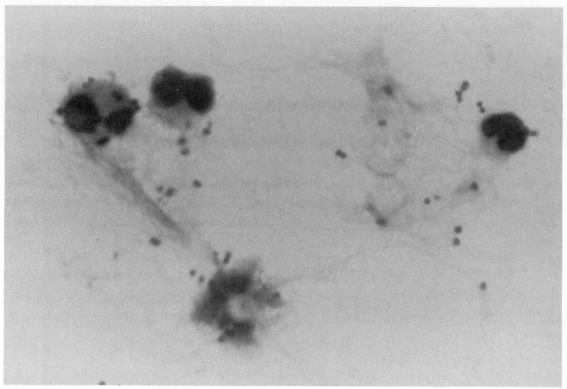

Figure 47.4. Gram stain of CSF from a patient with meningococcal meningitis. Gram-negative diplococci and polymorphonucelar leukocytes are evident.

admitted to the hospital. When Pvt. B. W. was diagnosed the next morning with the same illness, the remaining soldiers in the camp became alarmed. Their fears were calmed when the medical corps personnel explained that this meningococcal meningitis "epidemic" would be stopped by the prophylactic administration of antibiotics to all.

At about the same time, Pvt. V. L. was assigned to Fort Leonard Wood (Missouri). When he arrived there, he had a fever, slight headache, and some nausea. The next day, when putting on his boots, he noticed that his neck was stiff. When he went to the infirmary, he immediately had a lumbar puncture: the CSF pressure was 90 mm H_2O, nearly in the normal range, and the fluid contained 76 neutrophils/μl, 80 mg/dl of protein (an elevated value, see Table 47.3), and 66 mg/dl of glucose, in the normal range. He was observed in the hospital for three days and was discharged with a diagnosis of aseptic meningitis when his CSF proved to be sterile and his symptoms resolved.

Why did meningococcal meningitis, the illness of Pvt. B. W., produce alarm and called for preventive measures, whereas aseptic meningitis, that of Pvt. V. L., was just observed? How does the pathobiology of these diseases differ and how can they be differentiated?

Encounter and Entry

Meningococci are acquired by inhalation of aerosol droplets from asymptomatic human carriers. It is likely that in the outbreak at Ford Ord most of the recruits were exposed to the organisms from another individual, since meningococci are found in the oropharynx of about 10% of healthy people. This frequent degree of colonization does not, however, always correlate directly with outbreaks, because individual strains of meningococci vary considerably in virulence. The reason why so many people become colonized but only a few get sick is not truly known. The best hint comes from the observation that susceptible individuals lack antibodies against the meningococcal capsular antigen, whereas those who become carriers have such protective antibodies. There is also a striking association between congenital deficiency in the late components of the complement cascade and neisserial infection, with either meningococci or gonococci. These findings suggest that the immunological repertoire of an individual plays a role in determining who does and who does not manifest the disease.

Spread, Multiplication, and Damage

Meningococcal meningitis may be a distinct clinical event, as in the cases of the soldiers at Fort Ord, but it may also follow an overwhelming septicemia caused by these organisms. In such cases, the symptoms of meningitis only add to an already grave clinical picture; the presence of organisms in the blood in large numbers causes severe non-neural manifestations, such as shock and intravascular coagulation. These signs are due to the high blood content of Gram negative endotoxin. In such cases it is proper to speak of *meningococcal septicemia*, rather than meningococcal meningitis.

The clinical manifestations of acute meningitis, caused by meningococci, *H. influenzae*, or other bacteria, are fever, a stiff neck (nuchal rigidity), headache, and occasionally other focal CNS dysfunctions. These symptoms are due to the inflammatory response to meningeal invasion. Pus in the subarachnoid spaces may spread over the brain, the cerebellum, and the spinal cord. It tends to be particularly thick in pneumococcal and *Haemophilus* infections, which leads to blockage of various foramina and to an increased CSF pressure, resulting in headache and nausea. In meningococcal meningitis, the CSF pressure is usually only slightly elevated. The extent of inflammation varies considerably, with the intrinsic virulence of the strains and the immune state of the patient. Severe signs and symptoms of meningeal irritation, "meningismus", include involuntary extension of the neck and back to keep the dura from being stretched at the point where spinal nerves exit the spinal foramina. Additional symptoms, such as altered vision, may be caused by compression of the nerves that emanate from the base of the brain. Spasm or thrombosis of blood vessels may lead to small or large strokes.

In general, meningitis leaves fewer traces when caused by meningococci than by the other bacteria. *H. influenzae* meningitis is often followed by mental retardation and/or deafness. Some of these deficits are cortical, presumably due to decrease in cerebral cortical blood flow during the acute stages of the disease.

Diagnosis

An acute infection of the CNS presents a diagnostic problem of grave urgency. Saving the life of a child with meningococcal meningitis sometimes requires instituting proper therapy within minutes. Fortunately, examination of a Gram stain of the CSF obtained by lumbar puncture may rapidly give a presumptive diagnosis. Examination of the CSF is absolutely necessary when acute meningitis is suspected. Table 47.3 shows the pattern of inflammation in the CSF in various CNS infections.

The elements of the inflammatory response in the CSF may also be helpful in determining whether the infection is likely to be bacterial or viral and even in suggesting specific infectious agents. A large number of neutrophils points to a bacterial infection, whereas the predominance of lymphocytes suggests a viral etiology. Recall that the symptoms of Pvt. B.W. were almost identical to Pvt. V.L.; the nature of their illnesses was discerned by CSF examination. Gram stain examination of the spinal fluid should be a routine procedure because it reveals infecting bacteria in about 50% of the cases of meningitis.

Culture of CSF is the means of definitively establishing the etiology and is useful for making a specific choice of antibiotics (Table 15.2). More rapid tests are based on identification of unique microbial constituents in the CSF. Most of these tests are based on detecting a specific antigen, such as a bacterial or fungal capsular polysaccharide. Future methods may test for specific genes rather than their antigenic products.

Prevention and Treatment

Vaccination against meningococci is limited to high-risk groups, such as military recruits. Currently, U.S. military personnel receive a meningococcal vaccine when they arrive in a recruit camp. The vaccine contains capsular polysaccharides of type A and C meningococci, the most common types to cause meningococcal epidemics. An effective vaccine against type B meningococci, which cause the majority of cases of meningococcal meningitis in the United States, is not available. However, even if it were available, it would probably not be used because most of these cases are sporadic and do not occur often enough to warrant widespread vaccination. Chemoprophylaxis with rifampin or minocycline will eradicate nasopharyngeal carriage in 90% of the recipients.

To effectively treat bacterial meningitis, antibiotics to which the bacteria is susceptible must penetrate the CSF in an active form. β-lactams are usually administered for the common forms of bacterial meningitis. These drugs are highly polar and enter the CSF poorly by diffusion through the blood-brain and blood-CSF barriers. The average drug concentration in CSF normally achieved is 15% that of serum. However, β-lactams also enter the CSF through capillary leaks which are enhanced by inflammation, and these drugs may thus reach therapeutic levels in patients with meningitis. It has been estimated that in order for the drugs to be effective, it is necessary to achieve a CSF concentration that is 8 to 10 times that of the minimal bactericidal concentration (MBC) measured in the laboratory. The reason for this is not really known.

New β-lactams, such as cefotaxime and ceftriaxone, are very potent and produce CSF concentrations which exceed the MBC by 20-fold or more. As the inflammation resolves, the β-lactam concentration decreases, but is still adequate to sterilize the CSF. Other antibiotics such as chloramphenicol and tetracycline are lipophilic and diffuse readily across blood-brain and blood-CSF barriers. They achieve effective CSF concentrations independent of the presence or magnitude of the meningeal inflammation and are bactericidal against H. flu and meningococci. Chloramphenicol, however, may produce serious toxic side effects and its serum levels should be monitored (a practice that may be prohibitive in economically disadvantaged countries). Tetracycline may cause permanent discoloration of the teeth, mitigating its administration to young children.

An important aspect of the treatment of meningitis is to control the increased intracranial pressure. Cerebral edema may further decrease the already diminished cerebral blood flow and depress oxidative glucose metabolism. Death may ensue from compression of the brainstem into the foramen magnum (i.e., herniation). Supportive measures must ensure that the patient is adequately oxygenated and that blood glucose is in the normal range.

Viral Meningitis

Viremia gives viruses the opportunity to invade the CNS and cause so-called *aseptic meningitis*. This traditional term only means that the CSF is sterile on routine culture. The term is also used for infections by other agents that do not grow on the usual bacteriological media (e.g., fungi, leptospira, *Treponema pallidum*). Aseptic meningitis may also be caused by noninfectious etiologies such as certain cancers or cerebral collagen-vascular disease. In viral meningitis, the brain is usually involved as well, and the illness should therefore be described as a meningoencephalitis. However, the meningeal signs (stiff neck and headache) are more prominent than those of cerebral involvement.

Viral meningitis can be distinguished from bacterial meningitis because it produces a milder disease, a low to moderate inflammatory reaction in the CSF, consisting primarily of lymphocytes. Pvt. V.L. had the clinical disease and CSF findings typical of viral and not fungal meningitis (chiefly, a large number of leukocytes and normal glucose level; Table 47.3.) For this reason, antibiotics were not administered and he was only observed in the hospital. His improvement without antibacterial or antifungal treatment points further to a viral etiology. If Pvt. V.L. had not improved, another cause for his symptoms and the presence of leukocytes in the CSF would have had to be found.

In infants less than a year of age, it is frequently difficult to distinguish bacterial and aseptic meningitis. The newborn has a limited repertoire of responses, and the relative immaturity of its reticuloendothelial system may not permit an adult-type inflammatory response. The presence of bacterial polysaccharide in the CSF helps in making this distinction. However, the absence of bacterial antigens does not eliminate the diagnosis of pyogenic meningitis. As a result, most infants with the symptoms of acute meningitis and an increase of leukocytes in the CSF are treated with antibiotics.

Chronic Meningitis

Case

Ms. L., a 32-year-old, immigrated to the United States 1 year ago from the Solomon Islands, together with her husband and three children. Four weeks later her oldest child came home from day-care with chickenpox. Two weeks

Table 47.3
Usual composition of the cerebrospinal fluid in various infections

	None	Acute Bacterial Meningitis	Fungal and Viral Meningitis	Herpes Encephalitis	Brain Abscess
Leukocytes/μl	0–6	>1000	100–500	10–1000	10–500
Neutrophils, %	0	>50	<10	<50	<50
Red blood cells/μl	0–2	0–10	0–2	10–500	10–100
Glucose, mg/dl[a]	40–80	<30	≤40	>30	>40
Protein, mg/dl	20–50	>100	50–100	>75	50–100

[a] Diagnostic values are best interpreted as the ratio of glucose levels in the blood to those in the CSF.

later she and the rest of the family also developed the disease. As her rash faded, she developed a headache and again had fever. Over the next week she lost her appetite and vomited a few times. These symptoms persisted for an additional week and she became apathetic. When 4 days later she became stuporous, she was taken to a hospital.

The diagnosis of varicella (chickenpox) encephalitis was considered, but the fact that her chickenpox began a month ago made this unlikely because invasion by this virus would have occurred earlier, during active disease. On physical examination, she was deaf in her right ear and had paralysis of the right side of her face. A chest radiograph showed a right upper lobe pneumonia. A technetium-99 brain scan showed increased uptake at the base of her brain, and a cranial CT indicated increased intracranial pressure. On lumbar puncture, the CSF pressure was 310 mm H_2O (highly elevated) and the fluid contained 350 leukocytes/μl, of which 87% were lymphocytes, and a protein concentration of 68 mg/dl (elevated). A Gram and acid-fast stain did not show any organisms, but the CSF contained a lipid typical of tubercle bacilli, tuberculostearic acid, which allowed the diagnosis of tuberculous meningitis (see Chapter 22 for other procedures). Subsequently, Mycobacterium tuberculosis grew from her CSF, and was found to be susceptible to streptomycin, rifampin, and isoniazid. Ms. L. was treated with these agents for 6 weeks and was then discharged, to continue on oral rifampin and isoniazid for an additional 9 months (see Chapter 22 for a discussion of this therapeutic regimen).

Pathobiology

Ms. L. came from a geographic region where pulmonary tuberculosis is endemic. During primary infection, tubercle bacilli were deposited in many organs (including the brain), where they become contained within granulomas. Ms. L.'s chickenpox suppressed her cell-mediated immunity, and the tubercle bacilli were now able to multiply and cause inflammation. In the brain, granulomas located near the ventricles spilled tubercle bacilli into the CSF. The organisms then spread throughout the subarachnoid space, and, for reasons as yet unknown, became most prevalent in the basilar cisterns. As cell-mediated immunity returned, it elicited an intense delayed hypersensitivity-type reaction to the organisms. Granulomas formed around cranial nerves caused their dysfunction. In Ms. L.'s case, the nerves affected were cranial VII and VIII (as indicated by deafness and paralysis of the side of the face, respectively.) Inflammation of the meninges compromised her cerebral blood flow, leading to the stupor (which could have progressed to coma). In Ms. L.'s case, the CSF findings and indolent course were consistent with chronic meningitis and both fungi and *M. tuberculosis* had to be considered. The presence of a tubercular lipid (tuberculostearic acid) in the CSF made the diagnosis of tuberculous meningitis likely, and it was confirmed by the isolation from the CSF of *M. tuberculosis*.

ENCEPHALITIS

Encephalitis is almost invariably caused by a virus, with herpes simplex the most frequent in the United States, followed by the togaviruses (encephalitis viruses). These viruses are listed in Table 47.2 and described in detail in Chapters

31 and 55. They cause extremely serious illnesses which, if untreated, have mortality rates of 75% or greater. Fortunately, herpes simplex encephalitis can be treated if diagnosed early.

Herpes Simplex Encephalitis

Ms. H., a 19-year-old living in the inner city, was brought to the emergency room by her mother because she was "acting funny". Her mother reported that on arising she thought "there were devils in the room", and she nearly destroyed her bedroom trying to escape them. On her way to the hospital, Ms. H. hallucinated intermittently, telling her mother that she was smelling roses. In the prior 3 days she had some mild nausea and vomiting. In the emergency room, her urine was found to contain "angel dust" (phencyclidine) and she was admitted to the psychiatric ward. There she was noted to have a low-grade fever and received a phenothiazine tranquilizer (haloperidol). After 2 days she had a generalized seizure and then became comatose.

Since convulsions are not associated with phencyclidine intoxication and are not a side effect of phenothiazines, there was a good likelihood that Ms. H. had a CNS infection. Her fever and seizures made this suspicion more probable. CSF obtained by lumbar puncture contained 280 erythrocytes and 350 mononuclear leukocytes per microliter. The glucose content was in the normal range (48 mg/dl) and the protein concentration elevated (126 mg/dl; see Table 47.3 for normal values). A technetium-99 scan showed increased uptake in the left temporal lobe, indicating involvement of brain tissue (see under "Diagnosis"). In light of her recent neurologic history, these findings prompted a biopsy of the temporal lobe, a preferred site for herpes simplex. A tissue sample was sectioned and, upon examination by immunofluorescent microscopy, was positive for herpes simplex antigen. Herpes virus grew in cell cultures inoculated with the biopsy material. Ms. H. was treated with acyclovir for 2 weeks, but had many residual signs of neurological impairment, which needed extensive rehabilitation therapy.

Pathobiology

Herpes simplex encephalitis is not a frequent disease, although it is the most common of the severe encephalitides. It usually follows the chronic latent infection characteristic of this virus. Genital herpes may also produce infection of the lower spinal cord and meninges, but this is rare. It is not known why in some individuals the virus travels centripetally (up the nerve) from the trigeminal ganglia, instead of following the more usual centrifugal route. Fibers emerging from the trigeminal ganglia innervate the dura of the middle and anterior fossae and the meningeal arteries of the area. Herpes simplex viruses may use this route to spread to the meninges and meningeal arteries and, from there, to the meningeal nerves and the contiguous cortex. This postulated pattern may explain the frequent localization of herpes virus in the temporal and orbital frontal lobes.

The characteristic manifestations of viral encephalitis are cerebral dysfunction, e.g., abnormal behavior, altered consciousness, and seizures. Fever, nausea and vomiting are also common, possibly due to increased intracranial pressure. Thus, Ms. H. had many of the typical signs and symptoms of the disease. Many of the manifestations of herpes simplex encephalitis are due to necrosis of neurons, especially of the temporal and frontal lobes. This is accompanied by inflammation, with infiltration of mononuclear cells from the perivascular sheaths (Virchow-Robin spaces). Her sites of involvement included the portion of the temporal lobe responsible for the sense of smell, hence her olfactory hallucination (smelling roses). The lesions are usually on one side only, probably because the viruses ascend from one of the trigeminal ganglia only.

Diagnosis

Patients are suspected of having herpetic encephalitis if they have fever and focal cerebral cortical lesions, particularly in the frontal and temporal lobes. Diagnostic tests are necessary to document the clinical impression that there is inflammation (i.e., CSF pleocytosis—the increase in the number of cells in the CSF) and focal involvement of cerebral tissue. A radioactive brain scan with technetium is the most sensitive test to indicate brain tissue involvement. Technetium 99, an artificial radioactive element, is injected in the blood covalently bound to serum albumin. Leaking from cerebral capillaries is detected by technetium 99 spilling into tissues. If the area of brain that is destroyed by HSV is large enough, damage may sometimes be detected by cranial CT examination.

The only conclusive way to diagnose herpetic encephalitis is by a brain biopsy, as was done with Ms. H. However, in patients with a history and physical findings of herpes encephalitis, acyclovir (a relatively nontoxic drug) is usually administered without further studies. The value of a brain biopsy is demonstrated by the fact that in approximately one-fourth of adults suspected of having herpes encephalitis, pathological examination of biopsy material revealed other diseases, e.g., cancer, bleeding, fungal infections, which require other forms of treatment.

Brain tissue obtained on biopsy is examined by conventional microscopy and is tested for herpes-specific antigens. This is currently done using fluorescent conjugated monoclonal or polyclonal antisera directed against an HSV glycoprotein. Culturing HSV from brain tissue provides unequivocal evidence of encephalitis, but takes more time. Since HSV spreads by contiguous cell-to-cell contact (Chapter 31), it can rarely be cultured from the CSF.

Many clinical conditions mimic herpetic encephalitis, including enterovirus or arbovirus encephalitis, cerebral collagen vascular disease, tumors, and even cryptococcal meningitis. A brain biopsy may sound like a dangerous invasive procedure. In skilled hands, it carries relatively little risk.

Treatment

As stated above, in patients with encephalitis it is essential to determine if the disease is due to herpes simplex, because the morbidity and mortality of this disease can be decreased by drug treatment. Two antiviral agents, acyclovir and arabinosyl adenine, are available for the treatment of herpes encephalitis (Chapter 37). In a randomized chemotherapy trial, carried out chiefly with adult herpetic encephalitis patients, the mortality rate and the sequelae were reduced with acyclovir treatment (in one study the overall mortality rate was reduced from 70% to 20%). With either agent, the outcome is related to the severity of disease at the time antiviral chemotherapy is begun, thus the urgency to begin treatment. As with the bacterial meningitides, supportive care must not be neglected. Sequelae are due to destruction of cerebral gray matter. Such lesions in the temporal or frontal lobes may result in personality changes, whereas involvement of the white matter may lead to significant paralysis.

ABSCESSES

Brain abscesses typically follow two diseases: congenital heart disease and chronic parameningeal infections. In a patient with endocarditis, a septic embolus from the heart may rarely cause a brain abscess.

Case

Ms. T., a 29-year-old housewife, complained of earache. She had had many such episodes since childhood, especially of the left ear, but this one was associated with a headache that made her nauseous. She vomited once. After 4 days of these symptoms, she was driven to the hospital because she had developed a large "blind spot" in her right field of vision. At the hospital it was noted that she had a low-grade fever of 38.1°C. A CT scan of the head revealed a 4 × 3 cm mass in her left occipital lobe, consistent with an abscess (Fig. 47.5).

A neurosurgeon performed a needle aspiration of the abscess under CT guidance. A smear of the aspirate revealed Gram positive cocci, and the material grew Staphylococcus aureus when cultured. Ms. T. was treated with intravenous nafcillin and metronidazole for 4 weeks, during which period serial CT exams showed the abscess to be shrinking. She recovered completely, with the exception of a remaining small blind spot in the right visual field.

Pathobiology

The case of Mrs. T. may well have started with a chronic infection of the middle ear or mastoid. Her history points to that—particularly because of the long-term

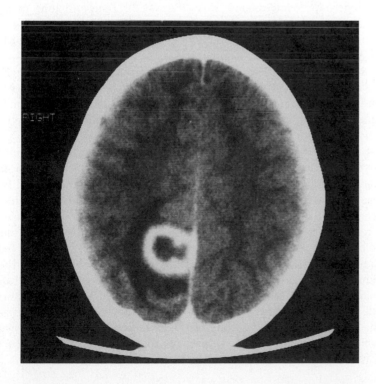

Figure 47.5. Computerized tomogram of the cranium of a patient with an abscess in left occipital lobe. The liquefied (necrotic) material in the abscess center appears dark. The white rim surrounding the abscess is its wall, which is visualized because of its vascularization and contiguous vasodilation. All the intracranial vasculature is visualized because gamma-ray absorbing material was infused intravenously at the time the radiograph was obtained.

earache. Chronic infections of the middle ear, the mastoid, or the sinuses often involve the bony structures that surround them, plus their vasculature. Veins that bridge the temporal bone and the cerebral cortex may become infected (septic thrombophlebitis), leading to a decrease in local blood supply and providing a reservoir of bacteria.

Abscesses may appear at many locations of the brain and the subdural or epidural meningeal spaces. Infarction of cerebral cortex during meningitis produces a subdural abscess that is poorly localized: this is called *subdural empyema*. If an empyema is not completely drained, it will slowly resolve, as will an abscess in other parts of the body. In contrast with intracerebral abscesses, those located on the outside of the dura mater (*epidural abscesses*) are invariably related to contiguous infection of bone, sometimes secondary to infection of the paranasal sinuses or mastoids.

Decrease in the blood supply to an area of the brain leads to a condition called *encephalomalacia*, the softening of the brain tissue that accompanies cell death. Bacteria that are transiently found in the circulation may lodge themselves in these softened and necrotic areas and cause abscess formation. Children with cyanotic congenital heart disease have multiple areas of encephalomalacia throughout their brain and many suffer from brain abscesses. In Ms. T.'s case, septic phlebitis of veins that pass from the temporal bone to the cortex not only produced encephalomalacia, but also supplied the bacteria that caused the abscess. Abscesses may also be a complication of meningitis, if cerebral vasculitis is severe enough to produce infarction of brain substance. This usually occurs in the watershed areas, on the margin between adjacent vascular territories where the vasculature least overlaps.

The symptoms caused by brain abscesses are due to increased intracranial pressure and to destruction of tissue at specific locations. When the frontal lobe is involved, there is diminished intellectual performance, memory deficits, drowsiness, and perhaps some memory loss (Fig. 47.3). Temporal lobe involvement results in visual field defects and occasionally in difficulty in speaking. In some patients, mastoiditis leads to cerebellar abscesses, resulting in incoordination, ataxia, and falling toward the affected side.

Acute abscesses in the CNS are frequently caused by a mixed bacterial flora consisting of strict and facultative anaerobes. They represent the mixture of bacteria found in the mouth, or in a parameningeal focus such as an infected middle ear, mastoid, or sinus. Staphylococci can also infect brain tissue if delivered to that location in a septic embolus from an infected heart valve.

Chronic abscesses may be located in either the meninges or the brain tissue. The most common causative agents are tubercle bacilli, the cryptococcus, and other fungi. Chronic abscesses are invariably due to metastatic spread from foci elsewhere, but sometimes the CNS manifestations may be the first indication of the presence of the organisms. These abscesses usually follow a course of remission and relapse. They are often associated with a loss of cell-mediated immunity, when the causative agents are no longer kept in check at the primary focus.

Brain abscesses may also develop from head injuries which allow the direct penetration of microorganisms. Some fractures of the temporal bone are said never to heal completely, and thus become a chronic portal of entry for bacteria from the middle ear and the mastoid. Invasion of the CNS may follow neurosurgical or orthopedic procedures of the brain or the spinal column. Brain abscesses that result from trauma or surgical procedures are usually due to *Staphylococcus aureus* or Gram negative bacilli.

Diagnosis

Diagnosis of brain abscess is aided by several imaging techniques. A brain scan with technetium 99 will show an area of increased radioactivity in the wall of the abscess (where the capillaries are inflamed and leaking) and an avascular central portion (the abscess cavity). This area often looks like a "donut" on the scan (Fig. 47.5). Cranial CT may also demonstrate the same structures: a fluid avascular abscess cavity and an overly vascularized (hyperemic) rim surrounding the cavity. Lumbar puncture is inadvisable in an individual suspected of having a brain abscess, as the increased intracranial pressure may cause brainstem herniation with lumbar decompression.

Aspiration of the abscess cavity yields material for cytological analysis, Gram stain, and culture. Anaerobes are common in brain abscess and the aspirate should immediately be cultured anaerobically. Often a smear will show the presence of lots of Gram positive cocci, Gram positive rods, and perhaps a few Gram negative rods, yet only *S. aureus* will grow in culture. In such a case, the bacteria that failed to grow can be assumed to be oxygen-sensitive anaerobes.

Treatment

Like abscesses elsewhere, brain abscesses must usually be drained to effect resolution. In addition, aspiration of the contents of an abscess helps lower the increased intracranial pressure and improve the patient's condition. Focal symptoms due to tissue destruction will not be improved, but the lesion can be contained from further increase in size by the administration of antibiotics.

Antibiotic therapy is not always effective in the treatment of brain abscesses. Inflammation of the meninges is usually too slight to enhance penetration of antibiotics into the CSF. In addition, most antibiotics function poorly in an abscess. Ideally, an antibiotic should be chosen based on the susceptibility of organisms isolated from the abscess cavity, but aspiration of material for culture and susceptibility testing is not always practical. Usually a β-lactam and a lipophilic antibiotic active against anaerobes are administered together.

CONCLUSIONS

The anatomic and physiological protective mechanisms of the central nervous system effectively limit access of microorganisms. On the other hand, if infective agents succeed in penetrating the tissues of the system, the same mechanisms tend to exacerbate the symptoms of disease.

The most frequent infections of the CNS are caused by relatively few agents. Typically, the organisms tend to cause specific disease manifestations: encephalitis is almost exclusively caused by viruses, acute meningitis by bacteria, chronic meningitis by tubercle bacilli and the cryptococcus. Bacterial abscesses, in contrast, are frequently caused by a mixture of bacteria derived from the normal flora of the mouth and oropharynx.

Infections of the CNS are often very severe and life threatening. Many require immediate action, based on acute clinical assessment and, when available, rapid diagnostic tests. The most important diagnostic procedure is the examination of the CSF for microorganisms, white blood cells, and the determination of the concentration of glucose and protein. Fortunately, there are drugs that are effective for many of even the most dangerous conditions, such as herpetic encephalitis.

SUGGESTED READINGS

Rosenblum ML, Hoff JT, Norman D, Edwards MS, Berg BO: Nonoperative treatment of brain abscesses in selected high-risk patients. *J Neurosurg* 52:217–225, 1980.

Sequiera LW, Carrasco LH, Curry A et al: Detection of herpes-simplex virus genome in brain tissue. *Lancet* ii:609–612, 1979.

Weiner LP, JO Fleming: Viral infections of the nervous system. *J Neurosurg* 61:207–244, 1984.

Whitley RJ, Alford CA, Hirsch MS et al.: (The NIAID Collaborative Antiviral Study Group.) Vidarabine versus acyclovir therapy in herpes simplex encephalitis. *N Engl J Med* 314:144–149, 1986.

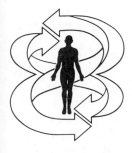

CHAPTER

Urinary Tract

48

M. Barza

From the distal urethra to the calyces of the kidney, the urinary tract is lined with a sheet of epithelium that is continuous with that of the skin. The epithelial surface is a potential pathway for entry of microorganisms from the outside world. The flow of urine and the sloughing of epithelial cells eliminate invading microorganisms and help to protect the urinary tract from infection. Nevertheless, bacteria often find their way into the urinary tract and cause disease. It is not surprising, therefore, that urinary tract infections (UTI) rank second in incidence only to infections of the respiratory tract. They rank first among the bacterial diseases of adults that come to the attention of physicians. For reasons that we will discuss, the majority of patients are women. As many as 20% of all women have an episode of urinary tract infection by the age of 30. There are an estimated 3 million office visits for this complaint each year in the United States alone. Recurrent episodes of urinary tract infections afflict about 1 in 10 women at some time in their life.

All portions of the urinary tract may be affected, but the most common UTI are infections of the bladder (*cystitis*) and the pelvis or the kidney (*pyelonephritis*). Infection of the urethra alone, or *urethritis*, is discussed with the sexually transmitted diseases (Chapters 14 on the gonococcus and 24 on chlamydiae). Prostatic infection is usually considered as separate from UTI, although chronic bacterial prostatitis may lead to recurrent UTI. *Renal abscesses* may occur as a result of ascending UTI or of bacteremia, and pyelonephritis may also result from bacteremia, without other involvement of the urinary tract.

As in other infectious diseases, the physician usually suspects urinary tract infection on the basis of characteristic symptoms and signs and confirms the

669

diagnosis by means of culture. In the case of UTI, however, culture poses some special problems that are not encountered in other sites. On the one hand, there are many patients who persistently excrete large numbers of bacteria in the urine but are asymptomatic: This is called "asymptomatic bacteriuria" and is clinically important in certain circumstances. On the other hand, the most convenient samples to obtain for culture are of voided urine, but such samples are usually contaminated to some degree by bacteria normally colonizing the distal urethra.

The distinction between true bacteriuria and the presence of contaminating bacteria in the voided urine of asymptomatic patients poses difficulties. One way to address the problem is to measure the number of bacteria per milliliter of urine, on the assumption that there will be more bacteria in the urine in true bacteriuria than with simple contamination. This approach has led to the definition of *true bacteriuria* by means of bacterial colony counts, a situation without parallel in other infections.

CASES

Bacterial Pyelonephritis in an Infant

David, a 3-month-old boy, was gaining weight poorly. On examination, the only other clinical or laboratory abnormality was the finding of 3×10^5 Escherichia coli per milliliter of urine. David was treated with intravenous ampicillin for 1 week and began to gain weight. However, after 6 weeks it was again noted that he was not gaining weight and had E. coli bacteriuria. Over the next 2 months the laboratory reported comparable bacterial counts with the same organism on two more occasions. Radiological studies showed that David had reflux of urine from the bladder into the ureter and scarring of the pelvis of the left kidney. No obstruction was seen. A tentative diagnosis of bacterial pyelonephritis was made. Treatment was given with intravenous ampicillin followed by oral ampicillin for 6 weeks in an attempt to eradicate the infection. This regimen was successful and David had no further problems with UTI.

Recurrent Cystitis

Ms. C., a 23-year-old woman, had five attacks of acute cystitis (painful urination, increased frequency and urgency) in the year since her marriage. The diagnosis was based on the clinical picture and the laboratory finding of significant bacterial counts in the urine. Three attacks were caused by E. coli, one by Staphylococcus saprophyticus, and one by Proteus mirabilis. Urinary colony counts in the various episodes ranged from 10^2 to 10^6/ml. Each attack responded either to trimethoprim-sulfamethoxazole or to ampicillin given for 1 week. Recurrences were noted at 1-week to 3-month intervals after stopping therapy. Treated with long-term antibiotic prophylaxis she did well and had no further recurrences.

Pyelonephritis and Bacteremia

Mr. P, a 65-year-old man, was admitted to the hospital with acute urinary tract obstruction due to prostatic hypertrophy. He was confused, had a temperature of 40.1°, and his blood pressure was lower than normal. Cultures of his urine and blood yielded Proteus vulgaris. A urinary catheter was placed to relieve the obstruction. He was diagnosed as suffering from bacterial pyelonephritis with secondary bacteremia. After treatment with antibiotics he underwent cystoscopy and resection of his hypertrophied prostate gland without further significant problems.

PATHOBIOLOGY OF UTI

As in other sites, host-parasite interactions in the urinary tract include the entry of microorganisms, their spread and multiplication, and the damage they cause (Fig. 48.1). But, in the urinary tract, *mechanical factors*, especially those that obstruct the normal flow of urine, play a particularly important role in disease. Cellular and humoral immunity are not as important in the defense against UTI as the normal flow of urine and other anatomic factors.

Entry

Access of infectious agents into the urinary tract is nearly always by *ascent from the urethra.* Bloodborne infections are relatively infrequent and are apt to

Figure 48.1. Pathogenesis of urinary tract infections.

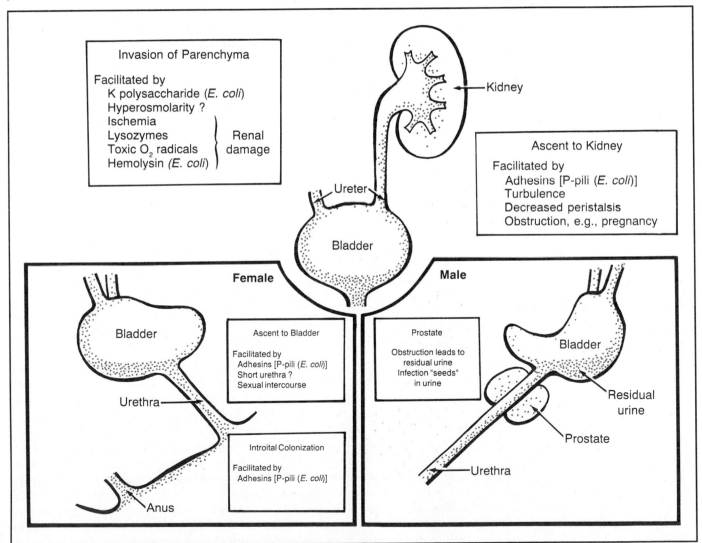

Invasion of Parenchyma

Facilitated by
K polysaccharide (*E. coli*)
Hyperosmolarity ?
Ischemia
Lysozymes ⎫
Toxic O$_2$ radicals ⎬ Renal damage
Hemolysin (*E. coli*) ⎭

Kidney

Ascent to Kidney

Facilitated by
Adhesins [P-pili (*E. coli*)]
Turbulence
Decreased peristalsis
Obstruction, e.g., pregnancy

Ureter

Bladder

Female

Bladder

Ascent to Bladder

Facilitated by
Adhesins [P-pili (*E. coli*)]
Short urethra ?
Sexual intercourse

Urethra

Introital Colonization

Facilitated by
Adhesins [P-pili (*E. coli*)]

Anus

Male

Prostate

Obstruction leads to residual urine
Infection "seeds" in urine

Bladder

Residual urine

Prostate

Urethra

Table 48.1
Causative agents of urinary tract infection

Uncomplicated	%	Complicated[a] or Nosocomial	%
Escherichia coli	80	Escherichia coli	20
Proteus mirabilis		Klebsiella	
Other Enterobacteriaceae		Enterobacteriaceae	
Staphylococcus saprophyticus	20	Pseudomonas aeruginosa	80
Streptococci (enterococci and group B streptococci)		Serratia	
Chlamydiae			

[a] Patients with structural or neurological abnormalities of the urinary tract.

result in renal abscesses rather than in ordinary UTI. Renal abscesses probably result from lodgement of bloodborne organisms in the glomeruli. Most ascending UTI are caused by enteric or skin bacteria, as in the three cases presented, followed in frequency by chlamydiae, the fungus *Candida albicans*, and, rarely by viruses, protozoa, or worms. The bacteria that most often cause UTI are of fecal origin; they are not however a random sample but are *a selected subset of the intestinal flora*. Strict anaerobic species of bacteria rarely cause UTI. More than 80% of acute UTI in patients without anatomic abnormalities are caused by certain strains of *E. coli*. Other members of the enteric bacilli and the group B and D streptococci are also prominent (Table 48.1). Some infections in women are caused by *S. saprophyticus*. The reason for the prominence of these species can be partially surmised: Adhesion to epithelial cells appears to be the most important single determinant of pathogenicity. Strictly anaerobic species of bacteria rarely cause UTI.

Some (but not all) prospective studies in women with recurrent urinary tract infections, such as Ms. C., indicate that shortly before the onset of bladder infections an increasing number of fecal bacteria colonize the epithelium of the vagina and around the urinary meatus. When the number of fecal bacteria at these sites becomes large enough, the organisms may enter the urethra and the bladder and overwhelm the normal defense mechanisms. However, large numbers of bacteria alone may not be enough to cause UTI; mechanical and other factors may contribute to causing infection. We shall consider how host and bacterial factors play a role in the entry phase of UTI.

Host Factors

The much greater prevalence of UTI among women than men has been attributed to the fact that invading microorganisms make a shorter trip up the female urethra to reach the bladder. Sexual intercourse contributes to UTI, perhaps by "massaging" bacteria upward into the bladder, hence the term "honeymoon cystitis". Celibate women, such as nuns, have a smaller frequency of bacteriuria than sexually active women. The use of contraceptive diaphragms also seems to predispose to UTI, possibly by making it more difficult to empty the bladder completely. Likewise, neurological disease affecting the bladder muscles impairs emptying of the bladder and also appears to contribute to UTI. Women who are particularly prone to recurrent UTI have been found to possess a greater than normal density of bacterial receptors on their uroepithelial cells. In other words, their epithelial cells are particularly "sticky" for bacteria.

Males are less prone to UTI, possibly because of their longer urethra and the presence of antimicrobial substances in the prostatic fluid. The greater frequency of UTI in older than in younger men correlates with the onset of prostatic hypertrophy, which leads to obstruction to voiding. Occasionally, the prostate gland itself may become infected and serve as a nidus from which bacteria may emerge periodically to cause relapsing infections. Mr. P.'s enlarged prostate was removed and could not contribute further to infection.

Bacterial Factors

Of the bacterial factors predisposing to UTI the best studied one is the ability of organisms to stick to the mucosa of the urinary tract. Adhesion to epithelial cells ensures that bacteria are not readily washed out by the flow of urine. Many causative agents of UTI have strong adhesins, usually in the form of pili (see Chapter 2). These protein appendages help overcome the repulsive forces between the surface of bacterial and epithelial cells, both types of cells being hydrophobic and negatively charged. In *E. coli*, the so-called *P pili* appear to play a role in the establishment of infection both in the bladder and in the kidney. In one study of women with recurrent UTI, P pili were present in 29% of random fecal isolates of *E. coli*, in 65% of isolates from patients with cystitis, and in 100% of isolates from patients with pyelonephritis.

Spread to the Kidney

The most serious consequence of bladder infection is the ascent of microorganisms to the kidneys to produce pyelonephritis. Any factor that contributes to the retrograde flow of urine may eventually contribute to the establishment of pyelonephritis. The more common examples of such predisposing factors include:

- *Reflux of urine* from the bladder into the ureters. This is a frequent problem in children and is caused by incomplete closing of the ureterovesical valves. It can lead to regurgitation of contaminated urine from the bladder into the ureter and the calices. Reflux is frequently corrected spontaneously as the child grows. This abnormality was probably a major contributory cause for the pyelonephritis in the case of baby David.

- *Other physiological malfunctions.* Neurological disorders lead to poor emptying of the bladder. The hormonal and anatomic effects of pregnancy cause dilatation and decreased peristalsis of the ureters. Diabetic patients are also prone to pyelonephritis for reasons that are not fully understood.

- *Urethral catheters.* These present at least two risk factors for cystitis and pyelonephritis: They serve as a conduit along which bacteria can spread, and as a nidus for persistent infection. Most patients who acquire UTI in the hospital become infected as the result of instrumentation of the urinary tract, especially from the use of an indwelling catheter. Scrupulous adherence to good technique, such as maintaining closed drainage and placing the collection bag below the level of the bladder, is helpful but cannot fully prevent these infections. The prevalence of bacteriuria in patients increases by about 5% for each day the catheter is in place. In these patients many of the infecting strains do not have adhesins: They are able to ascend along the catheter without having to adhere to the mucosa.

• *Urinary tract stones.* Once colonized by bacteria, stones serve as a nidus for relapsing infections of the bladder and the kidney. Bacteria may also contribute to the formation of such "infection stones". Species of *Proteus* split urea to form ammonium hydroxide, which raises the pH of the urine and facilitates the formation of "struvite" calculi (consisting of ammonium magnesium phosphate, which becomes increasingly insoluble as the pH rises).

Damage

Bacteria do not generally invade the mucosa of the lower urinary tract. The symptoms of cystitis and urethritis are caused mainly by superficial irritation. By contrast, bacteria which reach the parenchyma of the kidney produce the systemic effects of pyelonephritis, such as fever, chills, and leukocytosis. Pyelonephritis, is often accompanied by bacteremia. It has been suggested that hyperosmolarity in the renal pelvis diminishes the function of neutrophils and thereby facilitates invasion of the kidneys, but this is in dispute. Antibody is produced as the result of tissue invasion but probably plays little role in host defenses.

Strains of *E. coli* that possess certain capsular polysaccharides appear to be particularly invasive, perhaps because these polysaccharides inhibit phagocytosis. For reasons which are not clear, hemolysin production by some *E. coli* strains also appears to contribute to renal damage; and of course the endotoxin of Gram negatives may also contribute to inflammation and damage of the renal parenchyma.

BACTERIURIA AND COLONY COUNTS: A DIAGNOSTIC PROBLEM

As was mentioned in the introduction, laboratory confirmation of the diagnosis of UTI depends upon culture of the urine, but the interpretation of such cultures is made difficult because voided urine usually contains contaminating bacteria from the urethral meatus. Normal precautions of cleansing the external genitalia and collecting a "clean catch" midstream specimen reduce the degree of contamination but do not totally prevent the problem. Urine collected by needle aspiration of the bladder or by urethral catheterization contains fewer contaminants than voided urine (Table 48.2), but these procedures are not always practical. Certain species that are common members of the skin flora, including coagulase-negative staphylococci and diphtheroids, are more likely to be contaminants than are enteric Gram-negative bacilli, but this is not a reliable means to distinguish between true bacteriuria and contaminated urine. Repeated cultures may be obtained to determine the reproducibility of the findings but this is costly and time consuming.

For practical purposes, the distinction between *significant bacteriuria* and contamination of the urine is based on the enumeration of the number of bacteria in the urine. This approach relies on the experimental observation that there are usually more bacteria present in the urine of patients with "true bacteriuria" than in the urine of patients in whom the microorganisms are present only as contaminants. The following guidelines have been developed, which apply mainly to the Gram negative bacteria. Counts of fewer than 10^2 bacterial colonies per milliliter of urine are not considered clinically significant in the asymptomatic patient, whereas a level of 10^5 colonies per milliliter of urine or greater is considered

Table 48.2.
Definitions of "significant bacteriuria" in selected groups of patients

Population	Definition
Asymptomatic bacteriuria	$\geq 10^5$ cfu/ml
Acute pyelonephritis	$\geq 10^5$ cfu/ml
Women with acute dysuria	$\geq 10^2$ cfu/ml in women with abnormal pyuria (best shown for coliforms; not clear if same criteria applicable for staphylococci)
Patients with indwelling urinary catheters	$\geq 10^2$ cfu/ml

indicative of infection (Figure 48.2, Table 48.2). Among patients with symptoms of cystitis, even 10^2 colonies per milliliter is considered significant.

For many years there was confusion regarding the role of bacterial infection in patients with symptoms of cystitis but low urinary counts of bacteria. These patients were said to have the *acute urethral syndrome*. It is now recognized that these patients do not differ appreciably from those with cystitis and high bacterial counts in the urine. The reasons why some patients with cystitis have high and others have low bacterial counts in the urine are not known. Indeed, the same patient may have high counts on one occasion and low ones on another, as was the case with Ms. C., the patient described above. Of course, urine must be cultured as soon as possible after it has been obtained in order to avoid bacterial growth in vitro that would produce spuriously high counts.

As shown in Figure 48.3, asymptomatic bacteriuria is infrequent in both sexes at birth. The incidence of all urinary tract infections begins to rise in young women as they reach the sexually active years. By contrast, the frequency remains low in males until they reach the age when hypertrophy of the prostate becomes common (Fig. 48.2).

THE MAIN URINARY TRACT INFECTIONS

Most patients come to medical attention for UTI because they have symptoms. In young children such as baby David the symptoms may not call particular attention to the urinary tract. In adults the symptoms of UTI are usually related to the lower portion of the urinary tract (*cystitis*) or to the upper one (*pyelonephritis*).

Figure 48.2. Colony counts for women with and without bacteriuria. Results are similar for men except that colony counts from those without bacteriuria are lower using the clean-catch technique for urine collection. (Adapted from Fass RJ, et al: urinary tract infection. Practical aspects of diagnosis and treatment. *JAMA* 225: 1509–1513, 1973.)

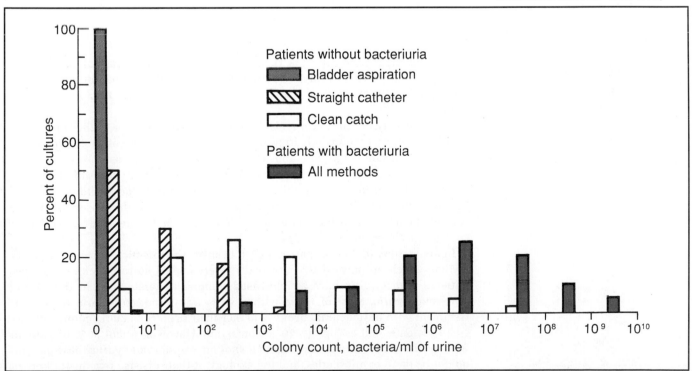

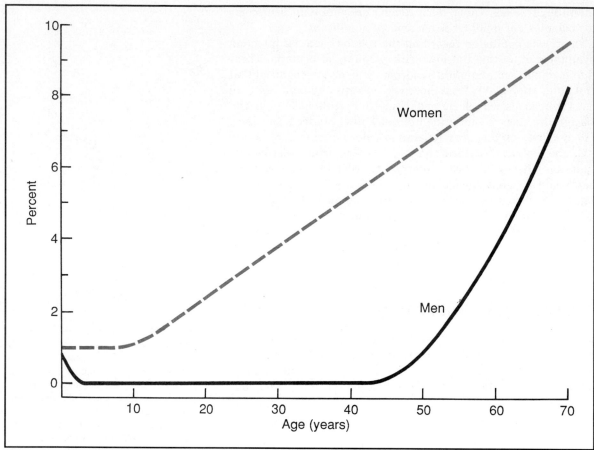

Figure 48.3. Prevalence of bacteriuria according to age and sex. (Adapted from Fass RJ, et al: Urinary tract infection. Practical aspects of diagnosis and treatment. *JAMA* 225:1509–1513, 1973.)

Cystitis

Patients with cystitis, like Ms. C., have dysuria (painful urination), urgency (the need to urinate without delay), and increased frequency of urination. These symptoms result from irritation of the mucosa of the lower urinary tract as a result of the infection.

Vaginitis may produce symptoms that are somewhat similar to those produced by UTI. Vaginitis may result from infection with *Trichomonas* or *Candida albicans*. "Nonspecific vaginitis" appears to be the result of complex interactions among various anaerobic bacteria, including the newly recognized *Mobiluncus* sp., and possibly *Gardnerella vaginalis*, a taxonomic cousin of *Haemophilus*. Although patients with vaginitis may experience pain on urination, the discomfort is perceived as external and there is usually no urgency or frequency of urination (in contrast to the symptoms of UTI).

In about 10% to 20% of patients with cystitis, the infection is caused by chlamydiae which are missed by the usual bacteriological culture techniques. Most patients with cystitis have an increased number of white cells in their urine, *abnormal pyuria*. Most of those with cystitis and abnormal pyuria respond to treatment with antibacterial drugs, whether their urinary bacteria counts are low ($<10^2$ colonies/ml) or high ($>10^5$ colonies/ml). However, about 30% of patients with cystitis and low bacterial counts *do not have abnormal pyuria*; these patients do not respond to antibiotics, and the etiology of their disease remains unknown.

Urethritis

Most of the infections that cause purulent urethritis *without* *cystitis* are sexually transmitted. Urethritis may be gonococcal or nongonococcal. Most cases of nongonococcal urethritis are thought to be caused by strains of *Chlamydia trachomatis*, certain mycoplasmas (e.g., *Ureaplasma urealyticum*) or combinations of these species, but there is disagreement on this subject. Furthermore, in some cases the causative agent of urethritis is simply not known. For some details, see Chapters 14 (gonococcus) and 24 (chlamydiae).

Pyelonephritis

In contrast to cystitis, pyelonephritis is an invasive infection that leads to fever, flank pain and tenderness; there is usually peripheral leukocytosis. These signs were seen in the case of Mr. P. The urine of patients with pyelonephritis often contains microscopic white blood cell casts, elongated structures composed of cells that were tightly packed in the tubules and excreted in a proteinaceous matrix. Their presence indicates involvement of the renal tubules. Some patients with pyelonephritis, like Mr. P, develop bacteremia, which may lead to shock and death. Renal abscesses are also occasional complications of bacterial pyelonephritis.

The Problem in Distinguishing Upper from Lower UTI

Clearly, upper and lower UTI differ in their potential to cause serious disease. As we shall see, they have also different implications for therapy, in that treatment of pyelonephritis is usually more intensive and carried out for a longer time than treatment of lower UTI. To distinguish between these infections is not always simple. Upper UTI is often accompanied by fever and flank pain. These symptoms strongly suggest involvement of the kidney. However, 30% to 50% of women with symptoms of cystitis alone have bacteria in the upper urinary tract even though they have no symptoms of kidney involvement. They may be suffering from a mild, subclinical pyelonephritis. Radiological studies sometimes help in pointing to upper UTI but are costly and not highly sensitive, and they also involve some risk.

Presently, the most accurate way to determine the site of involvement in UTI is to catheterize the ureter and obtain a sample directly. To try to avoid this costly and somewhat risky procedure, a test has been developed based on the assumption that invasion of the kidney leads to the production of specific antibodies, which will coat the bacteria in the urine. It is known as the *antibody-coated bacteriuria test*. Coating by antibodies can be seen in a smear of urine sediment stained with fluorescein-labeled anti-human gamma globulin antibody. Unfortunately, thus far the test has proven to be falsely negative in as many as 40% of patients with pyelonephritis and falsely positive in as many as 15% of patients without pyelonephritis. Men with bacterial prostatitis, for example, often have a positive reaction because this is a tissue invasive infection.

On practical grounds, the distinction between upper and lower UTI may have to be made empirically, based on the response to the administration of antibiotics (see below). In the absence of symptoms pointing to renal involvement or of factors predisposing to renal involvement, physicians will often treat patients for cystitis alone. Relapse of the infection may be the first clue to renal involvement, and may lead to more intensive treatment.

Recurrent Infections: Relapse vs. Reinfection

Among the most significant problems in the management of patients with UTI is the tendency of the infection to recur. Ms. C. exemplifies the situation. Recurrence may be either a *relapse*, i.e., the recrudescence of the original infection, or more commonly, reinfection, the occurrence of a new infection. Relapse is caused by the same strain of organism that caused the original infection and often occurs shortly after cessation of treatment. This suggests that the causative agent has persisted in the urinary tract or nearby—possibly because of an anatomic problem such as an obstruction or a stone. By contrast, reinfection may be caused by the original organism or by a different one, and can occur at any time after treatment is stopped. It does not suggest an anatomic abnormality. Ms. C. suffered from reinfections, as shown by the fact that the offending organism was different in each attack.

"Complicated" UTI and Nosocomial Infections

UTI occurring in patients with a structurally normal urinary tract is called *uncomplicated UTI*. Infections in patients with anatomic abnormalities, stones or indwelling catheters are called *complicated UTI*. The latter have a tendency to relapse unless the predisposing factors can be removed. In the case of Mr. P, resection of the prostate and removal of the catheter contributed to his cure. Nosocomial UTI, i.e., UTI acquired in the hospital, is usually the consequence of instrumentation, mainly catheterization of the bladder. The selective action of antibiotics commonly used in hospitalized patients tends to favor infection by species of bacteria which are relatively resistant to antibiotics.

TREATMENT AND PREVENTION

The basic tenets in the treatment and prevention of UTI follow the concepts of the pathogenesis of these infections (Table 48.3). The choice of antibacterial drugs should include the following considerations: Is the infecting agent sensitive to the drug or drugs? Can an effective drug concentration be achieved at the site of infection? What is the likely effect of therapy on the recurrence of infection?

Asymptomatic Bacteriuria

In the past it was thought that asymptomatic bacteriuria was an important contributor to chronic nephritis, renal failure and hypertension. Recent studies have generally failed to support this concept. It is currently believed that asymptomatic bacteriuria merits treatment in three groups of patients. One is pregnant women because, without treatment, 25% to 40% of them will develop pyelonephritis. The second group is children because reflux from the bladder to ureters may lead to ascent of the infection into the kidneys. The third group is patients who are about to undergo instrumentation of the urinary tract, because of their high risk of developing ascending UTI.

Cystitis

This is the most common type of UTI encountered by the physician. Most of the cases are caused by organisms that are relatively sensitive to antibacterial antibiotics. A single large dose or a few ordinary doses of a drug suffice to erad-

Table 48.3
Principles of Treatment of Urinary Tract Infection

Type of Infection	Treatment	Rationale
Cystitis	Single-dose Rx or short course (e.g., 3 days)	Effective for bacterial cystitis; will not be effective in pts with early pyelonephritis, chlamydial cystitis or infection caused by resistant bacteria, which will be detected by follow up culture or by relapse of symptoms
Acute urethral syndrome with "abnormal" pyuria	Single-dose Rx, if no response, 10 days of doxycycline or trimethoprim-sulfamethoxazole (TMP-SMX)	Coliforms or staphylococci respond to many agents, chlamydia (found in 20%) should respond to doxycycline or possibly TMP-SMX. Patients without abnormal pyuria do not respond to antibacterial drugs.
Pyelonephritis	At least 2 wks (some say 4–8 weeks) of full doses IV or by mouth. Tend to prefer bactericidal drug.	Not many data re importance of bactericidal vs. bacteriostatic drug or optimal duration of Rx but with shorter courses the relapse rate is high (e.g., 10%–50% relapse after 7 to 14-day treatment)
Asymptomatic bacteriuria	Mainly indicated for pregnant women, young children, or patients about to undergo instrumentation of the urinary tract	25%–40% of pregnant women with asymptomatic bacteriuria develop pyelonephritis if not treated
Recurrent infection		
Multiple reinfection	Individual attack usually responds well to short course treatment	Main issue is of prophylaxis: continuous or postintercourse
Relapse	Long-term treatment (e.g., 4–8 weeks)	Usually suggests tissue invasion or structural abnormality and usually merits IVP or other evaluation

icate most uncomplicated infections, presumably because of the high concentration of the drug in the urine and the lack of tissue invasion by the bacteria. It does not matter if the antibacterial agent is bacteriostatic or bactericidal. Short-course treatment has the advantage of lower drug cost, lower rate of side effects, and lesser chance of selection of resistant strains. This practice is not always followed, and Ms. C. was treated with week-long courses of drug therapy.

Pyelonephritis

These patients should be treated for longer periods of time than those with simple cystitis, i.e., 2 weeks or more. Longer treatment makes sense because these infections involve deeper tissues, from which it may be difficult to eradicate the bacteria. Indeed, treatment of patients with pyelonephritis for only 7 to 14 days results in failure rates of 10% to 50%. Physicians tend to prefer bactericidal over bacteriostatic drugs for the treatment of pyelonephritis, but this preference is not based on the results of controlled clinical studies.

Nosocomial UTI

UTI acquired in the hospital is often caused by bacteria that are resistant to orally administered antibiotics, and requires treatment with potent cephalosporins or aminoglycosides. Prophylactic administration of antibiotics in the catheterized patient is not recommended, because the result is usually simply to postpone the infection by a day or so and to select resistant bacteria. The usual indication to start treatment is the development of fever. As in the case of Mr. P., treatment in such patients will usually keep the infection under control but will not eradicate it. Eradication usually requires removal of the foreign body (e.g., the catheter).

Recurrent Infections

The greatest challenge in treating patients with UTI is not usually the management of the initial infection but the problem of recurrence. We have already emphasized the importance of distinguishing between relapse and reinfection, because the management of these two types of recurrences is different.

In patients with frequent reinfections, the major goal should be to interrupt the cycle of colonization of the introitus and infection of the bladder. Good success is achieved with drugs such as trimethoprim-sulfamethoxazole or some quinolones, which reach high concentrations not only in the urine but also in vaginal secretions. Special studies to search for anatomic abnormalities, by x-rays or ultrasound, for example, are not usually called for because the likelihood of finding abnormalities is very low. However, such studies may be indicated in very young patients or in those with unusual frequency of recurrence. It is worth instructing young girls with recurrent UTI to wipe the perineum from front to back rather than the reverse after defecation. This reduces contact of perianal bacteria with the urethra.

Relapse of infection, by contrast, signals either a structural abnormality (stone, obstruction, bladder dysfunction) or invasion of deep tissues (pyelonephritis, renal abscess, bacterial prostatitis) and merits not only long-term treatment with antibiotics but also urological studies to detect the abnormality.

CONCLUSIONS

The lining of the urinary tract is open to the exterior of the body, and, not surprisingly, often becomes colonized by fecal bacteria. Organisms successful at colonizing tend to be the ones capable of adhering to the epithelial cells and not readily washed away by the urine.

The defense mechanisms of this system of the body are different from those that operate at many other sites. Here neither white cells nor antibodies occupy center stage. Rather, the major role is played by mechanical factors, especially the normal flow of urine. Accordingly, interruptions in these defenses predispose persons to colonization and infection. A particularly important feature of these infections is that they recur unless the underlying predisposing factor is found and the condition corrected. An optimal approach to treatment and prevention must take these facts into account.

SUGGESTED READINGS

Brumfitt W, Gargan RA, Hamilton-Miller JMT: Periurethral enterobacterial carriage preceding urinary infection. *Lancet* 1:924–926, 1987.

Gillespie L: The diaphragm: an accomplice in recurrent urinary tract infection. *Urology* 24:25–30, 1984.

Kamaroff AL: Acute dysuria in women, *N Engl J Med* 310:368–375, 1984.

Nicolle LE, Harding GMK, Preiksaitis J, Ronald AR: The association of urinary tract infections with sexual intercourse. *J Infect, Dis* 146:579–583, 1982.

Stamey TA: The role of introital enterobacteria in recurrent urinary infections. *J Urol* 109:467–472, 1973.

Stamm WE, Counts GW, Running KR, Fihn S, Truck M, Holmes KK: Diagnosis of coliform infection in acutely dysuric women. *N Engl J Med* 307:463–468, 1982.

Stark RP, Maki DG: Bacteriuria in the catheterized patient. What quantitative level is relevant? *N Engl J Med* 311:560–564, 1984.

Strom BL, Colins M, West SL, Kreisberg J, Weller S: Sexual activity, contraceptive use, and other risk factors for symptomatic and asymptomatic bacteriuria. *Ann Intern Med* 107:816–823, 1987.

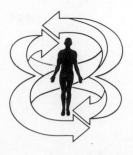

Skin and Soft Tissue

F.P. Tally

Inflamed hangnails, infected cuts, and athlete's foot happen to us so frequently that we scarcely take notice. These mild and usually inconsequential conditions represent one extreme of the infections of the skin. The other extreme include less frequent but potentially serious diseases, such as herpes zoster, candidiasis, or bacterial cellulitis. Infections of the skin may be caused by viruses, fungi, or bacteria. In addition, many diseases that affect other organs have cutaneous manifestations. Visible skin lesions may be the telltale sign of systemic infections by viruses (e.g., smallpox, measles, chickenpox), fungi (e.g., cryptococcosis, blastomycosis), or bacteria (e.g., syphilis, tuberculosis, scarlet fever, meningococcemia).

Primary infections of the skin and systemic infections with cutaneous manifestations are discussed throughout this book in the context of specific agents (for the main ones, see Chapters 11, staphylococci; 12, streptococci; 19, pseudomonas; 34, warts; 36, measles; 38, fungi). This chapter will be limited to bacterial skin infections, emphasizing those that reveal important pathobiological concepts. These infections frequently involve the "soft tissues" underlying the skin, subcutaneous fat, and superficial fasciae, which are also included in this discussion.

An understanding of the pathogenesis of skin and soft tissue infections requires knowledge of the anatomy and physiology of this part of the body. The skin is divided into three distinct layers, the epidermis, dermis, and fat layer (Fig. 49.1). The *epidermis* is a thin, self renewing epidermal sheet that covers the body. Over most of the body, it is about the thickness of two of the sheets of this book (0.1 mm) and is devoid of vessels and nerves. The basal cells of the epidermis, the

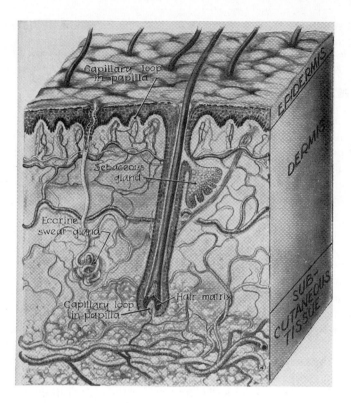

Figure 49.1. Schematic diagram of the skin. (From Pillsburg DM, Shelley WB, Kligman AM: *A Manual of Cutaneous Medicine.* Philadelphia, WB Saunders, 1961.)

keratinocytes, divide, differentiate, and eventually slough. As they rise from the basal layer to the surface, they become more stratified and produce a cornified layer of dead cells, the *stratum corneum.* This outermost epidermal layer consists of dead keratinocytes rich in the tough fibrous protein keratin and stuck together by intercellular neutral lipids. The stratum corneum is the major physical barrier that prevents environmental chemicals and microorganisms from entering the body. In addition to the keratinocytes, the epidermis contains minor cell types, the *Langerhans cells* and the pigment containing melanocytes. Langerhans cells are fixed tissue macrophages, a distal outpost of the immune system that serves to process antigens which breach the stratum corneum.

So-called *skin appendages,* including hairs, oil (sebaceous) glands and sweat glands, originate from the basal layer of the epidermis. They invaginate into the dermis and exit to the surface through the epidermis. Bacteria may bypass the stratum corneum by traversing these conduits.

The *dermis* is several millimeters thick and is separated from the epidermis by a basement membrane. The fibrous proteins *collagen* and *elastin* are embedded in a glycoprotein matrix and constitute the strong supportive dermal structure. Through it courses a rich plexus of blood vessels and lymphatics. Interruption of dermal blood flow predisposes to infection by restricting access of humoral and cellular defenses against invaders and by compromising the nutrition of the epidermal barrier.

Subcutaneous fat, the third layer of the skin, consists predominantly of lipid cells which play not only an aesthetic role, but are also effective as heat insulators, shock absorbers, and depots of caloric reserves. Below this layer is a *superficial fascia* that separates the skin from muscles. As described below, any or all these layers of "soft tissue" may be involved in a given infectious process.

ENCOUNTER

The skin is sterile only at birth. It is soon colonized by a flora that includes both anaerobic and aerobic bacteria, ranging from 10^2 to 10^4 colony forming units (cfu) per square centimeter of surface. Many factors affect the distribution, composition and density of this flora, few of which are understood. They include not only the environmental climate, which differs throughout the world, but also the microclimates of the body. The "tropical swamps" of the axilla and the groin are markedly different from the "deserts" of the back.

The two properties that make the skin hostile to bacterial growth are *exfoliation* and *dryness*. The constant sloughing of the stratum corneum dislodges many of the bacteria that adhere to its surface. The importance of dryness can be seen when occlusive dressings are applied: within two or three days bacterial counts may increase from 10^2 to more than 10^7 cfu/cm^2. Accordingly, bacterial counts are much higher in the moist areas than in drier regions. Other factors that contribute to limit bacterial growth are low pH, low temperature, and chemical composition. The skin has a pH of approximately 5.5, the result of hydrolysis of sebum lipids by the skin bacteria themselves. Growth of some microorganisms is further hindered by the skin's low temperature, with an average of about 33°C. Parts of the skin are also frequently salty due to the evaporation of sweat, which selects for salt-resistant species, such as *Staphylococcus epidermidis*. Some organisms are also inhibited by the lipid content of the skin surface.

The bacterial flora of the skin, like that of mucous membranes, also helps protect the host from invasion by pathogens and skin infections are more likely to occur when it is wiped out. The mechanisms involved are not known but may include saturation of binding sites, competition for nutrients, and production of bacteriocins and other inhibitory chemicals.

Members of the resident flora are of low virulence and rarely cause significant infections. Included are *resident bacteria*, capable of multiplication on the skin and regularly present, and *transient bacteria*, which survive on the skin for a time but cannot develop permanent residency. Members of the transient flora are deposited on the skin either from mucous membrane "fallout" or from the environment. Evidence is accumulating that specific adhesins are required for some bacteria to adhere to the skin before they are able to colonize it.

The dry and exposed areas of the skin are normally colonized with Gram-positive bacteria (including *Staphylococcus epidermidis*, micrococci, anaerobic Gram-positive cocci, and both anaerobic and aerobic diphtheroids). *Propionibacterium acnes*, a Gram-positive anaerobic rod, thrives in the sebaceous areas. Facultative and anaerobic Gram-negative rods more often colonize the axilla and groin regions and other moist areas, such as the web of the toes. For some unknown reason, in bedridden patients with serious medical illnesses, there is increased colonization of Gram-negative bacilli on the skin.

The most important organisms of the transient flora are the common pathogens of cutaneous infections, *Staphylococcus aureus* and *Streptococcus pyogenes*. These organisms are found more often on exposed skin than on areas normally protected by clothing. *S. aureus* is found commonly on the face and upper body rather than on the trunk and legs, probably because the reservoir for this organ-

Table 49.1
Members of the skin flora and the infections they cause

Resident Flora
    Propionibacterium acnes
    Staphylococcus epidermidis—infection around foreign bodies (prosthetic
        devices, etc.)
    Micrococci
    Anaerobic Gram-positive cocci
    Aerobic Gram-negative bacilli—(low numbers)
    Pityrosporum ovale (a yeast)
Transient Flora
    Bacteria
        Frequent:
            Staphylococcus aureus—abscesses, toxic shock and bacteremia
            Streptococcus pyogenes—cellulitis, lymphangitis
        Infrequent:
            Haemophilus influenzae—cellulitis
            Clostridia—gangrene
            Francisella tularensis—tularemia
            Bacillus anthracis—anthrax
            Pseudomonas aeruginosa—hot tub infection
            Pseudomonas cepacia—foot infection ("foot rot")
            Mycobacterium marinum—"fish tank cellulitis"
    Fungi
        Candida albicans—diaper rash, chronic paronychia
        Dermatophytes—tinea infections (ringworm)
    Viruses
        Frequent:
            Herpes simplex I & II—perioral ("cold sore"), genital infection
            Papilloma—warts
        Infrequent:
            Molluscum contagiosum—wart-like lesions

ism is the upper respiratory tract. Table 49.1 lists some of the important pathogens that transiently colonize the skin and the infections they cause.

ENTRY, SPREAD, AND MULTIPLICATION

Infectious agents enter the skin and its underlying soft tissues in many different ways:

• From the outside, via cuts, wounds, insect bites, skin disease or other breaks in the integrity of the stratum corneum;

• From within, from underlying tissue or carried by blood or lymph.

Once microorganisms have penetrated the skin, they may spread locally and invade the lymphatics or the blood stream. As a result, infections that are originally confined to the skin and soft tissues may ultimately cause complications in other areas of the body. An example of staphylococcal osteomyelitis following a skin abscess is discussed in Chapter 11.

In some bacteria, spreading is associated with specific virulence factors: an example is *hyaluronidase* (also called *spreading factor*), an extracellular enzyme made both by *S. pyogenes* and *S. aureus* (Chapter 11). Other enzymes, such as hemolysins, lipases, collagenase and elastases are elaborated by cutaneous pathogens and probably play a role in pathogenesis (see Chapter 7). In general, S. aureus infections tend to localize, i.e., form abscesses, whereas S. pyogenes infections spread more extensively through tissues.

What is the role of cellular and humoral immunity in the skin? Neutrophils are attracted to the infected area by chemoattractants elaborated by the bacteria, by tissue macrophages, and by activation of complement via the alternative pathway. A local antimicrobial effort is mounted by the epidermal macrophages, the Langerhans cells, through the elaboration of cytokines. Patients with acquired and congenital immunodeficiences have an increased frequency of certain skin infections, e.g, Candida, which suggests that both humoral and cellular immunity are important in skin defenses. When microorganisms breach the stratum corneum and begin to multiply, the host's traditional defenses are mobilized to the skin as elsewhere. When the defenses are defective, infections of the skin become frequent events.

DAMAGE

Cellular damage to the skin and soft tissues may be mediated by toxins, degradative enzymes, and the induction of the host cellular responses that destroy tissues. The kind of infection caused by the invasion of microorganisms in the skin depends on the level of penetration and on the host response. Infections of skin and soft tissue may be divided into three classes:

• Exogenous infections that result from direct invasion from the external environment.

• Endogenous infections due to invasion from an internal source, such as the blood or an infected organ; and

• Toxin induced skin diseases, caused by toxins produced at a distant site.

EXOGENOUS INFECTIONS

There is controversy about whether potent pathogens are able to directly penetrate the normal skin when present in high concentrations, or whether they enter via imperceptible microscopic lesions. When there are no noticeable mechanical interruptions, it takes a high number of potent pathogens to produce exogenous skin and soft tissue infection: experimental studies have shown that colonization of the skin by more than 10^6 S. aureus per square centimeter of skin is required to cause skin lesions. Normally, bacteria grow to such high densities only under special circumstances, such as when the skin gets very dirty or is kept moist for prolonged periods of time. Once the skin barrier is broken from trauma or surgery, infection may be caused by as few as 10 to 100 S. aureus per square centimeter. A number of conditions predispose one to skin invasion.

Excessive moisture may result from the use of occlusive dressings or from wet diapers in babies. Obese people accumulate moisture in their intertriginous folds. Immersion infection is seen in people who spend much time in wet or swampy areas and cannot allow their footwear to dry out, such as troops during training or combat. Moisture induces skin maceration and a breakdown of the stratum corneum. It is estimated that among U.S. foot soldiers in Vietnam, disability was more often due to skin infections than to combat-associated wounds. Staphylococci and streptococci are frequently responsible, but waterborne Gram negative bacteria may also be involved. The modern era has heralded a new type of immersion infection that is acquired by bathing in hot tubs containing high numbers of *P. aeruginosa* (Chapter 19).

Trauma is the most common factor leading to skin and soft tissue infection. It may be mild, as in a torn hangnail or cracks in the skin due to athlete's foot. Major forms of trauma that place the patient at risk include surgery ("organized trauma"), gunshot wounds, crush injuries (automobile accidents), or burns, with large areas of skin denuded and left open. Infections in surgical wounds are a major cause of morbidity in postoperative patients. Infections are also the primary cause of mortality in burn victims, once their acute problems of fluid balance are controlled.

Many procedures used in the hospital breach the skin, the most common being the use of *percutaneous* ("through the skin") *catheters*. The list of such devices has grown enormously: It includes central venous lines, peritoneal dialysis catheters, tubes to drain body cavities, temporary pacemaker lines, chemotherapy infusion lines, and parenteral nutrition lines. Indeed, the most common reason for premature removal of these catheters is bacterial infection. Another type of skin infection in hospitalized patients are the cutaneous lesions that develop secondary to pressure injury—the so-called bed sores. Constant pressure leads to skin necrosis and frequently to secondary infection.

Any condition that compromises the blood supply predisposes the skin to invasion by causing barrier breakdown and limiting defenses. This may occur following peripheral vascular disease, as in diabetics, elderly patients, or patients with vasculitis. In the diabetic patient, compromise of the vascular supply is often accompanied by peripheral sensory neuropathy; these patients are sometimes not aware of traumatic damage to their skin. Secondary infections may also follow certain noninfectious skin diseases known as atopic dermatitis or pemphigus vulgaris.

The skin responds to invading microorganisms in a limited number of ways, which fall into three general categories:

- *Spreading infections*, called impetigo when confined to the epidermis, erysipelas when involving the dermal lymphatics, and cellulitis when the major focus is the subcutaneous fat layer.

- *Abscess formation*, known as folliculitis, boils (furuncles), and carbuncles.

- *Necrotizing infections*, including fasciitis and gas gangrene (myonecrosis).

The organisms commonly implicated are listed in Table 49.2. Cellulitis is illustrated in the following case.

Table 49.2

Some frequent exogenous infections of the skin and soft tissues

Disease	Organisms
Folliculitis	Staphylococci, *Pseudomonas*
Abscesses	Staphylococci
Impetigo	Streptococci, staphylococci
Erysipelas	Streptococci
Lymphangitis	Streptococci
Cellulitis	Streptococci, staphylococci, *H. influenzae* (in children)
Synergistic cellulitis	Streptococci, enteric bacteria, anaerobes
Fasciitis	Streptococci, enteric bacteria, anaerobes

Streptococcal Cellulitis

Case

A 27-year-old emergency medical technician was seen for a slight infection around the nail of his left index finger (medically called paronychia). The lesion was drained and a culture of the pus grew a group A β-hemolytic streptococcus (S. pyogenes). The patient was not given antimicrobial agents because the physician believed that drainage was sufficient. Five days later the patient complained of fever and severe pain in the forearm, which had become swollen and reddish (erythematous). His temperature was 40.2°C and he was sweaty and hot. A patchy rash extended from the left upper arm to the shoulder. Lymph nodes in the axilla were enlarged and tender. The patient was admitted to the hospital with a diagnosis of streptococcal cellulitis. He

*was treated successfully with high doses of penicillin. Blood cultures drawn
before starting chemotherapy also yielded group A S. pyogenes.*

Comments

Cellulitis refers to an acute inflammatory process that involves subcutaneous
tissue, characterized by areas of redness, induration, heat, and tenderness. The
borders usually blend with the surrounding tissues, which distinguishes it from
erysipelas where the lesions are frequently sharply demarcated. Cellulitis may
spread very rapidly and is often accompanied by lymphangitis and inflammation
of the draining lymph nodes. More than 90% of cases are due to group A streptococci, *S. aureus*, and the rest to a variety of bacteria. In children, *Haemophilus
influenzae* type b is an important cause of cellulitis, and may be characterized by
a blue tint of the overlying erythema (such a case is described in Chapter 52).
Cellulitis associated with cat or dog bites or scratches is often due to *Pasteurella
multocida* (see Chapter 55). This organism is a normal inhabitant of the oral flora
of many domestic and wild animals. When injected into the skin through a bite or
scratches, it causes a rapidly spreading and painful cellulitis.

The pathological processes in cellulitis develop rapidly and may progress within 24 to 48 hours from a minor injury to severe septicemia. Characteristically, the
tissues contain few organisms, but have a marked inflammatory response, probably caused by the toxins and inflammation-provoking compounds elaborated
by the invading bacteria. The ability of group A streptococci to spread through
the tissues is aided by hyaluronidase and other spreading factors mentioned
above.

Impetigo is a characteristic infection of the epidermis, manifested by intra-
epidermal vesicles filled with exudate, which eventually result in a weeping and
crusting lesion (Fig. 49.2). It is caused either by group A streptococci or staphylococci and is a disease of children, seen mainly in exposed areas of the body
during warm and moist weather. It is not usually associated with systemic signs
or symptoms.

Figure 49.2.   A case of impetigo, showing a superficial crusting infection of
the face.

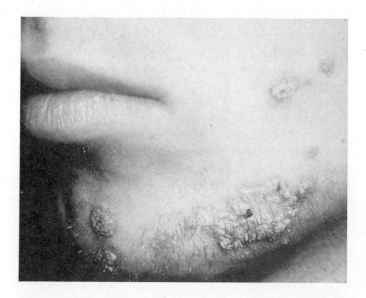

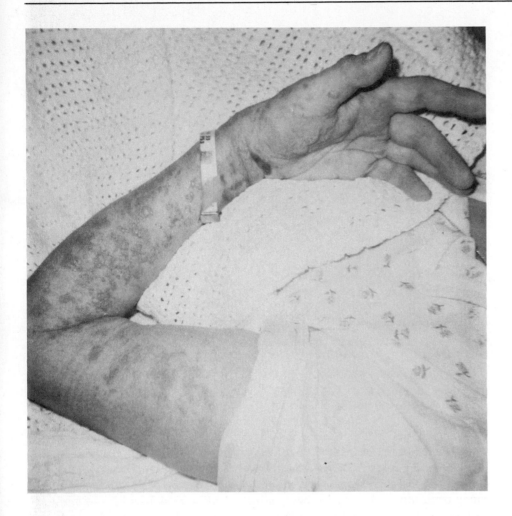

Figure 49.3. A case of erysipelas due to *Streptococcus pyogenes* in a patient with a preexisting skin disease (psoriasis).

Erysipelas is a more serious disease, characterized by tender superficial erythematous and edematous lesions. The infection spreads primarily in the superficial lymphatics of the dermis (Fig. 49.3). The rash is usually confluent but is sharply demarcated from the surrounding normal skin, and extends very rapidly. It is seen most frequently in adults with edema of the extremities and often occurs on the face. By far, the most common organisms that cause erysipelas are group A streptococci. Infection of the deep lymphatics, or *lymphangitis*, is also caused by group A streptococci. Erysipelas used to be one of the most serious complications of surgery and puerperal sepsis (postpartum infection, see Chapter 12), and had a high mortality rate. Its severity and incidence have markedly decreased over the last few decades. The decline can be explained only partially by the widespread use of penicillin to treat streptococcal infections.

Skin Abscesses

Case

A 37-year-old roofer came to the emergency room with a painful swelling on the left side of his neck and fever (Fig. 49.4). He had previously been healthy except for occasional boils. Three days before he noted a minor irritation

Figure 49.4. Skin abscess in the neck developing from an infected hair follicle of the beard.

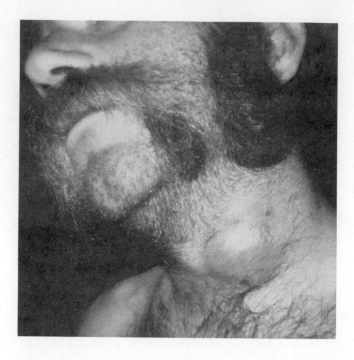

around some whiskers. The lesion progressed to the size of a walnut, which prevented him from buttoning his shirt. Physical examination revealed a febrile (temperature 38.8°C) healthy man in mild distress. On his left anterior cervical area at the beard line there was a 2 × 3 cm mass with a soft center, surrounded by a rash. Needle aspiration of the mass yielded about 1 ml of pus that, under the microscope, showed large Gram positive cocci in clusters and many neutrophils. A culture grew S. aureus. The abscess was incised and drained, and the patient was successfully treated with antibiotics.

Comments

Cutaneous abscesses usually begin as superficial infections in and around hair follicles, called *folliculitis.* This is a pustular eruption usually associated with S. aureus. In the follicle, bacteria are somewhat sequestered from defense mechanisms and are capable of forming microabscesses. If not controlled, these abscesses enlarge to become *furuncles,* better known as *common boils.* If a number of boils cluster together to form a large multifocal infection, the lesion is called a *carbuncle.* Furuncles may be a recurring and frustrating problem in patients, especially young ones, who are chronic nasal carriers of virulent S. aureus. Although these lesions are confined to the skin, they may be a source of bacteremia and complications, as in the case of osteomyelitis described in Chapter 11.

The pathological processes that lead to abscess formation involve a massive influx of neutrophils and walling off of the infected site. This is deposition of fibrin (fostered by staphylococcal coagulase), and stimulation of fibroblasts to produce a fibrous capsule. The result is a well-organized infection, containing necrotic white blood cells and huge numbers of bacteria— i.e., pus. The pathological steps that lead to abscess formation include tissue destruction by the invading organisms and by the massive release of lysosomal enzymes from lysing neutrophils, and deposition of fibrin (Chapter 11). The unique physicochemical characteristics of abscesses are discussed in the chapter on antimicrobial strategies (Chapter 28). Therapy of an abscess is usually two-pronged: removal of pus by incision and drainage, and when warranted, treatment with antimicrobial agents.

Necrotizing Infections

Case

A slightly feverish 57-year-old diabetic woman came to the emergency room after 2 days of pain in her right forefoot. When her pain started, she had noticed tenderness and serous (watery) discharge between her third and fourth toes. She had been bothered recently by an ulcer on the sole of her foot, apparently caused by constant scraping against her shoe. On physical examination she appeared ill and had a temperature of 39.8°C. Her whole right foot was swollen with patchy erythema, cyanosis, and signs of necrosis. There was crusting and oozing around her third and fourth toe (Fig. 49.5).

Cultures of the exudate and the blood were taken and the patient was started on antibiotics. After 24 hours she showed no clinical improvement and the infection continued to move up her leg. She was taken to the operating room, and multiple incisions revealed necrotic fasciitis extending to the upper thigh. As much necrotic tissue as possible was removed. Cultures from the wound grew out the anaerobic Gram negative rod Bacteroides fragilis and an enteric bacterium, Enterobacter. Her blood cultures were negative. She slowly recovered and underwent a second operation for closure of her wound.

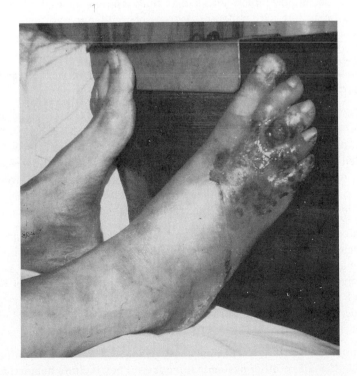

Figure 49.5. Necrotizing cellulitis of the foot due to a mixed anaerobic-aerobic infection. The patient was diabetic and the infection arose from an ulcer on the sole of the foot.

Comments

This is a case of *synergistic necrotizing fasciitis*, probably started by the entry of bacteria through the ulcer on the sole of her foot. Diabetics frequently suffer from poor skin circulation and lack of local sensation, which may have been the reason for the development of the ulcer. The infection spread rapidly along the superficial fascia that separates subcutaneous fat and muscle. The vessels and nerves that supply the skin course this fascia, and their destruction leads to the patchy necrosis and cutaneous anesthesia that characterizes such a rapidly spreading and dangerous infection.

Tissue necrosis occurs to some extent in most infections but the term *necrotizing infections* (or *gangrenous infections*) is reserved for those where extensive necrosis is the outstanding characteristic. Gas from bacterial metabolism is sometimes found in these lesions (Chapter 21). Necrotizing infections of the skin are often caused by *S. pyogenes*, or as in this case, by the synergistic combination of enteric Gram negative rods and strict anaerobes, such as *Bacteroides* or clostridia (Chapter 16). If a necrotizing infection is suspected, the diagnosis should be confirmed by inspection of the fascia on surgical exploration. This disease must be distinguished from the more severe clostridial gas gangrene or myonecrosis, which involves the muscle (Chapter 21). Antibiotic treatment of necrotizing fasciitis rarely works, probably because of the compromised blood supply; extensive surgical debridement is mandatory.

INVASION FROM WITHIN

The skin may become infected by microorganisms that spread from another infected site, either by direct extension from an underlying focus or via the blood stream. Such secondary infections occur in both immune competent and immunosuppressed hosts but with different degrees of incidence and severity. Some of the types of skin infections that occur from within are listed in Table 49.3. Systemic infections are manifested in a variety of ways:

- Abscesses. These may result from intravascular infections such as endocarditis, particularly when due to *S. aureus*.

- Necrosis. This manifestation is seen in chronic meningococcemia or in overwhelming meningococcal septicemia, where there may be large areas of confluent necrosis of the skin called *purpura fulminans*, the skin manifestation of disseminated intravascular coagulation (Fig. 49.6). Milder forms of necrosis are also seen, for example, in disseminated gonorrhea. In the immunocompromised host there is a unique skin lesion called *ecthyma gangrenosum*, usually seen with *Pseudomonas aeruginosa* septicemia. A case of this disease is presented below.

- Many infections are accompanied by *rashes*, or exanthems. These are seen in a large variety of infections, caused by rickettsiae, other bacteria, and viruses. They are subdivided as hemorrhagic rashes, often accompanied by necrosis (as in meningococcemia (Fig. 49.6), and macular (spotted) rashes (as in typhoid fever or Rocky Mountain spotted fever). Rashes are prominent in several viral infections, such as measles and rubella, and are known as the *viral exanthems* (Chapter 36 and Table 49.4).

- A large number of cutaneous lesions are themselves noninfectious but are secondary to septicemia or other systemic infections. They include hemorrhages, pete-

Table 49.3

Examples of sources of endogenous skin infections

Direct Extension
  Osteomyelitis—draining sinus
  Septic arthritis—draining sinus
  Lymphadenitis
    a. Tuberculosis
    b. Atypical mycobacteriosis
  Oral infection—dental sepsis
    a. Actinomycosis (lumpy jaw)
    b. Mixed cellulitis
  Intra-abdominal—necrotizing infection
  Herpes simplex
  Zoster—varicella
Hematogenous Spread
  Bacteremia
    Meningococcus
    Staphylococcus
    Pseudomonas
  Endocarditis
  Fungemia—*Candida*
  Viremia—varicella, measles
  Recurrent viral infections
    Herpes simplex
    Zoster
  Rickettsioses
    Rocky Mountain spotted fever
    Epidemic or endemic typhus

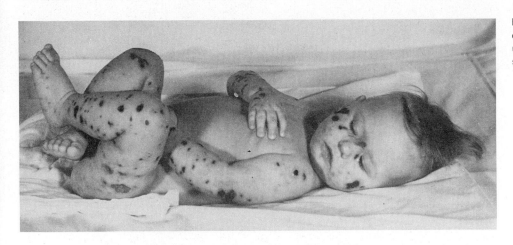

Figure 49.6. Hemorrhagic purpura due to disseminated intravascular coagulation in a child with meningococcal septicemia.

Table 49.4
Some viral diseases with cutaneous manifestations

Disease	Etiological Agent	Principal Cutaneous
Herpes simplex	Herpes simplex virus	"Cold sore" on lip Vesicles in genital area
Herpes zoster	Varicella virus	Shingles—vesicles over specific dermotome(s)
Chickenpox (varicella)	Varicella virus	Vesicles, becoming purulent, then dry, crusted lesions
Measles	Measles virus	Maculopapular rash
German measles	Rubella virus	Maculopapular rash
Smallpox (eradicated)	Smallpox virus	Uniform pustular vesicles

chiae, and special manifestations of subacute bacterial endocarditis called Osler nodes and Janeway spots (Chapter 51). They are due to vasculitis, probably caused by deposition of immune complexes.

Pseudomonas Ecthyma Gangrenosum

Case

A 52-year-old man underwent chemotherapy with cytotoxic agents for an aggressive lymphoma. As the result of the chemotherapy, his white blood cell count fell to fewer than 100 cells per microliter of blood. The patient suddenly developed shaking chills and fever, and complained of pain over his left shoulder. Examination of the area showed an erythematous round area with a central vesicle (Fig. 49.7). Because of the suspicion of Gram-negative bacteremia, the patient was started on broad-spectrum antimicrobial agents. Within a matter of a few hours, the lesion on the left shoulder developed a necrotic center with surrounding erythema, a lesion known as ecthyma gangrenosum. A biopsy of the lesion showed that it contained an infarcted blood vessel teeming with bacteria. Cultures of the biopsy material and the blood grew Pseudomonas aeruginosa. The patient responded to the antimicrobial chemotherapy, with resolution of fever and clearing of the skin lesions.

Figure 49.7. Ecthyma gangrenosum, a necrotic skin lesion due to *Pseudomonas aeruginosa*.

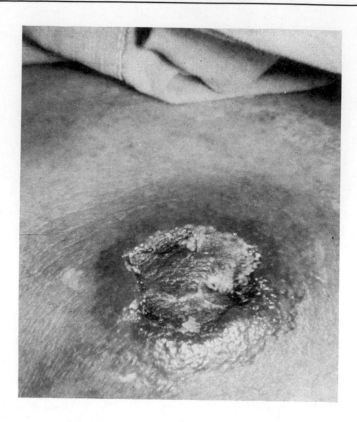

Comments

This case exemplifies a specific skin lesion resulting from seeding of the skin with *P. aeruginosa*. One of the characteristics of endogenous infection with this organism is arteritis resulting in infarction of the skin from vascular insufficiency. This organism grows in the infarcted area and causes necrosis by the production of exotoxin A and other toxins (see Chapter 19). Biopsy of the necrotic area revealed no neutrophil infiltrate because of the patient's granulocytopenia. Instead there was infarction of blood vessels by bacterial emboli, with destruction of the arterial wall and bacterial invasion of the surrounding tissues.

This characteristic lesion usually is diagnostic of Gram negative bacteremia, with *P. aeruginosa* the most common organism encountered. Other Gram negative rods may also be involved, e.g., *Aeromonas* and *Serratia*; occasionally, *Streptococcus pyogenes* also causes these manifestations. It is imperative that the physician treat early—before bacteriological confirmation—because the mortality rate in untreated granulocytopenic patients with Gram negative bacteremia is 50% within 24 hours.

CUTANEOUS RESPONSES TO BACTERIAL TOXINS

The skin responds to toxins elaborated during infections that take place at a distant site. An example is seen in scarlet fever, a pharyngitis caused by certain strains of group A streptococci that elaborate an exotoxin called *erythrogenic factor*. This toxin spreads through the blood stream and is responsible for the red rash, "strawberry tongue" and desquamation of the skin of the extremities.

Scarlet fever used to be a serious disease of childhood; the marked decrease in its severity over the last century has defied explanation.

Staphylococci cause two specific toxin-induced skin diseases: *scalded skin syndrome* and *toxic shock syndrome*. Staphylococcal scalded skin syndrome, a disease of infants, is due to the action of a toxin, *exfoliatin*, that separates the epidermis by destroying the intracellular connections (desmosomes). The result resembles skin scalded with hot water. The other staphylococcal toxin skin disease, toxic shock syndrome, is presented below.

Toxic Shock Syndrome

Case

A 24-year-old woman had an operation to repair an inguinal hernia. Five days later she developed shaking chills and a rash that started on her trunk and rapidly spread to the head and extremities. She became progressively sicker over the next 48 hours, developing a sore throat, headache, myalgias (muscle pains), vomiting, diarrhea, and postural dizziness (dizzy when upright, suggesting low blood pressure). She was neither menstruating nor using tampons. On physical examination she had a diffuse rash with some blanching on pressure. Her eyes were inflamed with conjunctivitis, and she had an erythematous pharynx and a "strawberry tongue". Her inguinal wound was draining a brown odorless material.

Laboratory examination revealed a high white blood cell count and elevated high serum creatinine (5.7 mg/dl), indicating acute renal failure. A Gram stain of the material from the wound showed Gram-positive cocci in clusters, and grew S. aureus. The organism tested positive for the toxic shock syndrome toxin. The patient ultimately showed desquamation of her hands and trunk (Fig. 49.8). She was placed on antibiotics and eventually recovered.

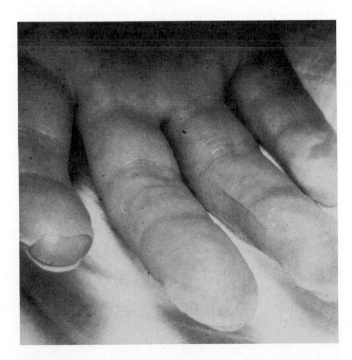

Figure 49.8. Desquamation of the skin of the hand in a patient with staphylococcal toxic shock.

Comments

This case is a typical clinical presentation of toxic shock syndrome (TSS). The disease is due to an exotoxin produced by *S. aureus* strains that cause minor infections, such as at small surgical wounds. This syndrome was first described in children in the early 1970s. It became widely known in the early 1980s when young menstruating women using "super tampons" developed this impressive syndrome: If untreated, TSS can be fatal. The tampons used facilitated the colonization of the vagina with *S. aureus*; the toxin was then absorbed to act systemically. Today tampon-associated TSS is rare; more commonly it occurs after an infection, as illustrated in this case.

CONCLUSIONS

The skin and its underlying soft tissues protect the body from hostile influences in the environment. To penetrate these barriers, infectious agents are most often helped by traumatic breaks, the bite of insects, or other skin diseases. Microorganisms may also lodge in the skin and soft tissues as the result of hematogenous or lymphatic dissemination. The resulting diseases are extraordinarily varied and are caused by a wide variety of mechanisms. Thus, the hallmark of infectious diseases of the skin and soft tissues is variety in the clinical presentation. The skin also acts as a diagnostic window for a multitude of diseases. The clinician can acquire a wealth of critical information by careful examination of the skin.

SUGGESTED READINGS

Noble WC: *Microbiology of the Human Skin*, ed 2. London, Lloyd-Luke, 1981.

Noble WC: *Microbial Skin Disease: Its Epidemiology*. London, Edward Arnold, 1981.

Swartz M: Skin and soft tissue infections. In Mandel GL, RG Douglas, JE Bennett (eds): *Principles and Practice of Infectious Diseases*, ed 2. New York, John Wiley & Sons, 1985.

Weinberg A, Swartz M: General consideration of bacterial diseases. In Fitzpatrick et al: *Dermatology in General Medicine*, ed 3. New York, McGraw-Hill, 1987, pp. 2089–2100.

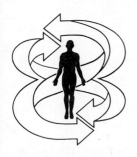

Bone, Joints, and Muscles

G. Medoff

BONE INFECTIONS

Infections of bone, or osteomyelitis, may result from bloodborne infections (hematogenous) or from the direct introduction of microorganisms from external (environmental) or contiguous sources (soft tissues or joints). A special type of the latter category is the infection of the bones of the feet that occurs in patients with diabetes. The pathophysiology of the diseases, the types of infecting agents, and the kinds of treatments and prognoses are frequently different. For this reason, they will be discussed separately.

A Case of Hematogenous Osteomyelitis

Oscar, a 15-year-old boy, received an injury to the lower part of his right thigh in a high school football game. The pain was so intense he had to leave the game. The pain then subsided for several hours but returned that night and he developed chills followed by a fever to 39.4°C. A physician who saw him the next day noted that the lower right thigh was hot, swollen, and tender. The knee joint was normal with full range of motion. The patient had a temperature of 38.3°C. The physician noted several small boils on the neck and chest of the patient. Some were scarred and crusted and the patient admitted squeezing them in the past 2 days. X-rays of the right femur showed soft tissue swelling without any abnormalities of the bone.

Oscar has acute hematogenous osteomyelitis and the most likely infecting organism is *Staphylococcus aureus*. This diagnosis becomes even more plausible when the pathophysiology of the infection is understood.

Which features of the history and physical examination of the patient point to this diagnosis?

1. The trauma to the leg suffered in the football game damaged the distal femur and probably resulted in rupture of small blood vessels and formation of hematoma or blood clot in the bone. The disruption in the normal anatomical barriers made the bone more susceptible to infection.

2. Manipulation of the boils by the patient probably resulted in bacteremia, with *S. aureus* a likely infecting organism. Bloodborne *S. aureus* could have then seeded the traumatized bone and caused the infection.

3. The history of chills and fever, as well as pain and inflammation over the area of trauma, indicates that an infection is in progress. The normal x-ray does not rule out osteomyelitis because it may take several weeks for the characteristic changes in the bone to appear (periosteal proliferation or elevation, loss of bone cortex, bone lysis, etc.). Why do you think this is so? Most likely it is because about 50% of bone must be destroyed before bone lysis can be detected on x-ray. A radionuclide bone scan would be more likely to be positive early in the disease because it measures inflammation, although not infallibly.

Pathophysiology of Acute Hematogenous Osteomyelitis

Bone has a high rate of synthesis and resorption, two processes that depend on a rich vascular supply. Many bloodborne infections therefore involve actively growing sites; this explains why hematogenous osteomyelitis occurs mostly in children and adolescents, at a time of life when long bones are growing rapidly. The most frequent sites are the growing ends (metaphysis, Fig. 50.1**A**) of long bones because this is the site of growth and of most rapid turnover. This is particularly true when this part of the bone has suffered severe trauma with disruption of blood vessels and hematoma formation.

The anatomy of the vascular supply of the metaphysis also predisposes this area to infection. The capillaries from the nutrient arteries of bone make sharp loops close to the growth plate and then expand to large sinusoidal vessels that connect with the venous network of the medullary cavity. The sudden increase in diameter of these vessels slows blood flow and results in sludging of red blood cells (Fig. 50.1**B**). This is a fertile area for the growth of bacteria because microclots form spontaneously in areas of slow blood flow. Clots retain bacteria and allow them to proliferate shielded from neutrophils. The result is inflammation, small areas of bone necrosis and an acid pH, all of which cause more tissue destruction and more bacterial growth. The endothelial cells in the capillary loop and sinusoids in the bone lack phagocytic properties, which also predisposes these areas to infection.

What Should the Physician Have Done?

The physician should have realized that the local pain and the systemic signs of infection (chills and fever) were indicative of a serious disease, acute osteo-

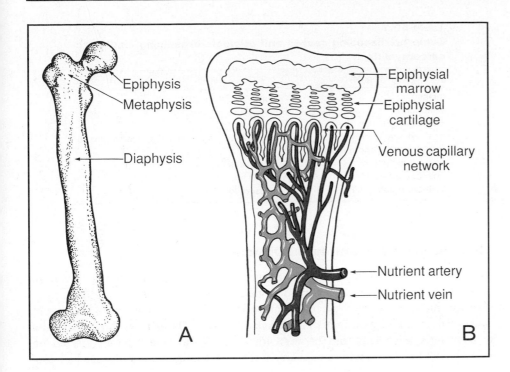

Figure 50.1. **A**, Femur showing epiphysis, metaphysis and diaphysis. **B**, Schematic representation of the vascular supply of a long bone.

myelitis, which calls for admission to the hospital; blood cultures should have been obtained and the patient should have been started on antibiotics. Since about 90% of the patients with this clinical presentation are infected with *S. aureus*, a penicillinase-resistant penicillin or a cephalosporin should have been used empirically. If the patient had specific predisposing conditions, other bacterial etiologies would have been more likely (e.g., *Salmonella* infection in patients with sickle cell disease, *Pseudomonas aeruginosa* in drug users). In this case aspiration or biopsy of bones for culture would be indicated to make identification of the organism more certain.

Treatment of osteomyelitis requires a high daily dose of antibiotic continued for 4 to 6 weeks. High doses are necessary to penetrate bone tissue, but we can only conjecture why treatment has to be continued for a prolonged period of time. The areas of bone necrosis that result from the infection are likely to shield the bacteria from body defenses. These areas have to be resorbed, which is a slow process. Meanwhile, antibiotics may help keep the bacteria in check and prevent them from spreading to adjacent areas.

If appropriate treatment is started early in the course of the infection, before very much bone necrosis occurs, patients respond quickly and cure can be achieved in greater than 90% of cases. If fever and pain continue for 24 to 48 hours after treatment is started, surgical drainage may be indicated. Blood cultures will be positive in about one third of cases, which may obviate the necessity of surgery to determine the infectious agent.

Although *S. aureus* is the most frequent infecting organism in hematogenous osteomyelitis, other organisms can also cause the disease. It is apparent from the clinical setting that these organisms may be involved in the infection. Table 50.1 lists other infecting organisms and the clinical situations which suggest them.

Table 50.1

Some predisposing causes and etiologic organisms leading to osteomyelitis

Predisposing Causes	Etiologic Organisms
Infancy	Group B streptococcus
Childhood	*Haemophilus influenzae*
Sickle cell diasese	*Salmonella* sp.
Immunosuppression	Opportunistic fungi, *Nocardia, Pseudomonas*
Residing in an endemic area	*C. immitis, H. capsulatum*
Trauma to the jaw	*Actinomyces israelii*
Animal exposure	*Brucella* sp.
Pulmonary tuberculosis	*M. tuberculosis*

The Course of the Untreated Disease

Unfortunately, the diagnosis was missed in our patient. Oscar was given an oral antibiotic by his physician and sent home. He was not seen again by a physician for another 2 weeks, when he returned to the emergency room because of continued fever and pain in his leg. A repeat x-ray of Oscar's leg showed definite osteomyelitis (Fig. 50.2) and he was admitted to the hospital and started on intravenous treatment with a cephalosporin. Unfortunately, his disease had pro-

Figure 50.2. X-ray showing changes in osteomyelitis (sclerosis and periosteal changes).

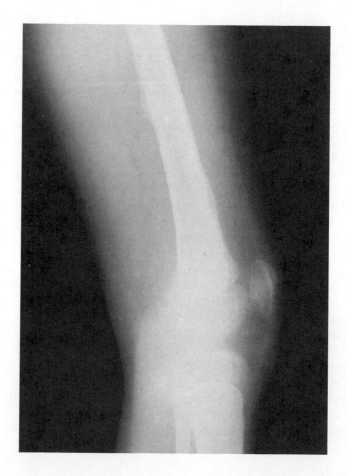

gressed into the subacute and chronic phase of osteomyelitis. By now the compromised blood supply resulted in small avascular pieces of bone, or *sequestra*. The blood supply was disrupted by the pressure caused by inflammation. The chance of medical cure had significantly lessened because of the delay in diagnosis. Over the next few years the patient had a slowly progressive infection with several acute flares each year. Over the next 10 years he spent many days in the hospital and had multiple surgical procedures to drain pus and cut away infected dead bone (Fig. 50.3). He suffered several fractures because of the weakened bone and finally, at the age of 25, had to have his leg amputated because it was feared that the infection would spread into his hip joint and pelvis. Thus an infection which should have been easily treated with antibiotics was converted into a more complex disease (chronic osteomyelitis) which required vigorous medical and surgical intervention, culminating in amputation of the leg to preserve the patient's life.

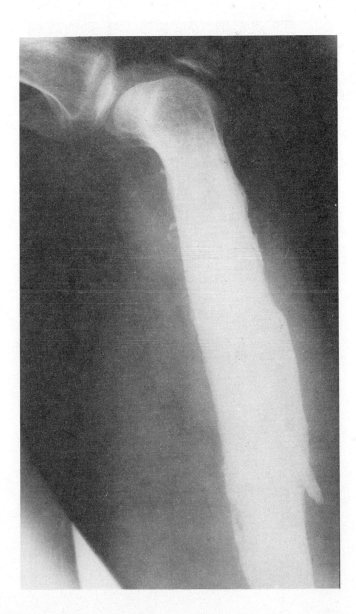

Figure 50.3. X-ray showing changes in more advanced osteomyelitis with extensive bone lesions.

Hematogenous Osteomyelitis at Different Ages

Infants

The clinical presentation of hematogenous osteomyelitis depends on the age of the patient. This is due to the changing characteristics of the bone in different age groups. In the infant, the bone is soft and the periosteum is loosely attached to the cortex. Infection can therefore spread and rupture through the thin cortical bone into the subperiosteal space. Subperiosteal abscesses are common in this age group and lead to a tremendous stimulation of periosteal bone formation at this inappropriate site, as periosteal cells transform into osteoblasts. This new bone formation is disorganized and produces a weakened bone called an *involucrum* (Fig. 50.4) Osteomyelitis in the infant can be a terrible disease early in life. The capillaries of the metaphysis extend into the epiphyseal growth plate and seriously affect growth of the bone. In addition, the infection can also rupture

Figure 50.4. Involucrum (arrow) secondary to extensive periosteal reaction.

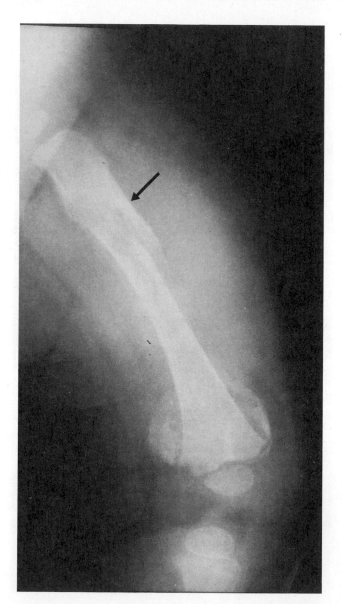

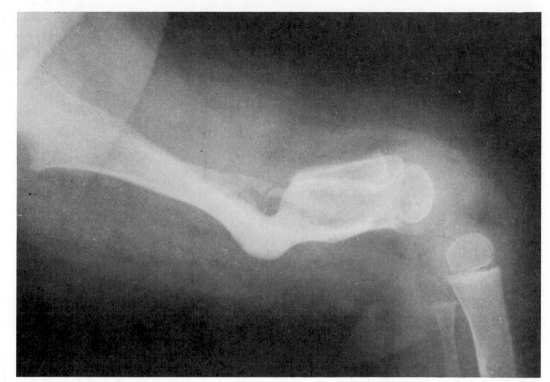

Figure 50.5. Deformity resulting from fracture secondary to osteomyelitis.

into the joint space and cause infectious arthritis. Consequently, osteomyelitis in infants can result in a severe destructive process with marked deformity of bone and abnormalities of growth that will affect patients for the rest of their lives (Fig. 50.5).

Children

Between age 1 and puberty, infection is generally contained in the metaphysis because the bone is more calcified and there are no vessels connecting the metaphysis and the epiphysis. Also, the periosteum is more tightly adhered to the cortex in this age group, so that rupture of infection into the subperiosteal space and formation of involucrum is less likely. Thus, the purulent infectious process will probably be contained in bone, but this has other consequences. Within the bone, pressure builds and results in occlusion of arterioles and clot formation in the capillaries.

Necrosis of bone is the end result of this process: the necrotic sequestrum. Such an area is no longer in contact with the vasculature and acts as a foreign body on which organisms can proliferate out of reach of host defenses and antibiotics. Ultimately, the sequestrum must be resorbed (by the body) or removed surgically if the infection is to be cured. With increasing age, this complication is even more likely because the bone is more calcified and the periosteum even more attached to bone. This is what happened to Oscar.

Adults

Hematogenous osteomyelitis also occurs in adults, in whom the most commonly involved bones are the vertebrae of the spine. The reason for the preferential involvement is unknown; it may relate to the degenerative changes and vascular proliferation in the disk space between the vertebrae that normally occur with age. The infection almost always begins in the disk space and then spreads to the two contiguous vertebrae. Abnormalities of the disk space with erosion of the vertebral plates on x-ray is always infectious and not a malignancy. This is one of the most reliable rules in radiology (see Fig. 11.2).

Staphylococcus aureus is still the most frequent infecting organism, but in vertebral osteomyelitis there is a high frequency of Gram negative bacterial infection. There are probably several reasons for this. First, Gram negative bacteremia resulting from sources in the bowel, gallbladder, and urinary tract is more frequent in the population over age 60. Second, the pelvic veins flow into the paravertebral plexus (Batson's plexus), and infection of bone may occur from drainage of infected pelvic organs (like the bladder and kidneys) which empty their blood into the complex ramifications and anastomoses of this venous system.

Diagnostic Approaches

Because of the variety of the etiologic agents, cultures and a determination of antibiotic sensitivity are imperative. If blood cultures are negative, tissue biopsies

Figure 50.6. Vascular supply of a vertebral body showing the ascending lumbar vein (*1*), the intraosseous vertebral venous plexus (*2*), the intervertebral vein (*3*), the traverse internal vertebral venous plexus (*4*), the posterior external vertebral venous plexus (*5*), the inferior vena cava (*6*), the anterior external vertebral venous plexus (*7*), nutrient branches from the segmental artery (*8*), and the spinal artery and its branches (*9*).

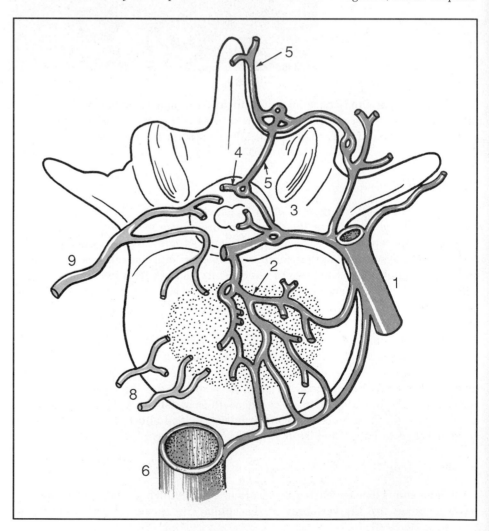

must be obtained for this purpose. Aspiration or needle biopsy of the disk space can be done with guidance from x-rays or a CT scan. Most of these infections respond to medical therapy, but the neurologic status of the patient has to be carefully followed since the infection may spread from the vertebral body into the subdural or subarachnoid space through the rich venous and arterial plexus of the paravertebral circulation (Fig. 50.6). Sensory or motor changes imply spread of the infection into the epidural space and may necessitate surgical drainage to prevent permanent damage to the nerves of the spinal cord. Thus, proper management of these cases requires a good understanding of anatomy, neurology, and pathophysiology.

Osteomyelitis Secondary to External or Contiguous Foci of Infection

Bone infection may also result from the direct introduction of microorganisms from external or contiguous sources. Penetrating trauma is an obvious example of this type of infection. Another type is postoperative infection, particularly when surgery involves placement of a foreign body like a prosthesis or fixation device, such as is done to stabilize a hip fracture (Fig. 50.7). This is often a difficult problem to treat both because the bone has been traumatized and the foreign body can act as an avascular sanctuary for the persistence of bacteria. The problem of whether or not to remove the fixation device or prosthesis

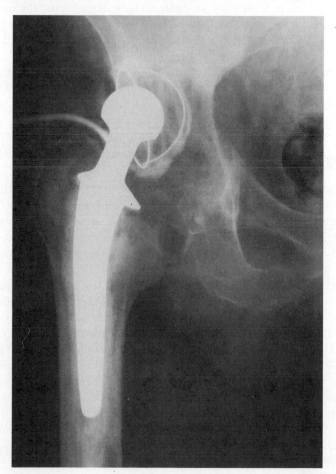

Figure 50.7. Osteomyelitis in bone with a prosthetic fixation device.

is a particularly complex one. On the one hand, the device is necessary for appropriate fixation of the bone (it has been put there for a good reason, i.e., to stabilize a fracture); on the other its presence may prevent the elimination of bacteria. These decisions require close interactions between surgeons and internists to determine if and when removal is appropriate.

Although *S. aureus* is still the number one infecting organism in this type of osteomyelitis, others are also common. Frequently, the type of pathogen reflects the circumstances of the trauma and the area of the body involved. Contamination of the wound with soil often leads to infection by Gram negative bacteria. Postoperative infections are frequently due to *S. aureus*. A wound may become contaminated with bacteria that are part of the fecal flora, particularly in an incontinent patient with a hip fracture.

Osteomyelitis in Diabetic Patients

A special category of osteomyelitis is that in diabetics because of the vascular insufficiency and nerve damage characteristic of diabetes. Skin and soft tissue ulcerations on the feet of such patients may penetrate into the bone (Fig. 49.5). These infections are usually caused by a mixed bacterial flora, with the actual species reflecting the area of involvement. *Staphylococcus aureus*, *Streptococcus* species, Gram negative bacteria, and anaerobic bacteria are all commonly involved. These infections are particularly hard to treat because the organisms grow in necrotic bone with poor vascular supply. Here again therapy involves the use of antibiotics effective against the specific organisms, plus careful surgical debridement. Because of the poor vascular supply to the bone in diabetics, phagocytic cells and antibiotics penetrate poorly into the infected area and therapy is often unsuccessful. Unfortunately, amputation is frequently the end result of what started as a trivial soft tissue infection of the foot. This is why prevention, by paying attention to foot care, is vital to the survival of a patient with diabetes. This point cannot be stressed too much.

INFECTION OF JOINTS

A swollen, red hot, painful joint in a patient with fever raises questions similar to those of osteomyelitis. First, is this an infection? Noninfectious inflammatory joint disease secondary to trauma, gout, pseudogout, or rheumatoid arthritis can also present in this manner. Second, if there is infection how did it get there? As in osteomyelitis, infection can be seeded from a bacteremic focus, be introduced directly into the joint by trauma, by a medical or surgical procedure, or can extend into the joint space from the bone. Third, what is the infecting organism? All three of these questions can usually be answered by obtaining a complete history, doing a careful physical examination and analyzing fluid obtained by aspiration of the joint. Examination of the joint fluid will provide confirmatory evidence.

Synovial fluid consists of water, electrolytes, and other low-molecular-weight substances filtered from plasma, as well as components synthesized and secreted by synovial cells. Serum proteins are present in normal synovial fluid, but in lower concentrations than in plasma. The absence of fibrinogen explains why normal synovial fluid does not clot. The inflammatory reaction in synovial fluid is due to the interaction of serum proteins, phagocytic host cells and microorganisms.

It is important to recognize that diagnosis of one joint disease does not preclude a second. Therefore a joint deformed by arthritis can become infected with bacteria, particularly if that joint has recently been operated on or if steroids have been injected into it. The key to understanding the disease process is to obtain joint fluid for analysis and culture.

The frequency with which bacterial agents cause septic arthritis varies with age. Once again *S. aureus* is the most common overall cause and affects all age groups. *H. influenzae* type b is most frequent in infants between the ages of six months and three years. The gonococcus is the leading cause in sexually active adults and accounts for 30% to 50% of hospital admissions for suppurative arthritis in adults under 30 years of age.

In 1975, a geographic clustering of arthritis cases in several rural communities in southeastern Connecticut, including the town of Lyme, led to the recognition of *Lyme disease*. The unraveling of the epidemiology of this disease is described in Chapter 60. Lyme disease is caused by a spirochete, *Borrelia burgdorferi* and is transmitted to humans by the deer tick. Joint manifestations develop in about half the cases of Lyme disease, usually with one or two large points involved. Since the original description, the disease has been shown to occur in widespread areas of the United States and Europe, and has to be considered in the differential diagnosis of joint infections, especially when distinctive skin lesion, neurologic, or cardiac manifestations are present in the patient.

The etiologic organism can be identified by Gram stain and culture. Even if the Gram stain is negative, antibiotic treatment should be started immediately after joint fluid and blood are obtained for culture to prevent continued infection and destruction of the structures in the joint. Table 50.2 lists the relative frequency of infecting organisms and the clinical situations in which they are most likely to occur. Certain organisms like the gonococcus, *S. aureus*, and several spirochetes have an unusual tropism for the joints. The reason for this is unknown.

In addition to appropriate antibiotic therapy given parenterally and in high doses, the infected synovial fluid should be drained. This can be done by repeated aspirations or by open surgical drainage. One resorts to the latter when the former fails. Open drainage is always done in septic arthritis of the hip joint. This is required to prevent necrosis of the head of the femur which results because the blood supply to this part of the bone is too tenuous. Once again, a review of anatomy helps in understanding the infectious process.

Table 50.2
Most frequent causes of bacterial arthritis by age

Organism	Neonates	Children 2 mos to 2 yr	Children 3–10 yr	Adults
Staphylococcus aureus	10–25%	1–10%	10–25%	25–75%
Streptococcus species (group A, viridans, microaerophilic, anaerobic *streptococcus pneumoniae*)	1–10%	10–25%	10–25%	10–25%
Group B streptococci	10–25%	Rare	Rare	1–10%
Haemophilus influenzae, type b	Rare	25–75%	1–10%	Rare
Neisseria	Rare	1–10%	10–25%	10–25%[a]
Gram negative bacilli	10–25%	1–10%	1–10%	1–10%
Anaerobes	Rare	Rare	Rare	Rare
Other	1–10%	Rare	1–10%	Rare

[a] Generally adults less than 30 years of age.

INFECTIONS OF MUSCLE (MYOSITIS)

All of us have experienced the muscle aches and stiffness (myalgia) that occur commonly when we have a viral illness ("the flu"). In fact, these myalgias are prominent features of a variety of infections such as viral illness, rickettsial infection, and even osteomyelitis and bacterial endocarditis. Fever is often accompanied by muscle pains or myalgias. It is rare that the infecting organisms are directly involved in myalgias. Most often, this muscle involvement is indirect, probably due to the accelerated catabolism of skeletal muscle, part of the so-called acute phase response that accompanies sepsis and trauma. This catabolism is probably mediated by several products of macrophages (monokines) including interleukin-1. The systemic symptoms resulting from these macrophage products are mediated by the increased synthesis of prostaglandin E_2, which in turn activates muscle proteases. The same substances lead to the production of fever in the hypothalamus. All this explains why inhibitors of prostaglandin synthesis, such as aspirin, make us feel better and help resolve both fever and muscle aches.

Specific Muscle Infections

Specific infections of skeletal muscle are uncommon. When they occur, they may be due to a wide range of organisms including bacteria, fungi, viruses, and parasitic agents. Muscles may be invaded either from contiguous sites of infection or by hematogenous spread from a distant focus. The kinds of infection and their frequency depend on the host, geographic area, eating habits, etc. of the patient.

Several of the clinical presentations are so distinctive that they readily suggest the etiologic agent. For example, the presence of gas in muscle makes one think

Table 50.3
Pathogenesis of muscle infections

Pathogenesis	Clinical Presentation	Principal Specific Etiologies
Localized and spread from a contiguous site	Gas gangrene	*Clostridium perfringens*, occasionally other clostridial species
	Synergistic myositis or gangrene	Mixed infections; anaerobic bacteria and enteric bacteria
	Muscle abscesses	*Staphylococcus aureus* Group A, hemolytic streptococcus, Gram negative bacteria
	Miscellaneous	Mycobacterium, nocardia, actinomyces, fungi
Hematogenous spread	Bacterial	Group A, β-hemolytic streptococcus, *S. aureus*, Gram negative bacteria
	Fungal	*Candida, Aspergillus, H. capsulatum, C. immitis*
	Mycobacterial	Typical and atypical mycobacteria, *Trichinella*
	Parasitic	*Dracunculus medinensis*, malaria, filariasis, etc.
	Viral	Influenza, echovirus, coxsackievirus, Epstein-Barr virus

of gas gangrene secondary to *Clostridium perfringens*. Generalized muscle pain and peripheral eosinophilia in a patient who has eaten undercooked pork should raise the possibility of trichinosis.

Table 50.3 lists several of the more common causes of infectious myositis and their specific clinical presentations. Therapy of nonspecific myalgia is usually symptomatic. When a specific etiologic agent is identified, therapy should be directed at this agent. Prompt drainage of abscesses and extensive surgical debridement may be necessary if necrotic tissue is present.

SUGGESTED READINGS

Smith JW: Infectious arthritis. In Mandell G, Douglas G, Bennett JE (eds): *Principles and Practice of Infectious Diseases*. New York, John Wiley & Sons, 1985, p. 697.

Swartz MN: Myositis. In Mandell G, Douglas G, Bennett JE (eds): *Principles and Practice of Infectious Diseases*. New York, John Wiley & Sons, 1985, p. 613.

Waldvogel FA, Medoff G. Swartz MN: Osteomyelitis: a review of clinical features, therapeutic considerations and unusual aspects (parts 1, 2, and 3). *N Engl J Med* 282:198, 282:260 and 282:316, 1970.

Waldvogel FA, Vesey H: Osteomyelitis: the past decade. *N Engl J Med* 303:360, 1980.

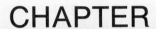

Blood and Circulation

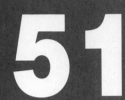

D. Durack

I nfections involving the bloodstream, the blood vessels, and the heart tend to be serious, often life threatening. They are of great concern because they are common and increasing in number. In recent years, the number of clinically significant bacteremias in the United States has risen to an estimated 300,000 cases annually. This is partly due to the large number of hospital-acquired infections associated with complex medical and surgical procedures.

Common terminology for the presence of microorganisms in the blood employs the name of the organism plus the suffix *-emia*: bacteremia, viremia, fungemia, parasitemia, meningococcemia, candidemia, etc. Confusion can arise because terms such as bacteremia, septicemia, and blood poisoning often are used interchangeably. *Bacteremia* covers the whole spectrum of conditions in which bacteria are found in the blood, from trivial to clinically serious. Septicemia implies the presence of severe symptoms and signs. The term "sepsis" is particularly unhelpful, being used loosely by some to mean any infection, with or without blood involvement, while others use it to denote a bloodborne infection.

All the elements of the circulatory system (heart, vessels, blood cells and plasma) can be subject to infections, with a characteristic pattern of entry, spread, and clinical manifestations for each. An enormous variety of microbial species can cause such infections. The most frequently isolated bacteria are Gram negative enteric bacilli, pyogenic cocci such as staphylococci, streptococci, and gonococci, and anaerobes such as clostridia and *Bacteroides*. Viruses and fungi may be transported via the bloodstream to seed other organs. Some protozoa are especially adapted to life in the circulation and carry out important parts of their life cycle in the blood. Examples are the agents of malaria, leishmaniasis, and trypanosomiasis. In this chapter we will discuss bloodstream infections due to bacteria only. Viremias, parasitemias, and fungemias are presented in the chapters dealing with the respective agents (mainly, viral hepatitis, 32; AIDS, 33; fungi, 38; blood protozoa, 40).

BACTERIAL SEPTICEMIAS

Described below is a case of a community-acquired bacterial septicemia caused by a Gram negative bacterium. Hospital-acquired (nosocomial) bacteremias are also often caused by Gram negative rods (see Chapter 19 for detailed examples of *Pseudomonas* septicemia). Gram positive bacteria also commonly cause septicemias (for an example, see Chapter 53, case 4).

Case

Ms. S., a 21-year-old woman, came to the emergency room complaining of fever, shaking chills, nausea, and faintness. She had not felt well for several days, with intermittent fever, nausea, headaches, and aching muscles. On examination, she looked pale and complained of pain when her physician pressed on her right costophrenic angle. She had a temperature of 41.2°C. Blood examination showed an increased neutrophil count (22,000/μl; normal is less than 9,000/μl). Her urinalysis showed 50 white blood cells per high power field.

While these tests were being done, Ms. S. vomited twice and had a chill followed by heavy sweat. Shortly thereafter she became confused and severely hypotensive, with a high respiratory rate and rapid pulse. She became increasingly short of breath. She was admitted to the intensive care unit, where hemodynamic measurements showed a high cardiac output and low systemic vascular resistance. Immediate intravenous fluid therapy quickly reversed impending shock. Then, she was given empirical antibiotic therapy and felt better by the next day. The laboratory reported that Escherichia coli had been isolated from her urine (at a count of 5×10^5 colonies/ml) and from two blood cultures taken on admission.

Encounter and Entry

Blood is a highly specialized tissue, and as a liquid, it has no shape and conforms to the boundaries of the vascular tree. As blood circulates, it carries microorganisms from place to place throughout the body. This can be either helpful or harmful to the host. It can be demonstrated experimentally that microorganisms are often cleared more rapidly from the blood than from other organs. For instance, it takes many more pneumococci or staphylococci to cause disease in a mouse when the organisms are injected into a vein than into the peritoneal cavity or under the skin. The bloodstream can carry opsonized bacteria to the spleen, liver, or bone marrow, where flow slows down in the sinusoids. Reticuloendothelial cells lining these channels can efficiently remove vast numbers of opsonized bacteria from the circulation.

From a microbe's view the bloodstream is a relatively inhospitable part of the body. Both constitutive and induced defense mechanisms are particularly well expressed in the circulation. Blood contains powerful antimicrobial systems, including leukocytes, immunoglobulins, and complement. The chemical systems act in the moving bloodstream; for example, antibodies and complement can attach to circulating bacteria. On the other hand, cellular defenses, such as neutrophils, act efficiently only after the blood has delivered them to a suitable site in another tissue.

The circulating blood can be considered to be sterile under normal circumstances. Nevertheless, in most people a few bacteria circulate briefly every day. These bacteria are members of the normal flora that "spill over" mechanical barriers such as the skin or mucosae. They are usually non-pathogens and are quickly cleared without any ill effect. On the other hand, pathogenic microorganisms are not always removed from the blood, but may persist there. Bacteria may travel throughout the body and seed various tissues to cause secondary infections. Important examples include meningitis, endocarditis, hematogenous osteomyelitis, brain and liver abscesses. Frequently, the organisms spread from an abscess or some other primary focus of infection (Table 51.1). Establishment

Table 51.1

Examples of sites of origin, precipitating factors, and likely organisms causing bacteremias

Origin of Organisms	Favored By	Typical Organisms
Normal flora		
Skin	Trauma, intravenous injections	*Staphylococcus epidermidis*, propionibacteria
Mouth	Tooth decay, periodontitis, dental procedures	Viridans streptococci
Gut	Neutropenia, portal hypertension	Gram negatives, enterococci, anaerobes
Genitourinary tract	Catheterization, delivery	Gram negatives, enterococci, group B streptococci
Transient flora		
Upper respiratory tract	Viral infections	Meningococci, *Haemophilus* species
Skin	Trauma	*Staphylococcus aureus*, group A streptococci
Gut	Achlorhydria	Salmonellae, *M. tuberculosis*
Environmental pathogens (primary bacteremia)		
Skin	Minor trauma, localized skin infections	Group A streptococci, *Staphylococcus aureus*
Vessels	IV injections	*P. aeruginosa, S. aureus*
Gut	Ingestion of large inocula	Salmonellae, brucellae
Throat	Viral infections	Group A streptococci, *H. influenzae N. meningitidis*
Environmental pathogens (secondary to foci of infection)		
Cellulitis, boils	Diabetes, neutropenia	*S. aureus*, group A streptococci
Phlebitis	Intravenous lines	*S. aureus*, Gram negative rods
Pneumonia	Hypogammaglobulinemia	*S. pneumoniae*, *K. pneumoniae*
Urinary tract infection	Instrumentation, stone	*E. coli, Enterococcus faecalis*
Genital tract infection	Delivery, sexual contact	Group B streptococci, *N. gonorrhoea*
Gastrointestinal tract	Trauma, perforation	*B. fragilis, Enterococcus faecalis*
Endocarditis	Prior heart disease	Viridans streptococci

of a clinically significant bloodstream infection requires one or more of the following conditions:

• Introduction of an inoculum large enough to overwhelm normal defenses;

• Preexisting impairment of defense mechanisms; and

• Adaptation of the invading organisms to survive in the blood.

These considerations also apply to the lymphatic system. Thus, organisms may be found in the lymph itself, may infect lymph nodes and vessels, or may be transported in lymph to other sites.

The patient described above, Ms. S., had Gram-negative septicemia. Gram-negative bacteria that cause septicemia usually are members of the normal gastrointestinal flora. They gain entry into the blood through some break or failure of the natural barriers, or as a complication of some preexisting infection, such as urinary tract infection, pneumonia, or abdominal infection (Table 51.1). In the case of Ms. S., the source was her infected urinary tract. Newborn infants with septicemia caused by group B streptococci (such as that described in Chapter 53, case 4) encounter the organism during the birth process. These organisms are present in the mother's vaginal canal, where they cause no disease. They quickly colonize the newborn baby's oropharynx, and probably enter into the bloodstream from that site.

Gram-negative septicemia is a major clinical problem. It has been estimated that in the United States alone there are more than 100,000 cases yearly, with a 20% to 50% mortality rate. In about one third of these cases, septicemia is accompanied by some degree of hypotension or shock, and in about 10%, by disseminated intravascular coagulation (see Chapter 7 on endotoxin). If severe, this condition is known as *septic shock*. This is a disease of modern medicine; very few cases were reported prior to 1920. Why is this so? Most likely, the reason is not increased pathogenicity of the etiologic agents, but the extraordinary repertoire of modern diagnostic and therapeutic techniques. Paradoxically, these technical advances can facilitate entry of bacteria into the bloodstream and render the host less able to clear the organisms. The following factors weaken or interfere with host defenses:

• Invasive techniques—intravenous catheters, arterial catheters, Foley catheters, and other medical devices often bypass host barriers and permit bacteria to enter the bloodstream.

• Immunosuppressive therapy—a wide range of powerful immunosuppressant drugs is being given to an ever larger number of patients for treatment of malignancies or inflammatory diseases, or for organ transplantation.

• Supportive measures—these keep patients alive for long periods despite severe or incurable underlying disease; and

• Antibiotics—use of high doses and long courses of multiple potent antibiotics promote selection of resistant organisms.

E. coli is the most frequent of the Gram-negative etiologic agents. Second is *Klebsiella*, followed by *Pseudomonas*, then many bacteria which may be acquired in a hospital setting (e.g., *Serratia, Enterobacter, Proteus*).

In people with intact immune systems, microorganisms usually must be introduced in relatively large numbers in order to infect the bloodstream. This may happen via trauma, by spread from other infections, or by accidental inoculation. Important examples are soft tissue or wound infections caused by group A streptococci or *Staphylococcus aureus*.

The size of the inoculum needed to produce septicemia may be lower among immunocompromised patients. For example, patients with multiple myeloma are relatively deficient in opsonizing antibodies of the IgG and IgM classes; they are predisposed to bacteremias with encapsulated bacteria such as *Haemophilus influenzae* or *Klebsiella pneumoniae*.

Damage

The manifestations of septicemia are due either to toxic bacterial products, to the host response, or to both. *P. aeruginosa*, *S. aureus*, and *Streptococcus pyogenes* are examples of organisms that produce exotoxins that cause damage to both red and white blood cells, as well as to cells in tissue (Table 51.2).

Central to our understanding of how Gram-negative bacteria give rise to the manifestations of septicemia is *endotoxin*, the lipopolysaccharide (LPS) of the outer membrane of these organisms (Chapter 7). The injection of LPS into animals reproduces many of the signs and symptoms of the disease in humans. The active portion of the molecule has been shown to be the lipid A moiety. Of the manifold activities of this compound, four seem to be particularly relevant to the pathophysiology of Gram-negative septicemia:

- *Vasodilatation and increased capillary permeability*. These changes may be of considerable magnitude and result in notable decreases in systemic vascular resistance, as in the case of Ms. S. This gives rise to a cardinal manifestation of the Gram-negative septicemia, *hypotension*. Leaky vessels in the lung may also lead to the so called *adult respiratory distress syndrome*. How are these changes mediated? A most important mediator appears to be a cytokine, *tumor necrosis factor* (TNF or cachectin, Chapters 4 and 7). The injection of this protein into animals produces a syndrome virtually indistinguishable from septic shock (see Chapter 4).

- Of particular importance is activation of complement by the alternative pathway, initiated by endotoxin. In Gram-negative septicemia, the degree of complement activation may be high. This leads to the release of mediators of inflammation, such as the anaphylatoxins C3a and C5a, which in turn release histamine from mast cells and basophils. Chemoattraction of white bloods cells by C5a may cause an abnormal accumulation of neutrophils in small vessels of the lungs,

Table 51.2
Examples of bacterial virulence factors important in infections of the circulatory system

Factor	Consequence	Examples
Pili	Attachment at mucosal surfaces	*E. coli, N. gonorrhoeae*
Slime layer	Colonization of surfaces	*Staphylococcus epidermidis*
Capsule	Resistance to phagocytosis	*Streptococcus pneumoniae, H. influenzae, K. pneumoniae*
Endotoxin	Activation of complement, clotting, kinins; fever, shock	Gram negatives
Hemolysins	Intravascular hemolysis	*S. aureus*, clostridia
Leukocidins, proteases	Killing of leukocytes and other cells	*S. aureus, Pseudomonas aeruginosa*

leading to decreased lung function and to poor oxygenation of the blood. Hageman factor (factor XII) also activates pre-kallikrein to kallikrein, which initiates the cascade leading to the production of bradykinin, a vasoactive peptide that leads to further vasodilatation and increased capillary permeability. Like histamine, this causes decreased systemic vascular resistance and leakage of fluid into the lung, thus contributing to the adult respiratory distress syndrome. This can cause respiratory failure, an important cause of death in patients with severe Gram-negative septicemia.

• *Intravascular clotting.* Endotoxin activation of Hageman factor results in turn in activation of the clotting cascade. This may result in consumption of platelets and formation of clots throughout the circulatory system. Eventually, when occlusion of small vessels leads to reduced blood flow, the function of major organs becomes affected. As clotting continues, clotting factors may be consumed more rapidly than they can be produced. This gives rise to the condition known as disseminated intravascular coagulation (DIC), which paradoxically is characterized by both continued thrombosis and uncontrollable bleeding (Chapters 4 and 7).

• *Fibrinolysis.* The Hageman factor also activates the fibrinolytic pathway by converting plasminogen proactivator into plasminogen activator. This contributes to DIC and to further hemorrhagic damage to infarcted tissues.

• *Fever.* TNF has an important role in the production of fever. It can itself produce fever but also induces the release of interleukin-1, the primary endogenous pyrogen (Chapters 4 and 7).

Finally, the stress of septic shock results in the release of other molecules, including ACTH, epinephrine, and the endorphins. The latter may lead to further vasodilatation, thus worsening hypotension.

The damage caused directly and indirectly by endotoxin, IL-1 and TNF helps us understand many of the clinical manifestations seen in Ms. S., the patient described above. Her classical signs of septicemia and septic shock—high fever, chills, hypotension—were easy to recognize. However, in many cases, the initial symptoms may be more subtle. Some of the early signs are apprehension, agitation, tachycardia, hyperventilation, and associated respiratory alkalosis. Early recognition is important because early therapy is the key to improved survival.

Gram-positive bacteria may also give rise to septicemic syndromes, with similarities to those due to Gram negatives. The most frequent source of the invading Gram-positive organisms is the skin, which at most sites is colonized chiefly by this group of bacteria. In people with an intact immune system, microorganisms must be introduced in large numbers in order to infect the bloodstream. This may occur via trauma or by drainage into the bloodstream of material from septic foci elsewhere in the body. Examples are wounds infected by group A streptococci or *S. aureus.*

Because Gram positives do not make endotoxin, one might expect lesser likelihood of shock in septicemias due to these organisms. This is partly true: only about 5% of the patients develop shock, as opposed to 25% with Gram negative septicemia. Nonetheless the two types of septicemias may produce shock and other manifestations; often they cannot be differentiated on clinical grounds.

How do Gram positives cause septic shock? This remains an open question. Some of the components that have been implicated are specific exotoxins, such as the α-toxin of *S. aureus*, which can cause aggregation of platelets and myocardial depression, and staphylococcal toxic shock toxin, which causes hypotension and other manifestations of shock (see Chapter 11). Some workers have suggested that portions of the Gram-positive murein or other cell wall components may substitute for endotoxin.

Diagnosis

The clinical manifestations of septicemia are highly variable. Typically, patients with this infection have a high spiking fever and are obviously ill. Severe, shaking chills followed by sweats are common. However, these findings may be intermittent, with regular or irregular periods of improvement. Some patients are virtually asymptomatic. Diagnosis of bacterial septicemia requires two basic steps: (a) suspicion of the diagnosis from a consideration of the setting, associated medical conditions, and the clinical findings, and (b) demonstration of the presence of bacteria in the blood, usually done by a blood culture. Occasionally bacteria can be seen directly in Gram-stained smear of buffy coat. Indirect evidence of septicemia may be obtained by the detection of bacterial antigens (such as pneumococcal polysaccharide) in blood, urine, or cerebrospinal fluid, using various serological means (see Chapter 59).

Prevention and Therapy

Prevention of septicemia is usually directed specifically towards persons who are known to be at risk. It is difficult to achieve, but can be prevented in some cases by the prophylactic use of antibiotics, infusion of immunoglobulins or leukocytes. Attention must be given to predisposing conditions which can cause bacteremia, such as dental procedures, abscesses, pneumonias, and urinary tract infections.

Treatment of a patient with septicemia usually has three priorities:

1. *To rapidly clear the blood of microorganisms* in order to prevent immediate major complications, such as hypotension, shock, acute renal failure, etc. This is usually attempted by the use of empirical antibiotic therapy, using drugs that are probably active against the most likely organisms. In immunologically normal hosts, bacteriostatic antibiotics are usually sufficient.

2. *To treat the original focus*, if known. Often this requires surgical intervention, such as draining abscesses, removing an infected gallbladder, and, in the case of gangrene, amputation of extremities.

3. *To treat systemic complications* such as hypotension or renal failure, and localized ones, such as seeding of the organisms at secondary sites. This may require intensive care, such as the administration of adrenergic drugs to support blood pressure, ventilation to support lung function, and dialysis to support renal function.

Critical factors in the treatment of septicemia are early clinical suspicion of the diseases, timely diagnosis, intensive supportive care, and antibiotic therapy. Antibiotics remain the most important specific therapeutic agents in treatment of these conditions. They should be administered at the first clinical suspicion of septic shock, without waiting for the result of bacteriological diagnosis. Therapy should consist of the administration of antibiotics active against the most likely etiological agents, enteric bacteria. Broad-spectrum antibiotic coverage usually includes an aminoglycoside and a β-lactamase-resistant β-lactam agent with anti-pseudomonal activity. The antibiotic regimen may have to be changed once the specific etiology is known.

The choice of supportive measure depends on the clinical complications encountered. Fever can be treated with antipyretics and cooling blankets. For *acidosis*, administration of bicarbonate is a helpful short term measure. Volume replacement is the key to treatment of shock in the early phases; pressor drugs may be necessary in later phases. Central venous monitoring is helpful in determining when volume replacement alone is no longer adequate and pressor drugs are needed. Adult respiratory distress syndrome may require the administration of oxygen and mechanical ventilation. For disseminated intravascular coagulation, the only truly proven therapeutic modality is control of the underlying infection. Transfusion of platelets, plasma, and red blood cells may be needed. Other therapeutic modalities include the use of steroids and passive immunization against *E. coli* endotoxin, both of which remain of doubtful benefit.

INFECTIVE ENDOCARDITIS

Case

Mr. K., a 49-year-old attorney, complained to his physician that he had had headaches, aching muscles, fever, and night sweats for 3 weeks. His health had always been good and he had played baseball for his college team. However, he had been refused admission to the Reserve Officer Training Corps at his college because of a "heart murmur". On further questioning, he reported that he had lost 10 lb over the previous 2 weeks, had poor appetite, suffered from two rather severe episodes of back pain that lasted several days, and generally felt "run down".

On examination, Mr. K. looked thin, pale, and slightly sweaty. His pulse rate was 110 per minute and his temperature 38.1°C. Three small hemorrhages were seen in the conjunctiva under his left lower eyelid, and several more on his palate. Auscultation of his chest revealed a heart murmur that suggested mild aortic valve incompetence. His urine was dark yellow with a positive test for blood; numerous red blood cells and a few red blood cell casts were seen under the microscope. These casts indicate that the RBC's originated in the kidney tubules. His blood count showed that Mr. K. was anemic (hematocrit 33%; normal is greater than 40%), had a normal leukocyte count and an elevated erythrocyte sedimentation rate (62 mm/hr; normal is less than 15). Analysis of his serum revealed the presence of rheumatoid factor and an increase in gamma globulins. Six blood cultures carried out on two successive days were all positive for α-hemolytic streptococci, later identified as Streptococcus sanguis. On the basis of the clinical and laboratory findings, the diagnosis of subacute bacterial endocarditis was made.

The Endocarditis

Infective endocarditis is the disease caused by infection of the endothelial surface of the heart, most often located on one of the valves. There are many forms of the disease, which can be classified in two ways:

• *By the time course.* Before antibiotic treatment became available, endocarditis was always fatal. It could be classified into acute, subacute, or chronic by the length of time from onset to death. If patients died within days or a few weeks. the disease had been acute; if they survived for 6 weeks to three months, subacute; if survival was longer, chronic. The acute form is typically caused by invasive organisms such as *S. aureus*, pneumococci, gonococci, or group B streptococci and often affects previously normal heart valves. Subacute or chronic endocarditis is usually caused by α-hemolytic streptococci originating from the mouth. This form commonly develops on a previously damaged heart valve. With treatment, the various forms of the disease are cut short, before they have run their course.

• *By the causative organisms.* This is a useful classification because it is specific. Predictions as to progress, outcome, and optimal therapy can be based on past experience with the etiologic agent. In practice, both classifications tend to be used together (see below).

Infective endocarditis is uncommon, but not rare. The yearly incidence is estimated to be approximately 10 cases per 1 million people. In the United States there are about 0.3 to 3 cases per 1000 admissions to large general hospitals. In the past, the leading predisposing cause was chronic rheumatic heart disease. Fortunately, this has become much less prevalent in the United States and has been replaced by other cardiac conditions: congenital heart disease, mitral valve prolapse, artificial heart valves, and degenerative valvular disease in the elderly.

Encounter and Entry

Infective endocarditis is often caused by members of the normal oropharyngeal flora, which is probably what happened to Mr. K. The α-hemolytic streptococci found in his case almost certainly originated from the mouth or throat, where they are prominent members of the normal flora. These organisms enter the blood through minor abrasions caused daily by food particles or by toothbrushing and flossing. In 30% to 70% of people, dental procedures caused small, transient "showers" of oral bacteria to enter the bloodstream. About 1 in every 5 or 6 patients with α-hemolytic streptococcal endocarditis have had dental work shortly before onset of the disease. Less commonly, organisms from the fecal and vaginal flora enter the circulation, with or without overt breaks in the epithelia. They are usually group D streptococci, the so-called enterococci (*Enterococcus faecalis*, *E. faecium*, *E. durans*). These organisms often cause prostatitis or urinary tract infections in elderly males; in such patients, cystoscopy or other procedures may lead to enterococcal bacteremia. A list of the most common etiologic agents is presented in Table 51.3.

The acute form of infective endocarditis in patients with no predisposing cause is usually caused by bacteria more virulent than the streptococci that infected Mr. K. *S. aureus* is the single most common cause of acute endocarditis in individuals with normal heart valves; other causes are the group B and D streptococci, pneumococci, and gonococci. Characteristically, this form of the disease is a destructive pyogenic infection that severely damages the heart valves, is likely to cause valve ring abscesses and has a devastating and rapid course.

Infective endocarditis is almost invariably preceded by bacteremia. An exception is postoperative endocarditis, where the infection may be initiated directly by contamination of prosthetic valves at the time of surgery. When this takes place by contamination of the valves at the time of surgery, *early prosthetic valve endocarditis* results (commonly arising less than 60 days after surgery). This deserves special consideration because of the nature of the organisms, and the poor

Table 51.3
Etiologic agents of endocarditis and their approximate frequency[a,b]

	Native Valve Endocarditis, %	Intravenous Drug Abusers, %	Early Prosthetic Valve Endocarditis, %	Late Prosthetic Valve Endocarditis, %
Streptococci (all)	65	15	10	35
Viridans, α-hemolytic	35	5	<5	25
S. bovis (group D)	15	<5	<5	<5
E. faecalis (group D)	10	8	<5	<5
Other streptococci	<5	<5	<5	<5
Staphylococci (all)	25	50	50	30
Coagulase-positive	23	50	20	10
Coagulase-negative	<5	<5	30	20
Gram negative aerobic bacteria	<5	15	20	15
Fungi	<5	5	10	5
Miscellaneous bacteria	<5	5	10	5
Polymicrobial infection	<1	5	5	5
Culture-negative endocarditis	5–10	5	<5	<5

[a] These are representative figures collated from the literature; wide local variations in frequency are to be expected.
[b] Adapted from Durack DT: Infective and non-infective endocarditis. In Hurst JW (ed): *The Heart*, ed. 6, New York, McGraw-Hill, 1986, pp 1130–1157.

prognosis. *S. epidermidis* is the most frequent infecting organism. Because this staphylococcus is often resistant to commonly used antibiotics, and is associated with the presence of a foreign body (valves, sutures), the cure rate is low. Surgical replacement of the infected valves is required in most cases. Endocarditis on a prosthetic valve caused by bacteremia occurring *after* the surgical implant is termed *late prosthetic valve endocarditis*. This form of valvular infection is more similar to endocarditis on a native valve, both in etiology and prognosis.

Bacteremia may result in various ways: as a frequent and spontaneous event in our daily lives; induced by the release of organisms from an infected focus at some site of the body, or arising from exogenous sources. Table 51.3 shows the approximate frequency of the various agents that cause endocarditis. It is apparent that the majority of cases of bacterial endocarditis are caused by Gram positive cocci. Therefore, the question of endocarditis should always be raised when bacteremia is caused by these organisms, and is much less of a consideration when bacteremia is caused by Gram negatives. Because the length of therapy and choice of antibiotics are so different in bacteremia and endocarditis, it is very important to differentiate between these two related entities. Special consideration must be given to endocarditis in intravenous drug users. They are prone to develop bacterial or fungal endocarditis due to frequent nonsterile injections using contaminated syringes, needles, or water. Such individuals have a high rate of endocarditis on right-sided heart valves, which is quite rare in nonaddicts.

Multiplication and Spread

Key factors that allow microorganisms to multiply in the bloodstream and cause endocarditis are their innate ability to withstand host defenses and their capacity to find a refuge from host defenses at sheltered sites. In general, Gram positives are the more common causes of endocarditis because they tend to adhere more avidly to collagen, fibrin, platelets, and heart valve surfaces. They are also generally more resistant to lysis by complement. In addition, the relatively high level of circulating antibodies to common Gram positive cocci makes them clump, which may render them more likely to stick to endocardial surfaces.

Bacteria that are not particularly well equipped to avoid or overcome host defenses, such as the α-hemolytic streptococci, may yet survive in the circulatory system if they can find a sheltered niche. This is probably what happened in the case of Mr. K. The heart murmur noted years earlier suggests that one of his heart valves may have been damaged, perhaps by rheumatic fever or a congenital defect. Underlying valvular disease contributes to bacterial colonization in several ways:

- Damaged or incompetent valves cause eddies and turbulence, which leads to deposition of fibrin and platelets on exposed collagen. Often, turbulence results in lower hydrostatic pressure on the far side of an anatomic abnormality through which blood passes under pressure. Therefore, colonization occurs more often on the atrial side of an incompetent mitral valve. The order of frequency of infection of the valves is mitral > aortic > tricuspid > pulmonic. Colonization may also take place in congenital heart lesions, such as the conditions known as ventricular septal defect, patent ductus, or coarctation of the aorta.

- On a damaged endocardium, bacteria may find shelter in vegetations, a special kind of blood clot. Here bacteria can multiply freely, being shielded from the defense mechanisms of the blood. From such sheltered sites bacteria may reseed the bloodstream, leading to a continuous bacteremia, which is typical of infective endocarditis. Not surprisingly, secondary (metastatic) infections may develop in other sites, especially if the organisms involved are inherently pathogenic.

After bacteria colonize the sterile vegetation, deposition of platelets and fibrin continues and the organisms grow at rates comparable to those in laboratory cultures. In experimental animals, a fully mature vegetation may be seen within 24 to 48 hours.

Microorganisms may also find sanctuary in the walls of blood vessels. The cells of vascular endothelia are weakly phagocytic and sometimes take up microorganisms from the circulation. This can lead to microbial multiplication in endothelial cells, as seen, for example, in Rocky Mountain spotted fever. The resulting vasculitis is the hallmark of this disease (Chapter 25).

Damage

The characteristic pathological feature of endocarditis is a vegetation on a valve (Fig. 51.1). Grossly, the lesions vary in size from a few millimeters to several centimeters. Vegetations are usually located at the line of closure of the valves. Vegetations may also spread along the valve surface to the adjacent mural endocardium or onto the chordae tendineae.

After some time, the presence of bacteria in the blood elicits the formation of specific and nonspecific immunoglobulins. This occurred in the case of Mr. K., who had rheumatoid factor in his blood, and is seen in 25% to 50% of subacute cases. When relatively large amounts of antigen are present, antigen-antibody complexes may form in sufficient quantities to cause immune complex disease,

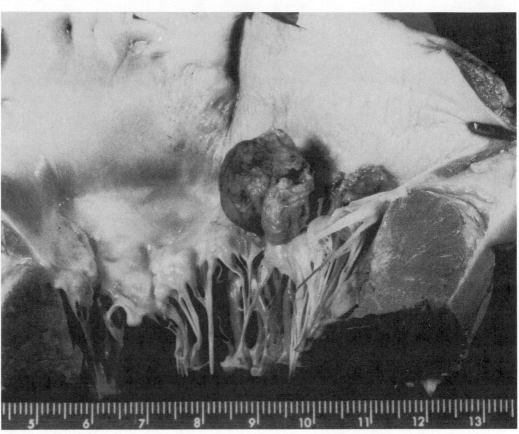

Figure 51.1. Vegetation on a heart valve from a patient with bacterial endocarditis.

for instance, in the joints or the kidney. Again, this happened to Mr. K.; he had immune complex glomerulonephritis, evidenced by the red cell casts in his urine.

Infection of the heart or the blood vessels eventually results in severe local damage. For this reason, infective endocarditis was invariably fatal in the pre-antibiotic era. Even today, Mr. K.'s subacute bacterial endocarditis could have caused his death through cardiac failure secondary to valvular damage. This is more likely if endocarditis is caused by antibiotic-resistant bacteria, or by fungi.

Tissue damage in endocarditis can result from the many different manifestations of the disease: direct invasion of heart tissue causes abscesses; embolization of vegetations occludes blood vessels and can cause tissue necrosis from vascular insufficiency; antigen-antibody complexes produce vasculitis, synovitis, glomerulonephritis, and skin lesions. Not surprisingly, infective endocarditis may also cause a wide variety of systemic and local manifestations; these are discussed in standard textbooks of medicine.

Involvement of the CNS may dominate the clinical course of endocarditis. It may be associated with cerebral emboli, pyogenic meningitis, abscess formation, or a diffuse vasculitis. Emboli of the vasa vasorum may lead to so-called mycotic aneurysms. Aneurysms of this sort may affect arteries at any site of the body, especially the ascending aorta.

Diagnosis

The clinical picture often suggests the diagnosis of infective endocarditis. The key to diagnosis is blood culture. Blood for culturing should be drawn with care, using techniques to avoid contamination by environmental or skin flora. Ten to 20 ml of blood is drawn, preferably on three different occasions over a period of hours. The samples are quickly injected into bottles containing 10 to 20 ml of bacteriological media containing an additive to prevent clotting and overcome the antibacterial factors present in the blood. This, together with dilution by the culture medium, should allow detection of most bacteria present in the sample of blood. To avoid false negative cultures due to antibiotics present in the blood, samples should be obtained before the administration of drugs whenever possible. Alternatively, β-lactamases or other antibiotic-removal compounds should be added to destroy residual antibacterial activity.

Therapy and Prevention

The key to proper treatment is to identify the etiologic agent and determine its drug sensitivity. When these are known, it is possible to achieve a cure with antibiotics in the great majority of cases. The rule is to use high doses of bactericidal antibiotics effective against the infective organisms for a prolonged period of time (4–6 weeks). The desired concentration of the drugs in serum should be high enough to achieve a bactericidal level when diluted 1:8. High doses of antibiotics are sometimes required to sterilize the relatively avascular vegetations. Some organisms, such as antibiotic-resistant Gram negative bacilli or fungi are difficult and sometimes impossible to eradicate with antimicrobial treatment alone. Surgery may be an essential part of the treatment, particularly in endocarditis on a prosthetic valve or in a patient who requires valve replacement for a destroyed valve causing congestive heart failure.

The value of prophylactic antibiotics to prevent endocarditis in patients at risk is uncertain. Such patients typically include those with heart valve lesions who are undergoing dental procedures that may lead to bacteremia. Carefully controlled studies have not been carried out, but most patients with α-hemolytic streptococcal endocarditis who had previous dental work had not received antibiotics. Based on this, it is recommended that patients with known rheumatic fever or heart valve malformations from other causes be given penicillin just prior to and immediately after such procedures as cleaning and extraction of teeth, or invasive maneuvers in the gastrointestinal or genitourinary tracts. Prophylactic use of antibiotics is particularly important in patients who have a prosthetic heart valve. Bacterial endocarditis in such patients has such a bad prognosis that attempts to prevent it are mandatory.

SUGGESTED READINGS

Durack DT, Beeson PB. Pathogenesis of infective endocarditis. In Rahimtoola SE (ed): *Infective Endocarditis*, New York, Grune and Stratton, 1978, pp 1–53.

Durack DT. Infective endocarditis. In Wyngaarden JB, Smith LH (eds): *Cecil Textbook of Medicine*. Philadelphia, WB Saunders, 1988, pp 1586–96.

Sheagren JN: Shock syndromes related to sepsis. In Wyngaarden JB, Smith LH (eds): *Cecil Textbook of Medicine*. Philadelphia, WB Saunders, 1988, pp 1538–41.

Wenzel RP: Prevention and treatment of hospital-acquired infections. In Wyngaarden JB, Smith LH (eds): *Cecil Textbook of Medicine*. Philadelphia, WB Saunders, 1988, pp 1541–49.

Young LS. Gram negative sepsis. In Mandell GL et al (eds): *Principles and Practice of Infectious Disease*. New York, John Wiley & Sons, 1985, pp 452–75.

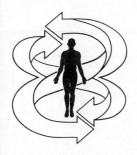

Head and Neck

A.L. Smith

Infections of the head and neck occur most commonly when organisms reach the soft tissue and interstitial spaces of this area by extension from contiguous mucosal surfaces. Less commonly, they may be seeded from the bloodstream. Regardless of the route by which the infectious agents reach the tissue, manifestations of head and neck infections come to medical attention because of signs and symptoms of inflammation. Infections of these parts of the body result in cellulitis, lymphadenitis, or abscesses of soft tissues. The resulting swelling may be readily recognized, for example, when it causes facial cellulitis, or when it affects a physiologic function (such as swallowing).

ENCOUNTER AND ENTRY

The air filled cavities of the head (sinuses, mastoids, middle ear) are lined with respiratory epithelium (Fig. 52.1). Infections of these spaces result when their normal drainage route becomes blocked. With blockage, the ciliated respiratory epithelium, which normally functions to remove bacteria by entrapping them in mucus and propelling the mucus blanket out, can no longer function. Once aerobic bacteria have reached their maximum growth, oxygen in the blocked cavity is depleted and anaerobes can grow. High densities of bacteria release fragments of cell envelopes (such as lipopolysaccharide or murein subunits), which elicit an inflammatory response, leading to swelling and more blockage. The inflammation produces the symptoms of such infections.

Frequently, when the infection involves soft tissue or lymph nodes, a previous viral or group A streptococcal infection served to disrupt the integrity of the

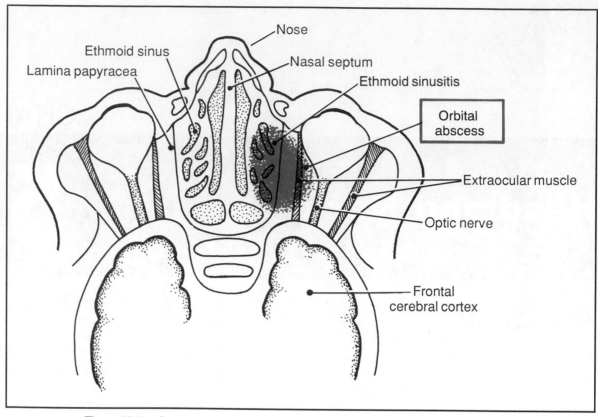

Figure 52.1. Superior view of the face sectioned through the level of the ethmoid sinus.

Table 52.1
Infections of the head and neck

Infections of air-filled cavities
 Otitis media
 Sinusitis
 Mastoiditis
Infections of structures contiguous to air-filled cavities
 Orbital cellulitis or abscess
 Cavernous sinus thrombosis or thrombophlebitis
 Lateral sinus thrombosis or thrombophlebitis
Infections of soft tissues
 Facial cellulitis
 Abscess of canine fossa
 Lymphadenitis
 Parapharyngeal abscess
  Paratonsilar
  Pteromaxillary
  Lateral neck
 Thyroiditis
Infections of embryonic remnants
 Branchial cleft cellulitis or abscess
 Thyroglossal duct cellulitis or abscess

epithelial surface. Histologic examination of respiratory mucosa during acute viral infections shows loss of ciliated epithelial cells and thinning of the mucosal layer. Extension of this process results in physical loss of continuity of the epithelium, allowing bacteria to enter the underlying soft tissue and produce cellulitis or overwhelm the defenses in the lymph nodes and produce lymphadenitis.

In sinusitis, the ostia may become blocked because of a viral upper respiratory infection, or more commonly by allergy, both of which produce edema. In the middle ear, eustachian tube dysfunction may occur congenitally (as in infants with cleft palate who lack the muscle to open the medial orifice of the eustachian tube), as a result of a viral upper respiratory tract infection, or allergy. Since the cavity of the middle ear is contiguous with the mastoid ear cells, every individual with acute otitis media also has mastoiditis, which is an acute inflammatory reaction in the mastoid ear cells.

The most common infections of the head and neck and their etiology are listed in Table 52.1. The bacteria that cause infections of the head and neck are those commonly isolated from the surface of the upper respiratory tract: *Streptococcus pneumoniae*, *Haemophilus influenzae*, *Staphylococcus aureus*, *Streptococcus pyogenes*, *Branhamella catarrhalis*, and anaerobic bacteria. Four clinical cases are discussed next.

OTITIS MEDIA

Emily, a 14-month-old baby, came down with the same "cold" that her sister Anna had for the past 3 days. She then stopped taking her bottle, became irritable, and developed a temperature of 39.8°C. She continued to feed poorly and had a low-grade fever and irritability, which prompted her mother to take her to a physician. In the doctor's office, the nurse used a tympanometer to measure the mobility of Emily's ear drum (see below), and told the mother that Emily had an ear infection. On further examination, the physician agreed, and prescribed the antibiotic amoxicillin.

Emily's mother had many questions:

1. Should Emily's sister Ann be brought in and checked for an ear infection?

2. Is an ear infection contagious?

3. How does a machine (the tympanometer) diagnose an ear infection?

4. Shouldn't a culture be obtained before antibiotics are prescribed? How can the doctor be sure that amoxicillin is the right antibiotic for Emily?

5. Are there complications of ear infections?

Otitis media is one of the most common infections seen by family physicians and pediatricians. The majority of the cases occur in children between 6 and 36 months of age, the average child having two episodes per year during the first 3 years of life. Why are children especially sensitive to this type of infection? A likely predisposing cause is that the eustachian tubes are distended in infancy. Supine feeding (the bottle at bedtime) permits reflux of pharyngeal contents into the lumen of the eustachian tubes, leading to inflammation and occlusion. Dysfunction of the eustachian tubes is also facilitated by upper respiratory infections of the abundant lymphoid tissue around the medial orifice, such as those caused by respiratory syncytial virus, influenza A or B, or adenovirus. Members of the normal upper respiratory flora (pneumococci, *H. influenzae*, and occasionally *S. aureus*, *Branhamella catarrhalis*, and group A streptococci) become entrapped in the middle ear and proliferate. An antecedent viral infection may also predispose to bacterial replication in the middle ear by direct damage to the respiratory epithelium.

The consequences of inflammation of the middle ear are consonant with the anatomy of this region. Early in the course of the infection, submucosal edema and hemorrhage lead to the outpouring of exudate into the lumen. A fluid-filled lumen makes the tympanic membrane relatively immobile and impairs hearing. Mobility can be measured by pneumatic otoscopy (changing the air pressure on the ear drum while looking at it), or by tympanometry (a technique that measures the ability of the ear drum to reflect sound at various air pressures). In the normal ventilated ear, tension on the tympanic membrane varies with the pressure exerted on it. With fluid in the middle ear, the tympanic membrane cannot stretch with changes in pressure and the acoustic impedance (or compliance) does not change.

Frequently in otitis media, the epithelium of the middle ear undergoes marked histological changes: mucus-secreting cells increase in numbers and even form glands. Mucin is secreted into the middle ear, possibly in an effort to entrap and "wash out" bacteria and inflammatory debris. These changes are elicited by bacterial cell wall material and secreted toxins. The usual exit route for fluids, the eustachian tube, may become occluded. Drainage of the fluid either by using drugs that restore eustachian tube function or by direct drainage through a tube inserted through the ear drum permits the metaplastic epithelium to return to normal and the middle ear to become ventilated.

The middle ear may become infected with any of the bacteria present in the upper respiratory tract. As with upper respiratory tract infections (e.g., sinusitis) the primary pathogens are pneumococci and *H. influenzae* (80% of the total). Antibiotics, alone or in combination, active against these two species have proven effective in the treatment of otitis media. Thus, empiric antibiotic administration directed against the most common pathogens is justifiable in this disease. It is not necessary to aspirate the middle ear fluid (a painful procedure) for culture and susceptibility testing.

Although most ear infections treated with antibiotics resolve without complications, chronic and recurrent episodes of otitis media may lead to sequelae such as brain abscess or meningeal epidural abscess. Usually the patient has had a perforated ear drum. In such cases, the pathogens include not only members of the upper respiratory flora, but occasionally enteric Gram negative bacilli that gain access to the middle ear through the perforated ear drum.

CELLULITIS IN THE ORBIT OF THE EYE

Betty, a 14-year-old girl, has had intermittent problems with allergies, manifested primarily as a runny nose, watery eyes, and episodes of fullness in the front part of her face and nose. One morning she developed fever, headache, cough, and had a foul taste in her mouth. She interpreted this as another one of her allergies and took an antihistamine pill and some antipyretics. However, the next morning she awoke with a severe headache, felt terribly ill, and could not open her left eye. Her pediatrician noted marked redness and swelling around her eye and a slight exudate from the eyelids. When she retracted her eyelids she found that Betty's left eye was slightly deviated down and laterally. She recommended that Betty should immediately see an ear, nose, and throat (ENT) physician as she probably had a serious illness, orbital cellulitis.

Betty wondered what was going on:

1. What is orbital cellulitis?

2. Why should she see an ENT physician if her problem was with her eye?

3. Was this not just another one of her allergies?

4. What about getting antibiotics?

Betty's orbital cellulitis—inflammation of the submucosal connective tissue of the eye socket—is a complication of acute sinusitis. The anterior and lateral borders of the ethmoid sinuses form the medial and superior borders of the orbit. The orbit is then separated from the ethmoid sinus by the lamina papyracea, which is literally a paper-thin piece of bone. Infection in the ethmoid sinus may break through this thin piece of bone and enter the orbit. If the infection is localized, it becomes an intraorbital but extraocular abscess (Fig. 52.1).

The physician quickly recognized the disease, because the region of the orbit affected (superior and medial) displaced the eye down and out. Had the eyeball been measured, the physician would have found that it was exophthalmic, i.e., it protruded out of the orbit. This may often not be appreciated without a measuring device. Exophthalmus is due to the edema in the orbit, literally making the cavity smaller and forcing the eye out. As might be expected, other signs of orbital cellulitis include limitation of the movement of the eye as the muscles become edematous and stretched. In addition, stretching of the optic nerve may decrease visual acuity, a very serious complication, and lead to blindness.

Since the source of orbital cellulitis is the sinus, the treatment of choice is surgical drainage. This will decompress the orbit and allow the eyeball to return to its normal place. Treatment of this infection should also include the administration of antibiotics. As with other infections of the head and neck, bacteria isolated from the infected sites represent the oral pharyngeal flora. In the more virulent infections, such as the one experienced by Betty, there is a higher probability that *Staphylococcus aureus* will be isolated. Here, the antibiotics to be administered should be active against *S. aureus* as well as members of the upper respiratory tract flora.

FACIAL CELLULITIS

Ryan, a 14-month-old baby, was not sleeping through the night and seemed hungry all the time; his mother started supplementing his food with a bottle of milk containing cereal. One afternoon, when he awoke from his nap, his mother noted that he was fussy, had a low-grade temperature, and had a slight swelling of his cheek. She thought he might have bumped it with the bottle as he frequently did when feeding himself in the crib. That evening when she put him to bed, he seemed a little improved but still irritable and his cheek was somewhat swollen and had a slightly purplish hue. His temperature seemed increased, but other than that he seemed well. The next morning, his mother thought that he was worse. She took his temperature and found that it was 41.6°C. She took him to the family doctor who told her that Ryan would need hospitalization for antibiotic administration for facial cellulitis.

His mother had many questions:

1. Was this cellulitis different from the kind that she had on her head following work in the garden?

2. Why did Ryan need to be hospitalized to receive antibiotics for cellulitis?

3. How did the bacteria get into Ryan's cheek?

4. Will the antibiotics cure Ryan?

Facial cellulitis in infants is almost exclusively an infection caused by *H. influenzae* type b. The pathogenesis is not entirely clear, but is probable that minor facial trauma allows blood to seep into the soft tissues. When transient *H. influenzae* bacteremia occurs, the organisms seed and grow in the traumatized subcutaneous tissue using the extravasated red blood cells as a source of nutrition (the organism is not called "hemo-philus" [blood-loving] for nothing: it requires, among other cofactors, heme for growth). Since the soft tissue was seeded via the bloodstream, the infant is at risk for other infectious complications of *H. influenzae* bacteremia (such as meningitis, septic arthritis, and osteomyelitis) and requires hospitalization for vigorous treatment and careful observation.

H. Influenzae does not make cell-damaging exotoxins, thus the inflammation in tissues is minimal. Often, as in Ryan's case, the distinction between a slight bruise on the face and cellulitis is difficult to make. The telling clue is that the swelling seems out of proportion to the magnitude of the facial trauma, and that the infant has a high fever. One of the reasons Ryan's physician suspected that the etiological agent was *H. influenzae* was the typical purplish (not reddish) hue of the inflamed region. The reason for this special coloration is not known, but it is characteristic.

H. influenzae cellulitis resolves with the administration of appropriate antibiotics. Because secondary diseases due to *H. influenzae* are serious, the usual treatment is to administer antibiotics intravenously until the cellulitis has resolved.

PARAPHARYNGEAL ABSCESS

Before going to bed one evening, Ms. J., a 19-year-old college student, noticed a "scratchy throat" with slight pain. Over the next 4 days she had an increasingly sore throat and her right ear began to ache. She thought she had a fever and took aspirin. On the morning of the sixth day of her illness, Ms. J. found that she could barely open her mouth to eat breakfast. When she did get food in, it was difficult for her to swallow. Her roommate noted that her voice was of lower pitch and decreased in volume, as though she had something hot in her mouth. She went to the infirmary, where the physician, after looking in her mouth, told her that hospitalization was necessary for additional tests, and possibly for surgery.

Ms. J. had many questions:

1. How could surgery help a sore throat?

2. Don't sore throats go away by themselves?

3. Does her roommate have to worry about catching this illness?

Ms. J. had symptoms that are typical of a *parapharyngeal abscess*. In her case, the most likely diagnosis was that of a *peritonsillar abscess:* This was evident by examination of the mouth. Tonsils lie between the two palatal pillars, with

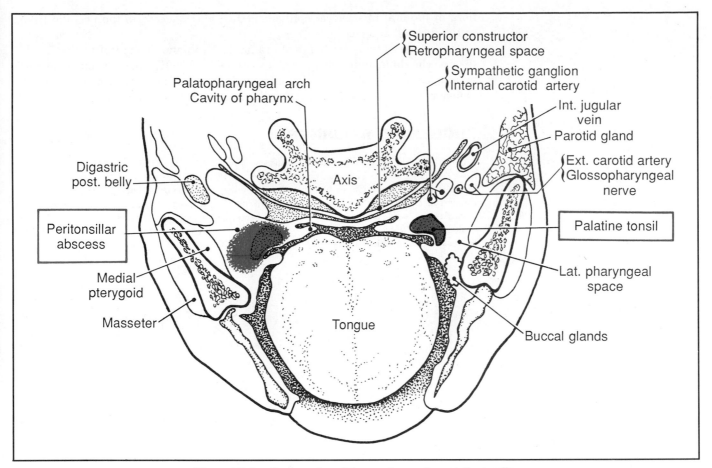

Figure 52.2. Cross section of the oropharynx through the tonsils.

their superior poles overlying a portion of the superior pharyngeal constrictor muscle and their medial portion, the medial pterygoid muscle (Fig. 52.2). These are two of the four muscles which function to open the mouth. Inflammation behind the tonsil adjacent to these muscles causes their dysfunction. Trismus, the inability to open one's mouth, is caused by dysfunction of the medial pterygoid, while the inability to initiate swallowing is due to dysfunction of the superior pharyngeal constrictor. Failure to elevate the palate results from edema in that area; this leads to a muffled, "hot potato" voice, even though the tongue is unaffected. Ms. J. could swallow, as there was no mechanical obstruction to a bolus of food entering her esophagus, but inflammation of the superior constrictor made it hard to initiate the process. When one looks in the mouth of patients with peritonsillar abscess, the tonsil appears medially and downward displaced and on palpation may feel as though it is floating. This is caused by the pus pushing it from behind.

Bacteria that cause this illness are, as in most head and neck infections, those commonly found in the oral pharynx. Most of these organisms commonly are commensals, but group A streptococci are responsible for approximately one-half of the cases of peritonsillar abscess. The infection seems first to cause a cellulitis of the peritonsillar tissues, followed by local necrosis. The aerobic and anaerobic flora of the oral pharyngeal epithelium then gains access to the necrotic tissue in the interstitial space.

The primary therapy is surgical drainage. Antibiotic therapy of choice for this disease should include a drug (such as penicillin G) active against common mouth anaerobes and aerobes but also effective against *S. aureus*. In most cases, the choice is a semisynthetic penicillin that is resistant to β-lactamase.

SUGGESTED READINGS

Brook I: Microbiology of retropharyngeal abscesses in children. *Am J Dis Child* 141:202, 1987.

Hora HJF: Deep neck infections. *Arch Otolaryngol* 77:129, 1963.

Meyerhoff WL, Giebink GS: Pathology and microbiology of otitis media. *Laryngoscope* 92:273, 1982.

Henderson FW, Collier AM, Sanyal MA, Watkins JM, Fairlough DL, Clyde WA, Denny FW: A longitudinal study of respiratory viruses and bacteria in the etiology of acute otitis media with effusion. *N Engl J Med* 306:1377, 1982.

Schlossberg D: *Infections of the Head and Neck.* New York, Springer Verlag, 1987.

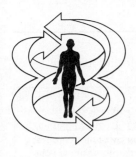

Congenital and Neonatal Infections

53

A.L. Smith
C. Meissner

Congenital infections are those present in the infant before birth. They develop during gestation and may persist after birth. They are also called *intrauterine* or *prenatal infections*. Most of them are acquired from the mother via the placenta. The causative agents include bacteria (e.g., syphilis), viruses (e.g., rubella, HIV, or cytomegalovirus), or animal parasites (e.g., *Toxoplasma*) (Table 53.1). Many of these agents produce benign, self-limited illnesses in adults, but in the developing infant they may cause serious disease. Neonatal infections are those acquired from the immediate surroundings, either from the birth canal during birth or within a few days to weeks after birth. To understand the basis of these infections we must reflect on the unique biological and immunological events that characterize embryonic and fetal development and the first month or so of life.

CONGENITAL INFECTIONS

Special Immunological Problems of the Fetus and the Pregnant Mother

The development of the mammalian fetus poses an immunological paradox: The immune system of the mother and that developing in the fetus must be kept in check to avoid mutual rejection. The mother must not treat her antigenically distinct fetus as she would an incompatible transplant. The fetal unit (fetus and placenta) aids by expressing relatively few transplant antigens on cell surfaces.

Table 53.1
Congenital infection

Organism	Placental Defense	Fetal Growth Retarded	Sequelae	Comment
Rubella	±	+ +	+ +	Illness may continue to progress after birth, producing lesions and embryopathy.
Cytomegalovirus	−	+ +	+	Most common congenital infection. If sequelae occur, deafness is most common.
Herpes simplex	−	−	+ +	Most disease in the neonate is not congenital.
Toxoplasma gondii	+ +	+	+ +	Infection must occur after conception or fetus not at risk.
Treponema pallidum	+	−	+ +	Infant can be treated in utero.
HIV	?	±	±	Normal maturation of immunocompetence may fail to occur.

The fetus, on the other hand, must not develop a "graft versus host" type of immune reaction. This mutual depression of the immune response places both the fetus and the mother at risk of infection. The consequent balancing act is usually but not always successful: Both fetus and mother may become infected—with congenital infection in the fetus and either asymptomatic or acute illness in the mother.

The humoral immune response of the fetus is detectable as early as 2 months of gestation but does not "ripen" until about 2 years of age. "Fetal immunodeficiency" is due to many factors, including the inability of fetal and neonatal mononuclear cells to produce macrophage activating factors. In the absence of cytokines (such as γ-interferon) neither a cytotoxic proliferative response nor an immune response can be mounted effectively. The defect is in the production of these intercellular signals, and partially in the cellular antimicrobial machinery itself. Placental or neonatal macrophages permit the intracellular replication of certain microorganisms (such as toxoplasma), whereas macrophages from adults kill them. In the mother, cytokines are present in the placental circulation but are not transported to the fetus. It would be detrimental if maternal factors were to activate the immune response of her "graft", i.e., the baby.

The fetus is protected by special defense mechanisms: The fetal membranes shelter it from external microorganisms and the placenta protects it from internal ones. The power of these defenses is illustrated by the increased incidence of fetal infections once the amniotic sac is perforated. The mother further protects the fetus by endowing it with considerable quantities of immunoglobulins, largely of the IgG class. At the end of pregnancy, the fetal concentration of IgG antibodies may be greater than the mother's: The placenta actively transports these molecules into the fetal circulation by a mechanism of receptor-mediated endocytosis. Conversely, a child born several months prematurely may not have inherited a full complement of maternal antibodies, which contributes to the increased risk of infection characteristic of such infants. IgM does not cross the placenta; thus if it is found in the newborn, it must have been synthesized by the fetus. Maternal IgG is slowly metabolized, with some maternal antibodies undetectable in the infant's serum 12 months after birth. However, certain antibodies, such as those against measles and HIV, may persist for as long as 12 to 15 months. In addition, breast milk contains IgA antibodies that appear to be protective against certain gastrointestinal invaders.

Special Consequences of Infections in the Fetus

Fetal infections that occur early in gestation (i.e., during organogenesis), carry with them the special danger of causing developmental abnormalities. For example, even minor cellular damage by rubella virus may have serious consequences in the fetus, probably because there are not many mechanisms to correct injury to developing fetal cells. Early in gestation, damage may be so severe that it kills the fetus, or it may be mild enough to be manifested only after the child has grown, or not at all. For example, infection with rubella virus may produce deafness, which is not easy to recognize in the first months of life. After the first trimester, when the early stages of organ development have passed, rubella virus is less likely to cause damage.

The fetus responds to infection in a limited number of ways, partly due to the immaturity of its immune system and partly because different organ systems mature at different rates. At different stages of development, fetal cells may be more or less sensitive to infection. For example, the heart develops in the early weeks of life, and rubella infection at this time may result in cardiac defects in a surviving infant. Similarly, the lens of the eye develops at 4 to 6 weeks of gestation, and rubella infection at this time may cause cataracts. As a consequence of the special sensitivity of developing organs, different infectious agents may provoke the same impairment. In fact, the manifestations of congenital infections tend to be so similar that it is generally difficult to pinpoint a specific etiologic agent on clinical grounds alone. Thus, infections with cytomegalovirus, rubella virus, or *Toxoplasma gondii* may all lead to fetal chorioretinitis, hepatitis, or encephalitis.

Case 1—Rubella

Ms. M., a 29-year-old registered nurse, was pregnant for the first time. During her sixth week of gestation she had her first visit to the obstetrician, who drew blood for serologic testing for rubella and toxoplasmosis. Two weeks later she was disappointed to find out that she had no detectable antibodies to rubella virus. After one more week (ninth week of gestation) she developed symptoms of the common cold, a runny nose and conjunctivitis with normal temperature. She noted three swollen lymph nodes in the back of her neck. These symptoms resolved quickly and she forgot to mention them to her obstetrician. The remainder of her pregnancy was uneventful.

Her son was born at term but showed characteristic signs of intrauterine infection. His birth weight was 2.1 kg (the normal range is 2.6 to 3.8 kg), which suggested intrauterine growth retardation. He had a cataract in his left eye and later was found to have moderate hearing impairment in both ears. He had no detectable heart or central nervous system abnormalities.

Mother and baby were tested for antibodies to rubella, cytomegalovirus, and toxoplasmosis. Both had a high titer to rubella but no antibodies to the other two agents. The infant's serum was found to contain a high titer of IgM *antibodies specific to rubella, which confirmed the diagnosis of intrauterine rubella.*

Ms. M. asked the following questions:

1. Were her early symptoms consistent with rubella?

2. Should she have received the rubella vaccine during her pregnancy?

3. What is the chance that she may transmit rubella to the fetus in future pregnancies?

Case 2—Toxoplasmosis

Drs. Sara T. and Dick T. had just finished their internal medicine residency and were to join a group practice in the fall. She was $3\frac{1}{2}$ months pregnant and was feeling wonderful now that her morning sickness had abated. To celebrate, they took a much needed vacation: 2 weeks in Paris. While there, Sara developed cervical and axillary lymphadenopathy with some fatigue. Several days later, she developed low-grade fever, myalgia, and headache and she sought medical attention. After obtaining blood from Sara and testing it, a Paris physician told her that she had toxoplasmosis and should receive treatment with spiramycin to "save the baby."

The couple considered the following questions:

1. What is the risk of toxoplasmosis to the developing baby?

2. Is spiramycin safe for the baby?

3. How did she catch toxoplasmosis?

To answer the questions presented by these two cases you would need to be familiar with the biology of congenital infections in general, and of rubella and toxoplasmosis specifically. Figure 53.1 shows in general terms the sequence of events in intrauterine infections.

The general features of rubella and toxoplasmosis are typical of many congenital infections: A susceptible mother acquires the infection during pregnancy, with only mild and nonspecific manifestations. Most frequently, the pregnancy is uneventful. At the time of birth, or shortly thereafter, it may become apparent that the infant has congenital malformations, is ill, or both. In many congenital infections, infants are born prematurely and have a birth weight that is inappropriately low for their gestational age.

Encounter and Entry

Congenital infections are almost invariably acquired by transmission from the mother. In this country approximately 75% of adult women are susceptible to infection with *T. gondii*. The remainder have already had the infection by the time they reach the childbearing years. Cysts of *T. gondii* are present in the muscles of many birds and mammals (Chapter 40). Toxoplasmosis is acquired by eating lightly cooked ("rare") meat, especially lamb or pork, or by inhalation of *T. gondii* cysts from stools of infected cats.

To affect the fetus directly, a pathogen must cross the placental barrier. Little is known about how this takes place, but it is surmised that in most cases it follows inflammation at the placental interface. To take *T. gondii* as an example,

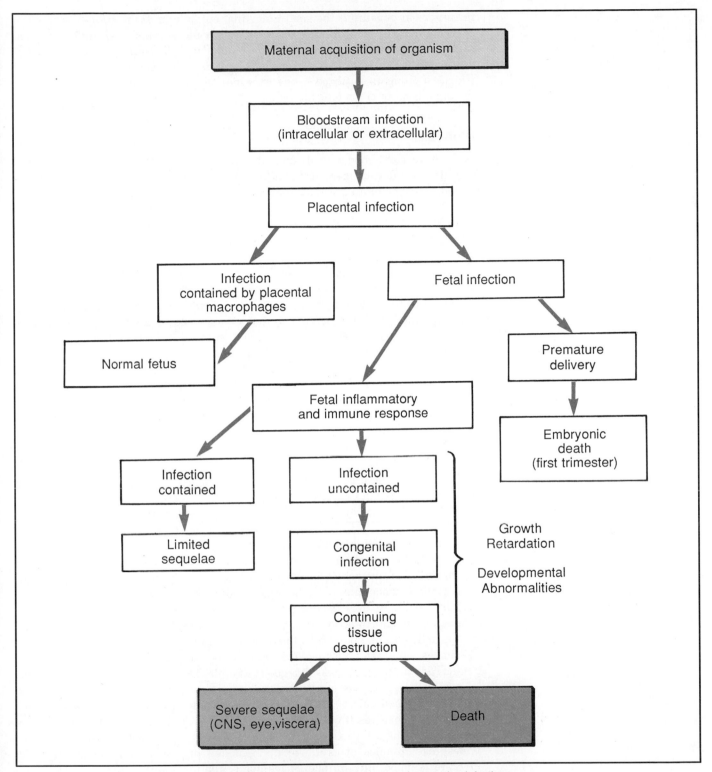

Figure 53.1. The sequence of events in intrauterine infections.

the organism penetrates the gastrointestinal epithelium of the mother, enters the systemic circulation, with the potential to invade a number of different cells. Intracellular replication of toxoplasma results in cell death, resulting in small necrotic foci. When this takes place in the placenta, it results in a *focal villositis*, which may remain localized to the maternal side of the placenta but may allow the organisms to cross into the fetus.

Damage

We have mentioned already that the manifestations of congenital infections may affect the development of the child and become evident only after the neonatal period. In congenital viral infections such as rubella, herpes simplex, or cytomegalovirus, sequelae in the infant are caused by death of infected fetal cells (Table 53.1). In congenital toxoplasmosis, sequelae appear to be due less to tissue destruction than to the host's inflammatory response and scarring of the damaged foci.

In some cases of congenital toxoplasmosis, the manifestations of infection may appear late. Lack of noticeable symptoms at birth does not ensure that there will not be sequelae. If the CSF of such infants is examined shortly after birth, it may show evidence of central nervous system invasion, containing many lymphocytes and an increased concentration of protein. In one study of 13 infants with congenital *T. gondii* infection who were asymptomatic at birth, 11 developed chorioretinitis between the ages of 1 month and 9 years. Three had functional blindness of one eye, one had severe neurologic sequelae, and 4 had minor neurologic sequelae. These data suggest that maternal *T. gondii* infection poses a serious risk to the fetus *even when it is asymptomatic both in mother and newborn*.

Diagnosis

The clinical picture of a newborn with irregular breathing, jaundice, poor feeding, lethargy, and temperature instability suggests that congenital disease is likely. In diagnosing congenital infections, the problem is frequently to distinguish whether the mother, the fetus, or both are infected. Traditionally, the distinction between maternal and fetal infection is based on measurements of antibody titers in the mother and the newborn infant. However, this is not straightforward: the presence of antibodies in the mother may simply indicate vaccination or a pregestational encounter with the organism. The same or slightly higher antibody titer in the infant may be the result of transplacental IgG transfer. A clearer indication of fetal infection is the presence of specific IgM (nonmaternal) antibodies in the infant. Likewise, if the titer of IgG antibodies in postnatally collected specimens increases with time, the baby is responding to an infection.

Once again, toxoplasmosis is a good example. The physician in Paris was able to quickly diagnose the mother's disease because physicians in endemic areas such as France are alert to the symptoms. (In France, young women are screened for toxoplasmosis, as it occurs there at a yearly rate of 1 per 1000 people, nine times higher than, for example, in Massachusetts. Apparently this is caused by widespread practice of eating of undercooked or raw meat.) Commonly used blood tests detect IgG antibodies against *T. gondii* (Chapter 40). These tests are so sensitive that antibodies can be detected within a week following infection; they then peak in the subsequent 2 months. The IgG antibody titer in the mother's serum usually stabilizes at 1:1000 6 to 8 weeks after infection (the figure means that antibodies can still be detected in vitro at a serum dilution of 1:1000). Thus, if a high titer is found in the first 2 months of pregnancy, it may represent infection prior to conception. In such cases the fetus is not at risk because the parasites will have been contained by the mother's immunological defenses prior to the onset of pregnancy.

Treatment

Ideally, antimicrobial drugs used to treat infections in pregnant women should have no teratogenic effects. One drug used for treating toxoplasmosis during pregnancy, spiramycin, is used in Europe and Canada, but is not licensed for use in the United States. Because *T. gondii* does not rapidly cross the placenta, early administration of spiramycin may prevent the infection before it passes to the fetus. Another drug active against *T. gondii*, pyrethamine, crosses the placental barrier and carries the risk of teratogenesis. The time of infection also influences the effectiveness of therapy. When mothers with acute toxoplasma infection are treated with spiramycin early after the onset of infection, the rate of fetal infection is reduced but not eliminated.

Prevention

Effective drugs against fetal rubella infections are not available, but the disease can effectively be prevented with a vaccine that contains live attenuated virus. It is administered as part of a trivalent viral vaccine called *MMR* (measles, mumps, rubella), the use of which is mandatory prior to kindergarten in several states in this country. Rubella infection is generally such a mild illness that the public health concern is primarily due to its teratogenic potential. Why is rubella vaccine given to boys as well as to girls? The reason is that widespread immunity to rubella in the population reduces the amount of circulating virus, and thereby reduces the chances that a susceptible person, pregnant or not, will encounter the virus.

Prevention of fetal toxoplasmosis requires that the pregnant mother avoid the agent. *T. gondii* cysts are acquired by eating undercooked meat from animals infected with the organism. Alternatively, oocysts passed in the stool of members of the cat family may be carried by inhalation. Pregnant women, especially if they have no antitoxoplasma antibodies, should attempt to avoid these sources of infection. A trip to the zoo and the lions' cage may pose some hazard and should be postponed until the child is born and is old enough to enjoy it.

INFECTIONS OF THE NEONATE ACQUIRED DURING OR SOON AFTER BIRTH

Being sterile at birth means being prone to infection by the first successful colonizers encountered. The newborn has no resident flora to discourage pathogenic bacteria. The newborn is not totally defenseless since it acquired maternal antibodies in the latter phase of gestation; however, its own immune system is still underdeveloped. This is a difficult period in life and the risks to the neonate are great indeed. Without proper attention to sanitary measures the rate of infant mortality may be prodigious. The expectation that most newborns will survive the first few years of life is of recent origin even in developed countries, and has yet to be realized in many of the developing ones.

Case 3—Neonatal Herpes

A 26-year-old pregnant woman was referred to a University Medical Center because she had a 5-year history of intravenous drug abuse, which placed her in a high-risk category. Her past history also included genital herpes, with her last episode 6 months prior to her current gestation. She was tested for antibodies to HIV because of her history of drug abuse, and none were found.

During a visit in her 32nd week she had no visible herpetic lesions but a swab of her cervix grew herpes simplex virus type II. The same virus was also cultured on a weekly basis until her 36th week of gestation, when the culture was negative. One week later she had a spontaneous onset of labor. At that time there were no visible herpetic vesicles on her cervix, vagina, or vulva, and a vaginal delivery was performed.

After birth, the baby boy was carefully examined for evidence of viral infection and drug withdrawal. Vesicular lesions developed on his trunk 9 days after delivery. He became lethargic, irritable, and febrile. A smear of material from the base of a vesicle ("Tzanck smear", see Chapter 59) was positive, and cultures of the spinal and vesicular fluid grew herpes simplex virus type II. Despite treatment with acyclovir, the child developed profound mental retardation.

Case 4—Group B Streptococcal Septicemia in a Neonate

A 21-year-old woman had twin boys via normal labor and delivery. During the first day of life, twin A developed mild respiratory distress that responded to oxygen therapy. However, at 30 hours of age he became lethargic and developed a temperature of 38.5°C. Cultures were taken and ampicillin and gentamicin were administered. The next day group B β-hemolytic streptococci were isolated from a blood culture. Prophylactic antibiotic therapy was administered to twin B after a sample of blood was drawn for culture. The next day this sample also grew group B streptococci. Both children received a 14-day course of ampicillin and were discharged from the hospital in excellent condition.

Encounter and Entry

The earliest source of environmental infection is the birth canal (Table 53.2). Thus, children born to mothers infected with chlamydiae or gonococci may become infected during birth, whereas infection by these organisms in the first weeks of life is unusual. Herpetic infection of neonates is most commonly acquired during or after birth since this virus is unlikely to cross the placental barrier. By contrast, cytomegalovirus has a greater ability to cross this barrier and is more likely to cause congenital infections. In case 3 the mother's previous and recent history suggest that the infant may have been infected by contact with virus present in the birth canal. However, the recent negative culture indicates that postnatal infection should not be disregarded as a possibility. In the immediate postnatal period, the nursery and its personnel become a source of other organisms. For example, herpetic whitlows on the hand of a nurse have been the source of nursery outbreak of herpes simplex infection.

Bacteria may colonize a newborn infant anywhere on the skin or mucous membranes. The umbilical stump may be an important portal of entry, allowing pene-

Table 53.2
Association of neonatal disease with microorganisms present in the birth canal*

Microorganism	Frequency of transmission, either transplacentally or during birth	
	Significant	Uncommon
Bacteria		
Group B streptococci	+	
Escherichia coli	+	
Listeria monocytogenes	+	
Gonococcus	+	
Chlamydia trachomatis	+	
Treponema pallidum	+	
Staphylococcus aureus		+
α-Hemolytic streptococci		+
Group A and D streptococci (enterococci)		+
Other Enterobacteriaceae		+
Meningococcus		+
Haemophilus influenzae		+
Campylobacter fetus		+
Anaerobes (*Bacteroides, Clostridia*)		+
Mycoplasma hominis		+
Viruses		
Cytomegalovirus	+	
Herpes simplex type II	+	
Hepatitis B	+	
Rubella	+	
HIV-1	+	
Fungi		
Candida albicans	+	
Protozoa		
Toxoplasma gondii	+	
Trichomonas vaginalis		+

*Adapted from Remington JS, Klein JD (eds): *Infectious Diseases of the Fetus and Newborn Infant.* Philadelphia, WB Saunders, 1983, Chap 1.

tration of microorganisms to the blood through the recently cut umbilical vessels. In some underdeveloped parts of the world the practice of packing the umbilicus with animal dung may result in clostridial infections such as tetanus.

Special Risk Factors of the Neonate and Its Defenses

Bacterial septicemia (case 4) usually develops in infants that have certain risk factors. Low birth weight and premature infants are at greater risk of infection than term infants, because of a less developed immune system. Two other factors include early rupture of membranes prior to delivery and obstetrical complications during delivery.

In addition to circulating antibodies, the newborn is supplied by the mother with protective factors in breast milk. Breast milk contain IgA type antibodies, white blood cells, and lysozyme. The growth of Gram negative enteric bacteria is suppressed in breast-fed babies, possibly by the encouragement of the growth of Gram positive lactobacilli and perhaps by presence of the iron-sequestering protein, lactoferrin. Epidemiological studies in India, for example, have shown that low-birth-weight babies fed breast milk developed fewer infections than those who were formula fed.

The importance of maternal antibodies in protecting a newborn is demonstrated in varicella infections acquired near the time of birth. An infant born to a mother who develops the vesicular rash of varicella at least 4 days before delivery is generally considered not to be at risk of developing severe neonatal varicella. However, if the rash develops less than 4 days before or up to 2 days after delivery, not enough time has passed for the mother to make antivaricella antibodies and to pass them to the infant. In such a setting, the untreated infant is at risk of developing an overwhelming infection. In such cases, varicella immune globulin may be administered to help modify the severity of the disease.

Damage

If the twins discussed in case 4 had not been treated promptly with antibiotics, it is likely that their infection would have progressed to a fatal outcome. The newborn also has a limited response to infection: respiratory distress, fever or temperature instability, poor feeding, and decreased activity. These symptoms occur with all neonatal infections—bacterial, viral, and fungal. Infants with such symptoms must be treated with antibiotics pending the result of laboratory studies. If these symptoms are seen within 3 days of birth, the disease is considered to have an *early onset* and is likely to be caused by organisms acquired during birth. When the disease has a *late onset* it is usually accompanied by meningitis, which is frequently caused by maternally acquired group B streptococci or by environmentally acquired organisms.

At present, the most common etiologic agents of neonatal septicemia in North America are *E. coli* and group B streptococci. Many of the *E. coli* strains isolated from neonatal meningitis cases have a specific capsular polysaccharide antigen called K1 (see Chapter 47). Other capsular types tend to be less virulent. The prognosis of untreated infants is poor, with a mortality rate of at least 70%. Even with treatment, many infants die. Neurological sequelae are particularly common in infants recovering from *E. coli* meningitis. They are less common in survivors of group B streptococcal meningitis.

Neonatal herpes, as in case 3, may lead to a life-threatening disseminated disease that involves the heart, brain, and other organs. Other viral infections of the neonate vary in severity and include those caused by cytomegalovirus, enteroviruses, hepatitis B, varicella, and respiratory syncytial virus.

Chlamydiae play an important role in neonatal infections, as they are a widespread cause of sexually transmitted diseases and are frequently acquired by the infant during birth. *Chlamydia trachomatis* may cause an eye infection called *inclusion conjunctivitis*, a purulent discharge seen within the first 3 weeks of life. About 10% of children born to mothers with chlamydial infection develop a syndrome of pneumonia, characterized by low-grade fever, cough, eosinophilia, and an increase in serum gamma globulin level. These features suggest that the infant's immune response to *C. trachomatis* may contribute to the symptoms. This pneumonia may have an incubation time of up to 4 months, a long time for a perinatally acquired illness. Antibiotic treatment shortens the clinical course and reduces the period over which infants shed the organisms.

The list of infectious diseases seen during this stage in life is long and includes those caused by many bacteria, viruses, fungi, and animal parasites. A few have distinct manifestations. An example is the scalded skin syndrome caused by certain strains of staphylococci (see Chapter 11). This exfoliation of the skin is a characteristic of infected infants: Adults with the same staphylococcal strains rarely have exfoliative lesions.

Diagnosis

The most frequent manifestations of neonatal septicemia are respiratory distress, poor feeding, lethargy, vomiting, and diarrhea, all of which may be due to noninfectious causes. Generally, the distinction between prenatal infection and that acquired during the birth process is difficult on clinical grounds. The mother's history may give important clues because neonatal septicemia may be associated with infection during gestation or previous complicated deliveries.

Treatment and Prevention

The diagnosis of neonatal septicemia calls for emergency measures: Treatment may have to be instituted before laboratory results are received. The antibiotics selected must be active against all the most likely pathogens. An aminoglycoside or a third-generation cephalosporin in combination with ampicillin are usually administered. Viral infections, such as herpes simplex, are treated with acyclovir or other antiviral drugs.

Preventive measures may be considered when risk factors are present, such as premature birth or low birth weight. Active vaccination is not generally effective (except for hepatitis B), partly because of the imperfect immunological development of the neonate and partly because of the time required to produce an effective antibody titer. Passive immunization with immunoglobulins may be effective in preventing certain infections, such as varicella or hepatitis B. The administration of penicillin to a mother during the last stages of pregnancy may be one method to reduce the incidence of infections due to group B streptococci.

SUGGESTED READINGS

Remington JS, Klein JD (eds): *Infectious Diseases of the Fetus and Newborn Infant.* Philadelphia, WB Saunders, 1983, Chap 1.

Wilson CB, Remington JS: Toxoplasmosis, in Kelley VC (ed): *Practice of Pediatrics.* Philadelphia, Harper & Row, 1986.

Wilson CB, Haas JE: Cellular defenses against *Toxoplasma gondii* in newborns. *J Clin Invest* 73(6): 1606–1616, 1984.

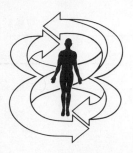

Infections of the Compromised Patient

54

W. Powderly

A person is considered to be compromised when suffering either from the disruption of specific defenses of a particular organ or system, or from systemic abnormalities of humoral or cellular immunity. In most cases it is possible to predict the general type of infection such a patient is likely to acquire, depending on which component of the defense mechanisms is disturbed. However, when the immune deficiency is general and profound the patient may acquire any of a number of widely differing infections. Several of these may even occur at the same time.

We have the opportunity to learn a great deal about the workings of the normal defense mechanisms by studying what happens when they become impaired. Ultimately, our knowledge of the relative importance of humoral and cellular immunity is derived from observing patients with immunodeficiencies. Thus, we note that persons with agammaglobulinemia are especially susceptible to extracellular bacteria that cause acute inflammation, whereas those with defects in cell-mediated immunity fall prey more readily to viruses, fungi, mycobacteria, and other intracellular agents of chronic diseases. The practical need to understand the risk factors associated with defects in defenses against invading microorganisms cannot be overestimated. Opportunistic infections have assumed immense importance in modern medicine, primarily because many of the major technological advances in therapeutics have been accompanied by iatrogenic disruption of body defense mechanisms.

In most instances, infections of compromised patients are caused by agents that are commonly known to be pathogenic. However, especially severe forms of immune compromise open the door to infections by organisms that are normally not considered to be virulent, including many that are common in the normal flora and the environment. Unexpected extremes have been reached in scattered cases of infections of heart valves and other vital tissues by mushrooms (in their mycelial form) and colorless algae! Note how this underscores how the definition of virulence must include not only obvious pathogenic properties of the micro-organism but also the range of susceptibility of the patient.

This chapter will recapitulate the consequence of risk factors mentioned throughout this book. Here we will present them according to the type of abnor-mality or defect in specific mechanisms.

CASE

A 17-year-old girl who came to the hospital with fever and bruising was eventually found to suffer from acute myelogenous leukemia. Remission of the leukemia was achieved with chemotherapy, and allogeneic (non-twin) bone marrow transplantation was attempted, in the hope of curing her leukemia. Five days after the transplantation, she had no detectable circulating white blood cells, and 2 days thereafter she became febrile. Blood cultures taken at this time were positive for Escherichia coli. She responded well to antibiotics and defervesced rapidly.

Eight days later she again became febrile, and blood cultures were positive for Candida albicans. Although she was placed on antifungals, she remained febrile for 4 days but rapidly defervesced upon removal of a venous catheter (that had been implanted in her subclavian vein for intravenous drug administration). At this time (19 days posttransplantation), white blood cells started to appear in her circulation, indicating that the transplanted marrow had successfully engrafted and was starting to function.

Thirty-one days after her transplantation she became short of breath, and chest x-ray showed a diffuse pneumonia. Examination of a tissue sample obtained at lung biopsy revealed the presence of Pneumocystis carinii. Treatment with trimethoprim/sulfamethoxazole was started and she responded slowly to therapy. She was discharged from the hospital 2 months after her transplantation, but 10 days later developed a painful cutaneous herpes zoster infection. She remained well for the next 3 months, although she had developed mild chronic graft-versus-host disease. She returned again to hospital 5 months after her transplantation, with a complaint of fever and shortness of breath. Physical examination and chest x-ray revealed a lobar pneumonia, and both blood and sputum cultures grew Streptococcus pneumoniae. She responded well to penicillin therapy and remained well thereafter.

Patients who have undergone bone marrow transplantation provide an extreme example of the profound disturbances of normal body defenses that predispose to infection. For example, disruption of anatomic barriers by radiation and chemotherapy, causing skin and mucosal ulcerations, provides sites of entry for invasive organisms. Severe neutropenia is characteristic of the immediate post-transplant period, and although granulocyte recovery begins in the third week after transplantation, qualitative defects remain for some time. Cellular immune function, which now depends on donor macrophages and T cells, remains abnor-mal for several months. It is also compromised by the use of immunosuppressive therapy to treat graft-versus-host disease. Although IgG and IgM levels may return to normal after 4 to 5 months, B cell function remains disturbed and antibody levels to specific organisms, such as pneumococci, may remain depressed for years.

With the example of this clinical case in mind, we will review the disturbances in specific body defense mechanisms and their consequences.

ABNORMALITIES OF LOCAL DEFENSE

We are protected from microbial invasion by the mechanical and biochemical barrier provided by skin and mucous membranes and by the presence of a normal commensal flora. Disruption of local mechanical barriers may occur as a consequence of instrumentation (e.g., intravenous or urinary catheterization), surgery, drugs, or burns. Under these circumstances, the infecting organisms are usually members of the commensal flora resident at site. Thus, breaching the skin with intravenous catheters may introduce S. epidermidis into the bloodstream, with subsequent septicemia (Chapter 51).

The consequences of immunological or biochemical impairment at the level of the integuments are less well understood. Thus, we do not know with certainty if secreted IgA immunoglobulins or lysozyme contribute to resistance to infection. We suspect, however, that people with IgA deficiency are more prone to sinusitis, pneumonia, or specific gastrointestinal infections (e.g., giardiasis). Persons with genetic defects in lysozyme have not yet been found.

Burns provide an extreme example of the critical role of the intact integument on resistance to infection. The necrotic skin tissue is an excellent culture medium for bacteria, thus increasing the size of the inoculum. In addition, the thermal injury itself leads to a poorly understood suppression of white blood cell function. It is not surprising then that skin and subcutaneous tissue infections and septicemias with S. aureus or Pseudomonas aeruginosa are major challenges in the management of patients with severe burns.

The normal bacterial flora may be disrupted in numbers and kinds of organisms as the result of antibiotic treatment, which may result in superinfection by organisms resistant to the drug. This happens particularly often in the intestine, sometimes as the result of antibiotic "prepping" of patients for abdominal surgery. Pseudomembranous colitis due to Clostridium difficile is a complication of such therapy (Chapter 21).

Some tissues possess additional local defense mechanisms. A good example is the lungs, where the combination of mucous production by goblet cells and ciliary activity of the respiratory epithelial cells serves to trap microbes and carry them out of the lungs. Disruption of this disposal system predisposes to pneumonia (Chapter 45). An extreme example of this occurs in cystic fibrosis, a chronic condition of genetic origin characterized by the production of abnormally thick mucus. These patients suffer from recurrent pneumonia and are often colonized by the opportunistic bacterium Pseudomonas aeruginosa. Most patients are unable to clear this organism from the respiratory tract and may die from respiratory failure due to repeated episodes of pneumonia.

DISTURBANCE IN PHAGOCYTIC NUMBERS AND FUNCTION

Once the first line of defense is breached, neutrophils assume a critical role in checking the spread of invasive disease. Defects in neutrophil activity, either qualitative or quantitative, predispose patients to infection with certain bacteria and

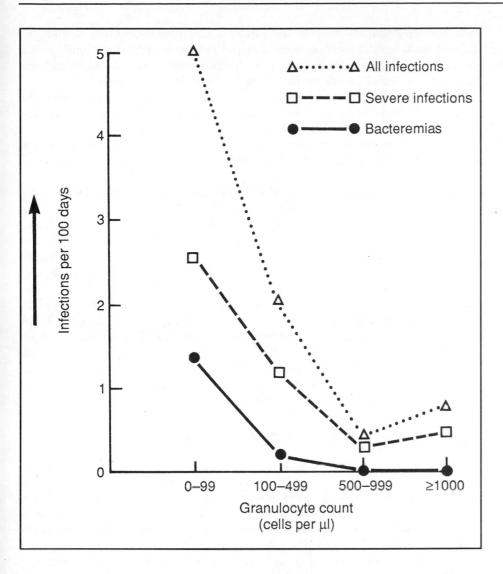

Figure 54.1. Relationship between the incidence of infection and the absolute neutrophil count in patients with acute nonlymphocyte leukemia. The incidence of infection rises as the neutrophil count decreases. (From Joshi J, Schimpff S: Infections in the compromised host. In Mandell G, Douglas G, Bennett JE (eds): *Principles and Practice of Infectious Diseases*. New York, John Wiley & Sons, 1985.

fungi (Table 54.1). These defects may involve a decreased number of phagocytic cells, impairment of their chemotactic response, and lowering of their ability to kill microorganisms.

Granulocytopenia (a decrease in the number of circulating neutrophils) clearly predisposes to infection. (In addition to the case described above, an illustrative case of infection in a granulocytopenic patient is described in Chapter 19). Myelosuppressive cancer chemotherapy is the most common cause of granulocytopenia in hospitals. Neutropenia also occurs in bone marrow failure due to aplasia, autoimmune disease, hematologic malignancy, or tumor invading the bone marrow. Serious infections usually accompanied by bacteremia are a frequent and often life-threatening problem in these hosts. The most important correlation is between the number of circulating neutrophils and the risk of infection. The rate of infection clearly increases as the number of neutrophils decreases (Fig. 54.1). Disturbances of the integrity of the skin and gastrointestinal tract, often the result of chemotherapy or radiation therapy, are also important in the pathogenesis of these infections. The organisms responsible are usually derived from the patient's own flora, particularly that of the bowel. Gram negative enteric bacilli and staphylococci are the most common bacterial pathogens. Prolonged antibacterial therapy predisposes to colonization by fungi, *Candida* and *Aspergillus* being important causes of fungal sepsis and mortality in this population.

Chemotactic dysfunction of phagocytes is uncommon and usually congenital in origin. Defective neutrophil chemotaxis may result from inadequate signaling of the neutrophil, abnormalities of neutrophil receptors for chemoattractants, or from disorders in cell locomotion. *Staphylococcus aureus* is the most important pathogen in these patients, who are usually seen with recurrent cutaneous or deep abscesses.

Most often, abnormalities in microbial killing power are inherited. Of the many disorders that have been described, the most common is *chronic granulomatous disease*, a condition in which neutrophils fail to mount a respiratory burst during phagocytosis. The reason for this deficiency is that the enzyme NADPH oxidase is defective, and hydrogen peroxide is not formed. Patients with this disorder are at risk of infection with catalase-positive organisms, especially *Staphylococcus aureus*. A Gram negative rod, *Serratia marcescens*, also causes infections in these patients, as do fungi (especially *Aspergillus*). These organisms are relatively resistant to the nonoxidative killing mechanisms of neutrophils. On the other hand, bacteria such as pneumococci and other streptococci that make their own hydrogen peroxide but have no catalase are likely to be killed by the defective neutrophils. The reason is that these neutrophils still contain myeloperoxidase. This enzyme can utilize hydrogen peroxide made by bacterial metabolism to produce lethal radicals (Chapter 4). In effect, these bacteria commit suicide.

ABNORMALITIES IN HUMORAL IMMUNITY

Immunoglobulin deficiency may be congenital (e.g., Bruton's X-linked agammaglobulinemia) or acquired (e.g., common variable immunodeficiency) (see Table 5.7). Acquired hypogammaglobulinemia may also arise as a consequence of conditions that lead to protein loss (nephrotic syndrome, intestinal lymphangiectasia), cancers of cell that make immunoglobulins (multiple myeloma, chronic lymphocytic leukemia), or burns. Defective B lymphocyte function also occurs as a consequence of bone marrow transplantation, as noted in the case above. The predominant infectious disease problem in these patients is recurrent upper and lower respiratory tract infection due to encapsulated bacteria. This reflects the important role of antibodies in opsonization of encapsulated bacteria.

Complement deficiencies are rare and are also characterized by predisposition to infection with encapsulated bacteria (see Table 4.5). *Neisseria* are a special problem for patients with deficiencies of any of the late complement components (C6, C7, C8, or C9), because complement-mediated lysis is required to kill these organisms. Many bacteria infect patients with defects earlier in the complement cascade (Table 4.5). Most clinically significant complement deficiencies are congenitally acquired.

The spleen is intimately concerned with adequate performance of the humoral arm of the immune system, both as a source of complement and antibody-producing B cells, and as the organ primarily responsible for the removal of opsonized microbes from the bloodstream. Defects in spleen function may be a consequence of splenectomy or of diseases such as sickle cell anemia. In these situations, patients are at risk of infection with encapsulated bacteria, such as pneumococci and *Haemophilus*. These bacterial infections may be fulminant in patients with splenic deficiency. Bacteremia and septic shock often result, and mortality is high unless appropriate therapy is introduced rapidly.

DISORDERS OF CELL-MEDIATED IMMUNITY

Defects in the function or number of macrophages and T lymphocytes lead to an increased risk of infection with bacteria that survive intracellularly, as well as with viruses, fungi, and protozoa (Table 54.1).

Patients with defective cell-mediated immunity may be divided in two groups, depending on whether their defect is congenital or acquired. Primary disorders of cell-mediated immunity are usually diagnosed in childhood and are lethal, with death usually arising from opportunistic infections before adulthood (Table 5.7).

Acquired defects in cell-mediated immunity are seen in an increasingly large population of patients treated in hospitals. The enormous success in transplant surgery is a consequence of the development of drugs (such as cyclosporin) that suppress the graft-versus-host response and prevent rejection of the transplant. These immunosuppressive drugs also interfere with normal cell-mediated immunity, and all these patients are at increased risk of opportunistic infection. Some immunosuppressive drugs, especially corticosteroids, are also used to treat a variety of inflammatory diseases. Cell-mediated immunity is also disordered in patients with lymphoma.

The most profound example of defective cell-mediated immunity occurs in AIDS (Chapter 33). Here, depletion of $CD4^+$ T helper cells due to HIV infection leads almost inevitably to death from uncontrolled opportunistic infection or malignancy.

Table 54.1
Common causes of compromise and their consequences

Impaired Function	Common Infecting Organisms	Sites Commonly Affected
Barrier		
Integument	Pyogenic cocci, enteric bacteria	Skin, subcutaneous connective tissue
Normal microbial flora	Pyogenic cocci, enteric bacteria, *Clostridium difficile, Candida albicans*	Skin, intestine
Phagocyte Functions		
Chemotaxis	*Staphylococcus aureus,* enteric bacteria	Skin, respiratory tract
Neutropenia	*S. aureus,* enteric bacteria	Skin, respiratory tract
Microbial killing	*S. aureus, Aspergillus*	Skin, visceral abscesses
Humoral Functions		
Hypogammaglobulinemia	Pyogenic bacteria	Any site
IgA deficiency	Pyogenic bacteria	Respiratory tract
Lack of spleen	Pneumococcus, *Haemophilus influenzae*	Septicemia
Complement deficiency		
C1q, C2, or C3	Pyogenic bacteria	Bacteremia, meningitis
C5, C6, C7, C8, or C9	*Neisseria*	Meningitis, arthritis
Cell-mediated immunity	Viruses, fungi, protozoa intracellular bacteria	Any site

Adapted from RB Johnston: Recurrent bacterial infections in children. *N Engl J Med* 310:1237–1243, 1984.

MANAGEMENT OF INFECTION IN COMPROMISED HOSTS: GENERAL CONSIDERATIONS

As with all infections, treatment in the compromised host should be directed against the specific infecting organism. However, defective host response heightens the risk of severe infection, and there may be urgent need to begin treatment presumptively, based on the most likely etiological possibilities. Knowing the type of immune defect, the site and clinical features of the infection, and some epidemiological features makes it often possible to predict the likely infecting organism. For example, in granulocytopenic patients, broad-spectrum antibiotics with activity against both Gram positive bacteria and Enterobacteriaceae and other Gram negative bacteria should be given at the first sign of infection, such as fever. Patients with decreased spleen function should be treated with drugs active against pneumococci and *H. influenzae*. A diffuse pneumonia involving most of the lung in a patient with AIDS is most likely due to *Pneumocystis carinii*. However, this is not always the case, and it is often necessary to specifically identify the causative organism so that appropriate treatment may be started or toxic therapy avoided. Specimens should be obtained prior to starting therapy, and there should be coordination between the clinician and the microbiological laboratory to assure the recovery and identification of opportunistic pathogens. Unless warned, the microbiological laboratory may consider *Staphylococcus epidermidis* a contaminant from the skin and not report it.

It is particularly important to attempt to reverse the immune defect: Whenever practical, iatrogenic causes should be eliminated. Catheters should be removed or at least changed; immunosuppressive drugs should be discontinued whenever possible. In some transplant recipients, it may even be necessary to allow the transplant to be rejected by suspending immunosuppressive therapy in order to permit an adequate host response to infection. In other cases, replacement therapy is of benefit. Passive administration of immunoglobulins decreases the incidence of infection in patients with hypogammaglobulinemia. Granulocyte transfusions may benefit some granulocytopenic patients with refractory Gram negative bacterial infections.

Preventive measures are also important in caring for these patients. Simple procedures such as care with use and insertion of catheters, careful handwashing, and appropriate isolation techniques may reduce the incidence of opportunistic infection acquired in hospitals. Some vaccines (e.g., against influenza virus or pneumococci) may be of benefit. It is essential to remember that live vaccines should not be given to immunocompromised hosts. Prophylactic antibiotics are rarely of benefit; major exceptions are the use of penicillin to prevent pneumococcal infections in children with sickle cell disease, and the use of trimethoprim/sulfamethoxazole to prevent *Pneumocystis* pneumonia in patients with severe defects in cell-mediated immunity.

SUGGESTED READINGS

Brown AE: Neutropenia, fever, and infection. *Am J Med* 76:421–426, 1984.

Buckley RH: Immunodeficiency disease. *JAMA* 258:2841–2850, 1987.

Grieco, MH (ed): *Infections in the Abnormal Host.* New York, Yorke Medical Books, 1980.

Rosen FS, Cooper MD, Wedgewood RJ: The primary immunodeficiencies. *N Engl J Med* 311:235–242, 311:300–310, 1984.

Rubin RH, Young LS: *Clinical Approach to Infection in the Compromised Host,* ed. 2. New York, Plenum, 1988.

Ven der Meer JW et al: Infections in bone marrow transplant recipients. *Semin Hematol* 21:123–140, 1984.

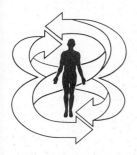

CHAPTER

55

Zoonoses

V.L. Yu
C. Meissner

Diseases that are transmitted from animals to humans are called *zoonoses* or *zoonotic diseases*. They are difficult to control because the existence of an animal reservoir makes it hard to eliminate them. Consider, for example, the problems involved in controlling rodents in the deserts of the southwestern United States that are infected with the plague, or large herds of wildebeest that carry sleeping sickness in Central Africa. Animal-related diseases have caused untold damage to people in the past and continue to be of enormous concern, especially in the tropical areas of the world.

Zoonoses are defined as those infectious diseases that are naturally transmitted between vertebrate animals and humans. The word is derived from the Greek, "zoon", meaning animal, and "nosos", meaning disease. The persons at greatest risk of acquiring zoonoses are of course those who work in close proximity to animals, like farmers, veterinarians, slaughterhouse workers, and animal researchers. The most common sources of zoonotic diseases are domestic animals, namely pets and farm animals. Over 100 million cats and dogs are kept as pets in the United States, and although they are rare, more than 30 human diseases can be acquired from them.

With the international movement of animals, importation of zoonotic diseases from one geographic locale to another takes place with increasing frequency. For example, Marburg virus disease was first documented in laboratory workers in Germany after they had contact with monkeys imported from Africa for use in vaccine research.

ENCOUNTER

Transmission of zoonotic agents from animals to humans has two scenarios:

• People are "dead-end hosts", accidental intruders in an animal-to-animal chain and cannot transmit the agent further.

• People acquire the agent from animals and can pass it to other people and/or animals.

In the first case the organisms are specifically adapted for transmission between animals. Humans may acquire the agent and even become very sick, but they do not provide a means for further transmission. Infection of people breaks a biological chain. An example is a disease of wild rodents called Colorado tick fever. The reason why the human is a dead-end host for the virus is that human-to-tick-to-animal transmission is a rare event.

In the second mode of transmission the organisms go from animals to humans and from them to other humans or even to other animals. The route of transmission may change in the process. For instance, plague bacilli enter the human body via flea bites, multiply, and may then go from person to person by inhalation of droplets produced by the cough of patients. Similarly, the virus of Korean hemorrhagic fever may be acquired by eating food contaminated with the excreta of rodents, but can then spread by the respiratory route. In salmonellosis the organisms enter humans by the ingestion of contaminated animal products and can then spread via the fecal-oral route to other people.

The pathogenesis of zoonotic diseases in the animal reservoir often helps one understand the nuances of their transmission to humans. The most successful organisms are those that cause an indolent, low-grade disease in the animal, but which are easily spread. They present great problems to the control of zoonotic diseases. An example is leptospirosis, a chronic, often asymptomatic infection of rats and domestic animals, especially dogs. The organisms multiply in the kidney tubules and are excreted in the urine. The disease can then be acquired by people who come in contact with contaminated urine, e.g., by swimming in an irrigation ditch. Similarly, cows infected with tuberculosis can shed the tubercle bacilli in their milk without undue signs of disease. In all these cases the animals have become shedders, because the agents have the ability to persist for long periods of time. Persistence is sometimes due to localization of the organisms at sheltered sites. Such sites are the kidney tubules in the case of *Leptospira* or the mammary glands for *Brucella*.

ENTRY

The zoonoses illustrate the diverse ways microorganisms gain access to the human host, in this case from animal reservoirs. The basic modes of entry are penetration of the skin, inhalation, and ingestion. Few microorganisms can penetrate the skin or mucous membranes directly, nor can they all traverse the distance between hosts. But evolutionary innovations have overcome these physical and biological barriers. Most of the time the organisms use an intermediary vector that can serve both the function of delivery and entry. For example, a tsetse fly that carries the trypanosomes of sleeping sickness bridges the distance between infected cattle and people, introducing the organisms when it bites.

In zoonoses transmitted by arthropod vectors, the microorganisms may undergo developmental changes within the vectors. Particularly elaborate examples are seen in the protozoa of malaria or sleeping sickness. In other zoonoses developmental changes take place within a vertebrate host, as in the case of tapeworms and other metazoan parasites. Finally, organisms involved in yet other zoonoses carry out developmental changes in the external environment, such as soil, bodies of water, food, or plants. For example, hookworm eggs hatch in soil and the larvae simply wait for a mammalian host.

The diversity of modes of transmission is well illustrated with a group of related diseases, the viral hemorrhagic fevers. These illnesses are found in tropical climates and have similar clinical manifestations; they include Lassa fever, Marburg virus disease, and Crimean-Congo hemorrhagic fever. In all three diseases the infection can be transmitted from person to person by direct contact. What is intriguing is how these viruses reach the human host from their animal reservoir. The Lassa virus is frequently present in mice and is transmitted to humans by ingestion of foodstuff contaminated with their urine. The Marburg virus is transmitted from monkeys to humans by direct contact. Finally, the Crimean-Congo hemorrhagic fever virus is transmitted from domestic animals to humans via tick bites.

Penetration Through the Skin

The epidermis of the skin may be breached in a number of ways to permit entry of microorganisms. One obvious mechanism is direct entry through minute abrasions or open wounds (Table 55.1). The organisms themselves may facilitate penetration of the skin. For instance, the fungi that cause athlete's foot produce an enzyme that hydrolyzes the keratin of the stratum corneum, whereas hookworms have "teeth" that allow them to chew their way through the epidermis. Microorganisms may also gain entry via arthropod vectors by sting or bite (Table 55.2). Finally, animals themselves may neatly solve the problem of entry by biting the victim (Table 55.3).

The anatomic sites that are usually penetrated by infectious agents are not only those that come in contact with the organisms, but also those that are more likely to experience abrasions or wounds. Thus, exposed extremities tend to be sites of infection in erysipeloid, anthrax, and cat scratch fever.

Arthropod Vectors

This fascinating mode of transmission is the most complex because it requires living intermediates. Some function as "flying syringes" (mosquitoes or biting flies), whereas others jump (fleas), or crawl (ticks or mites) (Table 55.2). Transmission by arthropod vectors can be either mechanical or biological. In mechanical transmission, the vector simply transports the organisms from animal to human; the pathogen undergoes no developmental change during transmission. Biting flies, for instance, often serve as mechanical vectors. After feeding on an infected animal, the insect digests the bloodmeal and contaminates its mouth and feces. When it moves to a human, microorganisms can be transmitted with the next bite. In an even more passive way, insects may transmit diseases without biting, just by contaminating foodstuff with organisms they carry on their legs. *Salmonella* may be transported in this manner by house flies that picked them up from feces of diseased animals.

Table 55.1
Direct skin penetration

Disease	Organism	Microbial Group	Animal Reservoir
Bacteria			
Anthrax[a,b]	*Bacillus anthracis*	Gram positive aerobic spore former	Domestic mammals (herbivores)
Brucellosis[a,b]	*Brucella melitensis*	Gram negative rod	Goats, sheep
	B. abortus		Cattle
	B. suis		Swine
	B. canis		Dogs
Erysipeloid	*Erysipelothrix rhusiopathiae*	Gram positive rod	Swine, poultry, fish
Leptospirosis[b]	*Leptospira interrogans*	Spirochete	Rodents, foxes, domestic animals
Melioidosis[b]	*Pseudomonas pseudomallei*	Gram negative rod	Rodents
Glanders[a]	*Pseudomonas mallei*	Gram negative rod	Equines, domestic mammals
Tularemia[a–c]	*Francisella tularensis*	Gram negative rod	Rabbits, rodents
Viruses			
Foot and mouth disease	Aphthovirus	Picornavirus family	Cattle
Orf (contagious ecthyma)	Parapoxvirus	Poxvirus family	Sheep, goats
Vesicular stomatitis	Vesicular stomatitis virus	Rhabdovirus family	Cattle, horses
Parasite			
Cutaneous larva migrans (creeping eruption)	*Ancylostoma caninum* (dog hookworm)	Nematode	Dogs, cats, carnivores
	Ancylostoma braziliense (dog and cat hookworm)	Nematode	
Fungi			
Dermatophytes	Zoophilic trichophytons, microsporums	Fungi	Dogs, cats, cattle
Miscellaneous			
Cat scratch fever[d]	Unknown	Gram negative rod suspected	Cats, dogs

Alternative portals:
[a] Inhalation
[b] Ingestion
[c] Arthropod vector
[d] Animal bite

In biological transmission, part of the developmental cycle of the microorganism must take place in an arthropod vector. This is most often seen with protozoa. For instance, in American trypanosomiasis (Chagas' disease) the organisms multiply and pass through developmental stages within reduviid bugs. After these vectors suck blood from infected animals, the ingested trypanosomes multiply in the gut and transform into flagellar forms. The insect feces then are infective. They enter the human host when the insect's feces are deposited at the site of the bite during feeding; the trypanosomes gain access when the host rubs them into the skin while scratching the insect bite.

Animal Bites

Animal bites introduce two kinds of floras into deep tissue: the flora that is present on the skin of the recipient, and, more often, that which is found in the mouth and teeth of the biting animal. Table 55.3 lists the more common pathogens that are transmitted by bites.

Table 55.2
Arthropod vectors

Disease	Vector	Organism	Microbial Group	Animal Reservoir
Bacteria				
Lyme disease	Tick	*Borrelia burgdorferi*	Spirochete	Rodents, deer
Plague, bubonic[c]	Flea	*Yersinia pestis*	Gram negative rod	Urban rats, rodents
Relapsing fever	Tick	*Borrelia* sp.	Spirochete	Rodents, wild mammals
Tularemia[a–c]	Tick, biting flies	*Francisella tularensis*	Gram negative rod	Rodents, wild mammals, birds
Rocky Mountain spotted fever	Tick	*Rickettsia rickettsii*		Wild rodents, dogs
Scrub typhus	Mite (chigger)	*Rickettsia tsutsugamushi*	*Rickettsia*	Wild rodents, rats
Murine typhus	Flea	*Rickettsia typhi*		Rats
Rickettsialpox	Mite	*Rickettsia akari*		Mice
Viruses				
Yellow fever	Mosquito	Flavivirus		Primates
Encephalitis Eastern equine Western equine Venezuelan equine	Mosquito	Alphavirus	Togavirus family	Birds, horses
Encephalitis St. Louis	Mosquito	Flavivirus		Birds
Encephalitis California	Mosquito	Bunyavirus		Mammals, wild rodents
Rift Valley fever	Mosquito	Bunyavirus	Bunyavirus family	Sheep, goats, cattle
Crimean-Congo hemorrhagic fever	Tick	Bunyavirus		Domestic mammals, rodents
Colorado tick fever	Tick	Orbivirus	Reovirus family	Rodents
Protozoa				
Babesiasis	Tick	*Babesia* sp.		Domestic and wild animals
Leishmaniasis (Kala-azar, cutaneous leishmaniasis)	Sandfly	*Leishmania* sp.		Dogs, foxes, rodents, wild mammals
American trypanosomiasis	Reduviid bug (kissing bug)	*Trypanosoma cruzi*		Dogs, cats, opossums, armadillos, wild mammals
African sleeping sickness	Tsetse fly	*Trypanosoma* sp.		Reptiles, cattle, wild animals

Alternative portals:
[a] Inhalation
[b] Ingestion
[c] Skin penetration

The most common pathogen associated with animal bites, especially by cats, is a bacterium, *Pasteurella multocida*, which can cause skin and soft tissue infections at the site of inoculation and can also cause disseminated infections following invasion into the bloodstream. A condition known as rat-bite fever can be caused by one of two organisms, a Gram negative called *Streptobacillus moniliformis* or a spirochete, *Spirillum minor*. Both organisms are members of the oropharyngeal flora of rats.

Viral diseases that can be transmitted through animal bites include rabies and a herpes virus of monkeys. The latter is usually transmitted by the bites of monkeys in a zoo or a laboratory. Both of these viruses are present in the saliva of the biting animal and both are neurotropic. They migrate to the central nervous system and cause paralysis, encephalitis, and even respiratory arrest.

Table 55.3
Animal bite

Disease	Organism	Microbial Group	Animal Reservoir
Bacteria			
Pasteurellosis[a]	*Pasteurella multocida*	Gram negative rod	Dogs, cats, birds, wild mammals
Rat bite fever[a,b]	*Spirillum minor*	Spirochete	Rats, mice, cats
	Streptobacillus moniliformis	Gram negative rod	Rats, rodents, turkeys
"DF-2"	DF-2 (dysgonic fermenter, type 2)	Gram negative rod	Dogs
Viruses			
Rabies	Rabies virus	Rhabdovirus	Domestic mammals, skunks, foxes, opossums, bats, cattle
Herpes B encephalomyelitis	Herpesvirus simiae (monkey pox virus)	Herpes virus	Monkeys
Fungi			
Blastomycosis	*Blastomyces dermatitidis*	Systemic pathogenic fungus	Dogs

Alternative portals:
[a] Skin penetration
[b] Ingestion

Inhalation

Zoonotic microorganisms may be inhaled in two ways: (*a*) from infected droplets aerosolized from the respiratory tract of animals, as in the case of bovine tuberculosis; or (*b*) from an inanimate reservoir, generally soil, that had been contaminated with excreta or carcasses of infected animals. Examples are anthrax or Q fever, which are caused by spore-forming organisms that are resistant in the environment. As can logically be expected, the primary clinical manifestation of zoonoses acquired by inhalation is pneumonia (Table 55.4). Disseminated infections occur after invasion of the bloodstream.

Ingestion

Most zoonoses that are acquired by ingestion are caused by bacteria or by animal parasites (Table 55.5). The bacterial diseases are acquired by ingestion of the organisms directly, usually in contaminated foodstuffs. An example is brucellosis, which often causes a chronic but mild disease of the mammary glands of cattle and goats and which can be transmitted to humans via unpasteurized milk.

Animal parasites are usually ingested as ova or cysts. In some cases these must be activated in the human host as part of the developmental cycle of the parasite. In others a cyst may contain viable organisms.

CLINICAL MANIFESTATIONS IN HUMAN HOSTS

The clinical manifestations of zoonotic infections generally depend on the portal of entry. If the route is inhalation, the primary disease is usually a pneumonia. If the organisms penetrate the skin, the primary manifestations are a cellulitis

Table 55.4
Inhalation

Disease	Organism	Microbial Group	Animal Reservoir	Inhalant
Bacteria				
Anthrax[a] (wool sorter's disease)	*Bacillus anthracis*	Gram positive anaerobic spore-forming rod	Goats, sheep	Spores from wool, animal hides
Tuberculosis	*Mycobacterium tuberculosis*	Acid-fast bacillus	Domestic mammals	Contaminated respiratory secretions
Q fever	*Coxiella burnetii*	Rickettsia	Domestic animals	Soil, fomites, contaminated with animal excretions
Ornithosis	*Chlamydia psittaci* (psittacosis)	Chlamydia	Parrots turkeys, birds	Dried excreta from infected birds
Fungi				
Histoplasmosis	*Histoplasma capsulatum*	Dimorphic fungus	Birds, bats	Microconidia from contaminated soil
Viruses				
Lymphocytic[a,b] choriomeningitis	Lymphocytic choriomeningitis virus	Arenavirus family	Mice, hamsters rodents	Infected aerosols

Alternative portals:
[a] Skin penetration
[b] Animal bite

near the site of entry, often followed by regional lymphadenitis (plague, tularemia, anthrax). This may proceed to dissemination via the bloodstream. Ingestion of the organisms leads to early gastrointestinal symptoms and later, systemic symptoms following dissemination through the bloodstream. For animal parasites, the clinical manifestations depend on the target organ favored by the released organism. In cysticercosis, central nervous system dysfunction results from encystment of the larvae in the brain; in trichinosis, myalgias result from the encystment of the larvae in skeletal muscles; in echinococcosis, abdominal pains result from enlarging cysts in the liver; in giardiasis, diarrhea and malabsorption result from invasion of the small intestine by trophozoites.

All these points are well illustrated in tularemia, since the causative bacillus, *Francisella tularensis*, can enter humans via multiple portals. When it penetrates the skin via minute abrasions, a papule develops at the site of entry and later ulcerates. This is followed by regional lymphadenopathy and fever (ulceroglandular form). The organisms can accidentally be inoculated into the skin or the conjunctiva during the skinning of an infected carcass, resulting in symptoms of conjunctivitis and cervical lymphadenopathy (oculoglandular form). The bacteria can also be inhaled as a result of a laboratory accident or via dust contaminated with excretions from infected rodents. The disease is then characterized by pneumonia, fever, and muscle aches (pneumonic form). Ingestion of infected meat leads to diarrhea, abdominal cramps, and fever (typhoidal form). Finally, the organisms may be transmitted by bites of ticks or flies, resulting in systemic manifestations

Table 55.5
Ingestion

Disease	Organism	Microbial Group	Animal	Ingestant (Contaminated Foodstuff)
Bacteria				
Brucellosis[a]	*Brucella melitensis* *B. abortus*	Gram negative rod	Goats, cattle	Dairy products
Campylobacter infection	*Campylobacter jejuni*	Gram negative rod	Domestic mammals fowl	Milk, water, meat, poultry
Listeriosis[a]	*Listeria monocytogenes*	Gram positive rod	Domestic mammals, rodents, birds	Vegetables, water, cheese
Salmonellosis	*Salmonella* sp. (not typhi)	Gram negative rod	Fowl, domestic mammals, turtles,	Milk, eggs, meat, poultry, shellfish
Tuberculosis[b]	*Mycobacterium bovis*	Acid-fast bacillus	Cattle	Milk
Virus				
Lassa fever[b]		Arenavirus family	Mouse	Contaminated food
Protozoa				
Giardiasis	*Giardia lamblia*		Wild animals	Cyst in water
Cryptosporidiosis	*Cryptosporidium*		Calves	Oocyst
Toxoplasmosis	*Toxoplasma gondii*		Cat	Oocyst from cat feces. Tissue cyst from uncooked meat
Helminths				
Tapeworms	*Taenia saginata*	Cestode	Cattle	Larva (cysticercus) in undercooked beef
	Taenia solium	Cestode	Pigs	Larva (cysticercus) in undercooked pork, Ova in soil
	Diphyllobothrium latum	Cestode	Fish	Larva in raw fish
	Echinococcus	Cestode	Dogs, sheep, reindeer, caribou, wolves	Ova
Anisakiasis	*Anisakis*	Nematode	Marine fish	Larva in undercooked fish
Trichinosis	*Trichinella spiralis*	Nematode	Pigs, domestic mammals, wild mammals, rodents	Larval cysts
Visceral larva migrans	*Toxocara canis* (roundworm of dogs)	Nematode	Dog	Ova in soil

Alternative portals:
[a] Skin penetration
[b] Inhalation

at various sites. If the portal of entry into the human host differs from that of the animal, the clinical manifestations will differ correspondingly. For example, ornithosis in birds results in diarrhea and systemic signs because the *Chlamydia* enter via the gastrointestinal tract. In humans, the same organisms cause pneumonia and cough because they usually enter via the respiratory route.

CONTROL

The control of zoonoses must be approached in a multidisciplinary manner because of the issues regarding the animal reservoir and the mode of transmission of the agents. The measures that must be taken range across human and veterinary medicine, sanitary engineering, and in some instances, entomology and wildlife zoology. Some appropriate interventions include: eradication of the infected animal reservoir (slaughter of infected domestic or wild animals), protection of the animals before they can become infected (improved sanitary practices, vaccination, antibiotics), killing the organisms before they can come in contact with humans (pasteurization of milk, cooking of food), or for zoonoses that depend on arthropod vectors, the eradication of flies, mosquitoes, etc. (insecticide application, sanitation). Experience has taught us that single approaches do not work as well as an integrated attack on several sanitary and medical fronts.

TWO MODELS OF ZOONOSES

The Plague

Case

Dr. Rieux felt his anxiety increasing after every visit. That evening a neighbor of his old patient in the suburbs started vomiting, pressing his hand to his groin, and running a high fever accompanied by delirium. The lymph nodes were much bigger. One of them was beginning to suppurate, and presently split open like an overripe fruit. Obviously, the abscesses had to be lanced. Two crisscross strokes, and the lymph nodes disgorged a mixture of blood and pus. His limbs stretched out as far as he could manage, the sick man went on bleeding. Dark patches appeared on the legs and stomach; sometimes a lymph node would stop suppurating, then suddenly swell again. Usually the sick man died, in a stench of corruption.

The local press, so lavish of news about the rats, now had nothing to say. For rats died in the streets; men in their homes. And newspapers are concerned only with the street. So long as each individual doctor had come across only two or three cases, no one had thought of taking any action. But it was merely a matter of adding up the figure, and once this had been done, the total was startling. In a very few days the number of cases had risen by leaps and bounds, and it had become evident to all observers of this strange malady that a real epidemic had set in. Dr. Castel, one of Rieux's colleagues and a much older man than he, came to see him.

"Naturally," he said to Rieux, "you know what it is."

"I am waiting for the post-mortems."

"Well, I know. And I don't need any post-mortems. I was in China for a good part of my career, and I saw some cases in Paris some twenty years ago. Only no one dared to call them by their name on that occasion. The usual taboo, of course; the public mustn't be alarmed, for that wouldn't do at all.

And then, as one of my colleagues said, 'It's unthinkable. Everyone knows it's ceased to appear in western Europe.' Yes, everyone knew that—except the dead men. Come now, Rieux, you know as well as I do what it is."

Rieux pondered. He was looking out of the window of his surgery, at the tall cliff that closed the half-circle of the bay on the far horizon. Though blue, the sky had a dull sheen that was softening as the light declined.

"Yes, Castel," he replied. "It's hardly credible. But everything points to it being the plague."

(From Albert Camus: The Plague, A. Knopf Publishing, New York, 1948)

The following questions may be asked of this narration:

1. Why were "limbs stretched out" in the patient described? What were the dark patches?

2. What is the meaning of the massive die-off of the rats?

3. How did this "strange malady" spread so quickly?

Historical Perspective

No infectious disease has caused more havoc to more people in the world than the plague. The first described pandemic occurred in the 6th century AD and killed an estimated 100 million people in its 50-year rampage. The second major pandemic, the Black Death, originated in Asia in the 14th century and spread to the Near East and Europe. In Europe alone, one fourth of the population died of the disease. The third pandemic originated in Burma in the 1890s, spread to Chinese seaports, and from there to other continents, including North America, via rat-infested ships. This pandemic led to the establishment of the organism in wild rodents of many countries. Sporadic cases arise from this reservoir. About 25 confirmed cases are reported each year in the United States, mainly in the western desert regions.

The Agent of Plague

The plague is caused by a Gram negative rod of the family *Enterobacteriaceae* called *Yersinia pestis*. Special stains bring out a bipolar appearance of the organism that makes it look like a safety pin.

Encounter

The disease is mainly transmitted by fleas from rodent to rodent and then to people (Fig. 55.1). Any of 1500 species of fleas may transmit the agent, but the oriental rat flea is the classic vector in human epidemics.

The plague has been detected in every continent except Australia. Most cases now occur in Southeast Asia. In the 1960s, outbreaks in South Vietnam took place as a result of the disruption caused by the war, which led to increased contact between people and an abundant rat population. In the United States there has been a modest increase in the number of cases reported in the past several decades.

Rodents are relatively resistant to Y. *pestis* and become the reservoir of the organisms between epidemics. Field mice, rats, hares and rabbits, as well as cats and dogs, are potential hosts for infected fleas. In the western United States, prairie dogs and squirrels have become important reservoirs as well. Infected fleas can

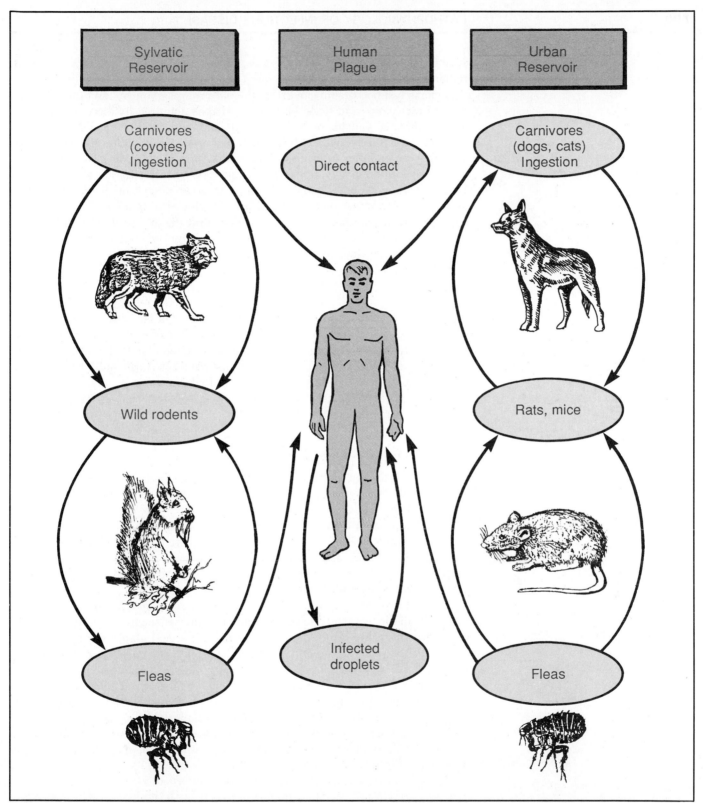

Figure 55.1. The spread of plague. Plague is perpetuated in rodent reservoirs and spread to humans via three cycles. Sylvatic cycle among wild rodents via transmission by fleas. Other mammals including skunks and coyotes may also acquire the organism by ingestion of infected animals. Urban cycle which is transmitted by the rat flea among urban rat populations. Human plague can be transmitted by contact with infected animal tissue, bite of the fleas, or by infected aerosols from other humans.

survive a year or more without access to a mammalian host and can then infect rodents that enter abandoned burrows.

Humans can become infected from this natural reservoir by the bite of infected fleas or rarely, lice and ticks. Plague can also be acquired by direct contact with dead or infected animals or with soil from contaminated burrows. Dogs and cats may transmit the disease via infected saliva or by the transfer of infected fleas.

Human populations in or near "enzootic" regions, where the reservoir animals become sick sporadically, are at particular risk when sanitation is disrupted or when the rodent population increases. The great plague epidemics have been associated with "epizootics", or episodes of high mortality among the rats. Fleas, deprived of their normal host by the massive rat die-offs, seek human beings in their stead. Explosive epidemics of primary plague pneumonia can also result from direct respiratory transmission of Y. *pestis* via aerosol droplets.

Entry

Y. *pestis* enters the body either by the bite of fleas or less commonly, by inhalation. The organisms make a coagulase that works together with an enzyme in the intestinal tract of some of the fleas to clot the ingested blood. The resulting fibrin-bacterial matrix blocks the lumen of the intestinal tract. As a result, the flea cannot feed, becomes hungry, and thus makes repeated and intensive attempts to feed. This increases the chances for transmission, especially because the flea regurgitates the organisms into the bite wound.

Spread, Multiplication, and Damage

Once inside human tissue, Y. *pestis* survives phagocytosis and multiplies within macrophages. During this time the organisms produce a capsule that allows them to resist further phagocytosis. The organisms multiply explosively and spread to regional lymph nodes via the lymphatics. These nodes become enlarged by the inflammatory response, edema, and hemorrhagic necrosis, leading to characteristic lesions, the "buboes", which give the disease the name bubonic plague. The organisms manufacture several virulence factors, including fibrinolytic enzymes, a coagulase, exotoxins, and the Gram negative endotoxin.

Bacterial invasion followed by inflammation takes place throughout the body, especially in the liver and spleen. Disseminated intravascular coagulation can produce thrombi in the capillaries of the kidneys, adrenal glands, skin, and lungs. "Black death" refers to the diffuse hemorrhagic changes in the skin plus the cyanosis caused by pneumonia. Symptoms may begin as early as two days after exposure and usually begin with fever, headache, generalized aches, and malaise. Patients with enlarging inguinal buboes characteristically flex or extend their extremities in an attempt to immobilize the lesions and to lessen the pain. The extreme tenderness appears early and is a diagnostic feature of the plague. The disease has also two other main manifestations, septicemic plague and pneumonic plague, both of which have high mortality.

Prevention

The plague can be prevented by controlling fleas with insecticides and rodents by extermination, and by improving sanitation by garbage disposal. Antibiotic therapy is quite effective, which makes quarantine of patients and their contacts less important today. Ships from ports known to be infected with the disease may be quarantined and their cargo fumigated. Circular shields placed around each hawser at the dock prevent rats from leaving and entering the ship.

Eastern Equine Encephalitis and Other Arbovirus Infections

Case

After graduating from college, Mr. R. was content to spend the month of July sunning himself on the beaches of Maryland. The weather was particularly hot and wet. His favorite spot was a pond in a wooded area where he could watch the horses of a nearby farm. One afternoon he suddenly became lethargic and fatigued and went home to bed. That evening he was awakened for supper by his father but felt confused and was not hungry. By 10 PM he had a fever of 40.7°C and refused to answer questions. Four hours later his father had difficulty arousing him and brought him to the emergency room of a local hospital. Several hours after admission he became unresponsive to simple commands. He gradually deteriorated, with periods of increasing stupor and paralysis of his limbs. He lapsed into coma two weeks after admission and died two weeks after that.

Sera obtained from Mr. R. showed a rise in antibody titer against Eastern equine encephalitis virus from less than 1:10 to 1:80. At autopsy, examination of his brain showed disseminated small foci of necrosis in both the gray and the white matter. Eastern equine encephalitis virus was isolated at the state laboratory by injecting brain tissue intracerebrally into suckling mice. Thus, the diagnosis of Eastern equine encephalitis could be made unequivocally on the grounds of the laboratory data and the clinical manifestations.

Eastern equine encephalitis (EEE) is an often fatal but fortunately rare disease. Between 1955 and 1985 there were a total of 178 cases in this country. It is an example of the many diseases carried by arthropods, the so called *arbovirus* or *arthropodborne infections*. The virus causing EEE is found among marsh birds that live in the fresh water swamps of the Atlantic and Gulf states and in regions around the Great Lakes. The reason this disease is rare in humans is that the mosquitoes that transmit this disease among marsh herons and egrets do not usually bite humans. Only when people-biting mosquitoes become involved are humans at risk. The likelihood that a person infected with this virus manifests clinical disease ranges from about 1 in 4 in children to as low as 1 in 50 in adults. The fatality rate among those that manifest symptoms is very high, from 50% to 80%. In children, mental retardation occurs in as many as half the survivors.

The Arboviruses

Arboviruses are a large group of viruses that share two characteristics: transmission by arthropod vectors and an RNA genome (Table 55.2). More than 100 different members are known to infect humans. Many cause encephalitis, while others produce yellow fever or dengue, diseases characterized by internal hemorrhages, severe pains of joints and muscles, skin rashes, etc. Diseases caused by arboviruses are distributed worldwide but are most prevalent in the tropics. They are sometimes named after the disease they cause but often after the place where they have been found (Semliki Forest virus, Rift Valley fever, Colorado tick fever, Venezuelan equine encephalitis, O'nyong nyong, etc.). They are diseases of wild and domesticated animals, with humans only accidentally infected.

The vectors include mosquitoes, ticks, and flies. Some diseases that are not transmitted by an arthropod vector are caused by viruses that are biochemically similar to members of this group. For example, the virus that causes rubella belongs to the same group as EEE virus, although it is transmitted directly from person to person.

Encounter

The natural life cycle for the viruses that cause EEE and other encephalitides is from bird to bird, via the bite of mosquitoes. It is not known if the virus overwinters in cold climates or if it is reintroduced each year by migrating birds. As the name implies, horses acquire EEE, but they seldom if ever play a role in the development of human infection. The virus is present in the horses' blood for so short a time that it is unlikely the horse would be bitten by a mosquito during the viremic phase. Horses, like humans, do not participate in the normal life cycle of the virus, but they are important *sentinel* animals, alerting that the virus has escaped its normal biological boundaries and is a threat to humans.

A certain period of time must pass before a mosquito that has acquired the virus can transmit it. Mosquitoes do not become sick with the virus, and once infected, can spread it for the rest of their lives (one season). The normal vertebrate host of the virus is also relatively unaffected, thus permitting a stable life cycle. The frequency of encounter is dictated by the proximity to humans of both the animal reservoir and the insect vector.

Entry, Spread, and Multiplication

EEE virus gains access to humans via the bite of infected mosquito. Virus-containing saliva is introduced into the capillary bed as the mosquito's proboscis penetrates the skin and endothelial cells of the capillary wall. The virus localizes in the vascular endothelium and the lymphatic cells of the reticuloendothelial system, where replication occurs. A primary viremia is induced as the virus is liberated from these infected cells. This period is of short duration, as seen in the case of Mr. R. About the time when his first symptoms abated, the virus had probably already disappeared from his blood.

This virus and many of its relatives are "positive sense" RNA viruses (Chapter 29). Their single-stranded RNA serves as messenger RNA and is transcribed directly into large proteins. These are cleaved after synthesis to make both regulatory proteins and the structural proteins of the virion. The viruses have a lipid envelope with surface glycoprotein spikes, which they acquire as they bud through the cytoplasmic membrane.

Damage

In many instances, infection by EEE and related viruses does not progress past the stage of replication in the vascular endothelium. If viremia does occur in a patient without a protective antibody titer, the virus may localize elsewhere, primarily in the central nervous system. The clinical manifestations seen in Mr. R's case are consistent with damage to various parts of the brain, as subsequently confirmed at autopsy.

It is not known how EEE virus crosses the blood-brain barrier, or why this happens in only some of the infected persons. Damage to brain and cerebellar tissue appears to be due largely to vascular involvement. Small hemorrhages are seen throughout these organs, with little preferred localization. Neurons are severely affected and many die, leading to extensive necrosis.

Diseases Caused by Other Arboviruses

In the United States, other encephalitides closely related to EEE are seen, called *St. Louis encephalitis* (SLE) and *Western equine encephalitis* (WEE). Of these, SLE is the most common, having caused about 5000 cases between 1955 and 1985. Occasionally SLE occurs in epidemics, including one in 1975 which resulted in some 1800 cases. Fortunately, it is a milder disease than EEE. *Japanese encephalitis* used to be relatively common in Japan, but its spread has been stemmed by the use of a killed virus vaccine administered to pigs and children.

The arbovirus disease of greatest historical importance is *yellow fever*. It has caused fearsome and extensive epidemics in Africa and the Americas. Despite the presence of suitable vectors and hosts, yellow fever has never taken hold in Asia. The devastating impact of yellow fever on the U.S. army in Cuba during the Spanish-American War led Walter Reed to his classic investigation into the etiology of the disease. His success in identifying a filtrable agent as the cause of yellow fever was the first proof that viruses cause human disease. Control of the disease is achieved by vaccination and by control of the vector, the mosquito *Aedes aegypti*.

Yellow fever continues to be a serious disease in much of western Africa and the Americas, where the mosquito has not been eradicated. An epidemic in central Nigeria in 1986 caused nearly 5000 deaths in the first 3 weeks of the outbreak. African monkeys, which remain asymptomatic after infection, are the reservoir in parts of Africa. In contrast, the virus may cause devastating epidemics in monkeys of Central and South America. As a consequence, outbreaks of yellow fever in monkeys are continually moving from one region of that continent to another.

Dengue is another arbovirus disease transmitted by the same mosquitoes. It is the most prevalent human disease caused by arboviruses and is found in tropical and subtropical regions of much of the world. Fortunately, it does not cause significant mortality. Clinical manifestations include sudden onset of fever, headache, pain behind the eye, and lumbosacral pain, often followed by a generalized rash. The incubation period may last up to 7 days, and North American travelers to endemic areas may become sick several days after returning home. This disease differs from other arbovirus infections in that it is not a zoonosis but is transmitted by mosquitoes directly from person to person.

Diagnosis

Diagnosis of diseases caused by any arbovirus on clinical grounds alone is difficult, because of the paucity of specific findings on physical examination. Proof of the etiology requires either isolation of the virus or demonstration of a rise in antibody titer during the illness. Both were accomplished in the case of Mr. R. The virus of EEE cannot usually be isolated from the blood of an infected person because the viremic phase is brief. Isolation of the virus from tissues such as brain should be attempted only in laboratories with appropriate containment facilities because of the danger of infection to laboratory workers.

The serological tests performed on Mr. R.'s serum sought specific antibodies against the virus using a *complement fixation* assay (Chapter 59). This is one of the oldest serological tests, dating from the early part of the century. As a test for syphilis it was known as the Wassermann test.

Therapy and Prophylaxis

Lack of specific therapy for these diseases increases the emphasis on their prevention. In endemic regions, community surveillance programs should be established to follow the density of vectors (i.e., mosquitoes) during the appropriate season of the year. At appropriate times, personal protection against mosquitoes should be emphasized (e.g., the use of repellents and bed nets). Because arboviruses cannot spread from infected patients directly, person to person contact is not a concern.

Vaccines against many of the arboviruses that cause encephalitides are either available or under development. Vaccination is an important consideration for travelers to areas where yellow fever is endemic. A live attenuated vaccine induces good immunity for at least 10 years.

SELECTED READINGS

Belsch RB (ed): *Textbook of Human Virology.* Littleton, MA, PSG Publishing Co., 1984, chap 21, Togaviruses.

Butler T: *Plague and Other Yersinia Infections.* New York, Plenum Press, 1983.

Last JM (ed): *Maxcy-Rosenau Public Health and Preventive Medicine,* ed 11. New York, Appleton-Century-Crofts, 1980.

McNeill WH: *Plagues and Peoples.* Garden City, NY, Anchor Press/Doubleday, 1976

Steele JH (ed): *CRC Handbook Series in Zoonoses, 1979–1982.* Boca Raton, FL, CRC Press.

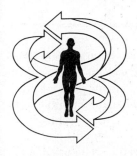

Fever of Unknown Origin

D.T. Durack

Fever is a universal and oft repeated experience for humankind. The phenomenon of raised body temperature is so familiar that everyone appreciates something of its significance. Most episodes of fever are trivial or transient, while some signify the presence of serious disease. This chapter discusses an important and diagnostically troublesome subgroup of fevers that persist for weeks without immediate explanation. This condition is termed fever of unknown origin (FUO).

PATHOPHYSIOLOGY

Body temperature depends on the balance between heat gained and heat lost. The main sources of heat are intermediary metabolism and, in warm climates, radiation, convection, and conduction from the environment. Heat is lost to the environment by radiation, convection and evaporation of sweat; some heat is lost in expired air. In homeothermic animals, normal body temperature is controlled within a narrow range by the thermoregulatory center, located in the brain in the preoptic hypothalamus, near the floor of the third ventricle. In healthy humans sleeping normal hours, diurnal variation results in lower temperatures between midnight and midmorning, and in higher temperatures in the late afternoon and evening.

External stimuli, such as pathogenic microorganisms, cause fever by a complex sequence of events. Microbes or their products act as *exogenous pyrogens*, which stimulate macrophages to release *endogenous pyrogen* into the bloodstream. This substance is interleukin-1 (IL-1), which mediates fever as well as many other important biologic responses (Chapter 4). IL-1 is the final common pathophysiologic pathway by which diverse stimuli cause fever. IL-1 circulates to the thermoregulatory center and "resets the thermostat" to a higher setting. (This step, mediated by synthesis of certain prostaglandins, may be interrupted by aspirin and other prostaglandin inhibitors.) The thermoregulatory center then stimulates vasomotor responses that *conserve* heat by constriction of blood vessels in the skin, and by shivering, which *produces* heat from rapid, uncontrolled muscular contractions called rigors. Conversely, the body can rid itself of heat by radiation through vasodilation of peripheral blood vessels and evaporation of sweat. Cyclic diurnal temperature variations still may be present in the feverish patient after the thermoregulatory center has reset, but the pattern is often exaggerated or distorted.

DEFINITION

Clinically significant fever may be defined as an oral temperature above 37.6°C (100.4°F) or a rectal temperature above 38.0°C (101°F). Because fever is such a common symptom, often with a trivial or easily diagnosed cause, a practical definition of FUO is needed. In the past, FUO was defined as continuous or intermittent fever of at least 38.0°C (100.4°F) for at least 3 weeks, which remained undiagnosed after at least 1 week of investigation in hospital. The most important of these criteria is the requirement for duration of 3 weeks or more; this eliminates most common, self-limited infections and transient postoperative fevers. Today, the requirement for 1 week of in-hospital investigation is no longer strictly necessary for the definition of FUO, because so many important diagnostic tests can now be performed on outpatients.

CASE

Mr. J., a 45-year-old married male who owned a filling station, developed persistent daily fevers to 39.9°C with heavy sweats. After 2 months, he had lost 7 kg despite reasonably good appetite. He felt rather weak, but continued to work. He had not traveled outside his home state of Virginia, and his family history was unremarkable except for pulmonary tuberculosis in an uncle 35 years ago. On examination the patient had a temperature of 39.1°C but otherwise looked well. Chest x-ray was normal except for a small calcified hilar lymph node. There was a soft heart murmur but no signs of heart disease. Blood counts showed a mild anemia. The erythrocyte sedimentation rate (rate of settling of red blood cells) was raised to 30 mm per hour (normal is <15 mm per hour). Such an increase is a nonspecific indication that an inflammatory process may be present. Urinalysis showed 30 red blood cells and 20 white blood cells per high-power field (both values abnormal), renal function was normal, and urine culture showed no significant growth after 2 days. He had not responded to three courses of different oral antibiotics prescribed by his local doctor for possible urinary tract infection.

Mr. J. was admitted to the hospital for further investigation. A skin test showed delayed hypersensitivity reactions to mumps, Candida, and tuberculin antigens. Six blood cultures were negative. Microscopic examination of a bone marrow aspirate was unrevealing and its culture was negative after 1 week. A liver biopsy was normal, also with negative culture. Repeat urinalysis again *showed some red and white blood cells, but urine culture was again negative after 2 days. X-ray of the kidneys by intravenous pyelogram showed mild irregularity and dilatation of the collecting system. The patient continued to have intermittent high fevers associated with heavy sweats while in the hospital.*

The following questions suggest themselves:

1. What are the most likely diagnoses?

2. What is the best sequence of investigations to establish a diagnosis?

3. Why is Mr. J. losing weight?

4. Is the disease likely to be fatal if untreated?

Mr. J. had a fever of unknown origin. A hidden disease process caused some of his macrophages to release IL-1 intermittently into the bloodstream. His body's homeostatic mechanisms responded by increased heat production and heat conservation, raising body temperature to an abnormally high level dictated by the thermoregulatory center. While his body temperature was rising, Mr. J. looked pale, felt cold, and experienced chills and rigors. When the temperature fell again, either naturally or due to antipyretic treatment with a drug like aspirin, Mr. J. experienced drenching sweats.

Several factors could contribute to weight loss, which often is prominent in patients with FUO. Poor appetite, nausea and vomiting may lead to various degrees of starvation. Fluid and electrolytes may be lost via sweating, vomiting, and diarrhea. Fever may accelerate protein catabolism. Very important to these processes is the synthesis of *tumor necrosis factor*, also called *cachectin*, by macrophages, especially in response to chronic infections (Chapter 4). This important biologic response modifier inhibits lipoprotein lipase and leads to severe protein catabolism. It is probably the leading reason for the weight loss in Mr. J., the patient described above.

CAUSES

The list of illnesses that can cause FUO is long. Nevertheless, patients with FUO can generally be classified into these few general categories: infections, neoplasms, rheumatic and collagen-vascular diseases, and miscellaneous other diagnoses (Table 56.1). Except in some specialized hospitals, the largest category is infections (30% to 35% of total). A small but important subgroup frustrates all investigative efforts, remaining undiagnosed. In the case above, the leading diagnostic categories seemed to be a hidden chronic infection or malignancy. The diagnosis of collagen-vascular diseases is unlikely due to absence of joint, muscle, or skin involvement. The slow tempo of disease, extending over more than 2 months, makes acute bacterial infections unlikely.

APPROACHES TO DIAGNOSIS AND MANAGEMENT

A patient with FUO presents a fascinating and often frustrating diagnostic puzzle. Optimal investigation and management require thoroughness, patience, and persistence. Myriad diagnostic tests are available. Rational selection of appropriate tests must be based on clinical findings or abnormalities found in initial laboratory tests (Table 56.2). For reasons of efficiency and economy, the investigation of a patient with FUO should progress in an orderly fashion through several sequential stages (Table 56.3). The speed with which these diagnostic steps are taken is determined by the tempo of the disease process.

Table 56.1

Main diagnostic categories and selected examples of underlying diseases

Main Diagnostic Approximate Categories	Selected Examples	Frequency, %
Infection	Abdominal abscesses	30
	Tuberculosis, infective endocarditis	
	Rheumatic fever	
	Urinary tract infections	
	Brucellosis, salmonellosis, Tularemia, Q fever, etc.	
Neoplasms	Lymphomas, e.g., Hodgkin's disease	30
	Carcinomas, primary or metastatic, etc.	
Collagen-vascular diseases	Vasculitides: temporal arteritis, giant cell arteritis, Wegener's granulomatosis, polyarteritis nodosa	15
	Systemic lupus erythematosus	
	Rheumatic fever	
	Rheumatoid and juvenile rheumatoid arthritis	
Miscellaneous	Pulmonary emboli	15
	Drug fever	
	Sarcoidosis	
	Atrial myxoma	
	Familial Mediterranean fever	
	Hepatitis: granulomatous; chronic infectious; active; alcoholic	
	Inflammatory bowel disease	
	Cyclic neutropenia	
	Subacute thyroiditis	
	Whipple's disease	
	Factitious fever	
	Habitual hyperthermia	
	Other	
Undiagnosed		10

From: Petersdorf, R.G. and Beeson, DB, 1961. Fever of unexplained origin. Medicine *40*: 1.

Patients with evidence of rapid progression should be admitted to a hospital for accelerated diagnostic testing. If, on the other hand, fever has been present for weeks without serious weight loss, weakness or other complications, investigations may begin in the outpatient clinic. The diagnostic sequence progresses to the next stage only when the present stage fails to yield the answer. In many cases, Stage 3 and especially Stage 4 are not reached, because a diagnosis was already made in an earlier stage.

Despite the increasing sophistication of diagnostic tests, the proportion of cases of FUO that remain undiagnosed—approximately 10%—has changed little over the past two decades. However, newer diagnostic tests (such as computerized tomography) have reduced the frequency with which, in the absence of a diagnosis, exploratory laparotomy (surgical opening of the abdominal wall) and/or a therapeutic trial must be performed.

The problems in diagnosing FUO are well illustrated by the case of Mr. J. The first stage of his evaluation revealed nonspecific findings: fever, weight loss, mild anemia, some red blood cells and leukocytes in his urine. Although these did not yield a diagnosis, they established that he had an active, chronic disease that was affecting his whole body. The presence of objective laboratory abnormalities such as anemia and increased erythrocyte sedimentation rate excluded a purely psychiatric cause of weight loss, such as depression.

Table 56.2
Examples of clinical and laboratory findings that may be useful in FUO, related to leading etiologic possibilities

	Differential Diagnosis	Useful Investigations
Lymphadenopathy	Cytomegalovirus, Epstein-Barr virus	Antibody titers
	Malignancies, especially lymphomas	Biopsies, computerized tomography
	Lymphogranuloma venereum	Biopsy, antibody
	Toxoplasmosis, tularemia	Antibody, biopsy
	Cat-scratch fever	Biopsy, special stains
Pneumonitis	Cytomegalovirus	Lung biopsy, serology
	Tularemia, psittacosis, Q fever	Serology
	Fungal infection	Biopsy
Heart Murmur	Rheumatic fever	Echocardiogram, antibody titers
	Infective endocarditis	Blood cultures, echocardiogram
	Atrial myxoma	Echocardiogram
Anemia	Infective endocarditis	Blood cultures
	Tuberculosis	Delayed hypersensitivity skin test; biopsies; cultures
	Malignancy	Biopsies of involved tissues
	Preleukemia	Bone marrow biopsy
Lymphocytosis	Tuberculosis	Skin tests; culture; staining
	Infectious mononucleosis	Epstein-Barr virus antibody titers
	Cytomegalovirus infection	Cytomegalovirus antibody titers, culture
Neutropenia	Systemic lupus erythematosus	Antinuclear antibody; anti-DNA;
	Tuberculosis	skin tests; culture; stains
	Lymphoma	Biopsy involved tissues
	Cyclic neutropenia	Repeat white blood cell count and differential 3 times/wk for 1 month
Monocytosis	Tuberculosis	Skin tests; culture; stains
	Brucellosis	*Brucella* titers, culture
	Hodgkin's disease	Biopsy of involved tissues
	Inflammatory bowel disease	Barium studies; endoscopy with biopsies
Elevated erythrocyte sedimentation	Infective endocarditis	Blood cultures
	Temporal arteritis	Biopsy temporal arteries
	Acute rheumatic fever	Antistreptolysin O; throat culture; joint aspiration
	Still's disease	Clinical diagnosis
	Lymphoma	Biopsy involved tissues
	Subacute thyroiditis	Antithyroglobulin antibodies
Hypercalcemia	Parathyroid adenoma	Endocrine consult
	Hypernephroma	Urinalysis; IV pyelogram
	Sarcoidosis	Chest radiograph; angiotensin-converting enzyme
Elevated alkaline phosphatase	Liver disease, obstructive or infiltrative, including infection or malignancy	Liver-spleen scan; liver biopsy for malignancy
	Hypernephroma	Intravenous pyelogram
	Subacute thyroiditis	Antithyroglobulin antibody titer
	Subacute osteomyelitis	Bone scan
	Still's disease	Clinical diagnosis
	Temporal arteritis	Biopsy
Low serum complement	Infective endocarditis	Blood culture
	Collagen-vascular diseases	Serologic studies
Rheumatoid factor	Infective endocarditis	Repeat titers, blood cultures
from: Petersdorf, Medicine *40*: 1,	Old age	Repeat titers
1966	Collagen-vascular disease	Serologic studies

The second stage of Mr. J.'s workup (in the hospital) again did not yield a diagnosis, but provided further useful information. His positive skin tests showed that (a) he was capable of mounting a normal cell-mediated immune response to ubiquitous antigens such as mumps and *Candida*, and (b) that he had encountered tuberculosis in the past. This latter observation fits with the history of tuberculosis in his uncle many years ago, and with the calcified lymph node seen in

Table 56.3
Four sequential stages in the diagnosis and management of FUO

Stage 1	Complete history, including travel, immunization, exposure; Detailed physical examination; Screening tests: blood count, sedimentation rate, urinalysis and urine culture, chest x-ray, blood cultures.
Stage 2	Review history, checking for omissions; Repeat detailed physical examination; Specific diagnostic tests: delayed hypersensitivity skin tests, urine culture for tuberculosis or CMV, serologic tests for infection and collagen-vascular diseases; echocardiogram; diagnostic imaging: upper and lower GI barium studies; intravenous urogram; lung scan, bone scan, CT scan, lymphangiogram; magnetic resonance imaging.
Stage 3	Invasive Tests: Bone marrow biopsy and culture, liver biopsy and culture, biopsy of abnormal tissues, endoscopy with biopsies, temporal artery biopsy, open lung biopsy, exploratory laparotomy.
Stage 4	Therapeutic trials: Prostaglandin inhibitors: aspirin, indomethacin. Corticosteroid therapy: prednisone, dexamethasone. Antituberculous therapy: isoniazid plus ethambutol. Antibacterial therapy: ampicillin plus gentamicin.

his chest x-ray. Could tuberculosis be the cause of his FUO? If so, it must be localized outside the lung because the chest x-ray did not reveal active pulmonary tuberculosis. The leukocytes present in Mr. J.'s urine could be due to renal tuberculosis, a diagnosis that would also explain his abnormal urogram.

The third stage of the investigation provided further important positive and negative findings. Histological examination of the bone marrow and liver biopsies showed no evidence of an occult malignancy, such as Hodgkin's lymphoma. An echocardiogram revealed no vegetations on the heart valves; this, together with negative blood cultures, made infective endocarditis unlikely.

At this point, a presumptive diagnosis was made of renal tuberculosis. Mr. J. was treated empirically with isoniazid and rifampin. At follow-up 6 weeks later, his fever had resolved and he felt well, although he still had a few leukocytes in his urine. The microbiological laboratory reported at this time that his urine culture had grown an acid fast organism, presumably *Mycobacterium tuberculosis*. Final identification of the organism, and thus confirmation of the diagnosis, followed 2 weeks later. Mr. J. completed 18 months of treatment with INH and rifampin, during which he felt well and had no further fevers.

SUGGESTED READINGS

Aduan RP, Fauci AS, Dale DC, et al: Prolonged fever of unknown origin. Clin Res 26:588A, 1978.
Dinarello CA, Wolff SM: Fever of unknown origin. In GL Mandell, Douglas Jr RG, Bennett JE (eds): *Principles and Practice of Infectious Diseases*, ed 2. New York, J Wiley & Sons, 1985, p 339.
Larson EB, Featherstone HJ, Pedersdorf RG: Fever of undetermined origin: Diagnosis and follow up of 105 cases, 1970–1980. *Medicine* 61:269, 1982.
Murphy PA: Temperature regulation and the pathogenesis of fever. In GL Mandell, Douglas Jr RG, Bennett JE (eds): *Principles and Practice of Infectious Diseases*, ed 2. New York, J Wiley & Sons, 1985, p 334.
Wolff SM, Fauci AS, Dale DC: Unusual etiologies of fever and their evaluation. *Annu Rev Med* 26:277, 1975.

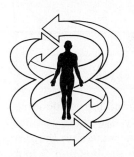

CHAPTER 57

Nosocomial and Iatrogenic Infections

D.R. Snydman

Approximately 5% of all patients develop an infection during their stay in the hospital. These hospital-acquired conditions are known as *nosocomial* infections. An infection that is the result of intervention by a physician, in or out of a hospital, is known as *iatrogenic*. Nosocomial infections often result in prolongation of hospital stay and represent an extraordinary cost in terms of morbidity and even mortality. It is estimated that about 5 billion dollars are spent each year for the management of hospital-acquired infections in the United States.

A number of factors related to hospitalization predispose patients to the risk of a hospital-acquired infection. The most important ones are those that violate the host's own defenses. Invasive procedures, often seemingly benign, result in new portals of entry for microorganisms from the patient's own flora or from the environment. Examples are the use of devices such as endotracheal tubes, mechanical ventilators, intravenous or intraarterial catheters, and surgical procedures in general.

Broadly speaking, the incidence of nosocomial infections is related to the severity of the underlying disease—i.e., patients who have a high likelihood of dying during their course of hospitalization run a higher risk of developing nosocomial infections. In contrast, patients who are admitted with less severe diseases have a smaller chance of acquiring infections in the hospital. This underscores the need for improved management of the severely compromised patient. Unfortunately, it is estimated that only about $\frac{1}{3}$ to $\frac{1}{2}$ of all nosocomial infections are preventable under the most favorable conditions.

AGENTS OF NOSOCOMIAL AND IATROGENIC INFECTIONS

Generally speaking, the organisms that cause nosocomial and iatrogenic infections are similar to those found elsewhere in the community. The most common causative agents are usually not especially pathogenic. In fact, sometimes they are even less pathogenic than those that cause disease outside the hospital, which illustrates the greater sensitivity of the hospitalized patient to infections.

A salient example is the emergence of *Serratia marcescens* as a hospital-acquired pathogen. This bacterium was thought to be so benign that it was used in the 1950s to trace the movement of air in a subway system, or to determine the movement of bacteria into the urethra through the catheter-meatal interface. This "nonpathogen" has become the source of significant nosocomial infections, although it rarely causes disease outside the hospital.

Like many pathogens associated with nosocomial infections, *Serratia* has acquired significant antibiotic resistance. Plasmid-mediated, multiple antibiotic-resistant Gram-negative bacterial strains are commonly encountered in nosocomial infections. Plasmid transfer occurs among different strains of the same species and even among different genera. Transfer of antibiotic resistance has been demonstrated in the urine of patients with Foley catheters and on their skin. Presumably, transfer of antibiotic resistance takes place in the gastrointestinal tract as well.

Table 57.1
Common hospital-acquired infections and frequently associated organisms

Infection	Most Common Organism
Surgical wounds	*Staphylococcus aureus*
	Escherichia coli
	Streptococcus faecalis
Pneumonia	*Klebsiella pneumoniae*
	Pseudomonas aeruginosa
	S. aureus
	Enterobacter sp.
	E. coli
Intravenous catheter	*S. epidermidis*
	S. aureus
	S. faecalis
	Candida sp.
Urinary catheter	*E. coli*
	S. faecalis
	Pseudomonas aeruginosa
	Klebsiella sp.

Table 57.2
Antimicrobial resistance of selected pathogens in large teaching hospitals in the United States[a]

Pathogen	Methicillin, %	Cefotaxime, %	Clindamycin, %	Gentamicin, %	Tobramycin, %
Staphylococcus aureus	7.8	10.6	12.3	Not tested	Not tested
Escherichia coli	Not tested	Not tested	2.1	2.01	1.8
Klebsiella pneumoniae	Not tested	Not tested	13.2	11.0	4.6
Serratia marcescens	Not tested	Not tested	12.7	13.3	12.5

[a] Data from the National Nosocomial Survey–1983.

Antibiotic-resistant pathogens have become so common that we regularly encounter methicillin-resistant *Staphylococcus aureus* and aminoglycoside-resistant Gram-negative bacteria in nosocomial infections. Examples of the incidence of antibiotic-resistant nosocomial pathogens are seen in Table 57.1. The pattern of antimicrobial resistance of selected pathogens in hospital settings is shown in Table 57.2.

ENCOUNTER

A hospital is a microenvironment where organisms can be transferred in a variety of ways from one individual to another, or from the hospital staff to the patients (Fig. 57.1). Transmission between individuals may be by direct hand contact, or indirect, by inhalation, ingestion, or puncture through the integument. Examples are infections due to methicillin-resistant staphylococci, which spread directly between patients or via hospital personnel. Tubercle bacilli are transmitted through aerosolization and inhalation. Food handlers may contaminate food eaten by patients, and physicians and nurses may introduce microorganisms into deeper tissues during operations or while dressing surgical or other wounds. Unusual epidemics can sometimes be traced to specific carriers among members of the hospital staff. For example, well-documented epidemics caused by group A streptococci have been attributed to carriers who had contact with patients in the operating room. In one epidemic the organisms were located in the carrier's vagina, from where they were presumably aerosolized through normal body movements.

Microorganisms that spread to patients may be endemic to the hospital environment. Notable examples include the fungi that cause aspergillosis, which may be

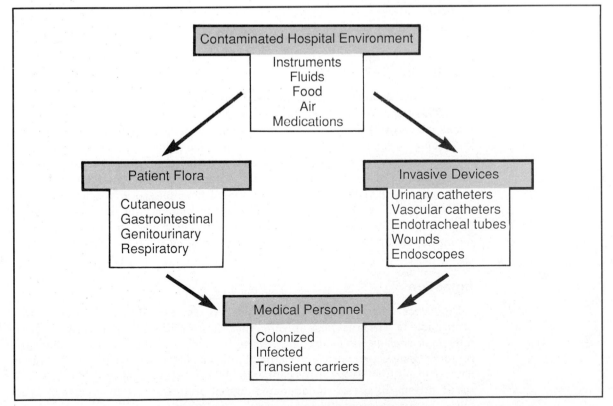

Figure 57.1. Sources of hospital-acquired infections.

present as more or less visible mildew on moist room walls or construction panels. Infections by exogenous organisms may also be acquired from improperly sterilized surgical instruments and even contaminated disinfectant solutions! Fortunately, these are rare events in a proper hospital setting.

Patients acquire nosocomial infections as the result of breaks in their own defenses and from their inability to combat infection. These breaks usually occur as the result of invasive diagnostic or therapeutic interventions that physicians perform on their patients. For these reasons, the most common nosocomial infections affect the urinary tract, because catheterization of the bladder is frequently used with bedridden patients. The commonly used Foley catheter bypasses the normal mucosal barriers and facilitates the entry of organisms that colonize the skin or the urinary introitus. The next most frequent type of infection is that of surgical wounds, followed by respiratory tract infections, each of which involves invasive procedures.

ENTRY

Skin Penetration

The skin barrier is breached by the use of intravenous catheters or devices used to measure intravascular pressure. The longer they stay in place, the higher the risk of both local infection and bacteremia. This underscores the need for vigilance in the care of patients with indwelling devices.

Another example of the role of the normal skin in protecting against microbial invasion is that of burn victims. Frequently patients who have extensive second- or third-degree burns will become colonized with bacteria, especially *Pseudomonas aeruginosa*. Necrotizing lesions at the site of skin damage are accompanied by sepsis, the major cause of death in burn victims.

Inhalation

The most common cause of nosocomial pneumonia is the use of an endotracheal tube. This bypasses the normal epithelial defenses and allows the entry of organisms via aerosols. In the early 1960s, when mechanical ventilation of the lungs was being developed, it was recognized that epidemics of Gram negative pneumonia occurred because nebulized mists contained bacteria-laden aerosols. An understanding of the problem brought about changes in design, which have virtually eliminated the ventilator as a source of hospital-acquired pneumonia. Patients with endotracheal tubes still develop pneumonia, but now the offending organisms tend to come from the patient's stomach or intestine and colonize the nasopharynx. From here, they may become aspirated into the lungs.

Ingestion

Epidemics of nosocomial infection sometimes result from the ingestion of pathogenic bacteria. The organisms are often those associated with community-acquired infections, such as *Salmonella*, hepatitis virus, and rotavirus, the latter being most frequent among neonates or infants. Epidemics of salmonellosis in hospitals usually result from eating foods contaminated during preparation. They have also resulted from the use of contaminated animal products used for diagnostic purposes, such as carmine dye.

The Inanimate Environment

The complexity of a hospital environment provides innumerable opportunities for the encounter of patients with microorganisms. Some of these are specific for these environments and not usually found elsewhere. An example is the use of contaminated intravenous solutions, which have caused many epidemics. Contamination rarely takes place at the point of manufacture; more commonly it occurs during the handling of bottles and infusion lines.

Instruments and dressings improperly sterilized before surgery also provide a possible source of infection. A whole technology has developed around the problems of determining if autoclaves and sterilizing ovens perform their expected task. Thus, it is customary to insert a vial containing bacterial spores with the material to be autoclaved, and to determine spore viability afterwards. Deviance from established procedures may well result in improper sterilization and in contamination of surgical or other wounds.

MODEL INFECTIONS

Urinary Tract Infection

Mr. H., a 67-year-old gentleman, underwent a transurethral prostatectomy for cancer of the prostate. Because of concern for postoperative bleeding from straining during urination, he had a Foley catheter placed into the bladder. Three days later Mr. H. developed a urinary tract infection with low-grade fever, some pain, and pyuria. Quantitative urine counts yielded 3×10^5 colonies of Escherichia coli per milliliter of urine. The organisms were resistant to all tested antibiotics except the aminoglycosides. Within 2 days, Mr. H. developed bacteremia with hypotension and shock. Physicians were eventually able to control the bacteremia with gentamicin therapy. Fortunately, Mr. H. recovered completely and was discharged.

How did Mr. H. acquire this infection?

This is a classic case of a nosocomial infection of the urinary tract. The use of Foley catheters for more than 1 or 2 days often results in contamination of the bladder, especially by fecal coliforms (Table 58.2). Nowadays catheters are usually provided with an expandable collection bag for the urine, thus making this a closed system. Nonetheless, the risk of bacteriuria is cumulative and still occurs at a rate between 5% and 8% per day. The risk of bacteriuria is related to the skill of the person inserting the catheter, the sex and age of the patient, and the duration of catheterization.

Nosocomial Wound Infection

Ms. Z., an 82-year-old lady with rheumatic heart disease, underwent a mitral valve replacement along with surgery for a coronary artery bypass graft. Her postoperative course was complicated by bleeding in the mediastinum, which necessitated more surgery. She did well after these operations and was discharged after 12 days. Three weeks later, Ms. Z. noticed some purulent drainage along the wound site on her chest. She continued to have pain but did not complain about it to her family, assuming that the pain was related to her healing process. When she returned to see the surgeon 1 month later, she reported her pain and low-grade fever. The surgeon noted that there was considerable drainage at the wound site. Probing the wound, he noticed a lot of pus.

Ms. Z. was hospitalized again for radical debridement (cleaning) of her chest wound. Cultures of the pus yielded Staphylococcus epidermidis. She was treated intravenously with vancomycin for 6 weeks and her wound was debrided with removal of the wires in her sternum. At the end of this period she required a plastic surgical procedure and a muscle flap to close the wound. After two more months of hospitalization, she was discharged and continued her convalescence at home.

How did Ms. Z. acquire the infection? What was the source of the organism?

This case illustrates the problem of surgical wound infections and the serious impact they can have on the patient's recovery. Wound infections of the mediastinum complicate between 1% and 5% of open heart surgery. If the infection reaches deep portions of the chest, its effect can be extremely serious. Patients frequently require multiple surgical interventions with removal of devitalized bone, cartilage, and other tissue.

Surgical wound infections are the most costly of all nosocomial infections. Some are clearly preventable. They are frequently due to *S. aureus* but the example used here illustrates that *S. epidermidis*, a normal skin commensal, may also be a significant pathogen (Table 58.2). In the case of Ms. Z. the source of the infection was probably her own skin flora. As with other infections, the establishment depends on the size of the inoculum, the pathogenic potential of the invading organisms, and the state of the host defenses. All these factors should be taken into account before planning surgical treatment. In cases where infection would be devastating, as in artificial hip implants, surgeons may go to great lengths, such as using laminar air-flow systems and prophylactic antibiotics.

Primary Bacteremia

Fifty-nine-year-old Mr. S. was hospitalized with acute myocardial infarction. His disease was so severe that he required a catheter to measure his cardiac pressure and output. Unfortunately, the catheter was left in place for several more days than was probably necessary. Six days after his infarction, Mr. S. developed fever, leukocytosis, and inflammation at the site of insertion of the catheter. Four blood cultures all revealed the presence of S. aureus. He was treated with intravenous antibiotics; however, a new cardiac murmur was noted 7 days into therapy. An echocardiogram revealed the development of a tricuspid valve vegetation. Mr. S. required 4 weeks of antibiotic therapy for his hospital-acquired, catheter-related endocarditis.

What was the source of the organism?

This case illustrates an example of primary bacteremia, which is defined as bacteremia which cannot be ascribed to another focus of infection. Primary bacteremia is frequently either the result of a contaminated intravenous line or associated with granulocytopenia in the immunosuppressed leukemic patient.

There are many different areas, from the bottle to the intravenous catheter, where contamination may occur during the course of intravenous therapy. The risk of intravenous catheter–related infection is generally influenced by the type of catheter and the duration of catheterization. Patients who have large bore catheters that require surgical insertion have the highest risk. If the catheter is left in place for 48 hours or longer, there is a 2% to 3% risk of bacteremia. In the example cited, the patient developed endocarditis, a rare but recognized complication. The usual pathogens tend to be *S. aureus*, *S. epidermidis*, a variety of Gram negative rods, or *Candida* (Table 57.1).

There have also been nationwide outbreaks of intravenous fluid-related infection due to contamination of intravenous bottles at manufacture. The pathogens that have been involved in these situations have usually been relatively nonpathogenic species of *Enterobacter*. These organisms are able to grow in sugar-water solutions at room temperature.

Another example of primary bacteremia is generally seen in leukemia or lymphoma patients who are granulocytopenic as a result of cancer chemotherapy. Patients will frequently become bacteremic, primarily from an intestinal focus. The usual pathogens in this setting are Gram negative rods, which may originate from the patient's endogenous flora or may be exogenously acquired in the hospital.

Nosocomial Pneumonia

Ms. J. was hospitalized for therapy of acute leukemia. Over a 3-week period her blood cell count remained low as a result of her chemotherapy. At the end of this period she developed a pulmonary infiltrate and sinusitis. She was treated with broad-spectrum antibiotics but failed to respond. Her lung involvement progressed and she was subjected to an open lung biopsy. A species of Aspergillus (A. fumigatus) *was cultured from this material. She was started on amphotericin B but became progressively more ill and died within a week.*

How did Ms. J. acquire aspergillosis? What was the source of the organisms?

Nosocomial aspergillosis, while not common, has recently been seen more often among immunosuppressed patients. A number of reported epidemics have been linked to hospital construction and contamination of air conditioning systems. Large numbers of fungal spores in the air lead to nasal or bronchial colonization. Immunosuppression and the resultant granulocytopenia, along with broad-spectrum antibacterial antibiotics, help the organism become established in the airways.

This is an example of a relatively uncommon form of acquisition of organisms that cause nosocomial pneumonia. More often, patients aspirate stomach or nasopharyngeal contents as the result of their debilitation. Infections acquired in this manner are frequently due to a mixed aerobic-anaerobic bacterial flora. Unfortunately, nosocomial penumonia is the least preventable of all hospital-acquired infections and is associated with the highest mortality rate.

CONTROL

Control of nosocomial infections requires awareness by all health care professionals. Handwashing between patient contact is a simple but much neglected procedure. It can decrease transmission of microorganisms between hospital staff and patients. The use of aseptic techniques during surgical and other invasive procedures, as stressed in surgical training, results in significant prevention of these infections.

Hospitals have instituted infection control committees, whose responsibility is to oversee all aspects of infection control within the institution. They supervise surveillance of hospital-acquired infections, establish policies and procedures to prevent such infections, and have the power to intervene when necessary in investigations of epidemics or other problems. Most hospitals have specific personnel, *infection control practitioners*, who are assigned these tasks and function as the "eyes and ears" of the committee. These individuals are responsible for tracing epidemics, monitoring the infection rate, and determining the level of isolation of patients. But, there is still a good deal to be learned. There is active interest in preventing infections in the increasing number of immunocompromised hosts and in working out effective means to prevent nosocomial pneumonias.

SUGGESTED READINGS

Altemeir WA, Burke JF, Pruitt Jr BA, Saudusky WR (eds): *Manual of Control of Infection in Surgical Patients*, ed 2. Philadelphia, J. D. Lippincott, 1984.
Bennett JV: In Brachman, PS (ed): *Hospital Infections*, ed 2. Little, Brown & Co., 1986.
Dixon RE (ed): *Nosocomial Infections*. New York, Yorke Medical Books, 1981.
Wenzel RP (ed): *Prevention and Control of Nosocomial Infections*. Baltimore, Williams & Wilkins, 1987.
Wenzel RP (ed): *CRC Handbook of Hospital Acquired Infections*. Boca Raton, FL., CRC Press, 1981.

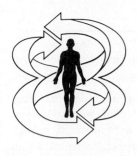

Foodborne Diseases

58

D.R. Snydman

Foodborne infections are a significant public health problem. In the United States, they are a major cause of morbidity, although an infrequent cause of mortality. In 1980 and 1981 there were 1180 outbreaks reported to the Centers for Disease Control from virtually all 50 states. The number of ill people reported to the health authorities in these outbreaks was more than 28,000. Surveillance suggests that the true scope of infection related to food probably is 10 to 100 times more frequent.

A foodborne disease outbreak is defined by two criteria: (a) two or more persons experience a similar illness, usually gastrointestinal, after ingestion of the same food; and (b) epidemiologic analysis implicates food as the source of the illness. There are certain exceptions to this definition. For example, one case of botulism constitutes an outbreak for the purposes of epidemiologic investigation and control.

Of all the diseases acquired by ingestion of contaminated food, the most common in the United States are those that are usually called food poisoning. They are defined as diseases caused by the consumption of food contaminated with bacteria or bacterial toxins. Bacteria cause approximately two-thirds of the foodborne outbreaks in the United States for which an etiology can be determined. However, it should be noted that only in 44% of such outbreaks is the etiology confirmed.

This chapter will deal with infectious diarrheas from bacterial food poisoning in general, and, more specifically, with its two main types:

• *Intoxications* due to toxin preformed in the food; examples of causative bacteria are *S. aureus*, *C. perfringens*, and *B. cereus*.

• *Intestinal invasive diseases*, such as gastroenteritis due to invasive organisms, e.g., *Salmonella* and *Campylobacter*.

The distinction between food poisoning caused by toxin-producing organisms and by invasive pathogens is important clinically and epidemiologically. In general, diseases due to toxin-forming organisms such as *Staphylococcus aureus* have a short incubation period and are characterized by upper gastrointestinal complaints, such as nausea and vomiting. Diarrhea is less frequent, and constitutional symptoms, e.g., fever and chills, are uncommon. In contrast, food poisoning from more invasive organisms, such as *Salmonella*, usually has a longer incubation period and is characterized by fever, chills and lower gastrointestinal complaints. Diarrhea, often bloody or containing pus or mucus, is more prominent than nausea or vomiting.

Therefore, we generally categorize food poisoning by whether intoxication or invasion is most prominent. There is some overlap in this classification scheme, since organisms such as *Shigella* or *Salmonella* may have invasive properties as well as being able to produce toxin.

Let us turn to outbreaks and cases in the United States (Table 58.1). The most frequently recognized agents of bacterial food poisoning are generally limited to a dozen organisms (Table 58.2). *Salmonella* outbreaks predominate among the confirmed outbreaks and constitute almost 33 percent of reported cases of foodborne illness. This is due in part to the ease of recognition and to the awareness of physicians and the public. *Staphylococcus aureus* is the next most frequent cause of foodborne outbreaks, associated with 25% of reported cases. *Clostridium perfringens*, *Shigella*, *Campylobacter*, *Bacillus cereus*, and other pathogens cause illness less frequently.

It is important to note that etiologic patterns vary throughout the world. They depend on many factors, such as food preferences, awareness by physicians and the public, and laboratory capabilities. For example, in the United States, food poisoning by *Staphylococcus aureus* and *Salmonella* represents more than 50% of the outbreaks. In contrast, *C. perfringens* is implicated in more than 90% of the recognized foodborne illness in England and Wales. Japan has yet different

Table 58.1
Confirmed foodborne disease outbreaks, by bacterial etiology, United States 1980–1981[a]

Bacterial Etiology	Outbreaks (%)	Cases (%)
Salmonella	105 (32.7)	4837 (32.0)
Staphylococcus aureus	71 (22.1)	3878 (25.7)
Shigella	20 (6.2)	1535 (10.1)
C. perfringens	53 (16.5)	1625 (17.4)
C. jejuni	15 (4.7)	649 (4.3)
E. coli	1 (0.3)	500 (3.3)
Y. enterocolitica	2 (0.6)	338 (2.2)
Streptococcus	3 (0.9)	331 (2.2)
B. cereus	17 (5.3)	161 (1.7)
C. botulinum	25 (7.8)	40 (0.3)
V. parahaemolyticus	6 (1.9)	25 (0.2)
V. Cholerae non-01	1 (0.3)	4 (0.03)
Others	2 (0.6)	88 (0.6)
Total	321	14011

[a] Data from the Centers for Disease Control, Atlanta, GA.

Table 58.2
Some characteristics of bacterial food poisoning

Organism	Mechanism	Frequency, %	Incubation Period, hr	Vehicles	Features
Staphylococcus aureus	Heat-stable toxin	15–20	1–6	Ham, pastry Baked goods	Vomiting
B. cereus	Heat-stable toxin	1–2	1–6	Fried rice	Vomiting
	Heat-labile toxin		8–24	Cream sauce	Diarrhea
Salmonella	Invasion	20–25	16–48	Chicken, beef Eggs, milk	Fever, diarrhea
Campylobacter	Invasion	5–10	16–48	Chicken, beef Milk	Fever, diarrhea
V. parahaemolyticus	Invasion (toxin?)	1–2	16–72	Shellfish	Fever, diarrhea
Y. enterocolitica	Invasion (toxin?)	1–2	16–72	Milk, tofu	Diarrhea
E. coli	Toxin	5–10	16–72	Salads	Diarrhea
	O157:H7 (vero toxin)	1–2	16–48	Beef Beef, poultry	Fever Diarrhea
C. perfringens	Toxin	5–10	8–12	Beef, poultry Gravy	Diarrhea

etiologic patterns, with *Vibrio parahaemolyticus* gastroenteritis representing more than 50% of the reported outbreaks

INTOXICATIONS

Case 1. *Staphylococcus aureus*

As the aircraft cruised at 35,000 ft, the cabin attendants passed out a lunch meal that included ham sandwiches. Two hours later two-thirds of the passengers aboard the jet plane developed nausea and vomiting. Diarrhea occurred in about one-third of those affected. The waiting lines for the facilities trailed down the aisle. As a result of such epidemics, rules for serving the cockpit crew different meals went into effect (without increasing the number of toilets).

We may consider the following questions:

1. What was the cause of the outbreak?

2. How could one meal have affected such a large number of individuals?

In the epidemic described, about two-thirds of the passengers were served ham sliced by a chef who had a pustular lesion on his hand. *S. aureus* was isolated from the lesion along with the identical strain from the ham. The passengers had ingested food contaminated with one of the many *S. aureus* toxins.

Encounter

Staphylococcal foodborne outbreaks are characterized by explosive onset 1 to 6 hours after consuming contaminated food. Attack rates are usually quite high since very small quantities of staphylococcal enterotoxin can cause illness. In outbreaks involving single families and uniform doses of enterotoxin, virtually 100% of individuals are affected. The enterotoxin is resistant to heat and is still present in food after cooking.

Outbreaks from staphylococci may occur at any time of the year, but most are reported during the warm weather months. Staphylococci are carried by so many people that food preparation in almost any setting may be involved. Most outbreaks are reported from large gatherings, i.e., schools, group picnics, clubs, and restaurants. Many different foods have been implicated: ham, canned beef, pork, or any salted meat, and cream-filled cakes or pastries such as cream puffs. Potato and macaroni salads are occasionally involved. Foods that have a high content of salt (ham) or sugar (custard) selectively favor the growth of staphylococci.

Foods that are involved in outbreaks have usually been cut, sliced, grated, mixed, or ground by workers who are carriers of enterotoxin-producing strains of staphylococci. Even though animal carcasses may be contaminated before processing, competitive growth from other members of the flora usually limits the staphylococci. Therefore, the primary mechanism of transmission is from the food handler to the food product.

Clinical Features

The symptoms of staphylococcal food poisoning are primarily profuse vomiting, nausea, and abdominal cramps, often followed by diarrhea. In severe cases, blood may be observed in the vomitus or stool. Rarely, hypotension and marked prostration may occur, but recovery is usually complete in 24 to 48 hours.

Diagnosis

Staphylococcal food poisoning should be considered in anyone with severe vomiting, nausea, cramps and some diarrhea. A history of ingesting meats of high salt or sugar content may be helpful. Usually the best epidemiologic clue, especially if a number of individuals are ill, is the short incubation period (1 to 6 hours). Of the bacterial foodborne diseases, only B. cereus has similar symptoms, with a short incubation period and a marked vomiting syndrome. Since the B. cereus vomiting syndrome is closely allied with rice, the epidemiologic distinction can usually be easily made.

The diagnosis can be confirmed by culturing the incriminated food, the skin or nose of the food handler, or occasionally the vomitus or stools of affected individuals. The recovered S. aureus may be phage-typed to prove identity between isolated strains (see Chapter 11). Detection of staphylococcal enterotoxin will be the ultimate means of making the diagnosis once an appropriate test becomes generally available.

Case 2. Clostridium perfringens

A group of college dormitory residents sat down for a turkey feast around 6 PM. They consumed turkey, giblets, gravy and "all the fixins". Around 2 AM the first of many awoke with severe intestinal cramps and watery diarrhea. Most of the students in the group became ill with similar symptoms around 6 AM. Several required hospitalization in the college infirmary. Fortunately, the wave of diarrhea resolved within 24 hours.

Let us consider the following:

1. What is the likely agent of this disease?

2. What is the pathophysiology of this type of diarrhea?

3. How could such an outbreak be prevented?

Encounter

The lengthy time of onset of symptoms, the clinical manifestations, and the fact that most of the persons present at the meal got sick point to *Clostridium perfringens* as a likely cause of the outbreak. *C. perfringens* food poisoning is the third most common cause of foodborne disease in the United States. Since this diagnosis is often difficult to establish, we must assume that these reports represent a small fraction of the actual cases that occur.

Epidemics of *C. perfringens* are usually characterized by high attack rates, affecting a large proportion of individuals. The incubation period in most outbreaks varies between 8 and 14 hours (median of 12 hours), but can be as long as 72 hours. For reasons that are not clear, more cases of *C. perfringens* food poisoning are reported in the fall and winter months. The nadir of reported cases is in the summer, in marked contrasts to outbreaks of *Salmonella* and staphylococcal food poisoning. It may be that the kinds of food usually implicated, such as stews, are eaten less frequently in the summer.

Outbreaks due to this organism are most frequently reported from institutions or large gatherings. The latter is probably a reporting artifact, since frequently only such groups recognize the illness as food poisoning. In the late 1940s it was discovered that *C. perfringens* caused outbreaks of severe and often lethal intestinal disease labeled *enteritis necroticans* which affected people in Germany and New Guinea (where it is termed "pig-bel", see below).

Pathophysiology

This form of food poisoning often takes place when poultry, meat or fish is precooked and then reheated before serving. Spores of the organisms resist the first heating and then germinate in the food. The second heating must be inadequate to kill them, therefore they are ingested either as spores or as vegetative cells. In the intestine, the organisms begin to sporulate, forming the toxin (Chapter 7).

Diarrhea is caused by a heat-labile protein enterotoxin with a molecular weight of approximately 34,000 (Chapters 7 and 21). The clostridial toxin differs from cholera toxin in several respects: Its activity is maximal in the ileum and minimal in the duodenum, just opposite to that of cholera toxin. Clostridial enterotoxin inhibits glucose transport, damages the intestinal epithelium, and causes protein loss into the intestinal lumen, none of which are observed with cholera toxin. Recently, *C. perfringens* enterotoxin has been detected in the stools of affected individuals. Enterotoxin activity disappears quickly from stool but can be measured in the serum.

Immunity in this disease is not well understood. In one study, 65% of Americans and 84% of Brazilians had anti-enterotoxin activity in serum. The significance of this finding is unknown at present: In none of the outbreaks studied to date was blood available that had been drawn before an outbreak, which would have permitted a correlation between anti-enterotoxin immunity and the disease. In animal studies, enterotoxin antiserum blocks the action of the toxin on ligated rabbit loops. It is not known, however, if the presence of antibody in serum has any affect on toxin activity in the intestine.

Clinical Features

C. perfringens food poisoning is generally characterized by watery diarrhea and severe crampy abdominal pain, usually without vomiting, beginning 8 to 24 hours after the incriminated meal. Fever, chills, headache or other signs of infection usually are not present.

The illness is of short duration, 24 hours or less. Rare fatalities have been recorded in debilitated or hospitalized patients who are victims of clostridial food poisoning.

Enteritis Necroticans

Enteritis necroticans ("pig-bel") is a very different illness characterized by high attack rates in children in New Guinea, coupled with a high mortality. Outbreaks of the disease have been clearly related to the consumption of pig in large native feasts. Improperly cooked pork is consumed in large quantities over 3 to 4 days.

This is a severe necrotizing disease of the small intestine. After a 24-hour incubation period, illness ensues with intense abdominal pain, bloody diarrhea, vomiting and shock. The mortality rate is about 40%, usually due to intestinal perforation. The disease is caused by a toxin known as β-toxin, a protein (molecular weight of 35,000) that is unusually sensitive to proteases and is thus rapidly inactivated by the intestinal enzyme trypsin. The disease usually affects people who eat large, high-protein meals that overwhelm their intestinal trypsin.

Diagnosis

The diagnosis of C. perfringens food poisoning should be considered in any diarrheal illness characterized by abdominal pain and moderate to severe diarrhea, unaccompanied by fever and chills. Usually many individuals are involved in the outbreak; the suspect food is beef or chicken that has been stewed, roasted, or boiled earlier, and then allowed to sit without proper refrigeration. The incubation period is 8 to 14 hours; occasional outbreaks have incubation periods as short as 5 to 6 or as long as 22 hours.

A form of food poisoning due to Bacillus cereus may have similar symptoms, and can only be ruled out by bacteriologic study. Enterotoxigenic E. coli may also produce these symptoms, although low-grade fever is often present. Vibrio cholerae produces more profuse diarrhea, which helps differentiate if from clostridial intoxication. Salmonella or Campylobacter infection is usually accompanied by fever, a longer incubation period, and more marked systemic signs.

Since C. perfringens may be isolated from normal stools, it is helpful to utilize an established serotyping schema to distinguish among about 20 different serotypes. In an outbreak, the same serotype of C. perfringens should be recovered from all cases and from the food they ate. If food specimens are not available, the diagnosis may be made by isolating organisms of the same serotype from the stool of most ill individuals but not from that of suitable controls. In the absence of either of these findings, culturing 10^5 or more organisms per gram of food is highly suggestive.

Case 3. *Bacillus cereus*

Case/Outbreak

Six medical students returned to class after a lunch break in Chinatown. Lunch consisted of hot and sour soup, spring rolls, fried rice, and three other Chinese entrées. Two hours later, while listening to Prof. S. expound on the hazards of mushroom poisoning, four of the six felt the urge to vomit and had to excuse themselves from class.

The following questions arose:

1. Which food is most likely to have contributed to this early onset form of food poisoning?

2. How could food become so generally contaminated?

Encounter

B. cereus has been increasingly recognized as a significant cause of food poisoning since about 1970. About 1% to 2% of all outbreaks in the United States are caused by this organism. Data from other countries are still generally sparse.

The incubation period for the outbreaks of emetic illness is usually 2 to 3 hours, whereas that for the diarrheal outbreaks is 6 to 14 hours. The clear-cut association between this vomiting syndrome and fried rice deserves emphasis. Most outbreaks of this syndrome in the United States and in Great Britain implicate this dish as the vehicle. The diarrheal illness, however, has been caused by a variety of vehicles including boiled beef, sausage, chicken soup, vanilla sauce, and puddings.

B. cereus is found in about 25% of foodstuffs sampled, including cream, pudding, meat, spices, dry potatoes, dry milk, spaghetti sauces, and rice. Contamination of food products generally occurs before they are cooked. The organisms will grow if the food is maintained at 30°C to 50°C during preparation. Spores survive extreme temperatures and, when allowed to cool relatively slowly, will germinate and multiply. There is no evidence that human carriage of the organism or other means of contamination play a role in transmission.

Contamination of rice by *B. cereus* is attributed to the practice common in oriental restaurants of allowing large portions of boiled rice to drain unrefrigerated to avoid clumping. The flash frying in the final preparation of certain rice dishes (e.g., fried rice) does not raise the temperature sufficiently to destroy the preformed heat-stable toxin.

Pathophysiology

Several extracellular toxins produced by strains of *B. cereus* may contribute to their virulence, including an enterotoxin that causes fluid accumulation in the rabbit intestine and stimulates the adenyl cyclase-cyclic AMP system in intestinal epithelial cells.

A second presumptive toxin has been isolated from a strain of *B. cereus* implicated in an outbreak of vomiting-type illness. Cell free culture filtrates from this strain do not produce fluid accumulation in rabbit intestine, do not stimulate the adenyl cyclase-cyclic AMP system, and only produce vomiting when fed to rhesus monkeys. This "vomiting toxin" is heat stable.

Clinical Features

Food poisoning due to *Bacillus cereus* has two main clinical manifestations, diarrheal and emetic. The diarrheal, long incubation form of the illness is characterized by diarrhea (96%), abdominal cramps (75%), and vomiting (23%). Fever is uncommon. The duration of disease ranges from 20 to 36 hours, with a median of 24 hours.

The emetic form of the illness has as predominant symptoms vomiting (100%) and abdominal cramps (100%). Diarrhea is only present in one-third of affected individuals. The duration of this illness ranges from 8 to 10 hours with a median of 9 hours. In both types of illness the disease is usually mild and self-limited.

The vomiting syndrome must be differentiated from *S. aureus* food poisoning. As stated above, the association with fried rice is epidemiologically useful in differentiating the two organisms.

FOOD POISONING DUE TO INVASIVE ORGANISMS

Case 4. *Salmonella* gastroenteritis

Forty-eight hours after eating poorly cooked chicken, Mr. T. developed fever, shaking chills, abdominal cramps and blood-tinged diarrhea. The illness lasted several days, and fever and diarrhea gradually abated. Mr. T. is a 65-year-old individual with a silent abdominal arterial aneurysm. Unbeknownst to him or his physician, the organisms causing his febrile diarrheic episode seeded the bloodstream and invaded the aneurysm. Ten days after the initial episode, Mr. T. developed more fever and chills, and his aneurysm expanded. Blood cultures were positive for Salmonella typhimurium. *Surgery and antibiotics were required. Fortunately, Mr. T. survived.*

This case underscores the invasive potential of several bacteria associated with food poisoning. A number of organisms are associated with invasiveness; particularly common agents are *Salmonella* and *Campylobacter*. More uncommon bacterial causes are *Vibrio parahaemolyticus*, *Yersinia enterocolitica* and a specific strain of *E. coli*. Invasiveness is generally associated with the presence of neutrophils in stool and systemic signs like fever, chills, myalgias, and headache. These organisms are discussed in Chapters 17 and 18.

Other Invasive Agents of Food Poisoning

Vibrio parahaemolyticus

The organism, like *Vibrio cholera*, is often associated with contaminated shellfish. The organism tends to behave as one of the "invasive" pathogens, rather than as a toxin-producing one, such as *Vibrio cholera*.

Yersinia enterocolitica

Y. enterocolitica is a Gram-negative rod that has recently been implicated as a cause of food poisoning. Contaminated milk has been one well-documented source. Infection due to this organism generally resembles the invasive variety although a heat-stable enterotoxin has been described. Tissue invasion, frequently mimicking acute appendicitis, is very common with this infection. At surgery the appendix of such patients may be spared but the mesenteric lymph nodes surrounding the appendix will be markedly inflamed (see Chapter 46).

Escherichia coli

Although E. coli is part of the host's normal flora there are some toxigenic and enteropathogenic strains which are associated with food poisoning. Toxigenic E. coli occurs in about 50% of traveler's diarrhea (Chapter 17). The organisms are ingested by travelers through contaminated salads, raw fruits, and vegetables. This syndrome is usually associated with watery diarrhea. Fever is less common. The organisms make both a heat-labile and heat-stable enterotoxin.

There is also a syndrome of bloody diarrhea, generally without fever caused by a "vero toxin" producing strain of E. coli (serotype O157:H7). The mechanism of action of this toxin appears to be identical to that of Shigella, the agent of bacillary dysentery. This organism has been epidemiologically connected to poorly cooked hamburger.

"Arizona"

The organism called "Arizona" is a motile Gram-negative rod closely related to Salmonella. It has been implicated in outbreaks of gastroenteritis and enteric fever. Various vehicles have included eggs or poultry as the contaminated products. Because of the similarities to Salmonella, contaminated animal products should be considered the usual vehicle.

The syndromes of "Arizona" infection are also very similar to salmonellosis. Gastroenteritis, enteric fever, bacteremia, or localized infection have been described. The incubation period is similar to Salmonella. Usually, symptoms develop 24 to 48 hours after ingestion of contaminated food. Fever, headache, nausea, vomiting, abdominal pain, and watery diarrhea may occur, as well as marked prostration. Symptoms may persist for several days. Therapy and prevention are also similar to those employed for salmonellosis.

Listeria monocytogenes

This organism is becoming increasingly recognized as a foodborne pathogen. Listeria monocytogenes is a Gram-positive, motile rod that is relatively heat resistant: It withstands pasteurization of milk. Listeria is widely distributed in nature, found in the intestinal tract of various animals and humans, as well as in sewage, soil, and water.

The syndromes usually associated with listeriosis include meningitis, bacteremia, or focal metastatic disease. Frequently gastrointestinal symptoms such as diarrhea precede the bacteremic disease. The organisms have a propensity to affect adults who are either immunosuppressed or pregnant. The evidence that Listeria is related to foodborne illness is accumulating from investigations of several recent epidemics. Contaminated cole slaw, raw and pasteurized milk have been implicated as vehicles for epidemic listeriosis. The source of sporadic Listeria infection is less well understood.

CONTROL AND PREVENTION

The common theme that ties all foodborne illnesses together is the improper handling of food prior to its consumption. In a study of factors responsible for

Table 58.3
Factors that contributed to foodborne disease outbreaks in the United States from 1961–1976[a]

Factor	Percent Implicated[b]
Inadequate refrigeration	47
Food prepared too far in advance of service	21
Infected person with poor personal hygiene	21
Inadequate cooking	16
Inadequate holding temperature	16
Inadequate reheating	12
Contaminated raw ingredient	11
Cross-contamination	7
Dirty equipment	7

[a] From Bryan F.L: Factors that contribute to outbreaks of foodborne disease. Food Protection *41*, 816–829, 1978
[b] Values total more than 100% because more than one factor may contribute to foodborne outbreak.

foodborne outbreaks in the United States over a 15-year period, it was shown that inadequate refrigeration is the single most frequent factor (Table 58.3). Usually other factors are also associated with a specific outbreak, such as advanced preparation of food without adequate storage, or improper reheating. To a lesser degree, contaminated equipment, cross-contamination, and poor personal hygiene of food preparation personnel may contribute to outbreaks. The ubiquity of *Salmonella*, *Campylobacter*, *B. cereus*, and *C. perfringens* makes it mandatory that food be cooked properly and stored at low temperature. It becomes obvious that control is based on inhibiting bacterial growth, preventing contamination after preparation, and killing potential pathogens with cooking. In general, foods should be heated to internal temperatures of 165°F, but lower temperatures for longer periods of time are also effective. (Would you like to think twice before ordering steak tartare, sushi, or other uncooked or undercooked meat or fish?) Once cooked or processed, foods must be held at temperatures of 40°F or below.

Although these control measures are standard, many places where food preparation takes place do not abide by them. It is through diligent efforts of public health officials that reported outbreaks are investigated and food preparation techniques corrected. Therefore, recognition and reporting of foodborne illness become essential in the control of the problem. Education of the public, nurses, physicians, and eating establishment personnel is crucial to the control of foodborne illness. Carriage of most of the organisms considered in this chapter is not a problem, with the exception of staphylococci. Since staphylococcal carriage is necessary for the development of this illness, food handlers must be educated to watch for boils and pustules.

TREATMENT

Since these illnesses are generally self-limited and for the most part toxin-mediated, antibiotics play no major role either in therapy or prophylaxis. Fluid replacement is a major consideration in all of these illnesses. Occasionally, with more invasive pathogens such as *Salmonella*, *Shigella*, *Listeria*, or *Campylobacter* antibiotic therapy may be necessary.

SUGGESTED READINGS

Centers for Disease Control: *Foodborne Disease Outbreaks.* Annual summary

Dack GM (ed): *Food Poisoning.* Chicago, The University of Chicago Press, 1956.

Fleming DE, Cochi SL, MacDonald KL, et al: Pasteurized milk as a vehicle of infection in an outbreak of Listeriosis, *N Engl J Med* 312:404–407, 1985.

Lowenstein MS: Epidemiology of *Clostridium perfringens* food poisoning. *N Engl J Med* 286:1026–1028, 1972.

Reimann H, Bryan FL (eds): *Foodborne Infections and Intoxication,* ed 2. New York, Academic Press, 1979.

Terranova W, Blake PA: *Bacillus cereus* food poisoning. *N Engl J Med* 289:143–144, 1978.

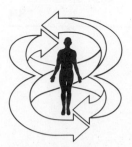

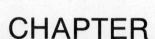

Diagnostic Principles

59

D.J. Krogstad

Proper use of the clinical microbiology laboratory to diagnose infectious diseases requires an interaction between the clinician and the microbiologist. A clinician must be aware of the sensitivity and specificity of the procedures employed and also recognize that specialized procedures usually take extra time (Table 59.1). The clinical value of laboratory testing is limited by mundane issues such as the turnaround time and the adequacy of specimen collection and transport, as well as by the state-of-the-art for each technique. Thus, the responsibility of the physician does not end with drawing a specimen and ordering microbiological tests.

Submitting a specimen for diagnosis should include relevant clinical information so that the specimen will be processed properly. For any clinical specimen, there are myriads of tests that can be carried out. Choices must be made to select the tests most relevant to the clinical situation. Unless the laboratory technologists are alerted to the need for performing special tests, they have no reason for doing so. Let the laboratory people know what you are thinking.

In turn, the laboratory microbiologist must be ready to assist the clinician in the interpretation of the result. This may include information about the significance of the results, especially with regard to antimicrobial susceptibility testing. For example, some hospitals have problems with certain organisms, such as methicillin-resistant *Staphylococcus aureus*. To help evaluate the epidemiological significance of finding such an organism, clinicians should be informed of the frequency of their appearance.

Sending a specimen to the laboratory also entails understanding the risks involved for the laboratory personnel. Certain organisms, such as the tubercle ba-

Table 59.1
Time required for the diagnosis of infectious disease

Minutes to 2 hours
 Morphology
  Gram stain for bacteria in CSF, sputum, urine or blood
  Acid-fast stain for mycobacteria
  India ink stain for *Cryptococcus* in CSF
  Lactophenol cotton blue staining for fungi
  Giemsa stain of sputum for *Pneumocystis*
  Giemsa stain for malaria
 Antigen detection (in CSF, blood or urine)
  Cryptococcal antigen
  Haemophilus influenzae type b antigen
  Neisseria meningitidis antigen
  Streptococcus pneumoniae antigen
6 to 48 hours
 Morphology
  Identification of parasites in stool or blood
 Culture
  Isolation and identification of bacteria from blood, CSF, sputum, wounds or urine
  Isolation and identification of certain viruses by their cytopathic effect on a monolayer
   (herpes simplex) or antigen detection (influenza virus from patients with pneumonia)
 Serology
  Measurement of antibody which was formed prior to the patient's current illness
 DNA probes
  Chlamydia
  Legionella
  Mycobacterium
  Mycoplasma
48 to 72 hours
 Susceptibility testing
  Antimicrobial susceptibility test results for aerobic and facultative bacteria
72 hours to 2 weeks
 Culture
  Isolation and identification of fungi, anaerobic bacteria and many viruses
2 weeks to 4 weeks
 Serology
  Appearance of antibody formed in response to the patient's acute illness
4 weeks to 8 weeks
 Culture
  Isolation and identification of slow growing organisms such as mycobacteria, some fungi, and
   viruses such as cytomegalovirus (CMV)

cillus, the agent of tularemia, *Francisella tularensis*, or the fungus *Coccidioides immitis*, represent serious hazards. Because of concern for such agents or for the possible transmission of HIV-1 virus, laboratory personnel routinely adopt precautionary measures in the handling of all clinical specimens.

 Four general types of procedures are used in the clinical microbiology laboratory:

• Morphology

• Culture (including drug susceptibility testing)

• Serology

• Nucleic acid probes.

MORPHOLOGICAL PROCEDURES

Morphological procedures characterize microorganisms by their appearance. Special staining properties are employed to differentiate organisms that are morphologically similar. One advantage of morphological identification is its speed, since most specimens can be stained and examined within 1 to 2 hours of their arrival in the laboratory. The disadvantage of morphology is that these procedures are relatively insensitive (yielding false-negative results) and non-specific (resulting in mistaken identities, false positives). Morphological examination may also provide valuable information regarding the adequacy of a specimen for culture. For example, a sputum culture is not reliable if the specimen contains large numbers of squamous epithelial cells, which suggests contamination with material from the upper respiratory tree.

Morphology is insensitive because organisms are often not present in sufficient numbers to be seen directly in the clinical specimens. It takes 10^5 to 10^6 or more bacteria per milliliter to be seen in a Gram stain. Morphology is often less specific than other techniques because of the subjective judgement required to distinguish among organisms. For example, most enteric Gram negative rods look alike and, therefore, it is often not possible to distinguish between harmless commensals and potential pathogens on morphological grounds alone. The technical competence to perform and interpret such studies correctly may vary widely among laboratories. The other methodologies described below are generally more objective and yield more specific results. Nonetheless, morphological examination retains a valuable role in diagnostic microbiology.

Bacterial Infections

The most useful morphological test in clinical microbiology is the Gram stain. In the office or the emergency room, a Gram stain may permit one to identify bacteria in specimens from patients with urinary or respiratory tract infections or meningitis, and thus to begin treatment immediately. These are errors that lead to false-negative results:

- Failure to concentrate dilute cerebrospinal fluid and other normally sterile specimens by centrifugation or filtration (except blood).

- Inadequate magnification during examination with the microscope. The high magnification oil immersion lens ($1000 \times$ total magnification) must be used to examine bacteria.

- Insufficient microscopic examination of the specimen. A minimum of 100 oil immersion lens fields should be examined before calling a specimen negative.

Common mistakes in carrying out the Gram stain include:

- Inadequate decolorization with alcohol or acetone, giving most or all bacteria the appearance of being Gram positive. The nuclei of neutrophils in the specimen should appear Gram negative. If they are Gram positive, the specimen has been inadequately decolorized.

- Over-decolorization changes Gram positives to Gram negatives. A simple control for this problem is to make a smear with known Gram positive bacteria on the same slide that contains the test smear and to stain the two together. If known cultures are not available, a control smear can be made by scraping the mucosa of the cheek: Most of the bacteria that adhere to epithelial cells are Gram positive.

• Precipitates of dye may be confused with microorganisms, usually Gram positives. These can be removed by filtering the crystal violet dye before use.

A negative Gram stain does not always exclude significant bacterial infection because, as stated above, it takes a large number of bacteria to be seen in a smear. This limitation should not deter anyone from using this procedure, because, used judiciously, it does prove extremely valuable in positive cases.

Other stains used commonly for the morphologic diagnosis of bacterial infection are acid-fast and auramine-rhodamine stains for mycobacteria. These techniques are particularly helpful since it takes so long to grow and identify mycobacteria (often 3 to 8 weeks). The auramine-rhodamine stain may be more sensitive than the traditional Kinyoun stain because it is read in a fluorescence microscope against a dark background. Auramine-rhodamine staining is also easier for color-blind observers who often cannot identify mycobacteria with traditional acid-fast staining (red against a blue background).

Fungal Infections

In the diagnosis of several fungal infections, morphological examination has two important attributes: on the one hand, the techniques are relatively insensitive because the number of fungal elements present in specimens may be quite low. On the other hand, morphology may be highly diagnostic because these organisms often display characteristic forms and shapes. For example, *Cryptococcus* is an encapsulated yeast that can be distinguished from other cells, such as white blood cells, both by its ample capsule and by the buds seen in India ink preparations. Cryptococcal meningitis may be diagnosed by direct microscopic examination of cerebrospinal fluid. The agent of cutaneous sporotrichosis may be seen by silver staining of skin scrapings or biopsies. Characteristic ovoid or cigar-shaped spores stained with lactophenol cotton blue stain may be seen in wet mounts of skin scrapings. Wet mounts with special dyes may reveal dermatophyte hyphae in skin scrapings or endospores in the sputum of patients with pulmonary *Coccidioides* infection. Spherules (50 to 100 μm in diameter) containing spores may be seen in the sputum of patients with coccidioidomycosis. On the other hand, sputum smears are rarely positive in pulmonary *Histoplasma* or *Blastomyces* infections.

Viral Infections

Material from skin lesions is often examined by the so-called *Tzanck preparation* for multinucleate giant cells due to herpes group virus infection. This test is performed by unroofing skin vesicles, scraping their base and staining a smear of the material with Giemsa or Wright stain. This test is useful when positive but is insensitive. For this reason, immunofluorescence with antisera to herpesviruses, as well as to cytomegalovirus, influenza, rabies, or others, is often used to make a presumptive diagnosis of viral infection. However, culture and immunologic staining for viral antigen in tissue often do not always correlate. A significant problem is that immunologic staining is less sensitive than culture.

Parasitic Infections

In these infections morphological examination plays a major role, because cultures are generally unavailable. Stool specimens are examined in saline (with or without iodine staining) to detect helminth eggs and larvae, and protozoan cysts. They are examined after fixation in polyvinyl alcohol and staining with Wheatley's trichrome stain for protozoan trophozoites. Giemsa stain is used to detect blood and tissue parasites such as malaria, toxoplasma, leishmania, and filaria.

The insensitivity of morphological identification is a constant problem in the diagnosis of parasitic infections. It is the reason why three or more stools are usually examined from patients who may have intestinal parasitic infection. The sensitivity of blood smears for the diagnosis of malaria and filariasis is increased by making thick smears of blood, i.e., by lysing the red blood cells before staining. This permits one to examine a 10-fold greater amount of blood per field. Another problem is that false positives may occur. In the United States, for example, only a relatively small number of technologists have enough experience to carry out these procedures and identify parasites with assurance.

CULTURE

Feasibility

Many but not all pathogenic microorganisms can be grown in the laboratory. Bacteria are generally the easiest microbial pathogens to grow. Most bacteria can be grown on artificial media within 24 to 72 hours at 35–37°C. Fungi and viruses generally require more time, usually several days to several weeks; also viruses require tissue culture because they cannot grow on artificial media alone. As stated above, most parasites cannot be grown in the laboratory and must be identified morphologically, often with the help of serologic testing.

Specimen Collection and Transport

The specimen collected must come from the site of infection. Common errors of diagnosis are, for example, to culture oral secretions rather than sputum in patients with pneumonia, or superficial skin organisms in a sinus tract rather than bone in patients with osteomyelitis.

If the pathogen is labile, the success of a culture may depend on variables such as temperature and transport time to the laboratory. For example, gonococci are sensitive to cold and require CO_2 for growth. Specimens plated on cold media (taken from the refrigerator and not warmed) or transported without CO_2 for 1 to 2 hours prior to plating, often yield false-negative results.

Sterile vs. Nonsterile Specimens

Cultures are most useful if the material that is cultured is normally sterile (blood, cerebrospinal fluid, synovial fluid, fragments of solid tissues). With such material, any growth is abnormal and suggests a clinically significant infection. Conversely, results with material from sites which are normally not sterile (sputum, urine, stool) are more difficult to evaluate. Evaluation of these results is usually based on quantitative cultures (e.g., urine, Chapter 48), on the identification of unusual organisms or changes in the normal flora (sputum), or on selective culture conditions that suppress the growth of normal flora (stool, Chapter 17).

In general, the techniques used to suppress the growth of normal flora also suppress the growth of pathogens to some extent. Therefore, cultures of material from nonsterile sites are less sensitive than those from sterile sites. Growth may also be inhibited by material in the culture system. For example, a detergent (sodium polyethylsulfonate or SPS) is used to inhibit blood clotting, to lyse white cells, and to inactivate complement and aminoglycosides in blood culture media. This compound also triggers the autolytic enzyme systems of some bacteria in the blood culture bottle and thus reduces the sensitivity of blood culture for bacteria with active autolytic enzyme systems, such as *Neisseria* (meningococci, gonococci). All these factors emphasize the need for letting the microbiological laboratory personnel know which organisms are suspected clinically.

Common Contaminants

Faulty specimen collection poses a particular problem in the interpretation of cultures from normally sterile sites. The most common contaminants are normal skin flora such as *Staphylococcus epidermidis* and diphtheroids. The presence of these organisms in cultures is often disregarded. However, they can produce significant infections and often cause catheter-related infections. Members of the normal skin flora are an important cause of prosthetic valve endocarditis and must not be disregarded in blood cultures from persons with prosthetic heart valves. Likewise, they can cause meningitis in patients with atrioventricular shunts, and bone and joint infections in patients with fixation devices or artificial joints. A diphtheroid called *Corynebacterium JK* is an important pathogen in immunocompromised patients. On occasion, normal skin flora may produce invasive disease even in normal hosts without prosthetic devices. Therefore, although most cultures that yield *S. epidermidis* or corynebacteria reflect contamination during specimen collection or in the laboratory, each apparent contaminant must be evaluated carefully in light of the patient's clinical situation.

SEROLOGY (IMMUNOLOGIC DIAGNOSIS)

Serologic diagnosis may be carried out in two ways:

• By detecting antibodies or cell-mediated immunity directed against an infectious agent.

• By detecting microbial antigens.

Most serologic diagnoses are based on antibody detection; antibody measurements have the disadvantage that 2 to 4 weeks or more must elapse to produce a clearly detectable antibody titer by most assays. Even IgM assays detect a positive response only after 7 to 10 days or more of active infection. Two other drawbacks of antibody detection are (a) a positive test only indicates exposure to the organisms and not necessarily active disease and (b) immunosuppressed patients may be unable to make measurable amount of antibody. A significant diagnostic indication is usually given by a *rise in antibody titer* that correlates with the course of the disease. In contrast, assays for antigen do not depend on the host immune response and may be positive early in infection (see below).

Serologic Procedures

Several types of serologic procedures are routinely used to diagnose infectious diseases in the clinical laboratory. Each of these procedures can be used to detect either antigen or antibody, depending on the reagents and methods employed.

Agglutination and Hemagglutination

Because antibodies have two or more antigen-binding sites, they form large aggregates when they react with antigen in excess. If the *antigen* molecules are

Figure 59.1. Agglutination. For antigen detection (*left*), latex spheres coated with a known amount of antibody (*shaded circles with Y-shaped antibody molecule on their surface*) are mixed with a specimen of patient serum which may contain antigen (*circles with Ag*). If antigen is present, the antibody-coated latex particles form a lattice connected by the antigen molecules (as long as the antigen is multivalent). The lattice is visible macroscopically as agglutination of the particles. For antibody detection (*right*), the patient's serum which is being tested for content of antibody molecules (*Y-shapes*) is mixed with a known amount of antigen (*Ag within shaded circles*) attached to latex spheres or red blood cells. If antibody is present, the particles will agglutinate.

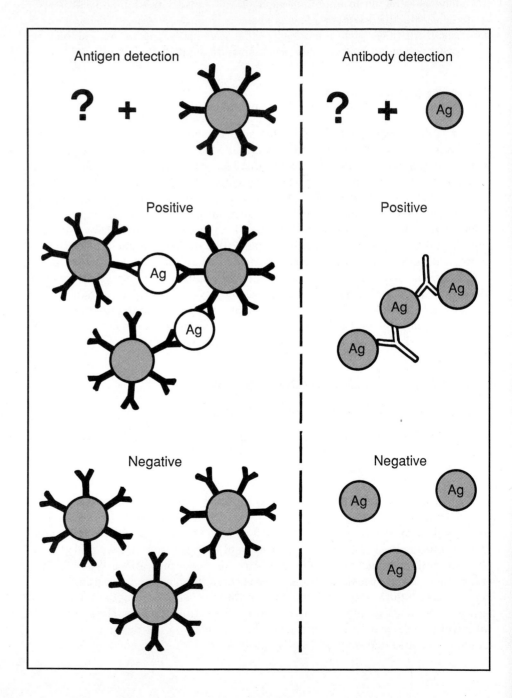

attached to a solid particle, such as a bacterium (naturally) or a latex sphere (artificially), the antigen-antibody reaction results in the visible clumping or agglutination of the particles. This reaction is the basis for many clinical tests, e.g., for detection of rubella antibody. If, on the other hand, *antibody* molecules are attached to latex spheres, agglutination is due to the presence of the corresponding antigen. An example of this approach is the test for cryptococcal antigen in cerebrospinal fluid or serum.

In lieu of latex particles, red blood cells may be used as inert carriers of antigens. Specific antibodies can then be detected by clumping (hemagglutination) of the red blood cells, as in a test for antibodies against the agent of amebiasis, *Entamoeba histolytica* (Fig. 59.1). In addition, hemagglutination can be used in non-serologic tests to detect the presence of certain viruses. Influenza or measles viruses, for example, bind to red blood cells via one of their surface proteins (hemagglutinins) and cause them to agglutinate (see Chapters 30 and 36).

Complement Fixation

When certain classes of antibodies bind to their corresponding antigens, they also react with complement (Chapter 5). This "fixation" of complement can be used in the laboratory to determine that an antigen-antibody reaction has taken place. Although it sounds intricate, this is one of the oldest and most sensitive serologic methods available (it was used for the original Wassermann test for syphilis, Chapter 23). Complement fixation is usually used to determine the presence of specific antibodies in patients' sera. How is complement fixation demonstrated? Two steps are required:

Step 1. Mix in a test tube the patient's serum, the antigen in question, and a limiting amount of complement (usually guinea pig serum). (One precautionary step must be taken: The patient's serum must previously be heated to 56°C to inactivate its complement.) If complement-fixing antibodies are present in the test serum, they will bind to antigen and react with the complement components present. How can one tell that this has happened? If the test is positive, all the complement in the test tube will be consumed (hence complement must be added in limiting amounts). If the test is negative, complement will not be fixed, but be free in solution.

Step 2. To tell if complement is free or fixed, add a known mixture of sheep red blood cells and an antibody directed against them (called hemolysin). If complement-fixing antibodies to the antigen are absent in the patient's serum, the guinea pig complement will not have been consumed, and will be available to react with the hemolysin-coated red blood cells. The result will be lysis of the red blood cells, which is easy to see with the naked eye. Conversely, if complement-fixing antibodies are present in the original specimen, little or no lysis of the red blood cells will occur (because most of complement will have been fixed in the first reaction; Fig. 59.2).

This technique has drawbacks because it requires rigorous quality control of the reagents as well as overnight incubation. Nevertheless, complement fixation is particularly useful for the detection of antibodies to measles and *Mycoplasma*.

Fluorescent Techniques

Antibodies or antigens may be conjugated to fluorescent dyes (e.g., fluorescein isothiocyanate) and used to visualize antigen-antibody reactions. The test material

Figure 59.2. Complement fixation. The patient's serum being tested for the presence of antibody molecules (*Y shape*) is mixed with the antigen (*Ag within circles*) and complement (*C' within circle*). If the patient serum contains complement-interacting antibodies (*upper panel*), complement will be "fixed", and become unavailable to lyse hemolysin (antibody) coated sheep red blood cells added later. Conversely, if the patient serum is negative for antibodies (*lower panel*), complement will be available to lyse the hemolysin-coated sheep RBCs. Thus, hemolysis indicates the absence of complement-fixing antibodies.

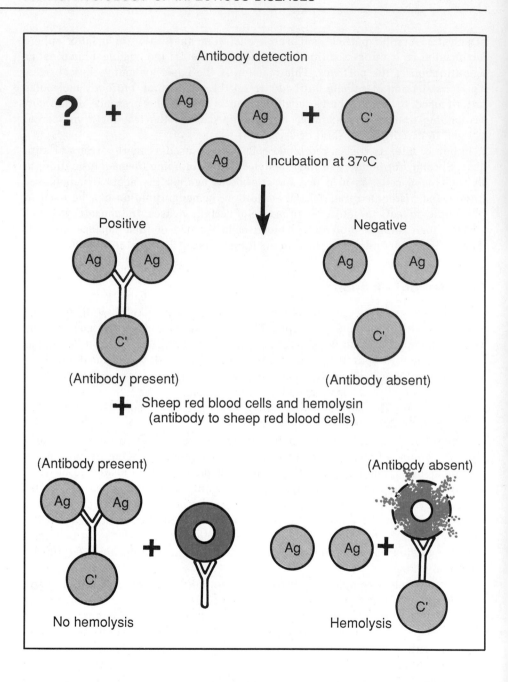

is deposited on a slide, either as a tissue section or as a smear, treated with the fluorescent "stain", rinsed, and then examined under an ultraviolet microscope (Fig. 59.3). The presence of antigen is detected with fluorescein-labeled antibody, that of antibody with an antibody directed against the one being sought (e.g., fluorescent-labeled goat antibody against human immunoglobulins). An example is seen in Figure 26.2, which shows *Legionella pneumophila* stained with specific fluorescein-labeled antibody. This technique has the added advantage of allowing the cytological localization of the test material.

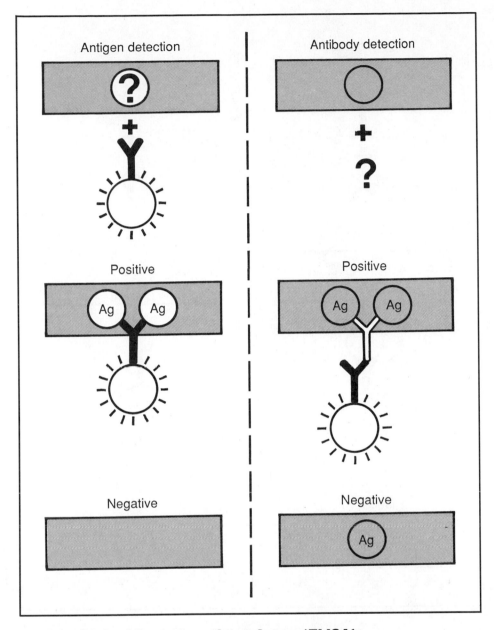

Antigen detection

?

+

Positive

Ag Ag

Negative

Antibody detection

+

?

Positive

Ag Ag

Negative

Ag

Figure 59.3. Fluorescent antibody test. For antigen detection (direct fluorescent assay, or DFA), material is placed on a microscope slide (for frozen tissue sections) or a microtiter well (*shaded rectangle*). Antibody labeled with a fluorescent compound is added and the preparation washed to remove unreacted antibody. For antibody detection (indirect fluorescent assay, or IFA), antigen is placed on a solid substrate (*Ag in shaded rectangle*) and exposed to the serum to be tested. After washing, a fluorescent antibody against human immunoglobulin is added. If antibody to the antigen of interest is present, fluorescence will be observed.

Enzyme-Linked Immunosorbent Assay (ELISA)

In the ELISA test (Fig. 59.4), an enzyme (rather than a fluorescent label) is linked to an antibody to allow its detection. As with fluorescence testing, ELISAs can be used to detect either antigens or antibodies. Antigen is detected using "solid phase antibody" attached to filter pads or to the wells of plastic "microtiter" plates. The test sample is added to a well, allowed to react, and then washed. If antigen is present, it will be bound to the antibody on the plastic. How can one tell this happened? The attached antigen molecules must have at least two reactive groups, and be available to react with more of the same antibody (in solution), which is linked to an easily detectable enzyme, such as alkaline phosphatase or peroxidase. After a second washing to remove unreacted enzyme-linked antibody,

Figure 59.4. ELISA (enzyme-linked immunosorbent assay). For antigen detection, antibody to the antigen being tested is attached chemically to a surface (such as that of a microtiter well) and incubated with the test specimen. After washing, a second antibody to the antigen is added (linked to an enzyme such as alkaline phosphatase or peroxidase). If a multivalent antigen is present, it will bind to the first antibody and later to the second (enzyme-tagged) antibody. The antibody-bound enzyme is allowed to react with a chromogenic substrate. A positive test is indicated by the presence of color, a negative by its absence. This method is known as a "sandwich" technique, because the antigen is sandwiched between two antibody molecules. For antibody detection, antigen is attached to a surface and exposed to the test serum. Enzyme-tagged antibody to human immunoglobulin is added and the enzyme allowed to react with a chromogenic substrate. As with antigen testing, a positive test is indicated by the presence of color and a negative, by its absence.

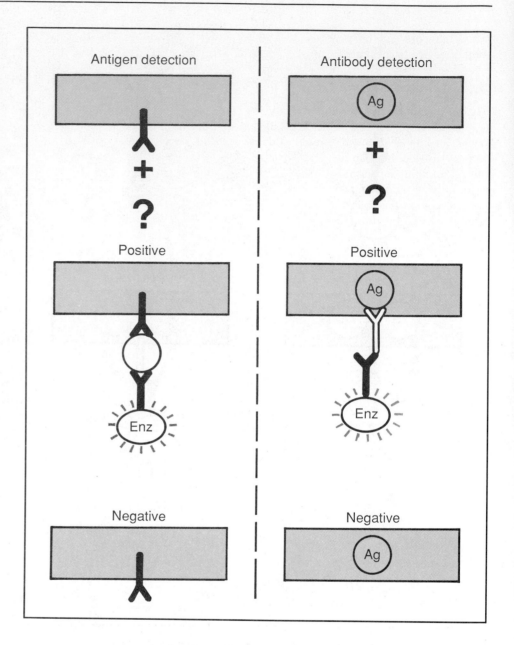

a chromogenic enzyme substrate is added to the well. A positive result—color formation—indicates that enzyme-linked antibody is bound, and that the antigen is present in the test sample. The result can be determined qualitatively (by the intensity of the color), or quantitatively using a spectrophotometer. Examples of the use of this technique are for the detection of group A streptococcal and rotavirus antigens.

For antibody detection, the antigen is attached to the well of the microtiter plate and exposed to a patient's sample, e.g., serum. The antibody being sought is detected using an enzyme-linked antibody directed against it. For example, mouse antibody against human immunoglobulins would detect a patient's antibody against the antigen fixed in the microtiter plate. ELISA tests are becoming more and more popular because they are simple and highly sensitive. The required reagents can be purchased as ready-to-use kits. Routine uses of these techniques are to measure antibody against *Toxoplasma* and cytomegalovirus.

Radioimmunoassays (RIA)

Radioimmunoassays are used mainly for antigen detection and are among the most sensitive tests available (Fig. 59.5). These assays are based on competition between a labeled known antigen and the same unlabeled antigen in the test sample. How is this done? Radiolabeled antigen (labeled with iodine-131 or iodine-125) is mixed with antibody and with the test sample and complexes are precipitated, either with 50% ammonium sulfate, or by adding a second antibody directed against the first one. If the specimen contains no antigen, all the radio-activity will be precipitated. If significant amounts of antigen are present in the

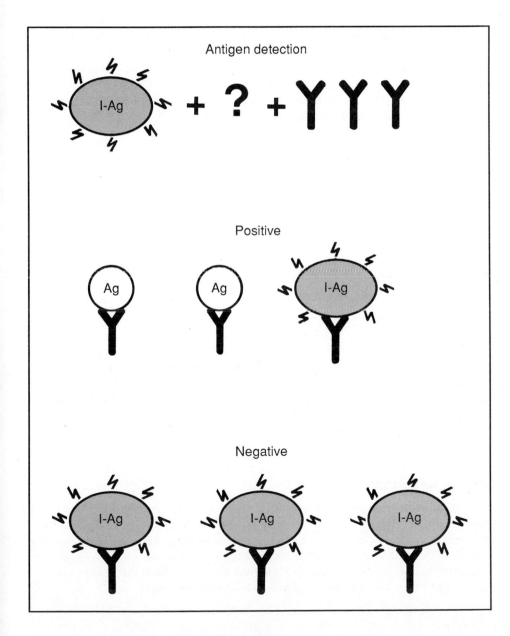

Figure 59.5. Radioimmunoassay (RIA). This is usually carried out as a competition assay: a known amount of antigen radiolabeled by iodination (^{125}I-*Ag within shaded circles*) is mixed with a known amount of antibody and the specimen being tested for that antigen. If the test specimen contains no antigen, all the radioactive antigen will combine with the antibody. This can be detected by precipitation with ammonium sulfate or a second antibody. Conversely, if antigen is present in the specimen, it will compete for antibody with the radioactive antigen and the number of radioactive counts precipitated will be reduced.

sample, they will compete with the radiolabeled antigen and reduce the proportion of radioactive counts in the precipitate. The test has many modifications, including the use of solid phases, as in ELISA testing. In the clinical laboratory, the great sensitivity of this test is often put to use to measure hormones and drugs. RIAs can also be adapted for antibody detection.

Some Problems Encountered in Serological Testing

There are many reasons why serological tests might give a wrong answer, either a false positive or false negative. Some are obvious, such as errors in procedure, inadequate reagents, etc. Other sources of error are less obvious. A few examples are discussed below.

IgM Testing

Several of the procedures outlined above can be used to detect IgM antibodies, which is sometimes helpful in determining the course of an illness (Chapter 5) or the infection of a fetus (Chapter 53). The methods used employ fluorescent testing or ELISA assays and use antibodies to the μ-chain of human IgM. Special precautions may need to be taken to prevent interference by large amounts of IgG antibodies that may be present in the same sample.

The Prozone Phenomenon

Assays that rely on agglutination or hemagglutination work best when there is more antigen that antibody (Fig. 59.6). Conversely, when there is an excess of antibody molecules, relatively little cross-linking occurs and the specimen may be reported to be negative for antibodies. This problem can be avoided by diluting the sample, thus reducing the ratio of antibody to antigen.

Bacterial Infections

Many bacterial infections are diagnosed readily by serology. Exceptions include organisms such as mycobacteria, for which serologic testing is not performed because antibody rises do not correlate with active disease.

Antigen testing is particularly helpful in the diagnosis of bacterial meningitis, since conventional serology (testing for antibody) is of limited value. Because only three bacteria cause most cases of meningitis (pneumococci, H. flu type b, and meningococci), it has been possible to produce kits which detect their antigens in the cerebrospinal fluid. Using these kits it is possible to identify the etiologic agents up to 24 hours before they can be detected by culture or Gram stain.

Fungal Infections

Patients with systemic mycoses often have positive antibody titers months before they manifest symptoms of the disease. However, patients with old, inactive infections also have such titers, and some persons with active disease are negative. Two antibody tests correlate well with active disease and are therefore useful in diagnosis: the complement fixation test for coccidiodomycosis and the immunodiffusion test for histoplasmosis and blastomycosis.

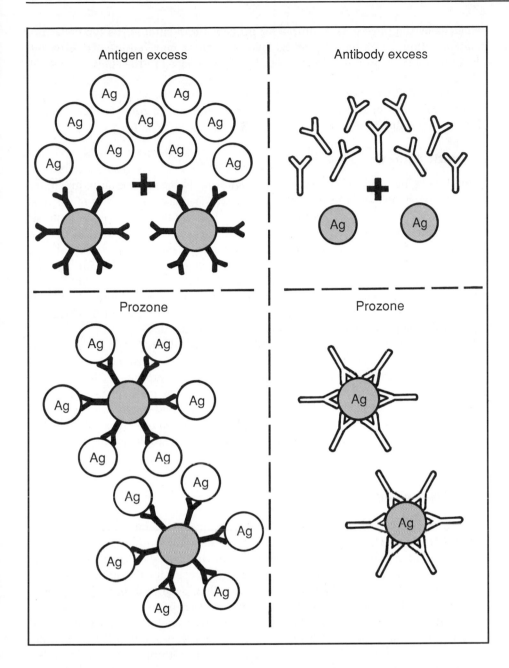

Antigen excess

Antibody excess

Prozone

Prozone

Figure 59.6. The prozone phenomenon. Antigen excess may produce a false-negative result in attempts to detect antigens by the agglutination method. If there are so many antigen molecules that antibodies on the latex spheres bind to separate ones, cross-linking necessary for lattice formation and agglutination will not occur. Antibody excess may also produce a false-negative reaction if each antigen molecule is bound to a separate antibody molecule. In both cases, the problem can be overcome by dilution of the test material.

The antigen test for cryptococcal infection is particularly helpful because cryptococci are often difficult to see in India ink stains of cerebrospinal fluid and because cultures may require 7 to 10 days to turn positive.

Viral Infections

Viral cultures are often expensive and may require 5 to 6 weeks to yield a result. Thus diagnoses of viral infections are often based on a rise in antibody titer. However, many viral infections are diagnosed retrospectively by serology; examples include influenza, rabies, enterovirus (polio, ECHO, and coxsackie) and cytomegalovirus infections. Cultures for influenza and enterovirus typically turn positive within 2 to 3 days; cytomegalovirus cultures may require 5 to 6 weeks. The importance of finding antibodies to HIV is discussed in the chapter on AIDS (Chapter 33).

Antigen detection tests are now available for rotavirus, herpesvirus and cytomegaloviral infections. An ELISA test for the detection of rotavirus infection is of particular value in children.

Parasitic Infections

Serology is particularly useful in the diagnosis of chronic parasitic infections for which morphology is insensitive and culture is unavailable. It is of greatest value in the assessment of persons who have had single exposures in endemic areas and otherwise would be expected to be seronegative. In contrast, it is usually of little value for residents of endemic areas, many of whom have been exposed to the agents without necessarily becoming ill. Serology is most useful for diseases that have systemic clinical manifestations without detectable evidence of infection in the gastrointestinal tract or the bloodstream. These include amebiasis (stool examination is usually negative when patients present with metastatic infection), echinococcosis, schistosomiasis, and leishmaniasis.

Unfortunately, serological tests are not useful for identifying several serious parasitic infections such as pneumocystis pneumonia, because most normal persons have antibody titers. In addition, many immunosuppressed patients cannot produce a rise in antibody titer. Similar problems are often observed in the diagnosis of toxoplasmosis, although infections in normal persons are regularly diagnosed by rises in antibody titer and by diagnostic IgM titers (see Chapter 53). Antigen detection correlates with acute infection in toxoplasmosis but is not available in most clinical microbiology laboratories.

NUCLEIC ACID PROBES

Recent studies have shown that detection of species-specific segments of microbial DNA by nucleic acid hybridization may be useful for diagnostic purposes. Generally, this method is highly sensitive, requiring some 10^5 molecules of the coded segment to yield a positive signal. The DNA used for detection of specific sequences is called the probe and must be labelled, usually in one of two ways: one is with radioactive isotopes, usually ^{32}P, the other by conjugating DNA with biotin. "Biotinylated" DNA can then be detected by the extraordinary affinity of the protein avidin for biotin. This method has the advantage that it does not depend on radioactivity handling and measurements, something that not all hospital laboratories are equipped to do. In general, radioactively labeled probes have produced better results with most clinical specimens because, at present, they provide greater sensitivity.

If a single copy of the sequence to be probed is present in the microorganism, 10^5 organisms are required for detection. The sensitivity of the method increases to less than 10^5 microorganisms if the nucleic acid segment is present in more than one copy per microbial cell, or if the sequence can be amplified in vitro. Nucleic acid probes have been used to detect *Leishmania*, which has 100 or more "minicircles" of DNA (plasmids) per cell. A probe directed against sequences in the minicircles allow one to detect 100 times fewer organisms, or as few as one thousand or less leishmanias per sample. Repetitive sequences in other organisms (without minicircle DNA) have been used to develop probes for malaria (*Plasmodium falciparum*), *Legionella*, *Mycoplasma*, *Chlamydia*, mycobacteria and cytomegalovirus. In vitro amplification of low copy number DNA sequences can be carried out by a DNA polymerase "chain reaction" that allows the production of large amounts of a specific DNA segment. The use of nucleic acid probes in diagnostic microbiology is being developed with considerable intensity.

SUGGESTED READINGS

Barker RH, Jr, Suebsaeng L, Rooney W et al: Specific DNA probes for the diagnosis of *Plasmodium falciparum* malaria. *Science* 231:1434–1436, 1986.

Lennette EH, Balows A, Hausler WJ Jr, Shadomy J, (eds): *Manual of Clinical Microbiology*, ed 4. Washington, DC, American Society of Microbiology, 1985.

Walls KW: *Immunodiagnosis of Parasitic Disease.* Orlando FL, Academic Press, 1986.

Wirth DF, Rogers WO, Barker RH, Jr et al: Leishmania and malaria: new tools for epidemiologic analysis. *Science* 234:975–979, 1986.

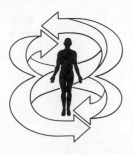

Principles of Epidemiology

60

D.R. Snydman

Epidemiology is the study of the determinants of disease in a population. It deals with both infectious and noninfectious etiologies. When infectious agents are involved, the aim is to understand their mode of transmission and what predisposes a population to a particular agent. The practical purpose of epidemiology is to control the spread of disease in a population, either by limiting microbial transmission or altering the susceptibility of a population. Commonly used measures include removing the source of the agent, controlling its transmission, and immunizing the population.

This chapter will consider epidemiological concepts and methods through the examination of an epidemiological "case", the investigation of a new disease. This will be followed by the consideration of general epidemiological issues.

AN EPIDEMIOLOGICAL "CASE"

In October 1975, the Department of Health of Connecticut received separate calls from two mothers living on rural roads in the towns of Lyme and Old Lyme. They reported that several children in their households and the neighborhood had what appeared to be arthritis. They had voiced their concern to local physicians and were not deterred by being told that arthritis is "not infectious".

Given the unusual nature of these reports, the epidemiologists considered the following questions:

1. Were these cases related?

2. Were there other similar cases?

3. Was this an infectious form of arthritis?

4. What forms of arthritis are infectious?

After discussing the cases with the parents and local physicians, the epidemiologists decided that this situation deserved looking into. What steps did they take and what principles did they apply to their study?

EPIDEMIOLOGICAL METHODOLOGY

The Connecticut epidemiologists undertook what is known as an *epidemic investigation*, the study of the extent, characteristics, mode of transmission, and etiology of a cluster of cases. It is perhaps the most self-evident of the methods used in epidemiology, but by no means the only one. Others, including *case-control studies*, *cohort studies*, and *epidemiological interventions*, are discussed below.

An epidemic investigation is undertaken when there is an increase in the number of cases of a disease over what is considered to be the norm or standard. In the Connecticut study, it was necessary to determine first if indeed this was an epidemic. The determination of an epidemic depends solely on the background incidence of the disease in the population and not on an absolute cut-off point. For example, prior to the advent of the polio vaccine in the 1950s there were about 50,000 cases of the disease in the United States annually. After the vaccine came into widespread use the number of cases dropped dramatically to about 10 per year. Therefore, one or two cases of polio might be considered to be an epidemic!

In addition to epidemics, there are endemic and pandemic diseases. An *endemic infectious disease* is one that is consistently found in the population, such as dental caries, gonorrhea, or athlete's foot. A *pandemic* is a worldwide epidemic; examples are the current AIDS pandemic, or the Spanish flu pandemic of 1918–1919.

Case Definition

The investigators of the Connecticut arthritis began by asking whether other individuals had the same disease. They first had to establish a set of clinical criteria known as the *case definition*. After all, many people have arthritis. From the mothers, physicians, and school nurses in the area they obtained a list of other individuals who may have had the same symptoms. After examining the patients and taking careful histories they included, as fitting the case definition, those with the following clinical picture: a sudden onset of swelling and pain in a knee or other large joint lasting a week to several months. Additionally, some patients remembered that their symptoms were preceded by an odd, large skin rash. Those affected had several attacks that recurred several times at intervals of a few months. Nearly half those affected also had fever and fatigue, and a few had a persistent rash.

Time, Place, and Personal Characteristics of Patients

Armed with a usable case definition, the investigators found other cases in Old Lyme and two adjacent towns. The best source of additional cases were the two determined mothers who had made the original phone calls. Between current and past episodes, they collected 51 cases that conformed to the case definition. They could now proceed to determine what epidemiologists call the time, place, and personal characteristics of these cases. The *time characteristics* include the time of onset of the disease and its *duration*. As shown in Figure 60.1, many of the Connecticut cases clustered in the late spring and summer months. The duration of each bout of the disease varied from a week to a few months, and 69% of the cases had recurrences of the symptoms. Not knowing at this time the etiology of the disease, they could not determine another important time characteristic, namely the *incubation period*, or the interval from exposure to the first onset of symptoms.

Place characteristics are primarily the site of residence and the area in which the affected cases lived. For occupation-related illnesses, this can also include the place of work. The cases were concentrated in three adjacent towns on the eastern side of the Connecticut River. Most of the patients lived in wooded areas near streams and lakes. *Personal characteristics* include the age and sex of the patients and any possibly genetic predisposition to the disease. Of the 51 cases, 39 were children, nearly evenly divided between the sexes. There was no discernible familial pattern. The epidemiologists now listed the cases by the time of onset and constructed what is called an *epidemic curve*. They gave this outbreak the name "Lyme arthritis", later modified to *Lyme disease*, which is its current eponym.

The epidemiologists now posed other questions: Was the outbreak a surveillance artifact based on the fact that many questions about arthritis were being asked

Figure 60.1. Time course of Lyme disease in Connecticut.

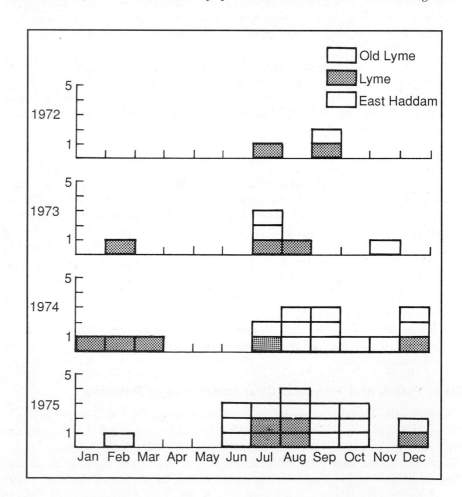

by outsiders? The simplest way to assess this was to go elsewhere and ask the same questions. The answer, from surveying towns across the Connecticut River, was that increased interest did not result in an increase in the number of cases of arthritis reported. The team then asked: Was this an infectious disease? The most common arthritic conditions of childhood, such as juvenile rheumatoid arthritis, are collagen vascular problems and not known to be infectious. Nonetheless, the clustering of cases, the fact that most of them began in the late spring or summer and that they were most frequently located in wooded areas along lakes or streams, suggested a viral illness transmitted by an arthropod. If so, would it be a new one?

Is Lyme Disease Communicable?

Many infectious diseases are *communicable*, e.g. measles, polio, or tuberculosis. Others, such as a ruptured appendix, urinary tract infections, or osteomyelitis, are not. Was Lyme disease communicable, or did it merely affect especially susceptible individuals? To answer this question, the investigators undertook a case control study, matching of the cases with a similar group of control or unaffected persons. After matching for age, sex, and any other relevant factors, the epidemiologists looked for any differences between the two groups that may give clues as to possible risk factors. They found one: those affected were more likely to live in a household with pets. One consequence is that they were more likely to come in contact with the ticks that dogs and cats pick up in the woods of that region. In a roundabout way, this clue became more credible when they remembered a suggestive clinical finding: about one quarter of the patients had reported that the symptoms of arthritis were preceded by an unusual skin rash. The rash had started as a red spot that spread to form a 6-inch ring. What was the connection? An astute dermatology consultant remembered that similar manifestations had been described in 1910 in Switzerland and attributed to tick bites. This rash went by the impressive name of "erythema chronicum migrans".

So far, the connection between the rash and Lyme disease depended on *retrospective* evidence. To make the connection stronger, it became appropriate to ask: Do patients with the signs of erythema chronicum migrans progress to develop Lyme disease? The team set up a *prospective study*, looking for patients with the rash and observing them for some time. Indeed, of 32 new cases of erythema chronicum migrans, 19 progressed to show the signs and symptoms of Lyme disease. The "tick connection" became even more plausible after a thorough entomological survey. Insects and ticks were collected from Lyme and surroundings, with the finding that adult ticks were 16 times more abundant on the east side of the Connecticut River than on the west side. This corresponded roughly to the proportion of incidence of cases of Lyme disease in the two areas. In addition, many more tick bites were reported by the arthritis patients than by their neighbors without the disease. Thus, the tick-rash-arthritis connection seemed more and more plausible. We will see that the final proof of this scheme awaited the discovery of the etiologic agent and the direct demonstration of its transmission via ticks.

At the same time, a *surveillance network* had been set up in Connecticut and part of the adjacent states to gather information about other cases. A careful study revealed that, contrary to the earliest reports, the disease was more frequent in adults than in children. Many arthritis patients had serious manifestations, such as neurological dysfunction and myocarditis. Thus, the disease turned out to be considerably more complex than described by the original case definition. This illustrates an important epidemiological point. An early case definition is, of necessity, tentative, and may be modified when the full spectrum of the disease becomes known.

The Search for the Etiologic Agent

So far the investigators could conclude with assurance that Lyme disease was an infection, most likely transmitted by ticks, It appeared to be a new clinical entity. However, up to this time the search for the etiologic agent had proved unproductive. Despite many attempts, no laboratory had succeeded in isolating a virus, which at the time seemed to be a good candidate for being the agent of the disease. On the other hand, the investigators collected anecdotal evidence that tetracycline, erythromycin, or penicillin were clinically effective. With time, more physicians reported on the beneficial effect of antibiotics, making a bacterial etiology more likely. At about this time, the Connecticut team asked for help from entomologists and microbiologists at the Rocky Mountain Public Health Laboratory in Montana who were experts on tickborne diseases. The Montana investigators examined ticks sent from the affected area and found that the gut of many specimens contained unusual spirochetes readily visible under the microscope. Were these the agents of Lyme disease?

Proving that a suspicious microorganism causes a given infection is not always easy, and this problem has periodically dogged microbiologists since the early days. Sometimes it is relatively easy to fulfill the so called *Koch postulates*: organisms seen in lesions are grown in the laboratory and inoculated in experimental animals, in whom they produce a disease similar to the original. In this instance, however, the microbiologists were aware that the cultivation of spirochetes is often problematic. In fact, the most notorious member of the group, the agent of syphilis, *Treponema pallidum*, cannot be readily cultivated in artificial media. Other spirochetes, such as the agents of leptospirosis and recurrent fever grow in the laboratory, but only under special conditions.

It was easier, then, to first try to infect laboratory animals directly, using the infected ticks. Indeed, rabbits on which the ticks were allowed to feed developed a rash resembling that of erythema chronicum migrans. With such ample material at hand, the microbiologists could experiment with different culture media and eventually succeeded in growing a spirochete. Was this the organism of Lyme disease? They demonstrated that this was the case because when they inoculated pure cultures into rabbits they obtained the same rash. Using an immunofluorescence assay, they found that the infected rabbits contained antispirochetal antibodies in their serum. They could now use this assay with humans, and found a high titer of antispirochetal antibodies in patients with Lyme disease but not in healthy individuals. Soon they completed the circle by isolating the spirochete from human cases. The spirochete was classified among the *Borrelia*, a group that includes the agent of another tickborne disease also found in the United States, recurrent fever. The agent of Lyme disease was given the name *B. burgdorferi*, in honor of the entomologist who discovered the organisms in the ticks.

With a simple diagnostic test at hand, investigators in many parts of the world could carry out serological surveys or *serosurveys*, that is, they determined the proportion of persons with antibodies to *B. burgdorferi*. In general, serosurveys allow recognition of a wide range of clinical manifestations, from asymptomatic cases to full blown disease. This is important because in most infectious diseases there are many more asymptomatic than clinically overt cases. Using these techniques, Lyme disease has been diagnosed in other parts of the United States, especially on the East and West Coasts, as well as in Canada, Europe, and Australia. It is considered a serious disease, especially because of its important and chronic neurological manifestations.

The original puzzle of "Lyme arthritis" had now been solved. A few years after the original phone calls, a new disease was described, its agent and mode of transmission identified, and preventive and therapeutic measures instituted. Note that it took the joint effort of epidemiologists, clinicians, entomologists, microbiologists, and alert and determined members of the public.

THE VARIOUS ROUTES OF TRANSMISSION

Humans as Reservoirs

We now turn from a specific example to a more general consideration of epidemiological principles. The first is the mode of transmission (Table 60.1). *Transmission from human to human* may take place from parent to offspring or between mature individuals. *Vertical transmission* refers to the passage of an agent from an infected mother to her fetus or infant. The most intimate mode is via the transplacental route. Examples of such congenitally acquired diseases are syphilis, and rubella. Newborns may also pick up chlamydiae, gonococci, cytomegalovirus, or hepatitis B virus during passage through the birth canal. Other organisms may be transmitted via mother's milk.

Horizontal transmission may be between individuals in close proximity or living far away, and includes intimate modes, such as sexual intercourse, or more casual ones, such as touching another person, breathing of aerosols, etc. The actual path of an organism from one person to another depends on the way the agent exits

Table 60.1
Examples of routes of transmission

Route of Transmission	Example	Factor	Route of Entry
Direct Contact			
Respiratory aerosol	Influenza	Crowding?	Lung
	Tuberculosis	Household	Lung
Nasal secretions	Respiratory syncytial virus	Household, nosocomial	Upper respiratory tract
Droplets	Meningococcus	Crowding, carriers	Skin
Skin	Streptococcus (impetigo)	Crowding, carriers	Skin
Semen	AIDS	Sexual contact	Mucous membrane
Respiratory			Upper respiratory
Transplacental	Hepatitis B	Carrier	Mother
Indirect Contact			
Blood	Hepatitis B	Transfusion, needle stick	Blood
	AIDS	Transfusion	Blood
Stool	Hepatitis A	Ingestion	GI tract
Animal	*Salmonella*	Ingestion	GI tract
Inanimate	*Legionella*	Water contamination	Respiratory
Arthropod Vector			
Tick	Lyme disease	Bite	Skin, blood
Mosquito	Malaria	Bite	Blood

the body of the donor. Thus, bacteria or viruses that infect the respiratory tract are often expelled as aerosols during coughing and even talking, and may be inhaled by bystanders. If the organism is resistant to drying, as is the case with the tubercle bacillus, the danger of inhalation may persist for a long time. Intestinal pathogens often cause diarrhea, which increases their distribution in the environment and, under conditions of poor sanitation, results in contaminated drinking water and foodstuffs.

Some diseases are acquired by breaching the skin or mucous membranes, by trauma, an insect bite, blood transfusions or contaminated hypodermic needles. Agents that are transmitted in this fashion include the AIDS or hepatitis B viruses. Many of the agents that are transmitted by insect vectors have different life cycles in the vector and in the host. Note that some of these organisms may be transmitted by more than one of these routes. Thus, the AIDS virus may be passed transplacentally, by sexual intercourse, or by the use of needles.

Nonhuman Reservoirs

Other diseases are acquired from nonhuman reservoirs. These include the zoonoses (Chapter 55), where the reservoir is an animal. Transmission from the animal may be direct, as in the bite from a rabid dog, or via insect vectors, as in the plague or the viral encephalitides. Lyme disease is also a zoonosis in which the natural reservoir is mammals such as deer that share the same ticks with humans.

For other diseases the reservoir is the inanimate environment and the organisms live freely in nature. For example, the clostridia of gas gangrene are commonly found in soil. However, humans or animals may contribute to the frequency with which the agents are found in nature. Thus, cholera bacilli grow naturally in warm estuaries, probably on the surface of shellfish. However, contamination from human feces may help the organisms become established, especially in a new area.

Incubation Periods and Communicability

The length of the incubation period differs considerably among infectious diseases, from a few hours to months and years (Table 60.2). It is influenced by many factors. For example, a large infective dose may shorten it and a small one lengthen it. To the epidemiologists, the incubation period is particularly important

Table 60.2
Examples of incubation periods

Disease	Range of Period
Staphylococcal food poisoning	1–6 hours
Clostridial food poisoning	12–24 hours
Hepatitis A	14–42 days
Hepatitis B	30–180 days
Gonorrhea	2–9 days
Salmonellosis	0.5–3 days
Epstein-Barr virus infection	21–49 days
Mycoplasma pneumoniae infection	8–21 days
Varicella	10–21 days
AIDS	21 days to 5 years or more
Leprosy	7 months–5 years

because during this time some diseases may be transmitted from asymptomatic patients. Control of transmission may, therefore, have to rely on special surveillance methods that include infected but asymptomatic persons. The periods of incubation and of communicability are not always the same. For example, the incubation period in hepatitis A most commonly lasts 3 to 4 weeks. However, individuals can communicate the virus only for 1 or 2 weeks prior to the onset of the disease.

The period of communicability may extend itself long after the disease symptoms abate, as in the case of chronic carriers. For example, hepatitis B carriers can usually transmit the virus for the length of time they carry it. In many of the preceding chapters, the carrier state has been discussed at some length (see the following chapters: 18 for *Salmonella typhi*, 14 for the gonococcus, 24 for chlamydiae, 31 for herpes viruses, 32 for hepatitis viruses, 33 for HIV).

Individual Susceptibility

Human beings differ in their predisposition to infectious diseases. We have all encountered individuals who seem more prone to respiratory or intestinal infections than the majority. For many of these persons we do not know the reason for this variability. They may have subtle deficiencies in certain of their defense mechanisms. When these deficiencies become severe and the risks more evident, the cause is often easier to ascertain. Chapter 5 discusses the consequences of the major kinds of innate and acquired immune deficiencies.

The epidemiologist must be aware of the different susceptibility of members of the population. Age, sex, nutritional status, previous exposure, immune competence, all contribute to a greater or lesser susceptibility to a particular infectious disease. Thus, children and older persons are frequently more susceptible to bacterial pneumonia or intestinal infections. The incidence of the carrier state of hepatitis B is greater in males than in females. It is also more frequent among individuals with Down's syndrome or those receiving hemodialysis.

Genetic factors are also known to play a role, although for the most part the data are inconclusive. The importance of these factors is often difficult to unravel from a myriad of socioeconomic factors, such as those that contribute to the state of health and nutrition. Nonetheless, the role of genetic factors has been well established in certain diseases. It was shown, for example, that among identical twins living apart if one contracted tuberculosis, the other had a much greater chance than average of getting the disease. Nonidentical twins did not show this pattern. One of the most intensively studied genetic effects is the decreased susceptibility to malaria of persons with the sickle cell trait (Chapter 40). It is also well established that non-Caucasians are more prone to the disseminated form of coccidioidomycosis than Caucasians.

PRACTICAL ASPECTS OF EPIDEMIOLOGY

In a civilized society, epidemiology is everyone's business. The practicing physician and all members of the health team must be aware of the public health implications of a given patient's infectious disease. In order to safeguard both the public interest and the rights of privacy of patients, a considerable body of local and national laws has been developed in most countries of the world. For instance, in the United States certain communicable diseases are notifiable, that is, physicians are obliged to report them to the U.S. Public Health Service. The information collected is published in a readily available pamphlet, the *Morbidity and Mortality Weekly Reports* (MMWR) which lists all routine information and calls attention to unusual occurrences. In addition, each state has its own surveillance mechanism and reporting requirements for the study of communicable diseases within its borders. Each has a state board of health and a reference laboratory, equipped to carry out special diagnostic tests that are often outside the scope of hospital laboratories.

CONCLUSIONS

Epidemiology may appear to be a remote discipline, practiced mainly by public health officials. In fact, it pervades all forms of medical practice and furnishes important clues for the diagnosis of infectious diseases. Thus, inquiry into time and place characteristics should be part of the usual process of taking a clinical history. Epidemiological information may reveal how people encounter disease agents and help reduce exposure and spread of infectious diseases.

SUGGESTED READINGS

Esdaile JM, Feinstein AR: Lyme disease: a medical detective story. 1985 Medical and Health Annual. *Encyclopedia Britannica*, pp 267–271.

Fox JP, Hall CE, Elebeck JR: *Epidemiology: Man and Disease.* London, MacMillan, 1970.

Rothman JK: *Modern Epidemiology.* Boston, Little, Brown & Co, 1986.

Sackett DL, Haynes RB, Tugwell P. *Clinical Epidemiology. A Basic Science for Clinical Medicine.* Boston, Little, Brown & Co, 1985.

Steere AC, Malawista SE, Snydman DR *et al.*: Lyme arthritis. An epidemic of oligoarticular arthritis in children and adults in three Connecticut communities. *Arth Rheumat* 20:7–17, 1977.

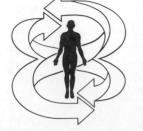

Nutrition and Infection

61

G.T. Keusch

Malnutrition is the most prevalent cause of acquired immunodeficiency in the world, leading to marked morbidity and mortality from infection. Malnutrition, impaired host defenses, and infection interact cyclically to produce progressive worsening of the host, resulting in death unless corrected (Fig. 61.1).

The initial manifestation of malnutrition is often an infection, typically manifested by loss of appetite (anorexia) and fever. Food intake usually drops off: even with a mild cold, people are usually satisfied with a cup of tea and a slice of toast and may become nauseated at the sight of normally mouthwatering food. At the same time, fever imposes greater demands for energy, since, on average, energy-consuming enzymatic reactions speed up by 13% per degree rise in temperature. In patients with severe septicemia, the resting metabolic rate rises as much as 35–40% above normal.

Greater energy demands during infections are accompanied by marked changes in host metabolism, regardless of the causative organism. The purpose of these changes appears to be preparing the host to survive the infection by consuming its own body stores of energy and protein, as if in anticipation of the decrease in food intake. As the host tissues are utilized, the individual loses weight and appears to become physically consumed in the process. These dramatic changes have been recognized since antiquity and are the reason why tuberculosis, for example, is popularly called consumption in several languages. Tuberculosis is a good example of a chronic infectious disease that causes wasting, although it is not necessary that the process be chronic. Acute infections also cause detectable catabolism of host tissue. Small losses may be induced even by attenuated live virus vaccines.

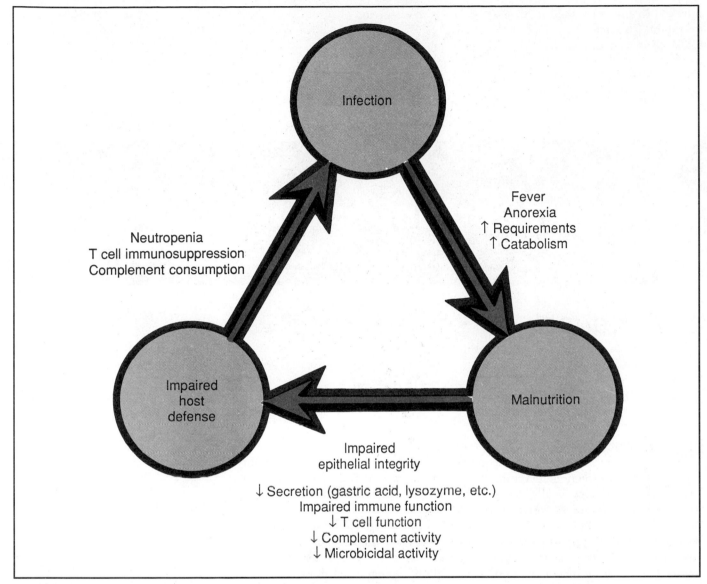

Figure 61.1. The triangle of interaction among malnutrition, infection, and host defenses. Malnutrition may be initiated by primary or secondary dietary deficiency (e.g., malabsorptive states), or by metabolic effects of infection. The consequences of this are impairment in host defenses, which in turn leads to an increased burden of infection and further malnutrition. (From Keusch GT, Farthing MJG: Nutrition and infection. *Annu Rev Nutr* 6:131–154, 1986.)

ENERGY METABOLISM

With decreased food intake and increased caloric demands, how does the host face the shortfall in energy? Glucose oxidation rate increases, even though the patient experiences hyperglycemia (typical of fasting) and a delayed glucose disappearance curve (as in diabetes). The readily available endogenous sources of glucose are the carbohydrate stores (e.g., liver glycogen), which suffice for some 24 hours only, and fat, a large store which is not as rapidly used in infection as it is during starvation. The only other large energy stores are the body proteins, which can be converted into energy by proteolysis, deamination of amino acids, and conversion of carbon skeletons into glucose. Gluconeogenesis, as this process is called, increases in the liver of infected patients, largely utilizing alanine as the substrate. Amino acids are lost because of deamination, which leads to loss of

nitrogen in the urine, and oxidation of their carbon skeleton, resulting in CO_2 excretion. This metabolic picture is fostered by elevated levels of insulin, glucagon, growth hormone, and corticosteroids, all of which are seen in the infected host.

PROTEIN METABOLISM

Gluconeogenesis is not the only process fed by proteolysis of host tissue. New protein synthesis also increases dramatically in the liver, using amino acids released from muscle. Some of the new proteins synthesized are components of the host defense response (see Chapter 4); examples are C3 and complement factor B (used in the alternative pathway of activation). Some of the proteins made in large amounts during infection are found in very low concentrations in the normal host. These include C-reactive protein and serum amyloid, which may have immunoregulatory functions. Still other proteins serve as transport or carrier proteins, such as haptoglobin or the copper-binding protein, ceruloplasmin, or function as enzyme inhibitors, such as α_1-antitrypsin or α_1-antichymotrypsin. At the same time, perhaps as a compensatory response, there is a reduction in the rate of synthesis of the hepatic export proteins, albumin and transferrin. The level of these proteins in serum drops to very low levels, inversely proportional to the severity of the stimulus, and may be predictive of the outcome of the infection.

Alterations in plasma proteins induced by inflammation are put to use in the diagnostic laboratory. For example, the increases in fibrinogen levels due to the acute phase response cause a change in the stacking of red blood cells as in a pile of coins ("rouleaux" formation), resulting in their more rapid sedimentation. An elevated "sed rate" is a simple and general marker of inflammation.

LIPID METABOLISM

In some infections, typically Gram negative bacterial septicemia, serum becomes milky due to an impressive increase in the concentration of triglycerides. This is due to a defect in lipid clearance by low density lipoproteins caused by the diminished activity of the clearance enzyme of adipocytes, lipoprotein lipase. In addition, the ability to store fats is inhibited, contributing to the excessive levels of lipids in serum. Although there are plenty of lipids around, they cannot be effectively used for energy production via oxidation of ketones. This is due in part to a so-called pseudodiabetic hormonal imbalance in the patient with bacterial septicemia.

MINERAL METABOLISM

A characteristic change in patients with severe acute infections is a drop in the serum level of iron and zinc, and an increase in that of copper. These changes are due to alterations in level of proteins that bind these cations. The increase in copper results from the increased production of the copper-binding plasma protein ceruloplasmin. The decrease in iron is due to the release of lactoferrin from leukocytes, resulting in the formation of lactoferrin-iron complexes that are taken up by the liver. There the complexes are converted to hemosiderin, a nonreutilizable form of iron that is unavailable for hematopoiesis and ultimately results in the anemia of chronic infections. The decrease in the zinc level results from the synthesis of metallothionin, an intracellular zinc-binding protein.

Figure 61.2. Schematic diagram of the tissue targets for interleukin-1 (IL-1) and/or tumor necrosis factor (TNF) in the metabolic response to infection. BCAA, branched chain amino acids; LPL, lipoprotein lipase; APP, acute phase proteins.

What is the effect of changes in the levels of these serum cations? Reduction in serum iron may have a protective effect by reducing the amount available for the growth of pathogens (see Chapter 2). The decrease of zinc in serum is accompanied by its increase in lymphoid cells where it may contribute to their proliferative ability in response to antigenic stimulation, since key enzymes in this process are zinc-containing metalloenzymes, for example, thymidine kinase. Ceruloplasmin oxidizes ferrous iron, increasing the availability of this cation for hematopoiesis.

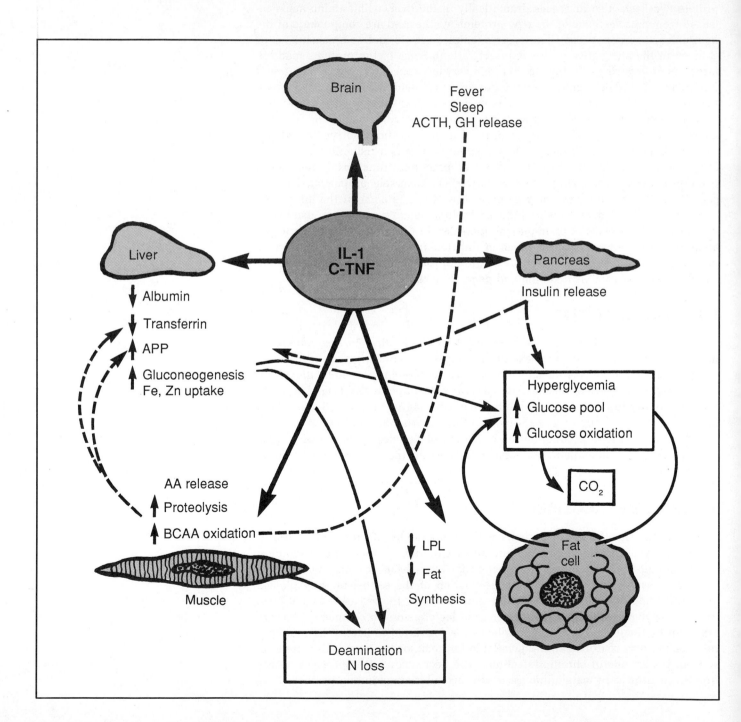

MECHANISMS OF METABOLIC CHANGES

Many of the metabolic alterations that accompany infections can be attributed to the action of at least two cytokines, interleukin 1 (IL-1) and tumor necrosis factor (TNF, or cachectin). Both these physiologically reactive proteins are made by activated macrophages in response to a variety of stimuli, such as the presence of endotoxin or the act of phagocytosis. IL-1 was first known as "endogeneous pyrogen", a leukocyte product that acts on the hypothalamic temperature regulation centers to produce fever (Chapters 4 and 56). It was later discovered that IL-1 mediates other responses, including the shift of zinc and iron from serum to tissues and the activation of T lymphocytes.

IL-1 has a wide range of activities that affect host metabolism and the immune response (Fig. 61.2). Acting at the crossroads of metabolic and immunologic responses to infection, IL-1 is critically important in the survival of the host under stress. When injected into experimental subjects, it reproduces the major metabolic changes associated with infection described above. IL-1 appears to act by activating the expression of selected genes to produce the proteins of the acute phase response, which are characteristic of the infected state (Chapter 4). It increases production of prostaglandin E2, which serves as a second messenger at tissue and cellular levels.

Tumor necrosis factor (TNF or cachectin) shares a number of biological properties with IL-1 and is an inducer of IL-1 (Fig. 61.2). It rapidly produces anorexia and weight loss when given to experimental animals. It produces severe depletion of the fat stores, inhibiting the production of lipoprotein lipase and lipid anabolic enzymes. TNF, much as IL-1, also causes fever, increases phagocytic activity of neutrophils, upregulates the expression of genes in the liver for acute phase proteins, and downregulates albumin and transferrin (chapter 4). In high doses, TNF causes a lethal shock syndrome, which is prevented by the administration of anti-TNF antibodies. Thus, like IL-1, TNF probably plays a role in the pathogenesis of septic shock. It is interesting that the production of both cytokines is downregulated at the transcriptional and translational level by glucocorticoids, which may exert a protective effect in the septic shock patient.

CONSEQUENCES OF METABOLIC CHANGES

The loss of protein and energy reserves that occurs during the febrile period of infections leaves the patient at an ebb of nutrient reserves. During convalescence, these must be restored. As a rule, replenishment takes about four times longer than loss. Thus, for one week of illness, about one month is required to replenish the patient, assuming that adequate nutrients are available. Stress-related malnutrition of this sort is not uncommon in the United States and other industrialized countries, but is generally not an insurmountable problem. Acute infection-related malnutrition can be reversed by resuming normal diet, and, if necessary, by enteral or parenteral nutritional rehabilitation in a hospital. In developing countries, however, the diet may be inadequate to allow repletion to occur in timely fashion, if at all. The high prevalence of infections in the young means that new diseases may ensue before the patient is nutritionally restored, adding new losses to the deficit left over from the previous episode. Repeated infections result in cumulative losses which lead to severe states of malnutrition.

In children, dietary intake is used not only for normal tissue maintenance and turnover, but for net growth as well. The stress of infection results in cessation of growth and in weight loss. In affluent societies, such growth faltering is quickly erased by rapid catch-up during convalescence. Growth rates may jump by as much as seven times normal during this period. In countries with inadequate diets and frequent infections, the host may never catch up, and this is the reason why adults may be short in stature (except, of course, in certain genetically short statured populations, such as the Pygmies). Body size may not matter, but infant mortality does. To combat the excessive mortality in children in developing countries, organizations such as UNICEF and the World Health Organization are attempting to promote child survival by reducing the incidence and impact of childhood infections and by improving infant nutrition and encouraging breast feeding.

EFFECT OF MALNUTRITION ON THE IMMUNE SYSTEM

"We are what we eat" is as true for the immune system as it is for the rest of the body. In the past two decades, the impact of malnutrition on the immune system has been demonstrated both in clinical and experimental studies. Most human malnutrition develops in populations that eat inadequate and monotonous diets lacking several nutrients, including energy sources, proteins, minerals, and vitamins. Only rarely are single nutritional deficiencies observed. This mosaic of deficiency diseases is commonly called protein-energy malnutrition (PEM). It usually includes deficiencies in iron, zinc, other trace minerals, vitamin A, and other both water- and fat-soluble vitamins.

PEM has a profound impact on certain host defense systems. Most consistent is the inhibition of cell-mediated immunity due primarily to a lack of mature functionally differentiated T lymphocytes (Fig. 61.3). The total number of lympho-

Figure 61.3. Localization of the specific effects of nutrients on the immunological network. Reproduced by permission from Keusch GT et al. Nutrition, host defense and the lymphoid system. PEM, protein-energy malnutrition. In Gallin JI, Fauci AS: *Advances in Host Defense Mechanisms*, vol 2. New York, Raven Press, 1983.

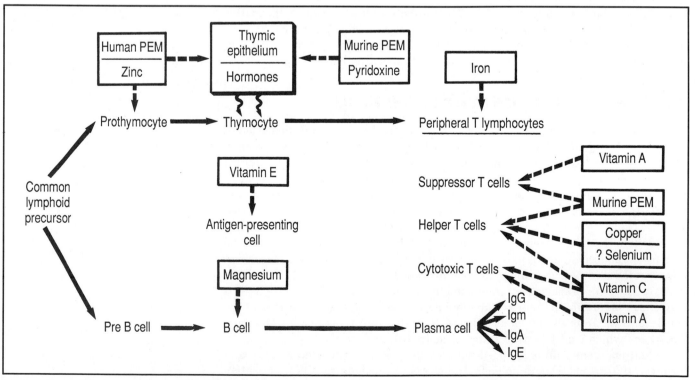

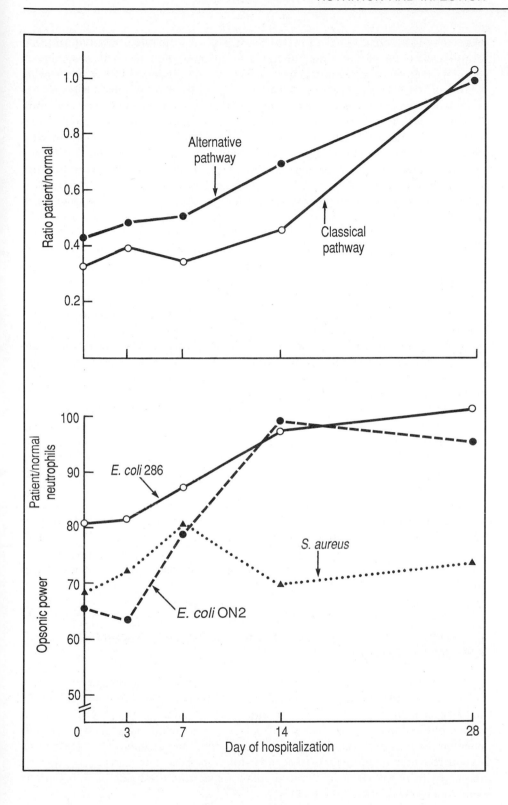

Figure 61.4. Complement and opsonic activity of serum from Guatemalan children with acute protein-energy malnutrition measured over 28 days of nutritional rehabilitation. Upper panel shows the level of complement activity via the classical pathway (*open circles*) and via the alternative pathway (*closed circles*). Lower panel shows levels of opsonization of *Escherichia coli* via the classical pathway (*closed circles*) and the alternative pathway (*open circles*). Opsonization of *Staphylococcus aureus* by antibody (not by complement factors) is also shown (*filled triangles*). These results indicate that the alternative pathway appears to be less affected by malnutrition than the classical pathway. Of the two, the classical pathway is more active in that it leads to a higher degree of opsonization. Note that opsonization of *S. aureus* by immunoglobulins is unaffected by the nutritional status. (From Keusch GT et al: Impairment of hemolytic complement activation by both the classical and alternative pathways in serum from patients with kwashiorkor. *J Pediatr* 105: 434–435, 1984.)

cytes may be normal, but the proportion of mature T cells is decreased and that of null cells is increased. Thus, functions that depend on mature T cells, such as proliferative responses to mitogens, are likely to be diminished. A manifestation of this deficit is a depressed response in PEM patients to skin test antigens that elicit a delayed hypersensitivity reaction, such as tuberculin. The defect in mature T lymphocytes is probably located in the thymus, which fails to induce differentiation of committed T cells (see Chapter 5 for details). It is not yet known with certainty at what level this deficit occurs, but there are suggestions that it may be due to a lack of thymic hormones which induce maturation of T lymphocytes. Defects in cell-mediated immunity are the likely reason for the susceptibility of PEM patients to intracellular infections such as tuberculosis and to progressive viral diseases such as measles.

Although B cells and immunoglobulin levels are normal in PEM patients, they show a diminished production of certain antibodies. Many antigens depend on T cells to help initiate the B cell response. Similarly, the switch from IgM to IgG production is T cell-dependent; a defect in this event may be reflected in the persistence of low affinity IgM antibodies. In malnourished patients some vaccines do not elicit a good antibody response (e.g., typhoid O antigen, live polio vaccines), whereas others do (e.g., tetanus toxoid, live smallpox vaccine). Thus, the nutritional state of a population must be taken into account when embarking on an immunization campaign since protective antibody responses may not occur. Another abormality in antibody response associated with malnutrition is the depression in the secretory IgA at mucosal surfaces.

In PEM patients the complement system is generally depressed. Both classical and alternative activation pathways are affected, especially the latter (Fig. 61.4). All complement components are reduced in plasma concentration, especially C3 and factor B. This depression may be due to more than one mechanism, including not only reduced synthesis but also greater consumption of complement components during the response to infection. Complement deficiency may condition the host to Gram negative bacterial infections (Chapter 4).

Phagocytosis and intracellular killing of microorganisms are close to normal in cells of PEM patients studied in vitro. However, there may be functional abnormalities in vivo because of deficits in the accessory humoral factors required for a normal phagocytic response, including complement and immunoglobulin opsonins.

CLINICAL CONSEQUENCES OF ACQUIRED IMMUNE DEFECTS IN PEM

An important principle in infectious diseases is that the success in combatting infection depends on the speed and the magnitude with which the host mobilizes defense mechanisms. Small defects in individual components may be unimportant alone, but together may lead to a sluggish response, which may make the difference between asymptomatic infection and severe illness. Generally speaking, the extent to which malnutrition causes disruption of host defenses is related to its intensity. In severe cases, children display a spectrum of clinical manifestations known as *kwashiorkor* (Fig. 61.5).

The clinician should be aware of the patient's nutritional status, whether in developing or in nutritionally affluent countries. For example, elective surgical patients should be screened for their cell-mediated immune status. When malnu-

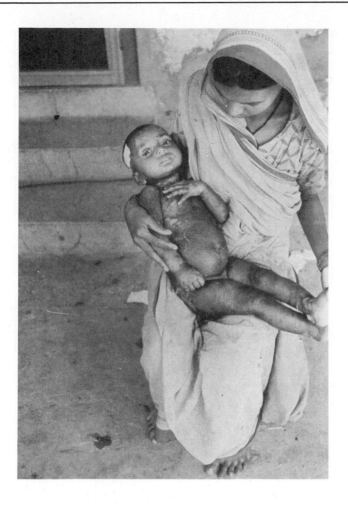

Figure 61.5 A young Bangladeshi child with acute kwashiorkor (a syndrome due to severe chronic protein deficiency) following shigella dysentery. His belly is bloated and the lower extremities edematous, masking a significant loss of lean body mass. Also typical are the scaling black "pellagroid" rash and the apathetic appearance.

trition is found, steps should be taken to correct the problem by appropriate nutritional rehabilitation. This will result in lower morbidity and mortality.

The effects of poor nutrition in early development are illustrated by a case below which shows the multifaceted manifestations of malnutrition on childhood infections.

CASE

Juanita R. was born in the highlands of a South American country of native Indian parents. Pregnancy, which was unsupervised, and birth, which was supervised by a traditional attendant, were uneventful. Juanita's birth was at full term and her weight, 2,540 g, was close to the village mean (which is at the 10% percentile of the figures provided for the United States by NCHS, the National Center for Health Statistics; Fig. 61.6). The baby took breast milk shortly after birth and had no problem feeding for the first 4 months, when weaning began.

A sample of cord blood had been obtained as part of a prospective research project. Analysis showed an elevated IgM and low IgA level, consistent with intrauterine antigenic stimulation of the fetus, suggesting prenatal infection (see Chapter 53 for details).

Figure 61.6. The growth curves for girls, indicating the National Center for Health Statistics percentile standards for the reference population (United States). Baby Juanita's progress is shown by the *squares*. C, conjunctivitis; U, upper respiratory track infection; B, bronchitis; I, impetigo; M, measles; D, watery diarrhea; BD, bloody diarrhea.

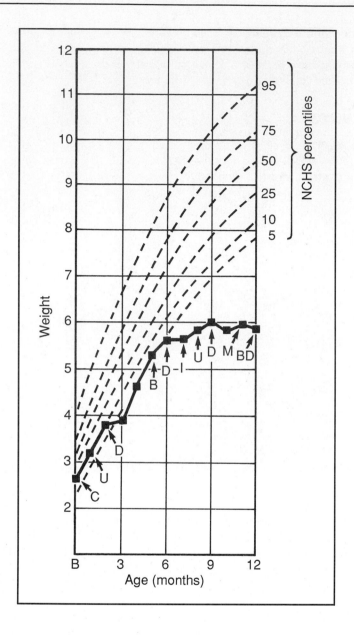

Juanita developed conjunctivitis at 3 weeks, a urinary tract infection at 5 weeks, and diarrhea lasting 10 days at age 2 months. Weight gain followed the village mean for 2 months and was parallel to the NCHS mean. Thereafter, infectious episodes, including diarrhea, acute respiratory illness, and skin infections, occurred with greater frequency and were associated with periods of deceleration in growth or actual weight loss (Fig. 61.6). At age 11½ months, Juanita developed bloody diarrhea, fever, and, in a few days, swelling around the eyes, abdomen, and the feet. She was brought to the hospital where acute dysentery and kwashiorkor were diagnosed. Antibiotics and an infusion of glucose were begun. Juanita's temperature diminished over the next few days, but the edema increased, she lost her appetite, and became increasingly lethargic. On the seventh day after admission, she became hypothermic, *hypotensive, and unresponsive. Her appearance was similar to that of the child shown in Figure 61.5. Had cultures been taken, it is most likely that Shigella flexneri would have been found in Juanita's stool and Escherichia coli in her blood. She died later that evening, on the day of her first birthday.*

COMMENTS

Baby Juanita's defenses faced formidable microbial challenges from the first moment of her life. She was soon caught in a downward spiral, with a series of infections contributing to her state of malnutrition. Juanita's condition was exacerbated by lack of an adequate diet after weaning, and she suffered from protein-energy malnutrition. Her clinical course could not be improved by access to appropriate medical care, especially antibiotics and symptomatic care. Most of the metabolic and immunological events characteristic of malnutrition contributed to the weakening of her defenses.

It seems fitting to end this book with the hope that preventable conditions such as Juanita's will become more and more exceptional rather than all too common events in human history.

SUGGESTED READINGS

Beisel WR: Metabolic effects of infection. *Prog Food Nutr Sci* 8:43–75, 1984

Keusch GT, Wilson CS, Waksal SD: Nutrition, host defenses, and the lymphoid system. In Gallin JI, Fauci AS (eds.): *Advances in Host Defense Mechanism*, vol 2. New York, Raven Press, 1983.

Keusch GT, Farthing MJG: Nutrition and infection. *Ann Rev Nutr* 6:131–154, 1986.

Keusch GT, Scrimshaw NS: Selective primary health care: strategies for disease control in the developing world. XXIII. Control of infection to reduce the prevalence of infantile and childhood malnutrition *Rev Infect Dis* 8:273–287, 1986.

Index

Page numbers in *italics* denote figures; those followed by "t" denote tables.